AF722582

Viruses, Vaccines and Antivirals

Viruses, Vaccines and Antivirals

Editor: Robin Keeney

AMERICAN
MEDICAL PUBLISHERS
www.americanmedicalpublishers.com

AMERICAN
MEDICAL PUBLISHERS
www.americanmedicalpublishers.com

Cataloging-in-Publication Data

Viruses, vaccines and antivirals / edited by Robin Keeney.
p. cm.
Includes bibliographical references and index.
ISBN 979-8-88740-560-5
1. Viruses. 2. Vaccines. 3. Viral vaccines. 4. Antiviral agents.
5. Virus inhibitors. 6. Virology. I. Keeney, Robin.
QR360 .V57 2023
576.64--dc23

© American Medical Publishers, 2023

American Medical Publishers,
41 Flatbush Avenue,
1st Floor, New York,
NY 11217, USA

ISBN 979-8-88740-560-5 (Hardback)

This book contains information obtained from authentic and highly regarded sources. Copyright for all individual chapters remain with the respective authors as indicated. All chapters are published with permission under the Creative Commons Attribution License or equivalent. A wide variety of references are listed. Permission and sources are indicated; for detailed attributions, please refer to the permissions page and list of contributors. Reasonable efforts have been made to publish reliable data and information, but the authors, editors and publisher cannot assume any responsibility for the validity of all materials or the consequences of their use.

Trademark Notice: Registered trademark of products or corporate names are used only for explanation and identification without intent to infringe.

Contents

Preface

Virus refers to a submicroscopic infectious agent that replicates solely within the living cells of an organism. Viruses infect all kinds of life, including animals and plants as well as microorganisms, such as bacteria and archaea. They are found in all the ecosystems that exist on Earth. Virology is a subspecialty of microbiology that studies viruses. A biological preparation that induces active acquired immunity against a specific infectious disease is defined as vaccine. It usually comprises an agent that resembles a disease-causing microorganism. It is commonly manufactured from weakened or deceased forms of the microbe, its toxins, or one of its surface proteins. Antivirals, or antiviral drugs, refer to a class of medications that are used to treat viral infections. These drugs do not destruct their target pathogen but prevent it from growing. Vaccines and antivirals play a significant role in controlling pandemics and eradicating viral diseases. This book is compiled in such a manner, that it will provide in-depth knowledge about viruses. Also included herein is a detailed explanation of the various concepts and applications of antivirals and vaccines. This book is appropriate for students seeking detailed information in this area of study as well as for experts.

This book is a comprehensive compilation of works of different researchers from varied parts of the world. It includes valuable experiences of the researchers with the sole objective of providing the readers (learners) with a proper knowledge of the concerned field. This book will be beneficial in evoking inspiration and enhancing the knowledge of the interested readers.

In the end, I would like to extend my heartiest thanks to the authors who worked with great determination on their chapters. I also appreciate the publisher's support in the course of the book. I would also like to deeply acknowledge my family who stood by me as a source of inspiration during the project.

Editor

1

Universal Vaccines and Vaccine Platforms to Protect Against Influenza Viruses in Humans and Agriculture

Daniela S. Rajão and Daniel R. Pérez*

Department of Population Health, University of Georgia, Athens, GA, United States

***Correspondence:**
Daniela S. Rajão
daniela.rajao@uga.edu

Influenza virus infections pose a significant threat to public health due to annual seasonal epidemics and occasional pandemics. Influenza is also associated with significant economic losses in animal production. The most effective way to prevent influenza infections is through vaccination. Current vaccine programs rely heavily on the vaccine's ability to stimulate neutralizing antibody responses to the hemagglutinin (HA) protein. One of the biggest challenges to an effective vaccination program lies on the fact that influenza viruses are ever-changing, leading to antigenic drift that results in escape from earlier immune responses. Efforts toward overcoming these challenges aim at improving the strength and/or breadth of the immune response. Novel vaccine technologies, the so-called universal vaccines, focus on stimulating better cross-protection against many or all influenza strains. However, vaccine platforms or manufacturing technologies being tested to improve vaccine efficacy are heterogeneous between different species and/or either tailored for epidemic or pandemic influenza. Here, we discuss current vaccines to protect humans and animals against influenza, highlighting challenges faced to effective and uniform novel vaccination strategies and approaches.

Keywords: influenza vaccines, universal vaccines, live attenuated vaccines, immune response, vaccine platform, poultry, swine, vectored vaccine

INTRODUCTION

Type A (IAV) and type B (IBV) influenza viruses are responsible for yearly epidemics of respiratory disease in humans. IAVs infect a broad range of avian and mammalian species, including humans. IBVs are considered primarily a human pathogen. According to the World Health Organization (WHO), ~300,000 deaths occur annually worldwide associated with seasonal influenza infections (World Health Organization, 2016). In the U.S., the Centers for Disease Control and Prevention (CDC) estimates that seasonal influenza affects at least 9 million people and results in 12,000–56,000 deaths annually (Centers for Disease Control Prevention, 2017d).

Human seasonal influenza infections vary in intensity, from typically mild respiratory disease with dry cough, nasal discharge, rhinitis and pharyngitis, fever, anorexia, and myalgia to occasionally more severe that can lead to secondary bacterial infections and deaths due to pneumonia (Taubenberger and Morens, 2008). Populations with compromised immunity are at the highest risk of severe and potential life threatening disease, such as chronically ill patients, pregnant women, children, and the elderly (Thompson et al., 2006). In general, H3N2 infections are usually associated with more exacerbated disease than infections with H1N1 or IBVs.

There is also the inherent zoonotic risk of IAV strains that circulate in avian and mammalian species, some of pandemic concern, which can result in atypical clinical symptoms and much greater burden to otherwise healthy people (Taubenberger and Morens, 2009). Most cases of H5N1 highly pathogenic avian influenza viruses (HPAIV) presented severe respiratory signs, and gastrointestinal symptoms can also be observed such as vomiting, watery diarrhea, and abdominal pain. Most patients infected with avian H7N9 viruses have had severe pneumonia, with fever, coughing and shortness of breath (Centers for Disease Control and Prevention, 2017e).

IAVs are among the most devastating pathogens for swine and poultry productions. Several genetically and antigenically diverse IAV strains are endemic in swine worldwide and continue to cause significant losses to the swine industry usually as a result of reduced weight gain, secondary infections, and sporadic abortion associated with hyperthermia. In pigs, IAV infections present similar characteristics as the disease in humans, with rapid onset of fever, lethargy, loss of appetite, and coughing (Van Reeth et al., 2012). Avian influenza viruses are endemic in large parts of the world, particularly Asia, the Middle East, and parts of Africa (World Health Organization/World Organisation for Animal Health/Food and Agriculture Organization (WHO/OIE/FAO) H5N1 Evolution Working Group, 2014). Outbreaks of HPAIV can have devastating consequences to an affected country, including direct costs related to the high mortality and indirect costs associated with eradication efforts, control and contention, and loss of markets. The latest outbreak of HPAIV in the U.S. Midwest in 2015 cost the country more than 3 billion dollars (Greene, 2015). In birds, mild forms of low pathogenic avian influenza can range from asymptomatic to mild to moderate respiratory clinical signs, with production losses as a result of lack of feed and water consumption, as well as drop in egg production (Swayne et al., 2013). HPAIV outbreaks are manifested by rapid onset of signs such as depression, neurological disorders, necrotic and swollen wattles and combs, and hemorrhage of the shanks (Swayne et al., 2013) with mortality rates reaching 100%, while some birds might die before showing any clinical signs.

Vaccination remains the most efficient and cost-effective means to prevent and control influenza in human and animal populations. Vaccines rely on the effective stimulation of the immune response against the virus, mostly against the surface glycoprotein hemagglutinin (HA), the primary immunogen of influenza viruses. Influenza vaccines were a high priority for the U.S. military since the Spanish influenza pandemic of 1918–1919 when 1 in every 67 soldiers died from influenza-related infections. However, it was not until 1946 that influenza vaccines became available for the general population (www.historyofvaccines.org). Despite many advances in terms of vaccine manufacturing and production, the technology available for influenza vaccines differs little from its origins and continue to face significant shortcomings about availability and/or efficacy. In this review, we will discuss the use of vaccines to prevent and control influenza in animals and humans. We will highlight challenges faced to establish an effective and standardized vaccination program and discuss new approaches that are being tested to address these issues.

INFLUENZA VIRUSES

IAV and IBV viruses are members of the *Orthomyxoviridae* family. IAV and IBV have in common a genome consisting of 8 single-stranded negative-sense viral RNA (vRNA) segments that encode for at least 10 viral proteins (Knipe et al., 2007; **Figure 1**). Each vRNA associates with the viral nucleoprotein (NP) and the three polymerase proteins (PB2, PB1, and PA–P-complex), forming the viral ribonucleoprotein complexes (vRNPs). The untranslated regions (UTR) at the 3′ and 5′ end of each segment serve as anchors for the P-complex to carry out transcription and replication in the nucleus of the host cells. The major surface glycoproteins, HA and neuraminidase (NA), plus neuraminidase gene region B (NB) in segment six in IBV, partake in virus attachment and release of progeny virus particles (Knipe et al., 2007). Also on the membrane, the matrix protein 2 (M2 in IAV and BM2 in IBV) acts as a unidirectional proton pump, which is essential early in the infection cycle by allowing the release of vRNPs from the endosome into the cytoplasm and subsequent migration to the nucleus. Matrix protein 1 (M1), NP, and nuclear export protein (NEP/NS2) take part in export of the progeny vRNPs out of the nucleus and assembly into novel virions at the cell surface along with HA, NA, and M2. The non-structural protein NS1 carries out multiple functions during infection with overall antiviral antagonistic activity (Knipe et al., 2007).

The HA is a type I glycoprotein present as homotrimers where each monomer consists of two di-sulfide-linked HA1 and HA2 subunits after cleavage of the HA0 precursor. The HA ectodomain also consists of a globular head domain, and the stalk or stem domain, which are responsible for receptor binding and membrane fusion, respectively (Knipe et al., 2007). The NA is a type 2 glycoprotein present as mushroom-shaped homotetramers. IAV are further classified into H (H1-18) and N (N1-11) subtypes according to the antigenic characteristics of the HA and NA, most of them detected in wild aquatic birds, considered the natural hosts of influenza. Only H1N1 and H3N2 subtypes currently circulate in humans. H1 and H3 subtypes combined with either N1 or N2 subtypes are endemic in pigs. In addition, permanent lineages of IAVs of the H3 subtype circulate in horses and dogs. A wider range of IAV subtypes have become established in land-based birds of the order *Galliformes* (e.g., chickens, quail, turkeys, guinea fowl, among others). Once in *Galliformes*, IAVs of the H5 and H7 subtypes can become HPAIVs due to accumulation of basic amino acids in the cleavage site of the HA0 precursor protein. IBVs are usually restricted to humans, and two antigenically distinct lineages circulate, the Victoria-like and the Yamagata-like lineages.

Influenza A and B viruses accumulate mutations due to the P-complex's lack of proof-reading activity. When these mutations occur in the HA and NA, they lead to antigenic drift, which over time results in escape from earlier immune responses. IAVs can also undergo antigenic shift, whereby a strain with a new HA subtype enters and transmits readily in an immunologically naïve population. Antigenic shift is possible through reassortment resulting from the exchange of gene segments between two or more strains. Reassortment plays a significant role in the evolution of IAVs in the

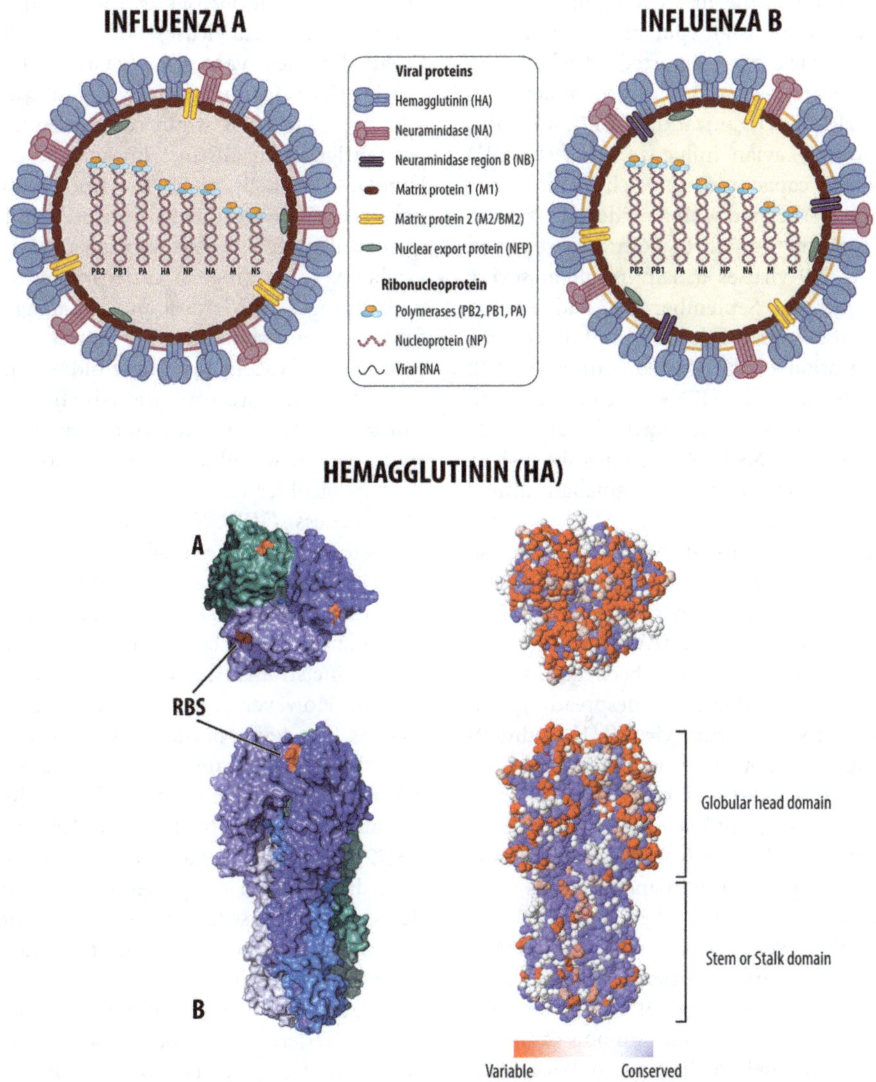

FIGURE 1 | (Top) Schematic structure and genome organization of influenza A and B viruses. Haemagglutinin (HA), neuraminidase (NA), matrix protein 2 (M2/BM2), neuraminidase region B (NB) are on the surface of the virus particle. Matrix protein 1 (M1) is associated with the membrane. Ribonucleoprotein complex formed by RNA segments, nucleoprotein (NP) and viral polymerases (PB2, PB1, PA). Non-structural nuclear export protein (NEP). **(Bottom)** The 3D molecular structure of the HA glycoprotein trimer from A/Hong Kong/1/68 (H3N2) (PDB 5T6N), top (A) and side (B) views (structure modified and colored using MacPymol, Schrodinger, LLC). Each monomer has a globular head domain and a stem/stalk domain. On the left panels each monomer is shown with a different color. The receptor binding site (RBS) is highlighted in red. On the right panels, residue conservation for every position in the protein sequence is shown in a color scale, and visualized using the 3D tool available at the Influenza Research Database (www.fludb.org).

natural reservoir and during the emergence of pandemic strains.

THE ANIMAL-HUMAN INTERFACE OF INFLUENZA ECOLOGY

IAVs that typically infect a particular host species can sometimes cross the species barrier and infect a new host. Animal species such as poultry and swine have significant interactions at the animal-human interface, providing ideal environments for zoonotic transmission events of IAV. These zoonotic transmissions pose a significant threat to public health, not only because of the disease severity and mortality seen in some cases, but also the risk of initiating a pandemic if these viruses become adapted to spread among humans. All human pandemics that happened in the last 100 years originated from viruses with gene segments from animal reservoirs (Taubenberger and Morens, 2009). Humans usually become infected with animal viruses as a result of close contact with a particular animal species. Some of the most prominent poultry-adapted IAVs have been responsible for zoonotic outbreaks and are, therefore, of great public health concern. The WHO considers Asian-origin poultry-adapted IAVs of the H5N1 and H7N9 subtypes among those with the greatest pandemic concern. Since the first detection of H5N1 HPAIV in 1997 and re-emergence as an epidemic in poultry in 2003, 860 human infections have been reported, of which 454 were lethal. Most these cases are the result of direct contact with infected poultry (World Health Organization, 2017). In 2013, a novel H7N9 low pathogenic avian influenza virus (LPAIV) emerged in poultry with the capacity to infect humans. Since then, H7N9 IAVs have been associated with 5 epidemic waves in humans in Mainland China, and the start of a 6th wave reported in October 2017. These H7N9 viruses usually result in severe acute respiratory disease, and until September 2017 had resulted in 1622 laboratory-confirmed human infections and 619 deaths (Food Agriculture Organization of the United Nations, 2017). On the fifth wave, HPAIV forms of the H7N9 were detected also associated with direct contact with infected birds (Iuliano et al., 2017). More importantly, some H7N9 HPAIV strains show signs of more efficient airborne transmission in mammalian animal models (ferrets) (Imai et al., 2017).

Despite the usual mild clinical signs, swine-origin IAVs also represent a real threat to public health due to limited population immunity and potential to become widespread. The 2009 H1N1 pandemic was a result of a swine-origin IAV with a unique combination of gene segments that had not been detected in pigs before, and quickly became globally widespread (Smith et al., 2009). After the 2009 H1N1 pandemic virus (H1N1pdm09) established itself in the human population, it transmitted back to pigs, where it continued to reassort with other IAVs of swine origin. In the U.S., one such reassortant known as variant H3N2 viruses, or vH3N2, containing the M gene from the H1N1pdm09 virus, spread to people resulting in 376 human infections since 2011 (Centers for Disease Control and Prevention, 2017c). Human infections with vH3N2 IAVs are linked with close contact with infected pigs at agricultural fairs (Epperson et al., 2013).

IAVs infect a range of hosts with the potential to jump between multiple species. Interspecies transmission among different animal species and/or from animals to humans or vice versa can have important economic and animal and/or public health consequences; so active surveillance programs are of essence for early detection of IAVs in new hosts. IAVs of swine-origins are often detected in commercial turkeys in the U.S. (Guo et al., 2015) while outbreaks of a H3N8 virus in 2004 and of a H3N2 virus in 2015 in North American dogs originated from IAVs circulating in horses and birds, respectively (Gibbs and Anderson, 2010; Schwartz, 2015). IAV transmission events from humans to swine are frequent and have influenced the diversity of viruses circulating in pigs: some of the most prevalent viral lineages that now circulate in pigs in the United States resulted from reverse zoonotic transmission of human H1N2 and H3N2 viruses to swine (Nelson et al., 2012).

THE CURRENT SCENARIO FOR VACCINE PRODUCTION

Vaccination against Influenza

Human influenza vaccines are formulated each year to protect against circulating IAVs and IBVs. The influenza vaccine can protect against influenza viruses that are antigenically the same or related to the viruses in the vaccine. Due to the mutating nature of influenza viruses, annual vaccination is recommended. Originally, these vaccines were available as trivalent inactivated vaccine (TIV) formulations (containing an A/H3N2, an A/H1N1, and an influenza B strain recommended by WHO). However, two antigenically distinct lineages of influenza B viruses have circulated globally since the mid 1980's with limited cross-protection between them (Ambrose and Levin, 2012). Therefore, quadrivalent inactivated vaccine (QIV) formulations are now available, containing an extra influenza B strain representing both lineages (B/Victoria and B/Yamagata). Recommendations for influenza vaccination vary between countries. Most countries recommend vaccination in children, the elderly, chronically ill, and health care professionals. In the U.S., CDC's Advisory Committee on Immunization Practices (ACIP) recommends routine annual influenza vaccination for all persons aged 6 months or older (Grohskopf et al., 2016). The U.S. Flu Vaccine Effectiveness (VE) Network coordinated by the CDC has estimated that the overall, adjusted vaccine effectiveness for influenza seasons from 2005-2016 was between 10 and 60%, with recent studies showing that vaccination reduced the risk of influenza illness by 40–60% when circulating viruses match the vaccine strains (Centers for Disease Control and Prevention, 2017b). However, vaccine efficacy can vary widely between seasons, depending particularly on how well matched are vaccine and circulating strains, and on characteristics of the person being vaccinated. For instance, during the 2014–2015 season, the overall vaccine effectiveness was 19%, and only 6% against the H3N2 component because two thirds of the circulating strains were drifted from the previous year (Zimmerman et al., 2016; Centers for Disease Control and Prevention, 2017b).

Vaccination of pigs is routinely used in several countries, but not all endemic countries vaccinate their herds. In swine, vaccination is typically done in gestating sows to transfer maternally derived antibodies (MDA) through colostrum to their litters, in two to three doses before farrowing (Rajao et al., 2014). Typically, vaccination of sows will protect the litter from clinical signs of disease, and MDAs persist until about 14 weeks of age in piglets (Markowska-Daniel et al., 2011). Occasionally and in herds with high virus circulation, vaccination in growing pigs can protect them against infection once MDA have weaned.

Vaccination is common in some countries where avian influenza viruses have become endemic to prevent and control at-risk populations, most commonly against H5, H7, and H9 viruses, particularly in Egypt, Vietnam, China, Indonesia, and Mexico (Domenech et al., 2009; Spackman and Pantin-Jackwood, 2014). Vaccination has also been successfully used as a control tool to aid in HPAIV eradication programs in poultry and wild birds in some countries, in situations where the regular stamping-out protocols are not enough to control spread and poses a threat to food supply reviewed in Spackman and Pantin-Jackwood (2014). Vaccination of poultry against influenza viruses is still seen with reluctance by many, due to the understanding that vaccines can protect against clinical signs but not infection and, therefore, mask outbreaks and may favor the spread of HPAIV.

The Immune Response Elicited by Vaccination

The local innate immune response is critical for limiting viral replication at the initial phase of infection. Particularly, alveolar macrophages (Kim et al., 2008), natural killer (NK) cells (Gazit et al., 2006), and neutrophils (Tate et al., 2009) have a crucial role in restricting viral spread and reducing disease severity. Infected cells recognize influenza virus RNA via pattern-recognition receptors (PRRs). Activation of PRRs stimulates production of pro-inflammatory cytokines and type I interferons (reviewed in Kreijtz et al., 2011). Inactivated vaccines are poor inducers of innate immunity to give immediate protection. However, a study has demonstrated that binding of UV-inactivated influenza virus to sialic acids (SAs) can trigger intracellular signals for activation of IFN-inducible genes and cytokine production in primary human dendritic cells (Ramos et al., 2011).

Immunization with traditionally inactivated influenza vaccines primarily induces virus-specific adaptive antibody responses. Antibodies against the HA protein, predominantly the globular head domain, are the major protective response against influenza since they usually correlate with surrogate *in vitro* assays such as the hemagglutination inhibition (HI) or virus neutralizing (VN) assays. HI-titers ≥1:40 are considered protective and the accepted standards used by regulatory agencies (Montomoli, 2008). A major hurdle to overcome is that the HA globular head is highly variable and harbors mutations that can lead to antigenic variation. Most HA-head-specific antibodies are only protective against closely antigenically related viruses. In contrast, the stalk domain is more conserved. Influenza infection can result in low levels of antibodies against the stalk region, but these antibodies can have broadly neutralizing activity (Ekiert et al., 2009). In pigs, however, vaccine-induced antibodies to a linear epitope located in the stalk domain increased virus fusion and enhanced respiratory disease, possibly involved with a negative effect (Khurana et al., 2013). However, in mice passive transfer of post-vaccination polyclonal sera resulted in reduced lung virus replication and weight loss compared to animals receiving pre-vaccination sera (Nachbagauer et al., 2014). Further studies are necessary to make clear the levels of HA stem-specific antibodies that correlate with clinical protections and/or if they can negatively influence clinical outcome. Antibodies against the other surface proteins, NA and M2, are not considered neutralizing by traditional assays but studies showed that they limit virus replication and spread *in vivo*.

The CD4+ T lymphocytes and CD8+ T cytotoxic lymphocytes (CTLs) mediate the cellular arm of the adaptive immune response against influenza and play an important role in viral clearance and cross-protective immunity. Virus-specific CD8+ T cells recognize influenza peptides presented by major histocompatibility complex class I (MHC-I) molecules present on the surface of infected cells, resulting in cell lysis. These CTLs are mainly directed against the relatively conserved internal proteins NP, M1, and the P-complex subunits, which confer a high degree of cross-reactive immune response to various influenza strains in humans and swine (Heinen et al., 2001; Hillaire et al., 2013). Not only these CTL aid in virus clearance, but also with protection against disease severity. CD8+ T cell activity correlated with lack of virus shedding, decreased risk of fever, and reduced influenza-like illness in people infected with the H1N1pdm09 virus (Sridhar et al., 2013). After infection in humans, memory CD8+ cell populations are found in lymphoid organs, in circulation or residing in the lungs, are long-lived, and can act upon subsequent infection (van de Sandt et al., 2015). In swine, memory T cells are CD4+/CD8+ double-positive, of which numbers increase in respiratory lymphoid organs and lungs after infection (Khatri et al., 2010). Antigen-presenting cells, such as dendritic cells (DCs), macrophages, and B cells, present peptide fragments of processed antigens on their surfaces in the context of MHC class II (MHC-II) molecules and activate CD4+ T cells. CD4+ T cells are predominantly helper cells, and offer co-stimulatory signals for the priming of B cells (Alam et al., 2014) and CD8+ T cells (Schoenberger et al., 1998) after. Pre-existing CD4+ T cells were also associated with disease protection and lower virus shedding during influenza infection (Wilkinson et al., 2012). Current traditional inactivated vaccines do not stimulate cellular immune responses and, therefore, are usually less effective against heterologous influenza infections, but novel technologies to stimulate T cell immunity are being tested (Soema et al., 2015b) and are discussed below.

Seasonal Vaccine Strain Selection and Production

Identifying circulating viruses, their spatial/temporal trends, and their antigenic relationships to other contemporary and vaccines strains are crucial for an effective influenza vaccine. Antigenic drift requires frequent vaccine updates to match circulating viruses and meet efficient coverage. The WHO's Global Influenza Surveillance and Response System (GISRS) monitors seasonal viruses' evolution by using data obtained year-round from more than 130 national influenza centers located in more than 100 collaborating countries. Meetings are held twice a year to select vaccine strains for the following influenza season. The meetings take place in February for the Northern Hemisphere and in September for the Southern Hemisphere, at least 6 months before their respective influenza seasons. Based on antigenic data from ferret antisera, paired serologic analysis of human samples, and virologic surveillance data, the GISRS recommends that vaccine strains are either maintained or updated to offer more effective protection. Usually following WHO recommendations, each country and its regulatory agencies decide about the influenza vaccines licensed in their territory. In general, each vaccine strain in the vaccine requires an update every 2–3 years, with at least one strain updated each year.

Vaccine Strains Selection and Production for Animal Use

Except for vaccine strain selection against equine influenza, for systematic vaccine strain selection or updates is lacking for other animal production systems. A panel of specialists coordinated by the World Organization for Animal Health (OIE) meets annually to analyze surveillance and epidemiological data related to worldwide circulation of IAVs in horses. Genetic sequences and antigenic data are used for recommendations of suitable vaccine strains for inclusion in commercial equine influenza vaccines (Paillot, 2014).

The U.S. Department of Agriculture (USDA) established a national swine IAV surveillance system in 2009. Similarly, efforts are also being made to intensify surveillance in European countries through the European Surveillance Network for Influenza in Pigs (ESNIP) (Anderson et al., 2013; Simon et al., 2014). Both of these efforts have generated consistent flow of genetic data that is useful for vaccine strain choice. Still lacking are collaborative panels to continuously analyze this surveillance data compared to antigenic characteristics of main circulating strains. Unlike IAVs in humans, IAVs in pigs do not follow common evolutionary trends and tend to adopt unique evolutionary pathways depending on the country, region, and even at the farm level. The high diversity and heterogeneous distribution of different viral lineages circulating in pigs represents a major obstacle for effective vaccine choices against swine influenza (Anderson et al., 2016; Lewis et al., 2016). Therefore, swine influenza vaccine manufacturers make independent decisions about the strains to include in their products, and those formulations are not often updated. Likewise, despite intense routine worldwide IAV surveillance in intensive poultry producing areas, the lack of structures to better assess the effects of the use of vaccines in the perpetuation and evolution of IAV in poultry often means that the available commercial vaccines available are not antigenically matched, resulting in less-than-optimal protection (Spackman and Pantin-Jackwood, 2014).

More recently, the OIE along with the Food and Agriculture Organization of the United Nations (FAO) launched a worldwide collaborative network of experts on animal influenza (OFFLU) to support the veterinary community to better manage and reduce the risk of IAVs of animal origin to animal and public health (http://www.offlu.net). This network aims to help recognized emerging strains, provide training and advice, to increase collaboration and data sharing within the scientific community, and to help promote animal influenza research and development.

CONVENTIONAL VACCINES AGAINST INFLUENZA

Most influenza vaccines on the market for humans and animals are inactivated influenza vaccines (IIV). For humans and horses there are also live-attenuated influenza vaccines (LAIV) available (**Table 1**). Regardless of the vaccine strain or manufacturing platform in which the vaccine is made, influenza vaccines are typically produced by growing the target viruses in chicken eggs, which is reliant on continual egg supply. For the most part, seed strains used for human vaccines are typically reassortants generated by the old-fashioned, classical co-infection method to get the target virus HA and NA gene segments in the background of six gene segments derived from an egg-adapted high growth master donor strain, usually A/Puerto Rico/8/34 (PR8) for IAVs and B/Lee/4/40 (B/Lee) for IBVs. Unfortunately, most recent influenza viruses do not grow well in eggs which affects the efficiency of the traditional reassortment method. More importantly, forcing these vaccine viruses to grow in eggs often results in egg-adapted changes associated with antigenic mismatches. In the case of HPAIVs, their inherent high lethality for chicken embryos makes them unsuitable as vaccine strains. Some of these limitations are overcome by reverse genetics techniques that allow generation of whole recombinant influenza viruses entirely from cloned DNA (Neumann et al., 1999; Hoffmann et al., 2000). Thus, reverse genetics allowed to increase the yield of some of the components of LAIV or to mutate the cleavage site of H5N1 HPAIVs and make them suitable for preparation of vaccine seed stocks for pandemic preparedness or as poultry vaccines. Whole wild-type viruses are predominantly used for traditional animal vaccines.

Inactivated Vaccines

Inactivated vaccines are the most commonly used products for influenza prevention due to the large history of manufacturing practices associated with relatively low production costs, safety, and effectiveness. There are four types of inactivated vaccines: whole inactivated virus vaccines (WIV), split virus vaccines, subunit vaccines, and virosomal influenza vaccines (reviewed in Soema et al., 2015a; **Table 1**). Typically, whole-virus killed vaccines produced in 9-11-day-old pathogen-free embryonated chicken eggs, chemically inactivated with formaldehyde or β-propiolactone, concentrated and purified. In split virus vaccines, the virus envelope undergoes disruption by diethyl ether or detergent treatment to expose all viral proteins (Neurath et al., 1971). Subunit vaccines have added purification steps to separate the nucleocapsid and lipids from the surface proteins HA and NA (Laver and Webster, 1976). Despite the loss in viral organization and some loss in immunogenicity, split virus and subunit vaccines are more commonly used against seasonal influenza in humans due to their reduced reactogenicity in comparison with the whole-virus products (Beyer et al., 2011). Virosomal vaccine formulations are mostly used in Europe and consist of unilamellar phospholipid bilayer vesicles carrying surface HA, NA glycoproteins that allow fusion to target cells (Holm and Goa, 1999; Herzog et al., 2009). Inactivated vaccines are usually protective against antigenically closely related strains, but small antigenic changes lead to potential loss of cross-reaction in the HI assay and associated with loss in protection, hence the continuous monitoring for antigenic evolution and updating of vaccine strains.

Most human seasonal TIV/QIV vaccines are available as single dose vaccines for people ≥9 years of age administered via an intra muscular (i.m.) injection, although intradermal (i.d.) formulations are also available. Current guidelines recommend that children 6 months old to <9 years old receive an extra dose administered 4 weeks after the first vaccination. Efficacy of existing vaccines is highly dependent on the age group, with much lower efficacy in children, the elderly, and adults with underlying conditions.

Most swine and poultry influenza vaccines used in the field are inactivated whole virus products combined with potent oil-in-water adjuvants delivered by the i.m. route (Swayne et al., 2011;

TABLE 1 | Summary of experimental and licensed vaccines against influenza viruses for humans and animals described in this review.

Vaccine platform	Vaccine type	Species	Efficacy	Status	References
Inactivated Influenza Virus (IIV)	Whole virus adjuvanted	Poultry, swine, equine, humans	Safe and immunogenic, homologous protection	Licensed	Swayne et al., 2011; Sandbulte et al., 2015
	Split, subunit	Humans	Safe and immunogenic, homologous protection	Licensed	Neurath et al., 1971; Laver and Webster, 1976; Beyer et al., 2011
	Virosomal	Humans	Safe and immunogenic, homologous protection	Licensed	Holm and Goa, 1999; Herzog et al., 2009
	Oil-in-water MF59 adjuvant	Humans	Safe and immunogenic, homologous protection	Licensed	Vesikari et al., 2009, 2011; Domnich et al., 2017
Live attenuated influenza virus (LAIV)	Cold-adapted	Humans, poultry, swine equine	Safe and immunogenic, homologous and partial heterologous protection	Licensed (human, horses), experimental	Song et al., 2007; Pena et al., 2011; Loving et al., 2013; Alam et al., 2014; Gauger et al., 2014; Santos et al., 2017b
	NS1 truncation	Humans, chicken, swine	Safe and immunogenic, homologous and partial heterologous protection	Experimental	Solorzano et al., 2005; Hai et al., 2008; Richt and Garcia-Sastre, 2009; Kappes et al., 2012; Pica et al., 2012; Shi et al., 2016
	Elastase-dependent	Swine	Safe and immunogenic, homologous and heterologous protection	Experimental	Masic et al., 2010
	Rearranged genome	Humans	Safe and immunogenic, homologous protection	Pre-clinical, experimental	Pena et al., 2013; Nogales et al., 2016; Harding et al., 2017
Viral vector vaccine	Modified vaccinia virus ankara (MVA) – conserved proteins	Humans, chickens	Broad cross-reactive response, partial/total homologous protection and partial cross-protection	Phase 1	Lillie et al., 2012; Boyd et al., 2013; Florek et al., 2014; Hessel et al., 2014; Ducatez et al., 2016
	Adenovirus	Human, chicken, swine	Partial homologous/heterologous protection	Phase 1, Experimental	Wesley et al., 2004; Boyd et al., 2013; Crosby et al., 2017
	Alphavirus	Humans, poultry, swine	Partial/total homologous and partial heterologous protection	Experimental	Vander Veen et al., 2012, 2013; Santos et al., 2017a
	Newcastle disease virus	Poultry	Homologous protection	Licensed (chickens), experimental	Liu et al., 2015; Kim et al., 2017
	Herpesvirus Turkey	Poultry	Homologous and partial heterologous protection	Licensed (chickens), experimental	Gardin et al., 2016
Nucleic acid-based	DNA	Humans, chicken, swine	Safe and immunogenic with prime-boost regimen	Phase 1, licensed, experimental	Ledgerwood et al., 2012; Crank et al., 2015; Borggren et al., 2016; Stachyra et al., 2017
	Messenger RNA (mRNA)	Humans, swine	Safe and immunogenic, homologous and heterologous protection	Phase 1, experimental	Petsch et al., 2012; Bahl et al., 2017
Recombinant, Protein-based and Virus-like particle vaccines	Baculovirus expression vector systems (BEVS)	Humans, chicken, swine	Safe and immunogenic, heterologous protection	Experimental	Crawford et al., 1999; King et al., 2009; Baxter et al., 2011; Hernandez et al., 2016
	Virus-like particles (VLPs)	Humans, chicken, swine	Safe and immunogenic, homologous and heterologous protection	Phase 1-2	Low et al., 2014; Pillet et al., 2016; Valero-Pacheco et al., 2016
	VLP-COBRA	Humans	Cross-reactive response, homologous protection	Pre-clinical	Carter et al., 2016

(Continued)

TABLE 1 | Continued

Vaccine platform	Vaccine type	Species	Efficacy	Status	References
	Headless	Humans	Broadly neutralizing antibody response, homologous and partial heterologous protection	Pre-clinical	Steel et al., 2010; Impagliazzo et al., 2015; Valkenburg et al., 2016
	Sequential immunization	Humans	Broadly neutralizing antibody response, heterologous protection	Pre-clinical	Krammer et al., 2013; Nachbagauer et al., 2014; Kirchenbaum et al., 2015; Ermler et al., 2017
	NA-based	Humans, chicken, swine	Cross-reactive response, homologous and partial heterologous protection	Experimental	Sylte et al., 2007; Van Reeth et al., 2009; Wohlbold et al., 2015
	M2e-based	Humans, swine	Broad cross-reactive response, heterologous cross-protection	Pre-clinical, phase 1, experimental	Turley et al., 2011; Lee et al., 2015; Kolpe et al., 2017; Tang et al., 2017; Tao et al., 2017

Sandbulte et al., 2015). Inactivation follows the same techniques as for human vaccines, using formalin, β-propiolactone or binary ethylenimine. The adjuvanted WIV vaccines usually stimulate robust antibody responses against the HA of antigenically similar strains. Just like in humans, circulation of antigenic different variants can decrease vaccine efficacy (Vincent et al., 2008; Grund et al., 2011). Originally, IAV vaccines available for use in swine were bivalent products, but some newer products contain 4–5 strains in response to antigenically distinct viruses circulating within the H1 and H3 subtypes (Sandbulte et al., 2015). Two doses are usually required for vaccination in swine, 2–3 weeks apart (Rajao et al., 2014). In poultry, a single dose is typically effective experimentally but in field conditions multiple doses are commonly applied (Kilany et al., 2010; Kapczynski et al., 2013). Typical large commercial poultry production systems have vaccination programs that include multiple vaccine boosts to protect against avian influenza over the entire production cycle.

Live-Attenuated Vaccines

Live-attenuated influenza vaccines (LAIV) are available in several countries for use in humans and horses. Experimental LAIVs are effective in swine and poultry (**Table 1**). LAIVs have an advantage over inactivated products because they mimic a natural route of infection but with very low rate of adverse reactions. In contrast to inactivated products, vaccination with live products provides both humoral and cell-mediated immunity, and they can induce mucosal IgA responses in the upper respiratory tract, hence providing more comprehensive cross-reactive and longer-lasting immune responses (Loving et al., 2012; Hoft et al., 2017). The major drawback of LAIVs is that they are usually poor stimulators of HI responses compared to inactivated vaccines, hence the HI titer cannot always be used as a correlate of protection for LAIVs. These vaccines are not recommended for use in immunocompromised people because of their inherent risk of developing disease. Other perceived risks associated with the use of LAIVs are vaccine strain reversion and recombination with circulating field strains; however, the different LAIV systems have been consistently safe and stable.

LAIVs for human use were independently obtained by the U.S. and Russia in the 1960's after serial passage in eggs resulting in viruses with cold-adapted, temperature-sensitive mutations that prevented their growth at temperatures higher than 35°C and thus restricting virus replication to the nasal cavity (Maassab et al., 1990). In the U.S., available LAIVs consist of reassortant viruses carrying cold-adapted, temperature sensitive (ts) mutations of the master donor viruses A/Ann Arbor/6/60 for IAV and B/Ann Arbor/1/66 for IBV (Maassab et al., 1990; Carter and Curran, 2011).

An intranasal cold-adapted LAIV produced by MedImmune (FluMist) was licensed in the U.S. in 2003. A quadrivalent version of FluMist received approval in 2012. Overall, adjusted vaccine effectiveness for LAIV against any influenza has been consistent with IIV (~50–60%), showing better effectiveness to some components than others in comparison to IIV (Ambrose et al., 2011; Caspard et al., 2017). After suboptimal protection observed against the H1N1pdm09 component in recent years in children aged 2–17 years (3%), CDC revoked its recommendation for the use of LAIV in the U.S. for the 2015–2016 and 2016–2017 seasons (Centers for Disease Control and Prevention, 2017a). The reasons for the recent lack of protection of the FluMist vaccine is not yet fully understood, and it is not known whether this is a characteristic specific to the H1N1pdm09 strain associated with reduced stability and/or infectivity (O'Donnell et al., 2014) or interference from other components in the vaccine. There is evidence that the LAIV contained a large amount of defective-interfering (DI) viral RNA, which could compromise virus replication in the respiratory tract and thus decrease the immune response to the vaccine (Gould et al., 2017). In contrast, the "Leningrad" LAIV available in Russia since 1987 for children over 3 years of age, adults and the elderly continues to show superior effective protection in children compared to inactivated vaccines (Ghendon et al., 1984; Rudenko et al., 2016). Since 2009, an agreement permitted WHO to grant sub-licenses of the Russian LAIV to manufacturers in developing countries, including China, India, and Thailand (Rudenko et al., 2016).

A modified live vaccine against equine influenza virus (EIV) is the only live-attenuated vaccine approved for use in animals.

The vaccine has a cold adapted and temperature sensitive virus derived from the wild-type A/eq/Kentucky/1/91 (H3N8) EIV strain and has been proven safe and efficacious for use in horses in the U.S. (reviewed in Paillot, 2014).

CURRENT CHALLENGES FOR VACCINE MANUFACTURING AND EFFECTIVE USE

The greatest challenge for vaccine manufacturing for both animal and human influenza is the high variability and rapid evolution of the virus that results on a constant chase for the vaccine virus to match the circulating strains. As a result, current vaccine programs are dependent on extensive surveillance, at a global scale for human vaccines and at a regional/local scale for animal vaccines. Since there are no standardized programs for vaccine selection in the veterinary field, vaccine strains are often mismatched and offer suboptimal protection that can promote, rather than stop, the spread of field strains. Additionally, pigs vaccinated with adjuvanted IIV and then challenged with a heterologous virus of the same subtype can show enhanced respiratory pathology due to strong stimulation of non-neutralizing antibody response, termed vaccine-associated enhanced respiratory disease (VAERD; Gauger et al., 2011). Furthermore, a suboptimal vaccine can result in escape mutants that will pose an increased threat to naïve populations.

Another obstacle for an effective vaccine is the timeline needed for vaccine manufacture and regulations for approval. The schedule for surveillance data collection for human influenza attempts to include the peak of the current season and increase the odds of correctly forecast which viruses are the most likely to circulate during the coming season. However, because manufacturers need to allow enough time for production to account for possible delays, this is not always the case and in some instances the distribution and antigenic make up of circulating viruses at the end of the season differs from the selected vaccine strain, which could result in a mismatch. From strain selection to vaccine distribution takes at least 6 months, without considering possible setbacks such as egg supply obstacles or problems in meeting biosafety and stability requirements. As for animal vaccines, strains are not updated as often and the process to license updated or new products could be even more time-consuming than for human vaccines. Recent changes implemented by the USDA Center for Veterinary Biologics now allow manufacturers to change or replace strains under an existing license without having to go through an entirely new licensing process (Center for Veterinary Biologics, 2007), which presents an advance on the path to advance vaccine programs.

The inherent variation in the immune status of a given population is also a major factor influencing vaccine safety and efficacy. For instance, high-risk groups, such as the elderly or immunocompromised people may not respond optimally to vaccination due to declined immune function (Kunisaki and Janoff, 2009; Lambert et al., 2012). An individual's previous immunity can have a major impact on the vaccine responses. It is well accepted that the first immunological encounter with influenza, either by natural infection or vaccination, will shape up future responses in the life of an individual, a process often called *original antigenic sin* and more recently as *antigenic imprinting*. The resulting secondary exposures tend to boost the antibody response to the priming exposure in total or partial detriment of the immunological response against the new strain, a process known as or *back-boosting* (Fazekas de St and Webster, 1966; Ma et al., 2011; Fonville et al., 2014).

In swine and poultry production systems, maternal derived antibodies in young animals can interfere with the active immune responses to vaccine depending on the age at vaccination (Loeffen et al., 2003; De Vriese et al., 2010). Other obstacles for implementation of vaccine programs in agricultural animals are the costs, the prohibitive withdrawal period post-vaccination, the difficulty to differentiate vaccinated from infected animals and the masking of clinical signs that can result in trade restrictions (Spackman and Pantin-Jackwood, 2014).

EFFORTS TO AVERT THE SETBACKS IN VACCINE USE

The limitations mentioned above highlight the need for new technologies and vaccine platforms that could improve vaccine production and availability, but also induce long-lasting broadly protective immunity. Alternative routes of delivery and different vaccination strategies could improve immune response to traditional vaccines. In addition, vaccines that target conserved regions of the virus and result in broader, longer-lasting immune response, termed "universal" vaccines, are also highly desirable and several different technologies developed in recent years show great promise as discussed below (**Table 1**).

New technologies to improve manufacturing processes, cut production time and costs, and increase production capacity are in demand. Large-scale cell-based production technology provides faster and easier production process, potential fewer issues with cell-adapted virus mutations and reduced risk of allergic reactions to egg-components. Influenza vaccines have been successfully evaluated in several continuous mammalian cell lines, such as Madin Darby canine kidney cells (MDCK), monkey kidney cells (Vero), and human embryonic retinal cells (PER.C6) (reviewed in Milian and Kamen, 2015). Cell-based vaccines produced in MDCK (Flucelvax and Celtura by Novartis) and Vero (Celvapan by Baxter Vaccines) cells received approval for use against human influenza in the US and Europe since 2009 (reviewed in Manini et al., 2017).

Adjuvants

Adjuvants increase the immunogenicity of vaccines, mainly by improving antigen processing and delivery to antigen-presenting cells and stimulating production of specific immunomodulatory cytokines and innate immune response (de Veer and Meeusen, 2011). Increasing the immunogenicity of vaccines leads to antigen sparing. Adjuvants are not widely used for influenza vaccines in humans, but are particularly desirable to increase vaccine efficacy in the elderly, children, and immunocompromised people. Some antigen formulations, such as peptides and DNA vaccines need adjuvants to improve immunogenicity. A diverse range of compounds serve as adjuvants for influenza vaccines, some licensed (aluminum salt or oil-in-water squalene-based emulsion), others in development (saponins, liposomes, cytokines, polymers) (reviewed in Soema et al., 2015a).

Aluminum salt is the most commonly used vaccine adjuvant for humans; however, it did not show a beneficial effect with the H1N1pdm09 vaccine (Manzoli et al., 2011) or with an avian H5N1 vaccine (Bernstein et al., 2008). The oil-in-water MF59 adjuvant first licensed by Novartis in 1997 in Italy for people ≥65 years of age is now approved in more than 30 countries, including the United States (Centers for Disease Control Prevention, 2016). The MF59-adjuvanted vaccine was highly effective and superior than non-adjuvanted vaccines in the elderly (>65 years) (Domnich et al., 2017). Importantly, M59-adjuvanted TIV is highly immunogenic and induces longer-lasting, broader immune response in children, and increased protection against influenza infection in pediatric populations compared to non-adjuvanted vaccines (Vesikari et al., 2009, 2011). AS03, an oil-in-water adjuvant containing α-tocopherol as an immunostimulant, has been licensed for use with avian-origin H5N1 and H1N1pdm09 split inactivated monovalent vaccines. The AS03-adjuvanted H1N1pdm09 vaccine has been extensively used in many European countries and in Canada; however it has been recently associated with increased number of narcolepsy cases in people <20 years of age (Persson et al., 2017).

In poultry and swine, the population targeted for vaccination is often composed of naïve animals. Most licensed influenza vaccines for use in poultry or swine use oil-based adjuvants to improve the immunogenicity and breadth of the immune response. In chickens, mineral and vegetable oil-based adjuvants (particularly Montanide ISA 70VG and Montanide ISA 71VG, SEPPIC) induced the highest antibody titers compared to other compounds (polymer, mineral nanoparticle, carbohydrate). Interestingly, protection of poultry against a H7N3 strain was not statistically different among various adjuvanted vaccine formulations (Lone et al., 2017).

Universally Protective Vaccines

New "universal" influenza vaccine approaches attempt to overcome the drawbacks of the highly changing nature of influenza viruses. The objective of these vaccines is to induce cross-protective broadly neutralizing immunity, which depends on stimulating both humoral and cell-mediated arms of the immune system. These "universal" vaccines rely on the concept of developing immune responses against conserved viral epitopes. Most of these strategies show great promise against IAVs and IBVs. The ultimate goal of these strategies is to avoid annual vaccine updates while prolonging the breath of immune responses and decreasing the need for re-vaccination. Broadly protective vaccine candidates that are under investigation target either the highly conserved epitopes of the HA, the NA or the extracellular domain of the M2 protein (M2e) to induce cross-reactive antibodies, and/or target internal proteins like NP and M1 to induce cross-protective T-cell response (**Table 1**, **Figure 2**).

Because these novel candidate "universal" vaccines focus on stimulating either T-cell and/or antibody responses against conserved epitopes other than the HA head, their protective responses cannot be evaluated nor quantified by standard methods. Historically, immunogenicity and vaccine protection parameters against influenza rely on the HI assay to measure neutralizing antibodies. An HI titer of 40 correlate with protection in healthy adults corresponding to a 50% reduction in the risk of contracting influenza. In children such risk reduction requires an HI titer of ~110 (Black et al., 2011). Other assays to measure immune responses to influenza viruses are available, such as NA-specific or cell-mediated responses, that could be used as surrogates of protection (McElhaney et al., 2013; Sridhar et al., 2013; Monto et al., 2015). Such assays are not routinely used and need further optimization and standardization. However, they could become extremely useful to predict protection, particularly in populations that show low HI response after vaccination like the elderly or for vaccines that do not elicit HI-antibodies.

Universal Vaccines Targeting HA-Specific Antibodies

Unlike the head domain, the stalk domain is much more conserved across HA subtypes and phylogenetically classified into two groups: group 1 that includes the H1, H2, H5, H6, H8, H9, H11, H12, H13, and H16 subtypes, and group 2 that includes the H3, H4, H7, H10, H14, and H15 subtypes. Antibodies against the HA globular head neutralize infection by either preventing binding to cellular receptors or membrane fusion (**Figure 2A**). Stalk-specific antibodies do not usually neutralize the virus (measured by using standard assays), but protect through inhibition of either entry, viral release, by mediating antibody dependent cell-mediated cytotoxicity (ADCC) or complement cytotoxicity (**Figure 2B**). Anti-stalk antibodies are naturally produced after infection but in low levels compared to those against the immunodominant globular head domain (Corti et al., 2011). Recently, a study found that high levels of HA stalk-reactive antibodies measured by ELISA and high ADCC activity correlated with protection against H1N1pdm09 challenge in mice with passive transfer of sera from H5N1 vaccinees (Jacobsen et al., 2017). Since HI responses against the H5N1 virus were below predictive protective values against the H1N1pdm09, the authors concluded that high levels of HA stalk-specific antibodies were responsible for protection and presented evidence for other parameters associated with correlates of protection.

By using a "headless" HA as antigen, vaccinated mice produced levels of anti-stem broadly neutralizing antibodies (bnAbs) that protected them against lethal homologous (Corti et al., 2011) or heterosubtypic challenge (Steel et al., 2010). The same "headless" HA approach reduced fever after sub-lethal homologous challenge in cynomolgus monkeys (Impagliazzo et al., 2015). In a distinct "headless" approach, mice vaccinated with a conformational polypeptide that mimics the H5 HA stem (mini-stem) resulted in protective responses against lethal challenge with both group 1 (H5 and H1) and group 2 (H3) influenza viruses (Valkenburg et al., 2016). Sequential immunization with chimeric constructs that express the same stalk but irrelevant divergent heads also induced broadly neutralizing, stalk-specific antibodies that protected mice against lethal heterologous challenge (Krammer et al., 2013; Ermler

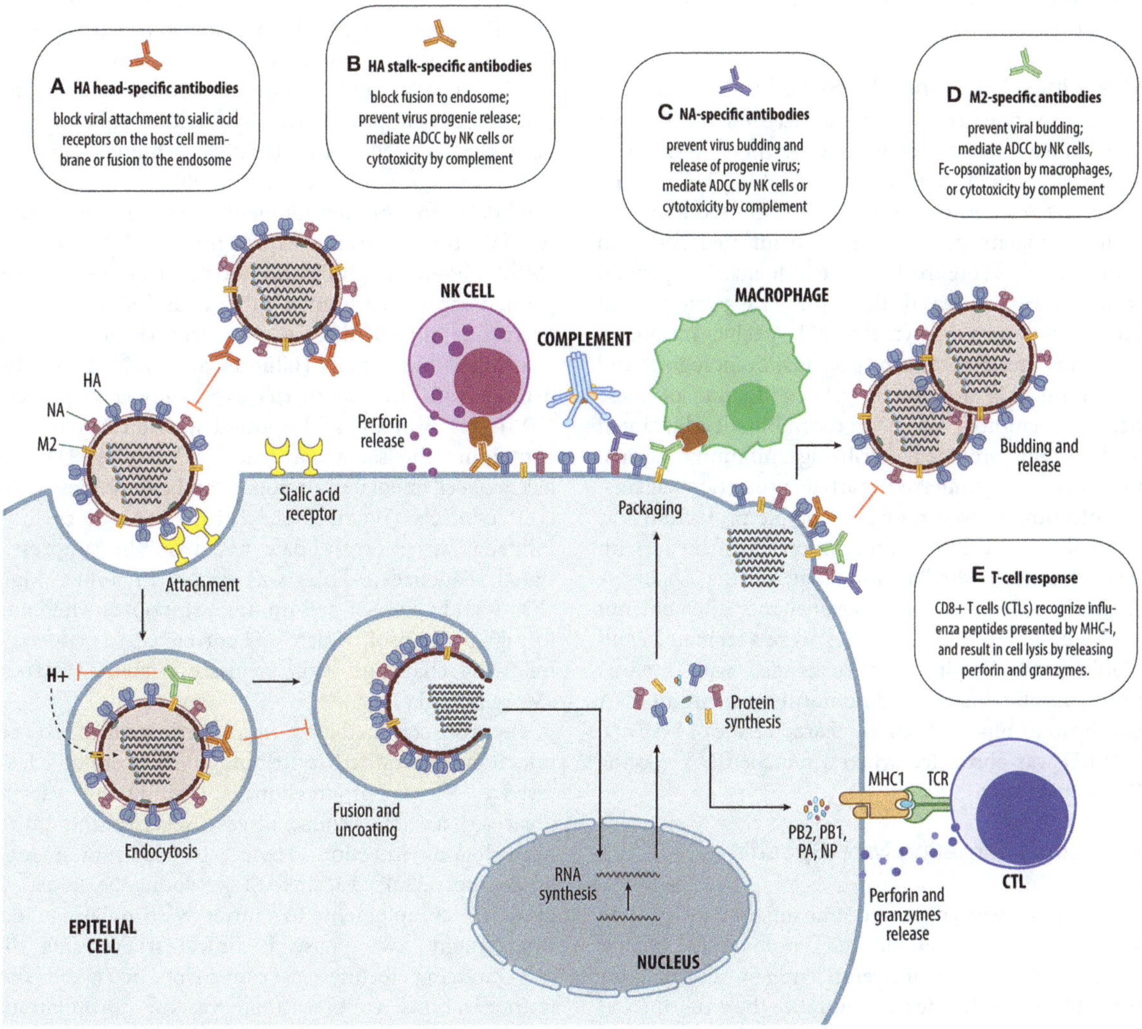

FIGURE 2 | Immune response elicited by different influenza vaccines. **(A)** HA-head-specific antibodies interfere or block virus binding to the sialic acid receptors on the cell surface and prevent virus entry to host cells. **(B)** HA-stalk-specific antibodies prevent virus fusion to the endosome, inhibit budding and release of new virus particles, and mediate antibody dependent cell-mediated cytotoxicity (ADCC) by natural killer (NK) cells or complement activation. **(C)** NA-specific antibodies inhibit budding and release of new virus particles, and mediate ADCC by NK cells or complement activation. **(D)** M2e-specific antibodies inhibit budding and release of new virus particles, and mediate ADCC by NK cells, Fc-opsonization by macrophages or complement activation. **(E)** CD8+ T cells (cytotoxic T lymphocytes, or CTLs) recognize influenza peptides presented by major histocompatibility complex class I (MHC-I) at the surface of infected cells via their T cell receptor (TCR), release cytotoxic granules containing perforin and granzymes, resulting in lysis of infected cells.

et al., 2017). Anti-stalk antibodies can also be stimulated with sequential immunizations with antigenically different strains within the same group (Nachbagauer et al., 2014; Kirchenbaum et al., 2015).

Interestingly, mice produce cross-reactive neutralizing antibodies directed to the globular head of the HA (Yoshida et al., 2009). More importantly, broadly neutralizing head domain antibodies have been characterized in humans, with activity against a single subtype (e.g., H1 for CH65, H3 for F045-092) or against multiple subtypes (e.g., C05, S139/1) (Whittle et al., 2011; Ekiert et al., 2012; Lee et al., 2012, 2014), suggesting that specific regions of the head domain are targets for "universal" vaccines. Despite the high variability between HA subtypes, attachment to sialic acid receptors on the host cells is a conserved activity (Weis et al., 1988). Antibodies that target highly conserved residues close to or at the receptor-binding site on the HA head result in receptor mimicry and prevent viral-host recognition. Recently, an antibody was shown to result in strong cross-protection against multiple lineages of influenza B in mice and ferrets (Shen et al., 2017).

Another HA-based strategy to develop "universal" vaccines is the Computationally Optimized Broadly Reactive Antigen (COBRA) technology, which uses consensus sequences to design vaccines that represent multiple circulating strains. A COBRA VLP-based H1 vaccine showed broad cross-reactivity to multiple H1 strains and protected mice against H1N1pdm09 challenge either in a monovalent cocktail or in prime-boost regimens (Carter et al., 2016).

Universal Vaccines Targeting NA-Specific Antibodies

Current influenza vaccines are not standardized for the amount of NA. The stability and correct folding of the NA in these vaccines is not well defined. Antibodies that inhibit NA activity interfere with virus release from the cell surface, reducing the amount of virus progeny produced by the infected cell, and may also mediate ADCC (**Figure 2C**). The influenza NA protein is antigenically more conserved than the HA protein, and several animal studies have shown that NA-specific antibodies may induce cross-protective immunity against homologous and heterologous strains that are closely related. In one of these recent studies, vaccination of mice with recombinant adjuvanted N1, N2, or IBV NA provided sterilizing immunity against homologous virus and conferred partial protection against heterologous infection; however, heterosubtypic protection was lacking (Wohlbold et al., 2015). Vaccination of chickens with a recombinant N2 with similar homology to the challenge virus and high NI activity protected against mortality but not morbidity (Sylte et al., 2007). When pigs were vaccinated with inactivated adjuvanted vaccine and challenged with a virus containing antigenically mismatched homosubtypic HA and NA proteins, they showed enhanced disease characteristic of VAERD. However, VAERD was abrogated when a matched NA vaccine was used (Rajao et al., 2016).

Universal Vaccines Targeting M2e-Specific Antibodies

M2 protein is a relatively conserved transmembrane protein of influenza viruses and its extracellular domain (M2e) has been extensively explored as a "universal"antigen candidate for vaccines. Anti-M2e antibodies do not neutralize the virus, instead these antibodies are thought to prevent viral budding, mediate killing of infected cells by NK cells or macrophages through ADCC, Fc-opsonization, or complement activation (El Bakkouri et al., 2011; **Figure 2D**). M2e is present on the virus' surface in low quantities and, thus, it is poorly immunogenic (Wu et al., 2007). However, strategies to improve immunogenicity, such as adjuvants, multimeric forms of M2e, co-immunization with other influenza vaccines, or fusion with carrier proteins (Kim et al., 2013; Lee et al., 2015; Tang et al., 2017) stimulate broad cross-reactive immune responses and provide protection against heterologous, hetorosubtypic challenge in mice (Lee et al., 2015; Tao et al., 2017). Human clinical trial demonstrated the safety and immunogenicityof different M2e vaccine candidates (reviewed in Turley et al., 2011; Kolpe et al., 2017). Surprisingly, pigs vaccinated with an M2e vaccine and challenged with a heterologous virus showed severe clinical signs compared to control animals (Heinen et al., 2002).

Universal Vaccines Targeting T-cell Responses

CD8+ cytotoxic T lymphocytes (CTLs) predominantly target conserved internal influenza virus proteins, such as the NP and M1, and, therefore, generate cross-reactive immune responses to influenza viruses of different subtypes (Gotch et al., 1987; Hillaire et al., 2013; **Figure 2E**). Vaccines focusing on the induction of CTL responses should provide a broader cross-protective response and are potential candidates for a more "universal" vaccine. The NP and M proteins were shown to contain highly conserved epitopes shared by various subtypes of influenza virus that are recognized by diverse human leukocyte antigen (HLA) backgrounds (Lee et al., 2008), and hence are potential candidates for the development of broadly protective vaccines. A MVA-based vaccine expressing the NP and M1 proteins (MVA-NP+M1) significantly boosted T-cell response in naturally primed vaccinated human subjects and vaccination was shown to reduce clinical disease and virus shedding in intranasally challenged individuals (Lillie et al., 2012). Similarly, chickens primed with an adenovirus expressing a fusion construct of NP + M1 proteins and boosted with an MVA vector vaccine containing the same construct (MVA-NP+M1) showed high levels of cell-mediated responses and showed less shedding than GFP controls (Boyd et al., 2013). A single-cycle "universal" influenza vaccine candidate based on the suppression of HA signal sequence (S-FLU) was shown to induce high levels of CD4+ and CD8+ T cell immune responses when administered to pigs by aerosol, which was correlated to reduced viral titers following challenge with a closely related H1N1pdm09 virus (Morgan et al., 2016).

Because cell-mediated immune responses do not prevent infection but rather contribute to accelerated clearance and restrict disease progression, CTL-inducing vaccines are a great aid to help reduce disease severity and mortality after heterologous infection. Hence, to reach their full potential as a "universal" vaccine they would be most efficient if used in complement to antibody-stimulating technologies. Interestingly, two phase I clinical trials using different T-cell inducing technologies in prime-boost or simultaneous immunizations with seasonal vaccine formulations resulted in stimulation of both T cell and antibody responses in the elderly (Antrobus et al., 2014; Atsmon et al., 2014).

Universal Vaccine Platforms

In the effort to achieve better vaccine products, a myriad of vaccine manufacturing platforms and technologies have been developed with potential application in different species and different epidemiological situations. An ideal "universal" vaccine approach would include not only a broadly protective vaccine methodology, but also a more standardized vaccine platform that can be applied indistinctively in multiple animal species or in different epidemiological scenarios. Ideally, these "universal" approaches could be complementary to each other and could be used for either endemic, epidemic, and/or pandemic influenza. Some possible approaches that could serve as "universal" platforms are summarized in **Figure 3** and will be discussed below.

Live-Attenuated Vaccines

As mentioned previously, cold-adapted/temperature sensitive LAIVs are already in use for humans and horses, and similar approaches have also been experimentally tested successfully in

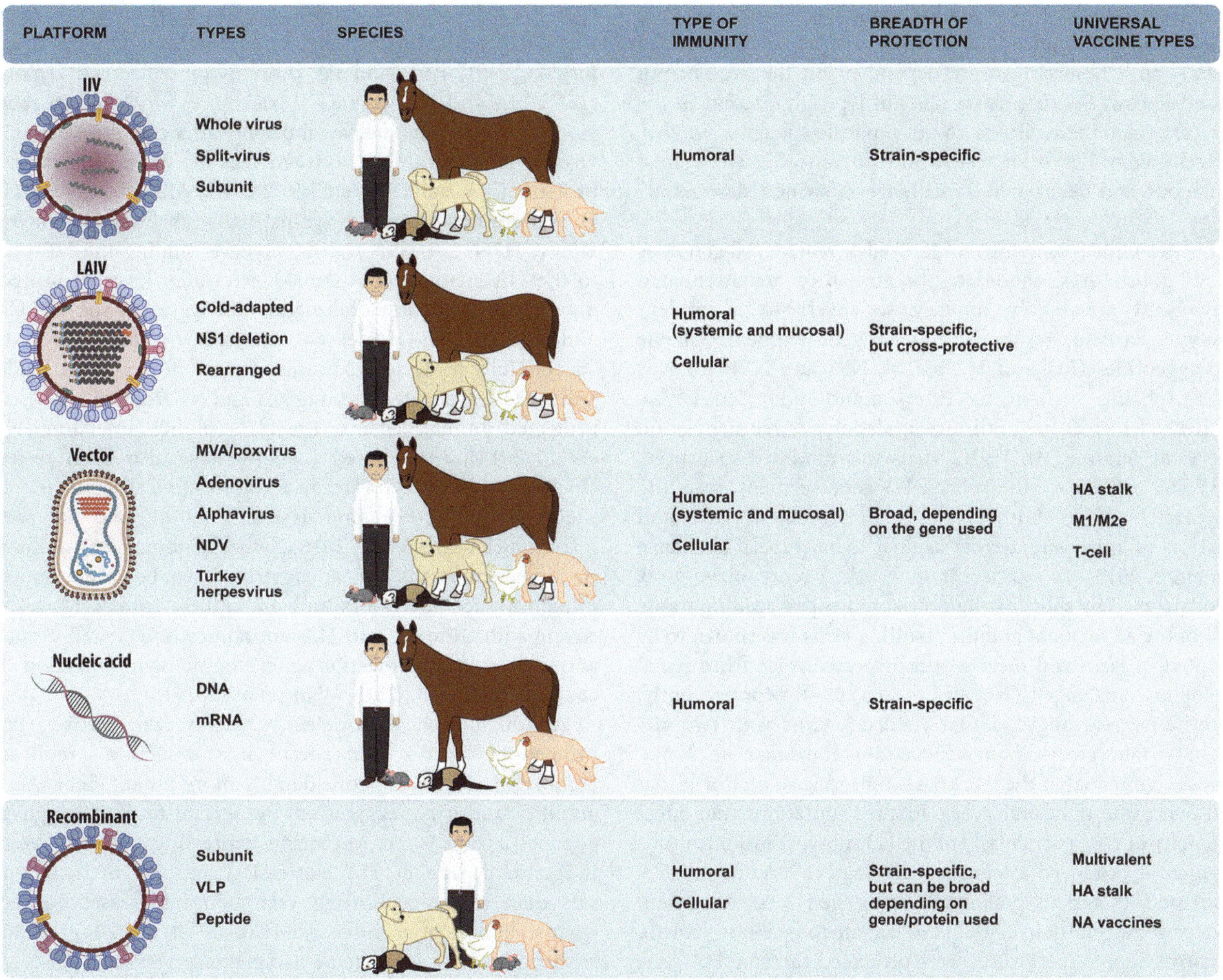

FIGURE 3 | Influenza "universal" vaccine platforms that are used in multiple species or epidemiological situations. Vaccine platform, types of technology, host species, type of immunity stimulated, breadth of protection, and types of universally protective vaccines within each platform are shown.

poultry and swine. In one approach, a combination of an HA tag at the C-terminus of PB1 along with temperature-sensitive mutations in PB1 and PB2 (tsHA LAIV) showed remarkable stability over multiple passages and in different IAV backbones of avian-, human-, and swine-origin. This strategy is safe and effective resulting in protection against low- and high-pathogenic influenza strains in chickens and against swine-origin IAVs in swine (Song et al., 2007; Pena et al., 2011). The tsHA LAIV has consistently shown cross protection after challenge with antigenically distinct viruses in swine and significantly more efficacious than inactivated products (Loving et al., 2013; Gauger et al., 2014). More recently, a prototypical influenza B virus engineered with a similar tsHA strategy resulted in a stable virus over multiple passages in tissue culture and eggs, and attenuated *in vivo*. In mice, a single intranasal dose of the IBV tsHA virus offered protection against lethal homologous and heterologous IBV challenges (Santos et al., 2017a).

Other strategies for the generation of attenuated virus have been described with great success in different species. NS1-truncated mutants can be used as LAIV candidates because they do not present the normal interferon-antagonist activity shown by viruses containing the wild-type NS1 protein (Richt and Garcia-Sastre, 2009). Several truncations of NS1 in both IAV and IBV strains resulted in virus attenuation and heterologous cross-protection (Solorzano et al., 2005; Hai et al., 2008; Pica et al., 2012). Additionally, this strategy has been proven to be immunogenic in young pigs, prime T cell response and result in partial heterosubtypic cross-protection (Kappes et al., 2012). In chickens, vaccination with a reassortant containing truncated-NS1 proteins harboring only 73 amino acids in addition to a modification in the HA to remove the polybasic cleavage site induced significant cross-protection against homologous and heterologous H5 clade viruses (Shi et al., 2016). Other modifications in the HA cleavage site can also result in attenuation of influenza viruses. By mutating one amino acid at the HA cleavage site, it is possible to engineer viruses carrying a cleavage site recognized by elastase instead of trypsin-like proteases, and these viruses are dependent on the presence of elastase to grow. Because elastase is not typically present in the respiratory tract, these viruses do not replicate efficiently *in vivo*. This technology has been tested and proven effective against homologous and heterologous challenge in swine (Masic et al., 2010).

Influenza viruses carrying reorganized or rearranged genomes serve as good LAIV candidates because they are attenuated *in vivo* and are highly unlikely to revert to a virulent phenotype. Particularly, the M and NS gene segments encode two polypeptides (M1 and M2 for M, NS1 and NEP for NS) by using splicing mechanisms (Paterson and Fodor, 2012; Wise et al., 2012), which allow for the manipulation and reorganization of the viral genome. An H9N2 virus was modified to express the H5 HA protein on the spliced NS gene segment, resulting in the expression of both H9 and H5 protein *in vitro* and protection of mice and ferrets against lethal H5N1 challenge (Pena et al., 2013). In a different approach, a reorganized virus was constructed by splitting the overlapping open reading frame (ORF) of the M segment and the resulting virus was shown to be attenuated *in vitro* and *in vivo* and protected mice from lethal homologous challenged (Nogales et al., 2016). More recently, an alternative rearranged design yielded a virus with two HA genes in the laboratory-adapted PR8 strain (Harding et al., 2017). The underlying goal of the work was to produce a platform that would overcome undesirable egg-adapted mutations that affect antigenicity of IAV, particularly of the H3 subtype. Modifications in segment 4 produced a segment carrying N1 NA and H1 HA genes from PR8 and a segment 6 carrying the H3 HA of a strain known to grow poorly in eggs and to mutate to facilitate growth. Alternative double HA viruses were produced carrying HA gene segments from current IAV and IBV vaccine strains. In general, double HA viruses grew to titers similar to the wt PR8 strain in eggs, carried no egg-adapted mutations and, as inactivated vaccines, produced protective anti-HA responses in mice against the corresponding HA genes (Harding et al., 2017). It remains to be determined whether such strategy would be amenable as an alternative LAIV in other animal species besides mice.

Virus Vectors

Vectored vaccines (adenovirus, poxvirus, alphavirus, etc.) are a non-replicating safe approach for different species that eliminates the risk of virus recombination. Vector vaccines can mimic the natural infection when delivered through the intranasal route, and the antigens of interest are expressed in the native conformation, which results in higher antibody specificity. Additionally, this approach can be rapidly produced, is fully scalable and does not require the use of eggs. Not all virus vectors can be used in common for all species, but the concept of vectored-vaccine production tends to be similar between different vector systems. Modified vaccinia virus Ankara (MVA, poxvirus) is a highly attenuated strain of vaccinia virus that originated from growth selection on chicken embryo fibroblasts (CEF), and is one of the most commonly used vectors for human vaccines. Goodman et al. (2011) showed increased CD4+ and CD8+ T cell response in mice by using a prime/ boost regimen with DNA and MVA-vectors containing human T cell epitopes for M1, NS1, PB1, and PA proteins or conserved regions of H5N1 HA and NA on an NP backbone, which led to reduced viral replication and delayed mortality after challenge with H1N1 viruses. Similarly, MVA vectored vaccines expressing conserved proteins (HA stalk, HA stalk/M2e, M1, M2, PB1) of an H5N1 virus were not protective against lethal challenge in mice with H5N1, H7N1, or H9N2 virus; however adding the NP protein to the HA stem or HA stem/M2e resulted in cross-protection due to the induction of broadly-reactive virus-specific CD4+ and CD8+ T-cells (Hessel et al., 2014). MVA-based H1N1pdm09 vaccine fully protected macaques from a homologous challenge and an MVA vaccine encoding HA and NP from an H5N1 cross-protected animals against the H1N1pdm09 infection (Florek et al., 2014). MVA-based vaccines have also been tested in chickens: a MVA-H9 vaccine reduced clinical signs and virus shedding against homologous challenge, but did not prevent infection (Ducatez et al., 2016). Other systems using alphavirus, parainfluenza virus, or adenovirus have been developed as influenza vaccine vectors and pre-clinical studies have shown strong induction of anti-HA antibodies and T cell responses and some showed protection against homologous infection (Yang et al., 2009; Li et al., 2015; Wang et al., 2017).

Although replication-defective vectors can mediate potent protection against influenza virus infection, replication-competent vectors are considerably more potent since they can amplify transgene expression by several-fold. A single-cycle adenovirus (Ad) vector vaccine expressing PR8 HA resulted in markedly higher HA expression and HI titers in cotton rats than a non-replicating vector, and increased protection against homologous infection (Crosby et al., 2017). Another replication-defective vaccine using adenovirus serotype 5 (Ad5) has been tested in pigs and resulted in moderate protection against heterologous challenge (Wesley et al., 2004; Braucher et al., 2012). A single-cycle, propagation-defective alphavirus-like replicon particle vaccine, based on an attenuated Venezuelan equine encephalitis virus, was recently approved to be used in swine (United States Department of Agriculture, 2014). This technology allows for rapid strain updates and the ability to generate custom made vaccines with circulating strains (autogenous). This alphavirus-replicon vaccine induced robust immune response against H1 or H3 viruses in pigs, and completely protected pigs against homologous challenge and partially protected against heterosubtypic infection (Vander Veen et al., 2012, 2013). A propagation-defective alphavirus-like replicon particle vaccine expressing an H5 HA, with a similar approach to the one approved for use in swine, was shown to provide partial protection in turkeys against a HPAIV H5N2 strain with homologous HA (Santos et al., 2017b). Newcastle disease virus (NDV)-vectored H5 and H7 vaccines induced high levels of HI antibodies and protected chickens from challenge with a H7N9 or HPAI H5N1 viruses, respectively (Liu et al., 2015). Although NDV-vectored vaccines were shown to be effective in protecting chickens against HPAIV infection, preexisting immunity to the NDV vector limits the protective efficacy of these vectored vaccines in the field (Spackman and Pantin-Jackwood, 2014). An alternative chimeric NDV-vectored with F and HN ectodomains replaced by those of avian paramyxovirus serotype-2 was shown to be safe, not cross-react with NDV, and to partially protect 1-day-old immunized chickens against H5N1 HPAIV challenge (Kim et al., 2017). Additionally, a recombinant turkey herpesvirus vector vaccine expressing the HA gene of H5N1 HPAIV consistently demonstrated a high degree of homologous protection as well as cross-protection against heterologous clades of the H5N1 HPAIV (Gardin et al., 2016). One of the advantages of using recombinant vectored vaccines against avian influenza for poultry is the possibility of using automated methods as a spray or in drinking water for mass-immunization, providing a rapid, efficient, and economical immunization method.

Nucleic Acid-Based Vaccines

Nucleic acid-based vaccines allow for the expression of target antigens *in vivo* and, therefore, induce both cellular and broad antibody immunity without exposing the host to a live virus. Hence, this technology provides a rapid, stable, highly scalable and safe alternative to traditional influenza vaccine production, without the need to grow virus in eggs (Kutzler and Weiner, 2008), and has been effectively tested in multiple host species. DNA vaccines against influenza are often based on expression of the HA protein, but the humoral immunogenicity is considered suboptimal in humans and large animals when compared to the traditional vaccine approaches. To increase their immunogenicity, further optimization has been proposed, including the use of adjuvants, different prime-boost combinations, or different delivery methods. In a recent study, by using the NK cell agonist α-Galactosylceramide as an adjuvant in mice, there was a significant increase in the IgG titers and IFN-γ levels compared with mice receiving the DNA vaccine alone (Fotouhi et al., 2017). Others have used the priming regimen to increase DNA vaccine immunogenicity. In a phase 1 trial in healthy adults, Crank and colleagues showed that a H1 DNA vaccine was safe but only modestly immunogenic as a single agent; however, antibody responses were significantly improved after boosting with a H1N1pdm09 monovalent inactivated vaccine (MIV) (Crank et al., 2015). Similarly, using a combined prime-boost regimen with DNA and protein vaccines significantly enhanced the humoral response of an H5 DNA vaccine in chickens (Stachyra et al., 2017). Alternative delivery systems, such as intradermal delivery, have been shown to improve levels of cross-reactive antibody and cell-mediated responses in pigs and humans (Ledgerwood et al., 2012; Borggren et al., 2016).

Messenger RNA (mRNA)-based vaccines, another variation of the nucleic acid-based technology, offers safety advantages in comparison to DNA-based vaccines since it harbors only components required for protein expression, is rapidly degraded and does not interact with the host genome. An intradermal mRNA vaccine encoding the full-length PR8 H1 protected young and old mice from lethal challenge with H1N1, H3N2, and H5N1 viruses, while the same mRNA vaccine encoding HA, NA and NP protected pigs from disease and reduced virus shedding after homologous challenge (Petsch et al., 2012). More recently, a modified mRNA vaccine encoding HA of H7N9 formulated with lipid nanoparticle generated robust immune responses in mice, ferrets, and nonhuman primates, protected mice from lethal H7N9 challenge and reduced lung virus titers in ferrets after homologous challenge (Bahl et al., 2017). The same vaccine platform encoding H10N8 HA was safe and immunogenic in humans in a randomized, double-blinded, placebo-controlled phase 1 trial (Bahl et al., 2017).

Protein-Based and Virus-Like Particle Vaccines

Vaccines produced using insect cell and baculovirus expression vector systems (BEVS) allows for expression of large quantities of HA and/or NA *in vitro*, relatively fast manufacturing cycles, lack of emergence of spurious adaptive mutations as seen in other systems, and ability to produce the vaccine without the need for high-level biocontainment. A trivalent recombinant HA vaccine has been licensed for use in individuals 18–49 years of age (Flublok by Protein Sciences Corporation) and was shown to be safe and immunogenic in healthy adults and the elderly, but not in children (King et al., 2009; Baxter et al., 2011). Recombinant baculovirus-expressed vaccines have been tested in swine and poultry, and thus could be used as a universal platform. A recent study showed that three recombinant H1 constructs, either displayed in the baculovirus envelope, displayed in a Feline Leukemia Virus (FeLV) gag virus-like particle (VLP), or purified as a subunit IgG fusion protein, protected pigs against heterologous, homosubtypic H1N1 challenge (Hernandez et al., 2016). Furthermore, recombinant baculovirus-expressed H5 and H7 proteins administered with a water-in-oil adjuvant protected chickens against a lethal homosubtypic infection and reduced viral shedding in some animals (Crawford et al., 1999).

Virus-like particles (VLPs) are recombinant virus particles formed solely by viral structural proteins that do not have any genomic component. Although these are non-replicating particles, they retain the morphology of the virus and, therefore, the antigenicity and can activate innate immunity. VLPs can be produced in several expression systems, including baculovirus-, insect cell-, bacteria-, or plant-derived systems (Low et al., 2014; Pillet et al., 2016; Valero-Pacheco et al., 2016; Li et al., 2017). In a double-blind, randomized phase I clinical trial, Low and colleagues showed that a non-adjuvanted H1NIpdm09 VLP vaccine was safe and resulted in seroconversion in more than 50% of the subjects with just one dose, and this percentage increased after boost (Low et al., 2014). A recent cross-sectional study demonstrated that subjects previously vaccinated with a H1N1pdm09 HA VLP vaccine in a phase 2, randomized, double blind, placebo-controlled study still had detectable levels of antibodies 24 months after vaccination (Valero-Pacheco et al., 2016). VLPs also represent a promising approach for broadly cross-protective "universal" vaccines, as shown by a recent phase I-II randomized clinical trial in which a quadrivalent VLP vaccine induced significant HI titers against all components of the vaccine and also cross-reactive HI responses against heterologous strains (Pillet et al., 2016). This cross-reactive response was also observed in chickens vaccinated with triple-subtype (H5, H7, and H9) VLPs that were protected against challenge with heterologous HPAI H5N2 and H7N3 and LPAI H9N2 (Pushko et al., 2017). Vaccination of chickens with adjuvanted VLPs expressing H9N2 HA and NA also induced robust HI antibodies and reduced viral shedding after homologous challenge (Li et al., 2017). In pigs, VLP antigens consisting of H1N1pdm09 HA, NA, and M1 proteins elicited robust levels of humoral and mucosal immune responses and protected pigs against homologous infection (Pyo et al., 2012).

CLOSING REMARKS

Current vaccines in use for humans and animals do not provide long-lasting broad protection. Novel strategies are available with the potential of providing "universal" broadly cross-protective and memory-stimulating immune responses against several or all influenza strains. Despite great progress in recent years, the "universal" vaccine technologies still present several obstacles on the path to licensing. To reach a full "universal" potential, vaccines should stimulate both antibody and T-cell immune responses to the more conserved epitopes of influenza viruses. One way to reach this full breadth of the immune system is to use live-attenuated vaccines or live vectored-vaccines to deliver these conserved proteins, while stimulating cellular and mucosal immunity. Questions remain regarding to the duration of the immunity of "universal" vaccines, how easily these strategies can be used in a field situation, if these vaccines will provide better protection than the current vaccines without the need for frequent updates, or if they should be used in combination with current technologies. More importantly, correlates of protection are not well defined for these novel technologies, and standardized assays to measure their protection levels need to be established.

Successful control of influenza can only be achieved through collaborative support between human and animal health. Any attempts in developing broadly cross-reactive vaccines should take under consideration the complex ecology of IAVs and how inter-related the viruses are between different species. Vaccine platforms that can be used indistinctively in various animal species and that can easily be accessed in different epidemiological scenarios (e.g., during a season, outbreak, or pandemic) could greatly improve vaccine production as such approach could create standardized regulations for vaccine licensing for different hosts and streamlined vaccine production processes. Such uniform approach is not necessarily novel. One could argue that production of inactivated vaccines follows similar paths irrespective of the targeted species. Thus, "universal vaccine platforms" for "universal vaccines" would ultimately be a great complement to drastically reduce the disease burden caused by influenza viruses in people and animals.

AUTHOR CONTRIBUTIONS

DR and DP have contributed in the conceptualization of the ideas, drafting the manuscript, critical revision of the manuscript, and final approval.

FUNDING

The authors were supported by the Center for Research on Influenza Pathogenesis (CRIP), a National Institute of Allergy and Infectious Diseases (NIAID) funded Center of Excellence for Influenza Research and Surveillance (CEIRS, HHSN272201400008C).

REFERENCES

Alam, S., Knowlden, Z. A., Sangster, M. Y., and Sant, A. J. (2014). CD4 T cell help is limiting and selective during the primary B cell response to influenza virus infection. *J. Virol.* 88, 314–324. doi: 10.1128/JVI.02077-13

Ambrose, C. S., and Levin, M. J. (2012). The rationale for quadrivalent influenza vaccines. *Hum. Vaccin. Immunother.* 8, 81–88. doi: 10.4161/hv.8.1.17623

Ambrose, C. S., Levin, M. J., and Belshe, R. B. (2011). The relative efficacy of trivalent live attenuated and inactivated influenza vaccines in children and adults. *Influenza Other Respir. Viruses* 5, 67–75. doi: 10.1111/j.1750-2659.2010.00183.x

Anderson, T. K., Macken, C. A., Lewis, N. S., Scheuermann, R. H., Van Reeth, K., Brown, I. H., et al. (2016). A Phylogeny-Based Global Nomenclature System and Automated Annotation Tool for H1 Hemagglutinin Genes from Swine Influenza A Viruses. *mSphere* 1, e00275–e00216. doi: 10.1128/mSphere.00275-16

Anderson, T. K., Nelson, M. I., Kitikoon, P., Swenson, S. L., Korslund, J. A., and Vincent, A. L. (2013). Population dynamics of cocirculating swine influenza A viruses in the United States from 2009 to 2012. *Influenza Other Respir. Viruses* 7, 42–51. doi: 10.1111/irv.12193

Antrobus, R. D., Berthoud, T. K., Mullarkey, C. E., Hoschler, K., Coughlan, L., Zambon, M., et al. (2014). Coadministration of seasonal influenza vaccine and MVA-NP+M1 simultaneously achieves potent humoral and cell-mediated responses. *Mol. Ther.* 22, 233–238. doi: 10.1038/mt.2013.162

Atsmon, J., Caraco, Y., Ziv-Sefer, S., Shaikevich, D., Abramov, E., Volokhov, I., et al. (2014). Priming by a novel universal influenza vaccine (Multimeric-001)-a gateway for improving immune response in the elderly population. *Vaccine* 32, 5816–5823. doi: 10.1016/j.vaccine.2014.08.031

Bahl, K., Senn, J. J., Yuzhakov, O., Bulychev, A., Brito, L. A., Hassett, K. J., et al. (2017). Preclinical and clinical demonstration of immunogenicity by mRNA vaccines against H10N8 and H7N9 influenza viruses. *Mol. Ther.* 25, 1316–1327. doi: 10.1016/j.ymthe.2017.03.035

Baxter, R., Patriarca, P. A., Ensor, K., Izikson, R., Goldenthal, K. L., and Cox, M. M. (2011). Evaluation of the safety, reactogenicity and immunogenicity of FluBlok(R) trivalent recombinant baculovirus-expressed hemagglutinin influenza vaccine administered intramuscularly to healthy adults 50-64 years of age. *Vaccine* 29, 2272–2278. doi: 10.1016/j.vaccine.2011.01.039

Bernstein, D. I., Edwards, K. M., Dekker, C. L., Belshe, R., Talbot, H. K., Graham, I. L., et al. (2008). Effects of adjuvants on the safety and immunogenicity of an avian influenza H5N1 vaccine in adults. *J. Infect. Dis.* 197, 667–675. doi: 10.1086/527489

Beyer, W. E., Nauta, J. J., Palache, A. M., Giezeman, K. M., and Osterhaus, A. D. (2011). Immunogenicity and safety of inactivated influenza vaccines in primed populations: a systematic literature review and meta-analysis. *Vaccine* 29, 5785–5792. doi: 10.1016/j.vaccine.2011.05.040

Black, S., Nicolay, U., Vesikari, T., Knuf, M., Del Giudice, G., Della Cioppa, G., et al. (2011). Hemagglutination inhibition antibody titers as a correlate of protection for inactivated influenza vaccines in children. *Pediatr. Infect. Dis. J.* 30, 1081–1085. doi: 10.1097/INF.0b013e3182367662

Borggren, M., Nielsen, J., Karlsson, I., Dalgaard, T. S., Trebbien, R., Williams, J. A., et al. (2016). A polyvalent influenza DNA vaccine applied by needle-free intradermal delivery induces cross-reactive humoral and cellular immune responses in pigs. *Vaccine* 34, 3634–3640. doi: 10.1016/j.vaccine.2016.05.030

Boyd, A. C., Ruiz-Hernandez, R., Peroval, M. Y., Carson, C., Balkissoon, D., Staines, K., et al. (2013). Towards a universal vaccine for avian influenza: protective efficacy of modified Vaccinia virus Ankara and Adenovirus vaccines expressing conserved influenza antigens in chickens challenged with low pathogenic avian influenza virus. *Vaccine* 31, 670–675. doi: 10.1016/j.vaccine.2012.11.047

Braucher, D. R., Henningson, J. N., Loving, C. L., Vincent, A. L., Kim, E., Steitz, J., et al. (2012). Intranasal vaccination with replication-defective adenovirus type 5 encoding influenza virus hemagglutinin elicits protective immunity to homologous challenge and partial protection to heterologous challenge in pigs. *Clin. Vaccine Immunol.* 19, 1722–1729. doi: 10.1128/CVI.00315-12

Carter, D. M., Darby, C. A., Lefoley, B. C., Crevar, C. J., Alefantis, T., Oomen, R., et al. (2016). Design and characterization of a computationally optimized broadly reactive hemagglutinin vaccine for H1N1 influenza viruses. *J. Virol.* 90, 4720–4734. doi: 10.1128/JVI.03152-15

Carter, N. J., and Curran, M. P. (2011). Live attenuated influenza vaccine (FluMist(R); Fluenz): a review of its use in the prevention of seasonal influenza in children and adults. *Drugs* 71, 1591–1622. doi: 10.2165/11206860-000000000-00000

Caspard, H., Mallory, R. M., Yu, J., and Ambrose, C. S. (2017). Live-attenuated influenza vaccine effectiveness in children from 2009 to 2015-2016: a systematic review and meta-analysis. *Open Forum Infect. Dis.* 4:ofx111. doi: 10.1093/ofid/ofx111

Center for Veterinary Biologics (2007). *Labeling of Equine Influenza and Swine Influenza Vaccines. Notice No 07-17.* Ames, IA: USDA Animal and Plant Health Inspection Service.

Centers for Disease Control and Prevention (2016). *FLUAD^{TM} Flu Vaccine With Adjuvant.* Available online at: https://www.cdc.gov/flu/protect/vaccine/adjuvant.htm (Accessed July 28, 2017).

Centers for Disease Control and Prevention (2017a) *ACIP Votes Down Use of LAIV for 2016-2017 flu Season.* Available online at: https://www.cdc.gov/media/releases/2016/s0622-laiv-flu.html (Accessed July 21, 2017).

Centers for Disease Control and Prevention (2017b). *August 24, 2017 Seasonal Influenza Vaccine Effectiveness, 2005-2017.* Available online at: https://www.cdc.gov/flu/professionals/vaccination/effectiveness-studies.htm (Accessed December 14, 2017).

Centers for Disease Control and Prevention (2017c) *Case Count: Detected, U.S. Human Infections with H3N2v by State Since August 2011.* Available online at: https://www.cdc.gov/flu/swineflu/h3n2v-case-count.htm (Accessed July 28, 2017).

Centers for Disease Control and Prevention (2017d). Estimated Influenza Illnesses, Medical Visits, Hospitalizations, and Deaths Averted by Vaccination in the United States. Available online at: https://www.cdc.gov/flu/about/disease/2015-16.htm (Accessed May 27, 2017).

Centers for Disease Control and Prevention (2017e). *Avian Influenza A Virus Infections in Humans.* Available online at: https://www.cdc.gov/flu/avianflu/avian-in-humans.htm (Accessed July 26, 2017)

Corti, D., Voss, J., Gamblin, S. J., Codoni, G., Macagno, A., Jarrossay, D., et al. (2011). A neutralizing antibody selected from plasma cells that binds to group 1 and group 2 influenza A hemagglutinins. *Science* 333, 850–856. doi: 10.1126/science.1205669

Crank, M. C., Gordon, I. J., Yamshchikov, G. V., Sitar, S., Hu, Z., Enama, M. E., et al. (2015). Phase 1 study of pandemic H1 DNA vaccine in healthy adults. *PLoS ONE* 10:e0123969. doi: 10.1371/journal.pone.0123969

Crawford, J., Wilkinson, B., Vosnesensky, A., Smith, G., Garcia, M., Stone, H., et al. (1999). Baculovirus-derived hemagglutinin vaccines protect against lethal influenza infections by avian H5 and H7 subtypes. *Vaccine* 17, 2265–2274. doi: 10.1016/S0264-410X(98)00494-0

Crosby, C. M., Matchett, W. E., Anguiano-Zarate, S. S., Parks, C. A., Weaver, E. A., Pease, L. R., et al. (2017). Replicating single-cycle adenovirus vectors generate amplified influenza vaccine responses. *J. Virol.* 91, e00720–00716. doi: 10.1128/JVI.00720-16

de Veer, M., and Meeusen, E. (2011). New developments in vaccine research–unveiling the secret of vaccine adjuvants. *Discov. Med.* 12, 195–204.

De Vriese, J., Steensels, M., Palya, V., Gardin, Y., Dorsey, K. M., Lambrecht, B., et al. (2010). Passive protection afforded by maternally-derived antibodies in chickens and the antibodies' interference with the protection elicited by avian influenza-inactivated vaccines in progeny. *Avian Dis.* 54, 246–252. doi: 10.1637/8908-043009-Reg.1

Domenech, J., Dauphin, G., Rushton, J., McGrane, J., Lubroth, J., Tripodi, A., et al. (2009). Experiences with vaccination in countries endemically infected with highly pathogenic avian influenza: the Food and Agriculture Organization perspective. *Rev. Sci. Tech.* 28, 293–305. doi: 10.20506/rst.28.1.1865

Domnich, A., Arata, L., Amicizia, D., Puig-Barbera, J., Gasparini, R., and Panatto, D. (2017). Effectiveness of MF59-adjuvanted seasonal influenza vaccine in the elderly: a systematic review and meta-analysis. *Vaccine* 35, 513–520. doi: 10.1016/j.vaccine.2016.12.011

Ducatez, M. F., Becker, J., Freudenstein, A., Delverdier, M., Delpont, M., Sutter, G., et al. (2016). Low pathogenic avian influenza (H9N2) in chicken: evaluation of an ancestral H9-MVA vaccine. *Vet. Microbiol.* 189, 59–67. doi: 10.1016/j.vetmic.2016.04.025

Ekiert, D. C., Bhabha, G., Elsliger, M. A., Friesen, R. H., Jongeneelen, M., Throsby, M., et al. (2009). Antibody recognition of a highly conserved influenza virus epitope. *Science* 324, 246–251. doi: 10.1126/science.1171491

Ekiert, D. C., Kashyap, A. K., Steel, J., Rubrum, A., Bhabha, G., Khayat, R., et al. (2012). Cross-neutralization of influenza A viruses mediated by a single antibody loop. *Nature* 489, 526–532. doi: 10.1038/nature11414

El Bakkouri, K., Descamps, F., De Filette, M., Smet, A., Festjens, E., Birkett, A., et al. (2011). Universal vaccine based on ectodomain of matrix protein 2 of influenza A: Fc receptors and alveolar macrophages mediate protection. *J. Immunol.* 186, 1022–1031. doi: 10.4049/jimmunol.0902147

Epperson, S., Jhung, M., Richards, S., Quinlisk, P., Ball, L., Moll, M., et al. (2013). Human infections with influenza A(H3N2) variant virus in the United States, 2011-2012. *Clin. Infect. Dis.* 57, S4–S11. doi: 10.1093/cid/cit272

Ermler, M. E., Kirkpatrick, E., Sun, W., Hai, R., Amanat, F., Chromikova, V., et al. (2017). Chimeric Hemagglutinin Constructs Induce Broad Protection against Influenza B Virus Challenge in the Mouse Model. *J. Virol.* 91, e00286–00217. doi: 10.1128/JVI.00286-17

Fazekas de St, G., and Webster, R. G. (1966). Disquisitions of Original Antigenic Sin. I. Evidence in man. *J. Exp. Med.* 124, 331–345. doi: 10.1084/jem.124.3.331

Florek, N. W., Weinfurter, J. T., Jegaskanda, S., Brewoo, J. N., Powell, T. D., Young, G. R., et al. (2014). Modified vaccinia virus Ankara encoding influenza virus hemagglutinin induces heterosubtypic immunity in macaques. *J. Virol.* 88, 13418–13428. doi: 10.1128/JVI.01219-14

Fonville, J. M., Wilks, S. H., James, S. L., Fox, A., Ventresca, M., Aban, M., et al. (2014). Antibody landscapes after influenza virus infection or vaccination. *Science* 346, 996–1000. doi: 10.1126/science.1256427

Food and Agriculture Organization of the United Nations (2017). *H7N9 Situation Update.* Available online at: http://www.fao.org/ag/againfo/programmes/en/empres/h7n9/situation_update.html (Accessed October 26, 2017).

Fotouhi, F., Shaffifar, M., Farahmand, B., Shirian, S., Saeidi, M., Tabarraei, A., et al. (2017). Adjuvant use of the NKT cell agonist alpha-galactosylceramide leads to enhancement of M2-based DNA vaccine immunogenicity and protective immunity against influenza A virus. *Arch. Virol.* 162, 1251–1260. doi: 10.1007/s00705-017-3230-7

Gardin, Y., Palya, V., Dorsey, K. M., El-Attrache, J., Bonfante, F., Wit, S., et al. (2016). Experimental and Field Results Regarding Immunity Induced by a Recombinant Turkey Herpesvirus H5 Vector Vaccine Against H5N1 and Other H5 Highly Pathogenic Avian Influenza Virus Challenges. *Avian Dis.* 60, 232–237. doi: 10.1637/11144-050815-ResNote

Gauger, P. C., Loving, C. L., Khurana, S., Lorusso, A., Perez, D. R., Kehrli, M. E., et al. (2014). Live attenuated influenza A virus vaccine protects against A(H1N1)pdm09 heterologous challenge without vaccine associated enhanced respiratory disease. *Virology* 471–473, 93–104. doi: 10.1016/j.virol.2014.10.003

Gauger, P. C., Vincent, A. L., Loving, C. L., Lager, K. M., Janke, B. H., Kehrli, M. E., et al. (2011). Enhanced pneumonia and disease in pigs vaccinated with an inactivated human-like (delta-cluster) H1N2 vaccine and challenged with pandemic 2009 H1N1 influenza virus. *Vaccine* 29, 2712–2719. doi: 10.1016/j.vaccine.2011.01.082

Gazit, R., Gruda, R., Elboim, M., Arnon, T. I., Katz, G., Achdout, H., et al. (2006). Lethal influenza infection in the absence of the natural killer cell receptor gene Ncr1. *Nat. Immunol.* 7, 517–523. doi: 10.1038/ni1322

Ghendon, Y. Z., Polezhaev, F. I., Lisovskaya, K. V., Medvedeva, T. E., Alexandrova, G. I., and Klimov, A. I. (1984). Recombinant cold-adapted attenuated influenza A vaccines for use in children: molecular genetic analysis of the cold-adapted donor and recombinants. *Infect. Immun.* 44, 730–733.

Gibbs, E. P., and Anderson, T. C. (2010). Equine and canine influenza: a review of current events. *Anim. Health Res. Rev.* 11, 43–51. doi: 10.1017/S1466252310000046

Goodman, A. G., Heinen, P. P., Guerra, S., Vijayan, A., Sorzano, C. O., Gomez, C. E., et al. (2011). A human multi-epitope recombinant vaccinia virus as a universal T cell vaccine candidate against influenza virus. *PLoS ONE* 6:e25938. doi: 10.1371/journal.pone.0025938

Gotch, F., McMichael, A., Smith, G., and Moss, B. (1987). Identification of viral molecules recognized by influenza-specific human cytotoxic T lymphocytes. *J. Exp. Med.* 165, 408–416. doi: 10.1084/jem.165.2.408

Gould, P. S., Easton, A. J., and Dimmock, N. J. (2017). Live attenuated influenza vaccine contains substantial and unexpected amounts of defective viral genomic. *R. N. A. Viruses* 9:E269. doi: 10.3390/v9100269

Greene, J. L. (2015). *Update on the Highly-Pathogenic Avian Influenza Outbreak of 2014–2015.* Washington, DC: Congressional Research Service.

Grohskopf, L. A., Sokolow, L. Z., Broder, K. R., Olsen, S. J., Karron, R. A., Jernigan, D. B., et al. (2016). Prevention and Control of Seasonal Influenza with Vaccines Recommendations of the Advisory Committee on Immunization Practices — United States, 2016–17 Influenza Season. *MMWR Recommend Rep* 65, 1–54. doi: 10.15585/mmwr.rr6505a1

Grund, C., Abdelwhab E.-S. M., Arafa, A. S., Ziller, M., Hassan, M. K., Aly, M. M., et al. (2011). Highly pathogenic avian influenza virus H5N1 from Egypt escapes vaccine-induced immunity but confers clinical protection against a heterologous clade 2.2.1 Egyptian isolate. *Vaccine* 29, 5567–5573. doi: 10.1016/j.vaccine.2011.01.006

Guo, X., Flores, C., Munoz-Aguayo, J., Halvorson, D. A., Lauer, D., and Cardona, C. J. (2015). Historical and Recent Cases of H3 Influenza A Virus in Turkeys in Minnesota. *Avian Dis.* 59, 512–517. doi: 10.1637/11166-051815-Reg

Hai, R., Martínez-Sobrido, L., Fraser, K. A., Ayllon, J., García-Sastre, A., and Palese, P. (2008). Influenza B virus NS1-truncated mutants: live-attenuated vaccine approach. *J. Virol.* 82, 10580–10590. doi: 10.1128/JVI.01213-08

Harding, A. T., Heaton, B. E., Dumm, R. E., and Heaton, N. S. (2017). Rationally designed influenza virus vaccines that are antigenically stable during growth in eggs. *MBio* 8:e00669-17. doi: 10.1128/mBio.00669-17

Heinen, P. P., de Boer-Luijtze, E. A., and Bianchi, A. T. (2001). Respiratory and systemic humoral and cellular immune responses of pigs to a heterosubtypic influenza A virus infection. *J. Gen. Virol.* 82, 2697–2707. doi: 10.1099/0022-1317-82-11-2697

Heinen, P. P., Rijsewijk, F. A., de Boer-Luijtze, E. A., and Bianchi, A. T. (2002). Vaccination of pigs with a DNA construct expressing an influenza virus M2-nucleoprotein fusion protein exacerbates disease after challenge with influenza A virus. *J. Gen Virol.* 83, 1851–1859. doi: 10.1099/0022-1317-83-8-1851

Hernandez, L. A., Miller, C. L., and Vaughn, E. M. (2016). Particle and subunit-based hemagglutinin vaccines provide protective efficacy against H1N1 influenza in pigs. *Vet. Microbiol.* 191, 35–43. doi: 10.1016/j.vetmic.2016.05.011

Herzog, C., Hartmann, K., Künzi, V., Kürsteiner, O., Mischler, R., Lazar, H., et al. (2009). Eleven years of Inflexal V-a virosomal adjuvanted influenza vaccine. *Vaccine* 27, 4381–4387. doi: 10.1016/j.vaccine.2009.05.029

Hessel, A., Savidis-Dacho, H., Coulibaly, S., Portsmouth, D., Kreil, T. R., Crowe, B. A., et al. (2014). MVA vectors expressing conserved influenza proteins protect mice against lethal challenge with H5N1, H9N2 and H7N1 viruses. *PLoS ONE* 9:e88340. doi: 10.1371/journal.pone.0088340

Hillaire, M. L., Vogelzang-van Trierum, S. E., Kreijtz, J. H., de Mutsert, G., Fouchier, R. A., Osterhaus, A. D., et al. (2013). Human T-cells directed to seasonal influenza A virus cross-react with 2009 pandemic influenza A (H1N1) and swine-origin triple-reassortant H3N2 influenza viruses. *J. Gen. Virol.* 94, 583–592. doi: 10.1099/vir.0.048652-0

Hoffmann, E., Neumann, G., Kawaoka, Y., Hobom, G., and Webster, R. G. (2000). A DNA transfection system for generation of influenza A virus from eight plasmids. *Proc. Natl. Acad. Sci. U.S.A.* 97, 6108–6113. doi: 10.1073/pnas.100133697

Hoft, D. F., Lottenbach, K. R., Blazevic, A., Turan, A., Blevins, T. P., Pacatte, T. P., et al. (2017). Comparisons of the humoral and cellular immune responses induced by live attenuated influenza vaccine and inactivated influenza vaccine in adults. *Clin. Vacc. Immunol.* 24, e00414–00416. doi: 10.1128/CVI.00414-16

Holm, K. J., and Goa, K. L. (1999). Liposomal influenza vaccine. *Biodrugs* 11, 137–144. doi: 10.2165/00063030-199911020-00007

Imai, M., Watanabe, T., Kiso, M., Nakajima, N., Yamayoshi, S., Iwatsuki-Horimoto, K., et al. (2017). A highly pathogenic avian H7N9 influenza virus isolated from a human is lethal in some ferrets infected via respiratory droplets. *Cell Host Microbe* 22, 615–626. doi: 10.1016/j.chom.2017.09.008

Impagliazzo, A., Milder, F., Kuipers, H., Wagner, M. V., Zhu, X., Hoffman, R. M., et al. (2015). A stable trimeric influenza hemagglutinin stem as a broadly protective immunogen. *Science* 349, 1301–1306. doi: 10.1126/science.aac7263

Iuliano, A. D., Jang, Y., Jones, J., Davis, C. T., Wentworth, D. E., Uyeki, T. M., et al. (2017). Increase in Human Infections with Avian Influenza A(H7N9) Virus During the Fifth Epidemic - China, October 2016-February 2017. *Morb Mortal Wkly. Rep.* 66, 254–255. doi: 10.15585/mmwr.mm6609e2

Jacobsen, H., Rajendran, M., Choi, A., Sjursen, H., Brokstad, K. A., Cox, R. J., et al. (2017). Influenza virus hemagglutinin stalk-specific antibodies in human serum are a surrogate marker for *in vivo* protection in a serum transfer mouse challenge model. *MBio* 8: e01463-17. doi: 10.1128/mBio.01463-17

Kapczynski, D. R., Pantin-Jackwood, M., Guzman, S. G., Ricardez, Y., Spackman, E., Bertran, K., et al. (2013). Characterization of the 2012 highly pathogenic avian influenza H7N3 virus isolated from poultry in an outbreak in Mexico: pathobiology and vaccine protection. *J. Virol.* 87, 9086–9096. doi: 10.1128/JVI.00666-13

Kappes, M. A., Sandbulte, M. R., Platt, R., Wang, C., Lager, K. M., Henningson, J. N., et al. (2012). Vaccination with NS1-truncated H3N2 swine influenza virus primes T cells and confers cross-protection against an H1N1 heterosubtypic challenge in pigs. *Vaccine* 30, 280–288. doi: 10.1016/j.vaccine.2011.10.098

Khatri, M., Dwivedi, V., Krakowka, S., Manickam, C., Ali, A., Wang, L., et al. (2010). Swine influenza H1N1 virus induces acute inflammatory immune responses in pig lungs: a potential animal model for human H1N1 influenza virus. *J. Virol.* 84, 11210–11218. doi: 10.1128/JVI.01211-10

Khurana, S., Loving, C. L., Manischewitz, J., King, L. R., Gauger, P. C., Henningson, J., et al. (2013). Vaccine-Induced Anti-HA2 Antibodies Promote Virus Fusion and Enhance Influenza Virus Respiratory Disease. *Sci. Transl. Med.* 5:200ra114. doi: 10.1126/scitranslmed.3006366

Kilany, W. H., Arafa, A., Erfan, A. M., Ahmed, M. S., Nawar, A. A., Selim, A. A., et al. (2010). Isolation of highly pathogenic avian influenza H5N1 from table eggs after vaccinal break in commercial layer flock. *Avian. Dis.* 54, 1115–1119. doi: 10.1637/9369-041310-Case.1

Kim, H. M., Lee, Y. W., Lee, K. J., Kim, H. S., Cho, S. W., van Rooijen, N., et al. (2008). Alveolar macrophages are indispensable for controlling influenza viruses in lungs of pigs. *J. Virol.* 82, 4265–4274. doi: 10.1128/JVI.02602-07

Kim, M.-C., Lee, J.-S., Kwon, Y.-M., Eunju, O., Lee, Y.-J., Choi, J.-G., et al. (2013). Multiple heterologous M2 extracellular domains presented on virus-like particles confer broader and stronger M2 immunity than live influenza A virus infection. *Antiviral Res.* 99, 328–335. doi: 10.1016/j.antiviral.2013.06.010

Kim, S. H., Paldurai, A., and Samal, S. K. (2017). A novel chimeric Newcastle disease virus vectored vaccine against highly pathogenic avian influenza virus. *Virology* 503, 31–36. doi: 10.1016/j.virol.2017.01.006

King, J. C. Jr., Cox, M. M., Reisinger, K., Hedrick, J., Graham, I., Patriarca, P., et al. (2009). Evaluation of the safety, reactogenicity and immunogenicity of FluBlok trivalent recombinant baculovirus-expressed hemagglutinin influenza vaccine administered intramuscularly to healthy children aged 6-59 months. *Vaccine* 27, 6589–6594. doi: 10.1016/j.vaccine.2009.08.032

Kirchenbaum, G. A., Carter, D. M., and Ross, T. M. (2015). Sequential Infection in Ferrets with Antigenically Distinct Seasonal H1N1 Influenza Viruses Boosts Hemagglutinin Stalk-Specific Antibodies. *J. Virol.* 90, 1116–1128. doi: 10.1128/JVI.02372-15

Knipe, D. M., Howley, P. M., Griffin, D. E., Lamb, R. A., Martin, M. A., Roizman, B., et al. (2007). "Orthomyxoviruses," in *Fields Virology, Vol.2, 5th Edn.*, eds P. F. Wright, G. Neuman, and Y. Kawaoka (Philadelphia, PA: Lippincott Williams & Wilkins), 1691–1740.

Kolpe, A., Schepens, B., Fiers, W., and Saelens, X. (2017). M2-based influenza vaccines: recent advances and clinical potential. *Expert Rev. Vacc.* 16, 123–136. doi: 10.1080/14760584.2017.1240041

Krammer, F., Pica, N., Hai, R., Margine, I., and Palese, P. (2013). Chimeric hemagglutinin influenza virus vaccine constructs elicit broadly protective stalk-specific antibodies. *J. Virol.* 87, 6542–6550. doi: 10.1128/JVI.00641-13

Kreijtz, J. H., Fouchier, R. A., and Rimmelzwaan, G. F. (2011). Immune responses to influenza virus infection. *Virus Res.* 162, 19–30. doi: 10.1016/j.virusres.2011.09.022

Kunisaki, K. M., and Janoff, E. N. (2009). Influenza in immunosuppressed populations: a review of infection frequency, morbidity, mortality, and vaccine responses. *Lancet Infect. Dis.* 9, 493–504. doi: 10.1016/S1473-3099(09)70175-6

Kutzler, M. A., and Weiner, D. B. (2008). DNA vaccines: ready for prime time? *Nat. Rev. Genet.* 9, 776–788. doi: 10.1038/nrg2432

Lambert, N. D., Ovsyannikova, I. G., Pankratz, V. S., Jacobson, R. M., and Poland, G. A. (2012). Understanding the immune response to seasonal influenza vaccination in older adults: a systems biology approach. *Expert Rev. Vacc.* 11, 985–994. doi: 10.1586/erv.12.61

Laver, W. G., and Webster, R. G. (1976). Preparation and immunogenicity of a purified influenza virus haemagglutinin and neuraminidase subunit vaccine. *Postgrad. Med. J.* 52, 373–378. doi: 10.1136/pgmj.52.608.373

Ledgerwood, J. E., Hu, Z., Gordon, I. J., Yamshchikov, G., Enama, M. E., Plummer, S., et al. (2012). Influenza virus h5 DNA vaccination is immunogenic by intramuscular and intradermal routes in humans. *Clin Vaccine Immunol* 19, 1792–1797. doi: 10.1128/CVI.05663-11

Lee, L. Y., Ha do, L. A., Simmons, C., de Jong, M. D., Chau, N. V., Schumacher, R., et al. (2008). Memory T cells established by seasonal human influenza A infection cross-react with avian influenza A (H5N1) in healthy individuals. *J. Clin. Invest.* 118, 3478–3490. doi: 10.1172/JCI32460

Lee, P. S., Ohshima, N., Stanfield, R. L., Yu, W., Iba, Y., Okuno, Y., et al. (2014). Receptor mimicry by antibody F045-092 facilitates universal binding to the H3 subtype of influenza virus. *Nat. Commun.* 5:3614. doi: 10.1038/ncomms4614

Lee, P. S., Yoshida, R., Ekiert, D. C., Sakai, N., Suzuki, Y., Takada, A., et al. (2012). Heterosubtypic antibody recognition of the influenza virus hemagglutinin receptor binding site enhanced by avidity. *Proc. Natl. Acad. Sci. U.S.A.* 109, 17040–17045. doi: 10.1073/pnas.1212371109

Lee, Y. N., Kim, M. C., Lee, Y. T., Kim, Y. J., Lee, J., Kim, C., et al. (2015). Co-immunization with tandem repeat heterologous M2 extracellular proteins overcomes strain-specific protection of split vaccine against influenza A virus. *Antiviral Res.* 122, 82–90. doi: 10.1016/j.antiviral.2015.08.001

Lewis, N. S., Russell, C. A., Langat, P., Anderson, T. K., Berger, K., Bielejec, F., et al. (2016). The global antigenic diversity of swine influenza A viruses. *Elife* 5:e12217. doi: 10.7554/eLife.12217

Li, X., Ju, H., Liu, J., Yang, D., Qi, X., Yang, X., et al. (2017). Influenza virus-like particles harboring H9N2 HA and NA proteins induce a protective immune response in chicken. *Influenza Other Respir. Viruses.* 11, 518–524. doi: 10.1111/irv.12472

Li, Z., Gabbard, J. D., Johnson, S., Dlugolenski, D., Phan, S., Tompkins, S. M., et al. (2015). Efficacy of a parainfluenza virus 5 (PIV5)-based H7N9 vaccine in mice and guinea pigs: antibody titer towards HA was not a good indicator for protection. *PLoS ONE* 10:e0120355. doi: 10.1371/journal.pone.0120355

Lillie, P. J., Berthoud, T. K., Powell, T. J., Lambe, T., Mullarkey, C., Spencer, A. J., et al. (2012). Preliminary assessment of the efficacy of a T-cell-based influenza vaccine, MVA-NP+M1, in humans. *Clin. Infect. Dis.* 55, 19–25. doi: 10.1093/cid/cis327

Liu, Q., Mena, I., Ma, J., Bawa, B., Krammer, F., Lyoo, Y. S., et al. (2015). Newcastle Disease Virus-Vectored H7 and H5 live vaccines protect chickens from challenge with H7N9 or H5N1 avian influenza viruses. *J. Virol.* 89, 7401–7408. doi: 10.1128/JVI.00031-15

Loeffen, W. L., Heinen, P. P., Bianchi, A. T., Hunneman, W. A., and Verheijden, J. H. (2003). Effect of maternally derived antibodies on the clinical signs and immune response in pigs after primary and secondary infection with an influenza H1N1 virus. *Vet. Immunol. Immunopathol.* 92, 23–35. doi: 10.1016/S0165-2427(03)00019-9

Lone, N. A., Spackman, E., and Kapczynski, D. (2017). Immunologic evaluation of 10 different adjuvants for use in vaccines for chickens against highly pathogenic avian influenza virus. *Vaccine* 35, 3401–3408. doi: 10.1016/j.vaccine.2017.05.010

Loving, C. L., Lager, K. M., Vincent, A. L., Brockmeier, S. L., Gauger, P. C., Anderson, T. K., et al. (2013). Efficacy of inactivated and live-attenuated influenza virus vaccines in pigs against infection and transmission of emerging H3N2 similar to the 2011-2012 H3N2v. *J. Virol.* 87, 9895–9903. doi: 10.1128/JVI.01038-13

Loving, C. L., Vincent, A. L., Pena, L., and Perez, D. R. (2012). Heightened adaptive immune responses following vaccination with a temperature-sensitive, live-attenuated influenza virus compared to adjuvanted, whole-inactivated virus in pigs. *Vaccine* 30, 5830–5838. doi: 10.1016/j.vaccine.2012.07.033

Low, J. G., Lee, L. S., Ooi, E. E., Ethirajulu, K., Yeo, P., Matter, A., et al. (2014). Safety and immunogenicity of a virus-like particle pandemic influenza A (H1N1) 2009 vaccine: results from a double-blinded, randomized Phase I clinical trial in healthy Asian volunteers. *Vaccine* 32, 5041–5048. doi: 10.1016/j.vaccine.2014.07.011

Ma, J., Dushoff, J., and Earn, D. J. (2011). Age-specific mortality risk from pandemic influenza. *J. Theor. Biol.* 288, 29–34. doi: 10.1016/j.jtbi.2011.08.003

Maassab, H. F., Heilman, C. A., and Herlocher, M. L. (1990). Cold-adapted influenza viruses for use as live vaccines for man. *Adv. Biotechnol. Process.* 14, 203–242.

Manini, I., Trombetta, C. M., Lazzeri, G., Pozzi, T., Rossi, S., and Montomoli, E. (2017). Egg-Independent Influenza Vaccines and Vaccine Candidates. *Vaccines (Basel)* 5:E18. doi: 10.3390/vaccines5030018

Manzoli, L., De Vito, C., Salanti, G., D'Addario, M., Villari, P., and Ioannidis, J. P. (2011). Meta-analysis of the immunogenicity and tolerability of pandemic influenza A 2009 (H1N1) vaccines. *PLoS ONE* 6:e24384. doi: 10.1371/journal.pone.0024384

Markowska-Daniel, I., Pomorska-Mol, M., and Pejsak, Z. (2011). The influence of age and maternal antibodies on the postvaccinal response against swine influenza viruses in pigs. *Vet. Immunol. Immunopathol.* 142, 81–86. doi: 10.1016/j.vetimm.2011.03.019

Masic, A., Lu, X., Li, J., Mutwiri, G. K., Babiuk, L. A., Brown, E. G., et al. (2010). Immunogenicity and protective efficacy of an elastase-dependent live attenuated swine influenza virus vaccine administered intranasally in pigs. *Vaccine* 28, 7098–7108. doi: 10.1016/j.vaccine.2010.08.003

McElhaney, J. E., Coler, R. N., and Baldwin, S. L. (2013). Immunologic correlates of protection and potential role for adjuvants to improve influenza vaccines in older adults. *Expert Rev. Vacc.* 12, 759–766. doi: 10.1586/14760584.2013.811193

Milián, E., and Kamen, A. A. (2015). Current and emerging cell culture manufacturing technologies for influenza vaccines. *Biomed. Res. Int.* 2015:504831. doi: 10.1155/2015/504831

Monto, A. S., Petrie, J. G., Cross, R. T., Johnson, E., Liu, M., Zhong, W., et al. (2015). Antibody to influenza virus neuraminidase: an independent correlate of protection. *J. Infect. Dis.* 212, 1191–1199. doi: 10.1093/infdis/jiv195

Montomoli, E. (2008). "Correlates of protection against influenza," in *Influenza Vaccines for the Future, 2nd Edn* eds R. Rappuoli and G. Del Giudice (Basel: Birkhauser), 199–222.

Morgan, S. B., Hemmink, J. D., Porter, E., Harley, R., Shelton, H., Aramouni, M., et al. (2016). Aerosol Delivery of a Candidate Universal Influenza Vaccine Reduces Viral Load in Pigs Challenged with Pandemic H1N1 Virus. *J. Immunol.* 196, 5014–5023. doi: 10.4049/jimmunol.1502632

Nachbagauer, R., Wohlbold, T. J., Hirsh, A., Hai, R., Sjursen, H., Palese, P., et al. (2014). Induction of broadly reactive anti-hemagglutinin stalk antibodies by an H5N1 vaccine in humans. *J. Virol.* 88, 13260–13268. doi: 10.1128/JVI.02133-14

Nelson, M. I., Gramer, M. R., Vincent, A. L., and Holmes, E. C. (2012). Global transmission of influenza viruses from humans to swine. *J. Gen. Virol.* 93, 2195–2203. doi: 10.1099/vir.0.044974-0

Neumann, G., Watanabe, T., Ito, H., Watanabe, S., Goto, H., Gao, P., et al. (1999). Generation of influenza A viruses entirely from cloned cDNAs. *Proc. Natl. Acad. Sci. U.S.A.* 96, 9345–9350. doi: 10.1073/pnas.96.16.9345

Neurath, A. R., Rubin, B. A., Sillaman, J., and Tint, H. (1971). The effect of nonaqueous solvents on the quaternary structure of viruses: a procedure for the simultaneous concentration, purification and disruption of influenza viruses. *Microbios* 4, 145–150.

Nogales, A., DeDiego, M. L., Topham, D. J., and Martinez-Sobrido, L. (2016). Rearrangement of influenza virus spliced segments for the development of live-attenuated vaccines. *J. Virol.* 90, 6291–6302. doi: 10.1128/JVI.00410-16

O'Donnell, C. D., Vogel, L., Matsuoka, Y., Jin, H., and Subbarao, K. (2014). The matrix gene segment destabilizes the acid and thermal stability of the hemagglutinin of pandemic live attenuated influenza virus vaccines. *J. Virol.* 88, 12374–12384. doi: 10.1128/JVI.01107-14

Paillot, R. (2014). A systematic review of recent advances in equine influenza vaccination. *Vacc. (Basel)* 2, 797–831. doi: 10.3390/vaccines2040797

Paterson, D., and Fodor, E. (2012). Emerging roles for the influenza A virus nuclear export protein (NEP). *PLoS Pathog* 8:e1003019. doi: 10.1371/journal.ppat.1003019

Pena, L., Sutton, T., Chockalingam, A., Kumar, S., Angel, M., Shao, H., et al. (2013). Influenza viruses with rearranged genomes as live-attenuated vaccines. *J. Virol.* 87, 5118–5127. doi: 10.1128/JVI.02490-12

Pena, L., Vincent, A. L., Ye, J., Ciacci-Zanella, J. R., Angel, M., Lorusso, A., et al. (2011). Modifications in the polymerase genes of a swine-like triple-reassortant influenza virus to generate live attenuated vaccines against 2009 pandemic H1N1 viruses. *J. Virol.* 85, 456–469. doi: 10.1128/JVI.01503-10

Persson, I., Granath, F., Askling, J., Ludvigsson, J. F., Olsson, T., and Feltelius, N. (2017). Risks of neurological and immune-related diseases, including narcolepsy, after vaccination with Pandemrix: a population- and registry-based cohort study with over 2 years of follow-up. *J. Intern. Med.* 281, 102–104. doi: 10.1111/joim.12581

Petsch, B., Schnee, M., Vogel, A. B., Lange, E., Hoffmann, B., Voss, D., et al. (2012). Protective efficacy of *in vitro* synthesized, specific mRNA vaccines against influenza A virus infection. *Nat. Biotechnol.* 30, 1210–1216. doi: 10.1038/nbt.2436

Pica, N., Langlois, R. A., Krammer, F., Margine, I., and Palese, P. (2012). NS1-truncated live attenuated virus vaccine provides robust protection to aged mice from viral challenge. *J. Virol.* 86, 10293–10301. doi: 10.1128/JVI.01131-12

Pillet, S., Aubin, E., Trépanier, S., Bussiere, D., Dargis, M., Poulin, J. F., et al. (2016). A plant-derived quadrivalent virus like particle influenza vaccine induces cross-reactive antibody and T cell response in healthy adults. *Clin. Immunol.* 168, 72–87. doi: 10.1016/j.clim.2016.03.008

Pushko, P., Tretyakova, I., Hidajat, R., Zsak, A., Chrzastek, K., Tumpey, T. M., et al. (2017). Virus-like particles displaying H5, H7, H9 hemagglutinins and N1 neuraminidase elicit protective immunity to heterologous avian influenza viruses in chickens. *Virology* 501, 176–182. doi: 10.1016/j.virol.2016.12.001

Pyo, H. M., Masic, A., Woldeab, N., Embury-Hyatt, C., Lin, L., Shin, Y. K., et al. (2012). Pandemic H1N1 influenza virus-like particles are immunogenic and provide protective immunity to pigs. *Vaccine* 30, 1297–1304. doi: 10.1016/j.vaccine.2011.12.083

Rajao, D. S., Anderson, T. K., Gauger, P. C., and Vincent, A. L. (2014). "Pathogenesis and vaccination of influenza A virus in swine," in *Influenza Pathogenesis and Control,* Vol. 1. eds R. W. Compans, M. B. A. Oldstone (New York, NY: Springer), 307–326.

Rajão, D. S., Chen, H., Perez, D. R., Sandbulte, M. R., Gauger, P. C., Loving, C. L., et al. (2016). Vaccine-associated enhanced respiratory disease is influenced by haemagglutinin and neuraminidase in whole inactivated influenza virus vaccines. *J. Gen. Virol.* 97, 1489–1499. doi: 10.1099/jgv.0.000468

Ramos, I., Bernal-Rubio, D., Durham, N., Belicha-Villanueva, A., Lowen, A. C., Steel, J., et al. (2011). Effects of receptor binding specificity of avian influenza virus on the human innate immune response. *J. Virol.* 85, 4421–4431. doi: 10.1128/JVI.02356-10

Richt, J. A., and Garcia-Sastre, A. (2009). Attenuated influenza virus vaccines with modified NS1 proteins. *Curr. Top. Microbiol. Immunol.* 333, 177–195. doi: 10.1007/978-3-540-92165-3_9

Rudenko, L., Yeolekar, L., Kiseleva, I., and Isakova-Sivak, I. (2016). Development and approval of live attenuated influenza vaccines based on Russian master donor viruses: process challenges and success stories. *Vaccine* 34, 5436–5441. doi: 10.1016/j.vaccine.2016.08.018

Sandbulte, M. R., Spickler, A. R., Zaabel, P. K., and Roth, J. A. (2015). Optimal Use of Vaccines for Control of Influenza A Virus in Swine. *Vacc. (Basel)* 3, 22–73. doi: 10.3390/vaccines3010022

Santos, J. J. S., Finch, C., Sutton, T., Obadan, A., Aguirre, I., Wan, Z., et al. (2017a). Development of an alternative modified live influenza B virus vaccine. *J. Virol.* 91, e00056–00017. doi: 10.1128/JVI.00056-17

Santos, J. J. S., Obadan, A. O., Garcia, S. C., Carnaccini, S., Kapczynski, D. R., Pantin-Jackwood, M., et al. (2017b). Short- and long-term protective efficacy against clade 2.3.4.4 H5N2 highly pathogenic avian influenza virus following prime-boost vaccination in turkeys. *Vaccine* 35, 5637–5643. doi: 10.1016/j.vaccine.2017.08.059

Schoenberger, S. P., Toes, R. E., van der Voort, E. I., Offringa, R., and Melief, C. J. (1998). T-cell help for cytotoxic T lymphocytes is mediated by CD40-CD40L interactions. *Nature* 393, 480–483. doi: 10.1038/31002

Schwartz, J. (2015). *Midwest Canine Influenza Outbreak Caused by New Strain of Virus.* Available online at: http://mediarelations.cornell.edu/2015/04/12/midwest-canine-influenza-outbreak-caused-by-new-strain-of-virus/ (Accessed July 07, 2017).

Shen, C., Chen, J., Li, R., Zhang, M., Wang, G., Stegalkina, S., et al. (2017). A multimechanistic antibody targeting the receptor binding site potently cross-protects against influenza B viruses. *Sci. Transl. Med.* 9:eaam5752. doi: 10.1126/scitranslmed.aam5752

Shi, S., Chen, S., Han, W., Wu, B., Zhang, X., Tang, Y., et al. (2016). Cross-clade protective immune responses of NS1-truncated live attenuated H5N1 avian influenza vaccines. *Vaccine* 34, 350–357. doi: 10.1016/j.vaccine.2015.11.045

Simon, G., Larsen, L. E., Dürrwald, R., Foni, E., Harder, T., Van Reeth, K., et al. (2014). European surveillance network for influenza in pigs: surveillance programs, diagnostic tools and Swine influenza virus subtypes identified in 14 European countries from 2010 to 2013. *PLoS ONE* 9:e115815. doi: 10.1371/journal.pone.0115815

Smith, G. J., Vijaykrishna, D., Bahl, J., Lycett, S. J., Worobey, M., Pybus, O. G., et al. (2009). Origins and evolutionary genomics of the 2009 swine-origin H1N1 influenza A epidemic. *Nature* 459, 1122–1125. doi: 10.1038/nature08182

Soema, P. C., Kompier, R., Amorij, J. P., and Kersten, G. F. (2015a) Current and next generation influenza vaccines: Formulation and production strategies. *Eur. J. Pharm. Biopharm.* 94, 251–263. doi: 10.1016/j.ejpb.2015.05.023

Soema, P. C., van Riet, E., Kersten, G., and Amorij, J. P. (2015b) Development of cross-protective influenza a vaccines based on cellular responses. *Front. Immunol.* 6:237. doi: 10.3389/fimmu.2015.00237

Solórzano, A., Webby, R. J., Lager, K. M., Janke, B. H., Garcia-Sastre, A., and Richt, J. A. (2005). Mutations in the NS1 protein of swine influenza virus impair anti-interferon activity and confer attenuation in pigs. *J. Virol.* 79, 7535–7543. doi: 10.1128/JVI.79.12.7535-7543.2005

Song, H., Nieto, G. R., and Perez, D. R. (2007). A new generation of modified live-attenuated avian influenza viruses using a two-strategy combination as potential vaccine candidates. *J. Virol.* 81, 9238–9248. doi: 10.1128/JVI.00893-07

Spackman, E., and Pantin-Jackwood, M. J. (2014). Practical aspects of vaccination of poultry against avian influenza virus. *Vet. J.* 202, 408–415. doi: 10.1016/j.tvjl.2014.09.017

Sridhar, S., Begom, S., Bermingham, A., Hoschler, K., Adamson, W., Carman, W., et al. (2013). Cellular immune correlates of protection against symptomatic pandemic influenza. *Nat. Med.* 19, 1305–1312. doi: 10.1038/nm.3350

Stachyra, A., Pietrzak, M., Maciola, A., Protasiuk, A., Olszewska, M., Smietanka, K., et al. (2017). A prime/boost vaccination with HA DNA and Pichia-produced HA protein elicits a strong humoral response in chickens against H5N1. *Virus Res.* 232, 41–47. doi: 10.1016/j.virusres.2017.01.025

Steel, J., Lowen, A. C., Wang, T. T., Yondola, M., Gao, Q., Haye, K., et al. (2010). Influenza virus vaccine based on the conserved hemagglutinin stalk domain. *MBio* 1, e00018–00010. doi: 10.1128/mBio.00018-10

Swayne, D. E., Pavade, G., Hamilton, K., Vallat, B., and Miyagishima, K. (2011). Assessment of national strategies for control of high-pathogenicity avian influenza and low-pathogenicity notifiable avian influenza in poultry, with emphasis on vaccines and vaccination. *Rev. Sci. Tech.* 30, 839–870. doi: 10.20506/rst.30.3.2081

Swayne, D. E., Suarez, D. L., and Sims, L. D. (2013). "Influenza," in *Diseases of Poultry, 13th Edn.* eds D. E. Swayne, J. R. Glisson, L. R. McDougald, L. K. Nolan, D. L. Suarez, and V. L. Nair (Ames, IA: Wiley-Blackwell), 181–218.

Sylte, M. J., Hubby, B., and Suarez, D. L. (2007). Influenza neuraminidase antibodies provide partial protection for chickens against high pathogenic avian influenza infection. *Vaccine* 25, 3763–3772. doi: 10.1016/j.vaccine.2007.02.011

Tang, X., Yang, Y., Xia, X., Zhang, C., Yang, X., Song, Y., et al. (2017). Recombinant Adenoviruses Displaying Matrix 2 Ectodomain Epitopes on

Their Fiber Proteins as Universal Influenza Vaccines. *J. Virol.* 91:e02462–02416. doi: 10.1128/JVI.02462-16

Tao, W., Hurst, B. L., Shakya, A. K., Uddin, M. J., Ingrole, R. S., Hernandez-Sanabria, M., et al. (2017). Consensus M2e peptide conjugated to gold nanoparticles confers protection against H1N1, H3N2 and H5N1 influenza A viruses. *Antiviral Res.* 141, 62–72. doi: 10.1016/j.antiviral.2017.01.021

Tate, M. D., Deng, Y. M., Jones, J. E., Anderson, G. P., Brooks, A. G., and Reading, P. C. (2009). Neutrophils ameliorate lung injury and the development of severe disease during influenza infection. *J. Immunol* 183, 7441–7450. doi: 10.4049/jimmunol.0902497

Taubenberger, J. K., and Morens, D. M. (2008). The pathology of influenza virus infections. *Annu. Rev. Pathol.* 3, 499–522. doi: 10.1146/annurev.pathmechdis.3.121806.154316

Taubenberger, J. K., and Morens, D. M. (2009). Pandemic influenza–including a risk assessment of H5N1. *Rev. Sci. Tech.* 28, 187–202. doi: 10.20506/rst.28.1.1879

Thompson, W. W., Comanor, L., and Shay, D. K. (2006). Epidemiology of seasonal influenza: use of surveillance data and statistical models to estimate the burden of disease. *J. Infect. Dis.* 194 (Suppl. 2), S82–S91. doi: 10.1086/507558

Turley, C. B., Rupp, R. E., Johnson, C., Taylor, D. N., Wolfson, J., Tussey, L., et al. (2011). Safety and immunogenicity of a recombinant M2e-flagellin influenza vaccine (STF2.4xM2e) in healthy adults. *Vaccine* 29, 5145–5152. doi: 10.1016/j.vaccine.2011.05.041

United States Department of Agriculture (2014). *Veterinary Biological Products: Licensees and Permittees.* Ames, IA: USDA APHIS Center for Veterinary Biologics.

Valero-Pacheco, N., Perez-Toledo, M., Villasis-Keever, M. A., Nunez-Valencia, A., Bosco-Garate, I., Lozano-Dubernard, B., et al. (2016). Antibody persistence in adults two years after vaccination with an H1N1 2009 pandemic influenza virus-like particle vaccine. *PLoS ONE* 11:e0150146. doi: 10.1371/journal.pone.0150146

Valkenburg, S. A., Mallajosyula, V. V., Li, O. T., Chin, A. W., Carnell, G., Temperton, N., et al. (2016). Stalking influenza by vaccination with pre-fusion headless HA mini-stem. *Sci. Rep.* 6:22666. doi: 10.1038/srep22666

van de Sandt, C. E., Hillaire, M. L., Geelhoed-Mieras, M. M., Osterhaus, A. D., Fouchier, R. A., and Rimmelzwaan, G. F. (2015). Human Influenza A Virus-Specific CD8+ T-Cell Response Is Long-lived. *J. Infect. Dis.* 212, 81–85. doi: 10.1093/infdis/jiv018

Van Reeth, K., Braeckmans, D., Cox, E., Van Borm, S., van den Berg, T., Goddeeris, B., et al. (2009). Prior infection with an H1N1 swine influenza virus partially protects pigs against a low pathogenic H5N1 avian influenza virus. *Vaccine* 27, 6330–6339. doi: 10.1016/j.vaccine.2009.03.021

Van Reeth, K., Brown, I. H., and Olsen, C. W. (2012). "Influenza virus," in *Diseases of Swine, 10th Edn.*, eds J. J. Zimmerman, L. A. Karriker, A. Ramirez, K. J. Schwartz, and G. W. Stevenson (Ames, IA: Wiley-Blackwell), 557–571.

Vander Veen, R. L., Loynachan, A. T., Mogler, M. A., Russell, B. J., Harris, D. L., and Kamrud, K. I. (2012). Safety, immunogenicity, and efficacy of an alphavirus replicon-based swine influenza virus hemagglutinin vaccine. *Vaccine* 30, 1944–1950. doi: 10.1016/j.vaccine.2012.01.030

Vander Veen, R. L., Mogler, M. A., Russell, B. J., Loynachan, A. T., Harris, D. L., and Kamrud, K. I. (2013). Haemagglutinin and nucleoprotein replicon particle vaccination of swine protects against the pandemic H1N1 2009 virus. *Vet. Rec.* 173:344. doi: 10.1136/vr.101741

Vesikari, T., Groth, N., Karvonen, A., Borkowski, A., and Pellegrini, M. (2009). MF59-adjuvanted influenza vaccine (FLUAD) in children: safety and immunogenicity following a second year seasonal vaccination. *Vaccine* 27, 6291–6295. doi: 10.1016/j.vaccine.2009.02.004

Vesikari, T., Knuf, M., Wutzler, P., Karvonen, A., Kieninger-Baum, D., Schmitt, H. J., et al. (2011). Oil-in-water emulsion adjuvant with influenza vaccine in young children. *N. Engl. J. Med.* 365, 1406–1416. doi: 10.1056/NEJMoa1010331

Vincent, A. L., Lager, K. M., Janke, B. H., Gramer, M. R., and Richt, J. A. (2008). Failure of protection and enhanced pneumonia with a US H1N2 swine influenza virus in pigs vaccinated with an inactivated classical swine H1N1 vaccine. *Vet. Microbiol.* 126, 310–323. doi: 10.1016/j.vetmic.2007.07.011

Wang, X., Fu, W., Yuan, S., Yang, X., Song, Y., Liu, L., et al. (2017). Both haemagglutinin-specific antibody and T cell responses induced by a chimpanzee adenoviral vaccine confer protection against influenza H7N9 viral challenge. *Sci. Rep.* 7:1854. doi: 10.1038/s41598-017-02019-1

Weis, W., Brown, J. H., Cusack, S., Paulson, J. C., Skehel, J. J., and Wiley, D. C. (1988). Structure of the influenza virus haemagglutinin complexed with its receptor, sialic acid. *Nature* 333, 426–431. doi: 10.1038/333426a0

Wesley, R. D., Tang, M., and Lager, K. M. (2004). Protection of weaned pigs by vaccination with human adenovirus 5 recombinant viruses expressing the hemagglutinin and the nucleoprotein of H3N2 swine influenza virus. *Vaccine* 22, 3427–3434. doi: 10.1016/j.vaccine.2004.02.040

Whittle, J. R., Zhang, R., Khurana, S., King, L. R., Manischewitz, J., Golding, H., et al. (2011). Broadly neutralizing human antibody that recognizes the receptor-binding pocket of influenza virus hemagglutinin. *Proc. Natl. Acad. Sci. U.S.A.* 108, 14216–14221. doi: 10.1073/pnas.1111497108

Wilkinson, T. M., Li, C. K., Chui, C. S., Huang, A. K., Perkins, M., Liebner, J. C., et al. (2012). Preexisting influenza-specific CD^{4+} T cells correlate with disease protection against influenza challenge in humans. *Nat. Med.* 18, 274–280. doi: 10.1038/nm.2612

Wise, H. M., Hutchinson, E. C., Jagger, B. W., Stuart, A. D., Kang, Z. H., Robb, N., et al. (2012). Identification of a novel splice variant form of the influenza A virus M2 ion channel with an antigenically distinct ectodomain. *PLoS Pathog* 8:e1002998. doi: 10.1371/journal.ppat.1002998.

Wohlbold, T. J., Nachbagauer, R., Xu, H., Tan, G. S., Hirsh, A., Brokstad, K. A., et al. (2015). Vaccination with adjuvanted recombinant neuraminidase induces broad heterologous, but not heterosubtypic, cross-protection against influenza virus infection in mice. *MBio* 6:e02556. doi: 10.1128/mBio.02556-14

World Health Organization (2016). *Influenza (Seasonal).* Available online at: http://www.who.int/mediacentre/factsheets/fs211/en/ (Accessed 27 May 2017).

World Health Organization (2017). *Cumulative Number of Confirmed Human Cases for Avian Influenza A(H5N1) Reported to WHO, 2003-2017.* Available online at: http://www.who.int/influenza/human_animal_interface/2017_09_27_tableH5N1.pdf?ua=1 (Accessed December 11, 2017).

World Health Organization/World Organisation for Animal Health/Food and Agriculture Organization (WHO/OIE/FAO) H5N1 Evolution Working Group (2014). Revised and updated nomenclature for highly pathogenic avian influenza A (H5N1) viruses. *Influenza Other Respi Virus.* 8, 384–388. doi: 10.1111/irv.12230

Wu, F., Huang, J. H., Yuan, X. Y., Huang, W. S., and Chen, Y. H. (2007). Characterization of immunity induced by M2e of influenza virus. *Vaccine* 25, 8868–8873. doi: 10.1016/j.vaccine.2007.09.056

Yang, S. G., Wo, J. E., Li, M. W., Mi, F. F., Yu, C. B., Lv, G. L., et al. (2009). Construction and cellular immune response induction of HA-based alphavirus replicon vaccines against human-avian influenza (H5N1). *Vaccine* 27, 7451–7458. doi: 10.1016/j.vaccine.2009.05.014

Yoshida, R., Igarashi, M., Ozaki, H., Kishida, N., Tomabechi, D., Kida, H., et al. (2009). Cross-protective potential of a novel monoclonal antibody directed against antigenic site B of the hemagglutinin of influenza A viruses. *PLoS Pathog.* 5:e1000350. doi: 10.1371/journal.ppat.1000350

Zimmerman, R. K., Nowalk, M. P., Chung, J., Jackson, M. L., Jackson, L. A., Petrie, J. G., et al. (2016). 2014-2015 influenza vaccine effectiveness in the united states by vaccine type. *Clin. Infect. Dis.* 63, 1564–1573. doi: 10.1093/cid/ciw635

2

Does Mucosal B1 Activation Result in the Accumulation of Peak IgM During Chronic Intrarectal SIVmac239 Exposure to Protect Chinese-Origin Rhesus Macaques from Disease Progression?

Zhe Cong[1†], Ling Tong[1†], Yuhong Wang[2], Aihua Su[1], Ting Chen[1], Qiang Wei[1], Jing Xue[1] and Chuan Qin[1*]*

[1] *Beijing Key Laboratory for Animal Models of Emerging and Remerging Infectious Diseases, NHC Key Laboratory of Human Disease Comparative Medicine, Institute of Laboratory Animal Science, Chinese Academy of Medical Sciences and Comparative Medicine Center, Peking Union Medical College, Beijing, China,* [2] *Department of Gerontology and Geriatrics, The First Affiliated Hospital of Harbin Medical University, Harbin, China*

Correspondence:
Jing Xue
xuejing@cnilas.org;
jessie830817@163.com
Chuan Qin
qinchuan@pumc.edu.cn

Human immunodeficiency virus (HIV) infection is characterized by a dynamic process and highly variable progression. Although extensive comparisons have been reported between the minority of non-progressors (NPGs) and the majority of progressors (PGs), the underlying mechanism is still unclear. One reason for this is that the initial onset of infection is very difficult to track, particularly when men who have sex with men (MSM) are predominantly responsible for the transmission of human HIV. To find potential early protection strategies against later progression during chronic mucosal exposure, 10 Chinese-origin rhesus macaques (ChRhs) that underwent repetitive simian immunodeficiency virus (SIV) intrarectal exposure were longitudinally tracked. The results of the periodic detection of peripheral blood mononuclear cells (PBMCs) and colorectal mucosal lamina propria mononuclear cells (LPMCs) with immunoglobulins in rectal fluid were compared between non-progressive and progressive subgroups, which were classified based on their circulating viral loads. As a result, four NPGs and six PGs were observed after disease onset for 2 months. Upon comparing the mucosal and systemic immune responses, the PBMC response did not differ between the two subgroups. Regarding LPMCs, the increased activation of B1a/B1 cells among B cells and a peak in IgM in rectal fluid was observed approximately 10 days after the first exposure, followed by consistently low viremia in the four non-progressive ChRhs. In the six progressive ChRhs, neither B cell activation nor a peak in IgM was observed, while a robust elevation in IgG was observed, followed by consistently high viremia post exposure. Based on the PBMC-LPMC disparity between the subgroups of monkeys, we hypothesize that early B1 activation in LPMCs that result in an IgM peak might attenuate the entry and acquisition of SIV in the mucosa, resulting in very low dissemination into blood. Our models have suggested that the use of early surveillance both systemically and in the mucosa to comprehensively determine virus–host interactions would be informative for mucosal vaccine development.

Keywords: PBMC, LPMC, SIV, IgM, B1 cells, Chinese-origin rhesus macaques, disease progression

INTRODUCTION

A tiny proportion of humans exposed to human immunodeficiency virus (HIV) retain a long-term non-progressive status and are known as "long-term non-progressors" (LTNPs) or "elite controllers" (ECs). Compared to the majority of those infected with HIV, who produce a strong virus-specific immune response and show obvious disease characteristics, LTNPs demonstrate extraordinarily low viral loads and do not progress to illness despite a lack of antiretroviral treatment (Sahu et al., 2001, 2005). More than 90% of new HIV infections occur by sexual transmission through mucosal contact (Tebit et al., 2012). Men who have sex with men (MSM) have the highest risk of HIV transmission and continue to transmit new HIV infections worldwide. Repetitive mucosal exposures in MSM could substantially enhance the frequency of mucosal immunity (Hladik and McElrath, 2008). Therefore, spontaneous LTNPs or ECs who are also MSM could provide a natural model of HIV-host immunity interactions. However, despite intensive studies comparing "dichotomized" infectors (Bendenoun et al., 2018), the mechanisms of "natural" protective mechanisms have not been clarified (Gurdasani et al., 2014). When considering the scenario, mucosal immunity as the first barrier (Miller et al., 1989; Xu et al., 2013) is the primary step in HIV infection, even in cases where infection occurs by the intravenous route (Bolton et al., 2012; Sutton et al., 2016). Therefore, early mucosal immunity, which could potentially confer some protection to non-progressed MSM infectors, has not been revealed because it is extremely difficult to detect the primary response to mucosal exposure during HIV transmission. In the present study, we employed Chinese-origin rhesus macaques (ChRhs) to generate spontaneous viral controllers with repeated low-dose simian immunodeficiency virus (SIV) exposure by the mucosal route. The animals were observed and the number of SIV RNA copies was detected periodically. NHP monkeys were divided into non-progressors (NPGs) and progressors (PGs) based on the degree of viral replication. By tracking primary mucosal immunity, immune responses occurring from the entry point in the rectal mucosa to the peripheral blood were compared in parallel to find some informative clues about how the first barrier of mucosal immunity performs in future non-progressive controllers.

MATERIALS AND METHODS

Animals and Ethics Statement

Two- to 4-year-old male and female ChRhs (*Macaca mulatta*) were housed and cared for in accordance with the Care and Use of Laboratory Animals of the Institute of Laboratory Animal Science and the recommendations of the welfare report for the use of non-human primates in research[1] in an Association for the Assessment and Accreditation of Laboratory Animal Care (AAALAC)-accredited facility. All macaques used in this study tested negative for the major histocompatibility complex class I (MHC-I) Mamu-A*01, Mamu-A*02, Mamu-B*08, and Mamu-B*17 alleles (Silver and Watkins, 2017) to reduce the bias introduced by MHC-enhanced control on SIV replication (Silver and Watkins, 2017). All animal procedures and experiments were performed according to protocols approved by the Institutional Animal Care and Use Committee (IACUC) of the Institute of Laboratory Animal Science, Chinese Academy of Medical Sciences (No. ILAS-VL-2012-002 and No. ILAS-VL-2015-003). All animals were anesthetized with an intramuscular injection of 10 mg/kg ketamine hydrochloride prior to sample collection, and the experiments were performed in the biosafety level 3 laboratory.

Animal Model and Longitudinal Tracing

Ten ChRhs were exposed intrarectally to SIVmac239 at a median tissue culture infectious dose ($TCID_{50}$) of 100 twice a week for 5 weeks. The SIVmac239 strain used was kindly gifted by Dr. Preston Marx at the Aaron Diamond AIDS Research Center of the United States. For the longitudinal tracking of virus-host immunity, peripheral blood, intestinal biopsy specimens, and rectal fluid were collected prior to and after the designated virus exposure. The animal model and longitudinal sampling schedule are shown in **Figure 1**. During the 60-day observation period, peripheral blood mononuclear cells (PBMCs) were collected at four time points. Colorectal mucosal lamina propria mononuclear cells (LPMCs) were biopsied by using an endoscope four times before or after PBMCs collection for the sake of animal welfare (McGary et al., 2017). Rectal fluid was collected at eight time points. The viral load in peripheral blood was intensively detected at twelve time points in each exposed monkey.

qRT-PCR Assay

Plasma RNA was extracted and purified using a QIAamp Viral RNA Mini Kit (Qiagen, Valencia, CA, United States). The quantification of plasma viral RNA in each sample was performed by quantitative real-time reverse transcription-PCR (qRT-PCR) using primers specific to a conserved region in the SIVmac239

[1] http://www.acmedsci.ac.uk/more/news/the-use-of-non-human-primates-in-research/

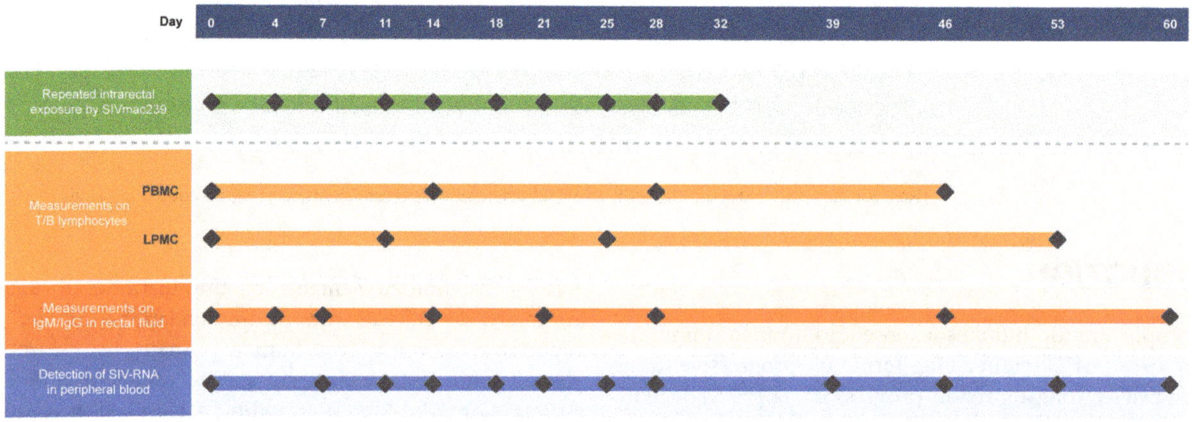

FIGURE 1 | Generation of the model using 10 ChRhs with periodical detection in the circulation and gut. Ten ChRhs were intrarectally exposed to low doses of SIVmac239 twice a week 10 times (along the green bar). T and B lymphocytes were measured at four time points in PBMCs or LPMCs at a short interval to minimize the impairment of the animals (along the light orange bar). Eight measurements of IgM and IgG were carried out in rectal fluid (along the dark orange bar). The plasma viral loads were detected 10 times (along the blue bar).

genome. The primers and probes used for vRNA amplification were gag91 forward (GCAGAGGAGGAAATTACCCAGTAC), gag91 reverse (CAATTTTACCCAGGCATTTAATGTT), and pSIVgag91-1 (5′-FAM-ACCTGCCATTAAGCCCGA-MGB-3′) (Chong et al., 2018). The limit of detection was 100 copy equivalents of RNA per ml of plasma. Three test reactions were performed for each sample.

Flow Cytometry to Measure T/B Cell Shifting in PBMCs/LPMCs

Gut biopsies were performed as previously described (Xue et al., 2013), and the biopsy tissue was then treated with 5 mM EDTA and 60 U/ml collagenase. LPMCs were enriched for lymphocytes by Percoll density gradient centrifugation, and PBMCs were isolated using conventional Ficoll Hypaque density gradient centrifugation (GE Healthcare, Uppsala, Sweden). Polychromatic flow cytometry was performed to stain the T lymphocyte panel or B lymphocyte panel. For the T lymphocyte panel, 50 μl of EDTA-anticoagulated whole blood or 1×10^6 primary cells derived from the lamina propria were stained with the monoclonal antibodies CD3-PE/Cy7 (SP34-2), CD4-Percp/Cy5.5 (L200), and CD8-APC/Cy7 (RPA-T8) from BD Biosciences (San Jose, CA, United States). The $CD4^+$ T cell counts were determined with BD Truecount tubes according to the manufacturer's instructions (BD, San Jose, CA, United States). For the B lymphocyte panel, PBMCs or LPMCs were incubated with CD3-PE/Cy7 (SP34-2) from BD Biosciences (San Jose, CA, United States); CD20-FITC (2H7), CD43-APC (10G7), and CD27-APC/Cy7 (O323) from Biolegend (San Diego, CA, United States); and CD5- PerCP/Cy5.5 (5D7) from Invitrogen (Carlsbad, CA, United States) to determine the following B cell subsets (Brocca-Cofano et al., 2017): B cells, $CD3^-CD20^+$; B1 cells, $CD3^-CD20^+CD43^+CD27^+$; and B1a cells, $CD3^-CD20^+CD43^+CD27^+CD5^+$. All the samples were analyzed by flow cytometry (FACSAria; BD, CA, United States).

Purification of IgM and IgG in Rectal Fluid

IgM in rectal fluid was purified with HiTrap™ IgM Purification HP according to the manufacturer's instructions (GE, Boston, MA, United States) (Hara et al., 2013). IgG in rectal fluid was purified with Protein A agarose resin. Briefly, the Protein A agarose resin was washed and equilibrated with PBS at pH 7.5. Then, filtered rectal fluid from each monkey was loaded onto the column at a flow rate of 0.2 ml/min. The adsorbed materials were eluted with 0.1 M glycine buffer at pH 2.5 after washing the column with PBS at a flow rate of 1 ml/min. The eluted fractions were neutralized with phosphate buffer at pH 8.5 and the effluents were monitored by UV spectrometry at 280 nm.

Statistical Analysis

Mann–Whitney *U*-tests were used to compare the plasma viral loads of non-progressive and progressive monkeys. Comparisons between two subgroups were determined using the unpaired *t*-test (Welch). Correlations between two variables were assessed by the Spearman correlation. All statistical analyses were performed with GraphPad Prism 6.0 software (GraphPad Software Inc., San Diego, CA, United States).

RESULTS

Generation of a Chronic Progression-Dichotomized Model Using 10 Homogenous ChRhs

To track the immune responses of monkey models between NPGs and PGs in parallel, 10 ChRhs were inoculated intrarectally with SIV (McDermott et al., 2004). The age, weight, white blood cell count in peripheral blood, and daily function score (Deng et al., 2019) were comparable to those at baseline (data

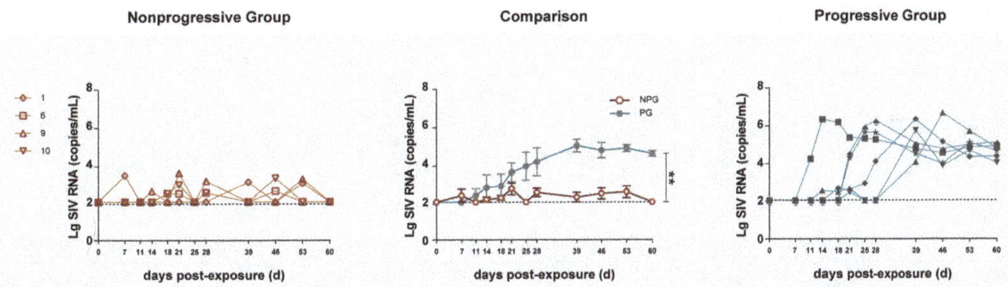

FIGURE 2 | Tracking plasma viral loads by detecting SIV RNA in non-progressive and progressive monkeys. The log of the geometric mean of the number of plasma SIVmac239 copies was compared between four non-progressive monkeys (orange line) and six progressive monkeys (blue line). The plasma viral loads are shown as log10 copies/ml. The assay had a sensitivity of 100 viral RNA copies per ml of plasma (black dotted lines). According to the Mann–Whitney *U*-test, the viral load in progressive monkeys was significantly increased compared with that in non-progressive monkeys (**$P < 0.01$).

not shown). The methods of repetitive mucosal exposure and sampling of peripheral blood, gut tissue, and rectal fluid were carried out on schedule (**Figure 1**). According to viral copy detection in peripheral blood, six ChRhs (Nos. 2, 3, 4, 5, 7, and 8) developed into chronic SIV PGs with stable high viremia and mild variation. By using peak plasma viremia to determine the degree of viral replication, the average number of copies was determined to be approximately 10^6 copies/ml with a range from 5.55 to 6.59 $\log_{10}$ RNA copies/ml. The remaining ChRhs (Nos. 1, 6, 9, and 10) were found to be NPGs, as the peak plasma viremia of SIVmac239 in these monkeys was consistently lower than 10^4 copies/ml throughout the entire observation period (**Figure 2**). During the follow-up observation period of 1 year, viremia in the four non-progressive monkeys remained as low as approximately 2–4 $\log_{10}$ RNA copies/ml (data not shown). Therefore, the non-progressive monkeys successfully mimicked the "long-term HIV controllers," and the progressive monkeys mimicked the chronic HIV infectors.

T/B Lymphocyte Activation in PBMCs and LPMCs in Non-Progressive and Progressive Monkeys

Longitudinal changes in the $CD4^+$ T cell counts, $CD8^+$ T cell counts, and $CD4^+/CD8^+$ T cell ratios in peripheral blood were demonstrated in the four non-progressive monkeys and six progressive monkeys (**Figure 3**). Comparisons between the two subgroups revealed no changes in the $CD4^+$ T cell counts, $CD8^+$ T cell counts, or $CD4^+/CD8^+$ T cell ratios at any of the four detection times between NPGs and PGs ($P > 0.05$). A notably higher average $CD4^+/CD8^+$ T cell ratio was observed in NPGs at baseline, although statistical significance was not maintained ($P = 0.068$), indicating that measurement of the baseline T lymphocytes in peripheral blood could not be used to predict the outcome of the shift in T lymphocyte activation. For LPMCs, four monkeys among the NPGs and six monkeys among the PGs also showed a similar tendency in terms of the T lymphocyte shift after repeated low-dose SIV challenge (**Figure 4**). The percentages of $CD4^+$ T cells, percentages of $CD8^+$ T cells, and $CD4^+/CD8^+$ T cell ratios were comparable between NPGs and PGs at each observation point ($P > 0.05$).

Next, the activation of B lymphocytes was examined between the two subgroups. In PBMCs, the B cell subset shift remained stable, including that of B1 cells among B cells and B1a cells among B1 cells, between NPGs and PGs. In addition, compared to the shifting of T cell subsets, the longitudinal shifting of B cell subsets was more stable, indicating that B lymphocyte activation in PBMCs was minimally impacted during SIV mucosal exposure in ChRhs (**Figure 5**). However, in LPMCs, the percentage of B1a cells among B1 cells and that of B1 cells among B cells from mucosa was significantly increased in non-progressive monkeys compared with progressive monkeys at the first detection. Additionally, dramatically increased B1/B and B1a/B1 cell ratios were observed in the early stage (approximately 11 days after the initial challenge) in the NPGs compared to the PGs (**Figure 6**). The increased numbers of B1a/B1 cells in LPMCs from NPGs were observed for 25 days after the initial exposure. At 53 days post exposure, a non-significant difference in the B cell shift was shown between the two progression-distinct subgroups. Longitudinally, the peaks in the increased B1 and B1a cells indicated the transient activation of B lymphocytes in LPMCs during the early stage in the four non-progressive monkeys.

Expression of IgM and IgG in Rectal Fluid From 10 Monkeys

In NPGs, IgM in rectal fluid precipitously increased to an average of 0.56 mg/ml with a range of 0.397–0.958 mg/ml at 14 days postexposure and gradually decreased to baseline levels at 21 days postexposure. Undetectably low IgM levels were observed during the entire observation period in the six PGs. An elevated IgG level in rectal fluid was shown at 46 days postexposure, and this level plateaued until 60 days (**Figure 7**).

B1 cells have been identified as a major source of infection-induced local IgM (Choi and Baumgarth, 2008; Baumgarth, 2011). To reveal the correlation between B cell activation in LPMCs, at 14 days postexposure the level of IgM in rectal fluid, viral replication in peripheral blood, B1a/B1 ratio, and IgM levels were individually correlated with the peak viral load in ten monkeys, including both NPGs and PGs. A temporally significant correlation was observed between the B1a/B1 ratio in LPMCs ($P < 0.05$, $R = -0.6848$) or the level of IgM in rectal

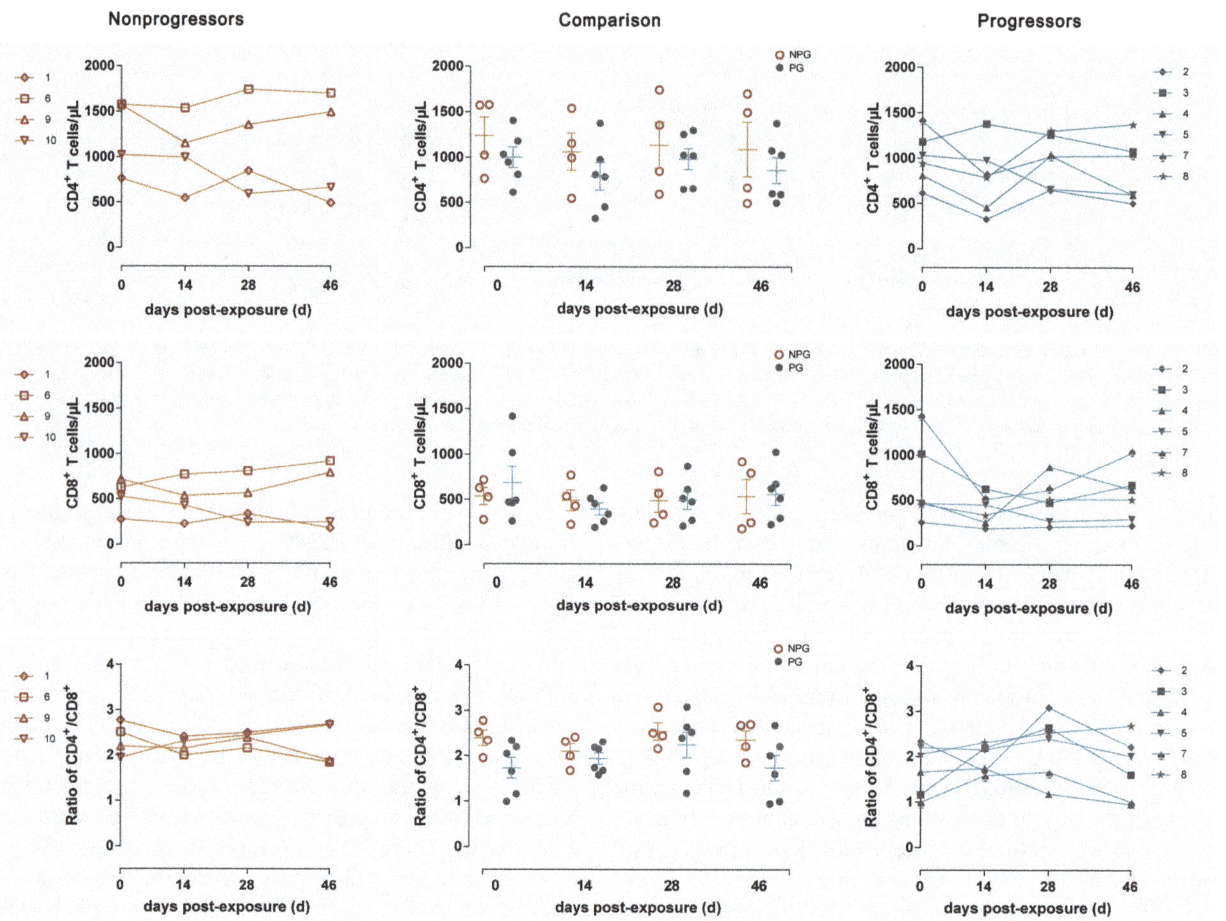

FIGURE 3 | Changes in T lymphocytes among PBMCs between non-progressive and progressive monkeys. The CD4+ T cell counts, CD8+ T cell counts, and CD4+/CD8+ ratios were measured in peripheral blood at four time points in four non-progressive monkeys and six progressive monkeys. No significant differences were found between the two subgroups at any time point, indicating that no notable T cell changes occurred in PBMCs from ChRhs subjected to repetitive SIV mucosal exposure (unpaired *t*-test, Welch's correction, $P > 0.05$).

fluid ($P < 0.05$, $R = -0.7781$) at 14 days postexposure and the peak viral load during the observation (**Figure 8**). As B1 cells contribute substantially to mucosal defense against pathogens, the presence of both negative correlations indicated that stepwise activation of B1 cells with subsequent peak IgM production in LPMCs might be responsible for the suppressed viral load in non-progressive monkeys. Therefore, we hypothesized that transient mucosal B1 cell activation along with peak IgM production in LPMCs impeded viral progression in SIV-infected monkeys.

DISCUSSION

We tracked the stepwise progression/non-progression of chronic mucosal exposure to SIV in ChRhs, which could mimic the most prevalent route of HIV transmission. It has been documented that ChRhs are relatively resistant to SIV-related progression, with approximately 30% of infected monkeys maintaining very low viral loads for several years (Ling et al., 2002). Therefore, the progression-dichotomized statuses of these homogenous monkeys could be easily predicted. In the present study, monkeys with genes highly associated with SIV spontaneous controllers, such as the MHC-I alleles Mamu-A*01 (Pal et al., 2002; Lim et al., 2010), Mamu-A*02 (Loffredo et al., 2004), Mamu-B*08 (Loffredo et al., 2007), and Mamu-B*17 (Yant et al., 2006), were removed from the study. Therefore, the MHC-dependent disparity has been minimized. As no well-acknowledged criteria for the viral load defining ECs/LTNPs/PGs status have been established in the ChRh model, as they have in HIV-infected humans, we simply classified the monkeys as either NPGs or PGs in the ChRh model. The dose used in this study could be considered low according to our experience. Indeed, even a $TCID_{50}$ of 50,000 could produce non-progressive controllers. As low- and high-dose challenges produced a similar PG/controller ratio (McDermott et al., 2004; Tasca et al., 2007; Xiao et al., 2012; Greene et al., 2014), the initial acquisition very likely played a predominant role in later outcomes. Based on the longitudinal viral load trajectories, four monkeys were observed

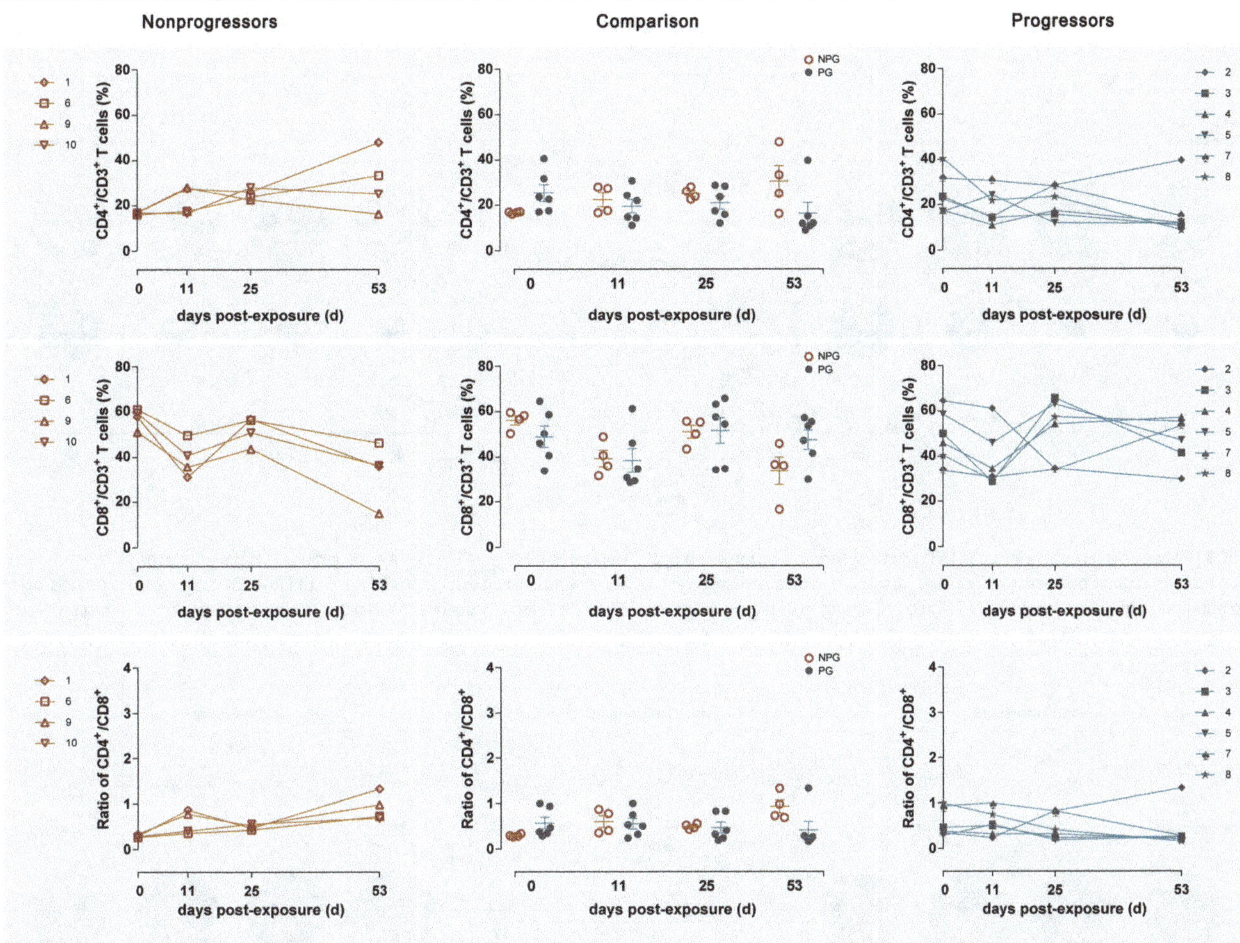

FIGURE 4 | Changes in T lymphocytes among LPMCs in non-progressive and progressive monkeys. The CD4+ T cell percentages, CD8+ T cell percentages, and CD4+/CD8+ ratios were measured in LPMCs obtained at four time points in four non-progressive monkeys and six progressive monkeys. No significant differences were found between the two subgroups at any time point, indicating that no notable T cell changes occurred in LPMCs from ten ChRhs subjected to repetitive SIV mucosal exposure (unpaired *t*-test, Welch's correction, $P > 0.05$).

to be NPGs, while six monkeys were classified as PGs among the 10 ChRhs. Therefore, we could use the present SIV ChRh model to mimic the general immunity disparity between the minority of NPGs/ECs and the majority of PGs in humans with HIV. Another characteristic of our model was that it could be used to track the very early stage of chronic mucosal infection with parallel detection in LPMCs and PBMCs. In humans, it is very difficult to track the onset of a chronic infection by observing both systemic and mucosal immunity (Lama et al., 2016). Here, we intensively tracked both PBMCs and LPMCs for T and B cell activation as well as IgM and IgG expression from rectal fluid, as it has been shown that the levels of immunoglobins in rectal fluid could robustly reflect the concentrations in mucosal tissues (Cottrell et al., 2016). A notable limitation was that IgA could not be detected despite numerous attempts to purify IgA from monkeys.

Our tracking observation resulted in an interesting difference between NPGs and PGs in the early stage post exposure. B1 cell activation (Choi and Baumgarth, 2008; Baumgarth, 2011), along with a precipitous increase in IgM, was observed in LPMCs at only approximately 9–11 days after the initial exposure in the four non-progressive monkeys. Our results are consistent with the phenomenon that early treatment with anti-HIV neutralizing antibodies potently induces sustainable immunity and subsequent progression (Nishimura et al., 2017). Although neutralizing antibodies showed a superior ability to block viral infection compared to that of non-neutralizing antibodies (Cheeseman et al., 2017), a paradoxical phenomenon showed that non-neutralizing antibodies were much more commonly detected in HIV ECs than neutralizing antibodies (Theze et al., 2011). In addition, a mucosal vaccine was found to have protective efficacy independent of anti-HIV neutralizing antibodies (Sui et al., 2019). Therefore, determination of the extent to which the early IgM peak contributes to the substantial suppression of viral dissemination within the mucosa in NPGs requires further experiments. As a non-specific antibody, natural IgM has been shown to robustly neutralize viruses within the mucosal epithelial barrier *in vitro* (Devito et al., 2018).

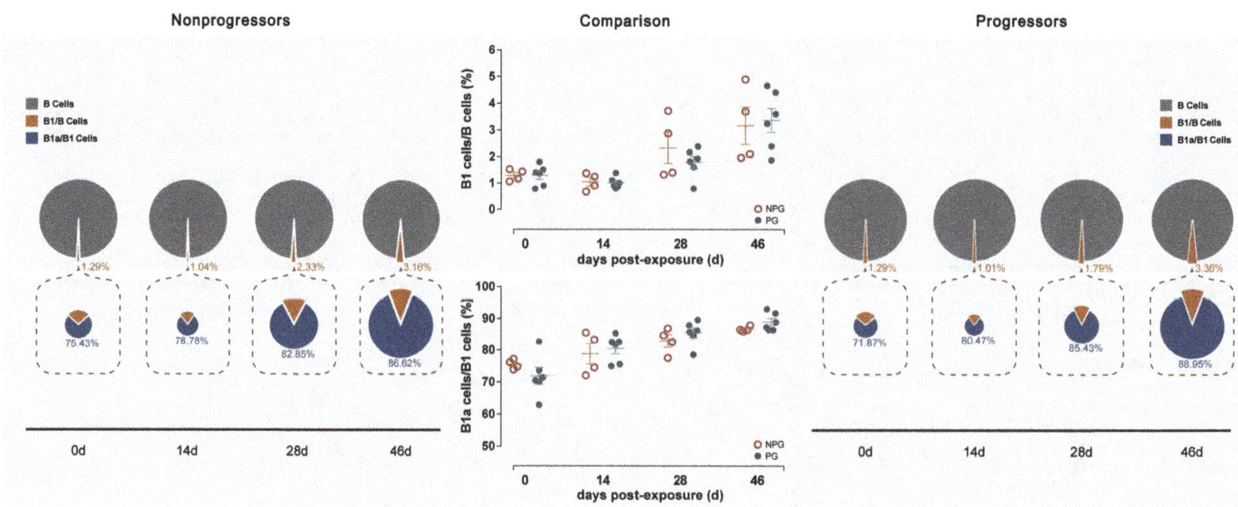

FIGURE 5 | Changes in B lymphocytes in PBMCs between non-progressive and progressive monkeys. B cell subsets, including B1/B and B1a/B1, were measured from PBMCs at four time points in four non-progressive monkeys and six progressive monkeys. The percentages of B1/B and B1a/B1 cells were compared between the two subgroups at each time point. No significant changes in B cells occurred in PBMCs in ten ChRhs under repetitive SIV mucosal exposure (unpaired *t*-test, Welch's correction, $P > 0.05$).

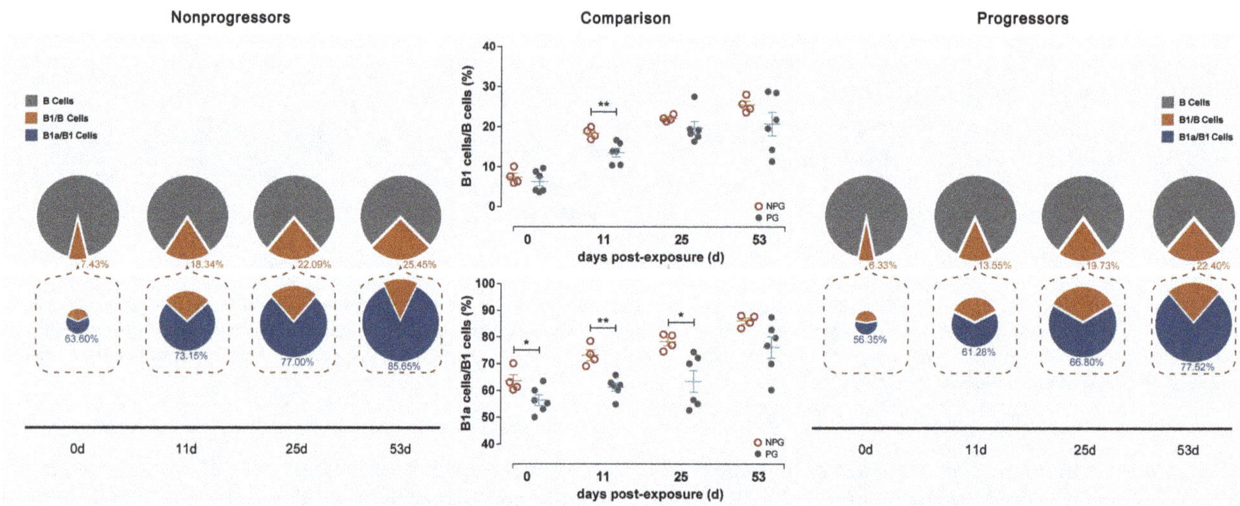

FIGURE 6 | Changes in B lymphocytes among LPMCs in non-progressive and progressive monkeys. B cell subsets, including B1/B and B1a/B1 cells, were measured among LPMCs obtained at four time points in four non-progressive monkeys and six progressive monkeys. The percentages of B1/B and B1a/B1 cells were compared between the two subgroups at each time point. Notably, increased ratios of B1/B and B1a/B1 cells were found in the four non-progressive monkeys during the early stage after initial exposure (unpaired *t*-test, Welch's correction, $^{*}P < 0.05$, $^{**}P < 0.01$).

After a peak in IgM was induced in LPMCs, viremia remained consistently low in the four NPGs, and the timing was consistent with that of the viremia peak during infection via the intrarectal route (Haseltine, 1989). Over 14 days, a stepwise route of infection from the mucosal epithelial barrier to the peripheral blood via profound mucosal immunity was observed (Miller et al., 2005; Haase, 2010). In this scenario, we supposed that the peak in IgM that occurred after approximately 10 days might have been an accumulative response to repetitive SIV exposure. Within the mucosa, gut-associated lymphoid tissue (GALT) made up of organized lymphoid nodules and multifunctional LPMCs could mount profound immunity responses both cellularly and humorally. Therefore, the LPMC response showed a sufficiently high efficacy to produce an EC without this response being mirrored in the blood (Shacklett and Ferre, 2011). Moreover, colorectal tissue was proven to be a consistent viral reservoir in long-term non-progressive ChRhs (Ling et al., 2010). Therefore, the disparity between the responses of NPGs and PGs has strongly demonstrated the fact that "outcomes depend on a race between expansion of infection and the immune response generated to contain it" (Li et al., 2009) in the early stages of viral infection.

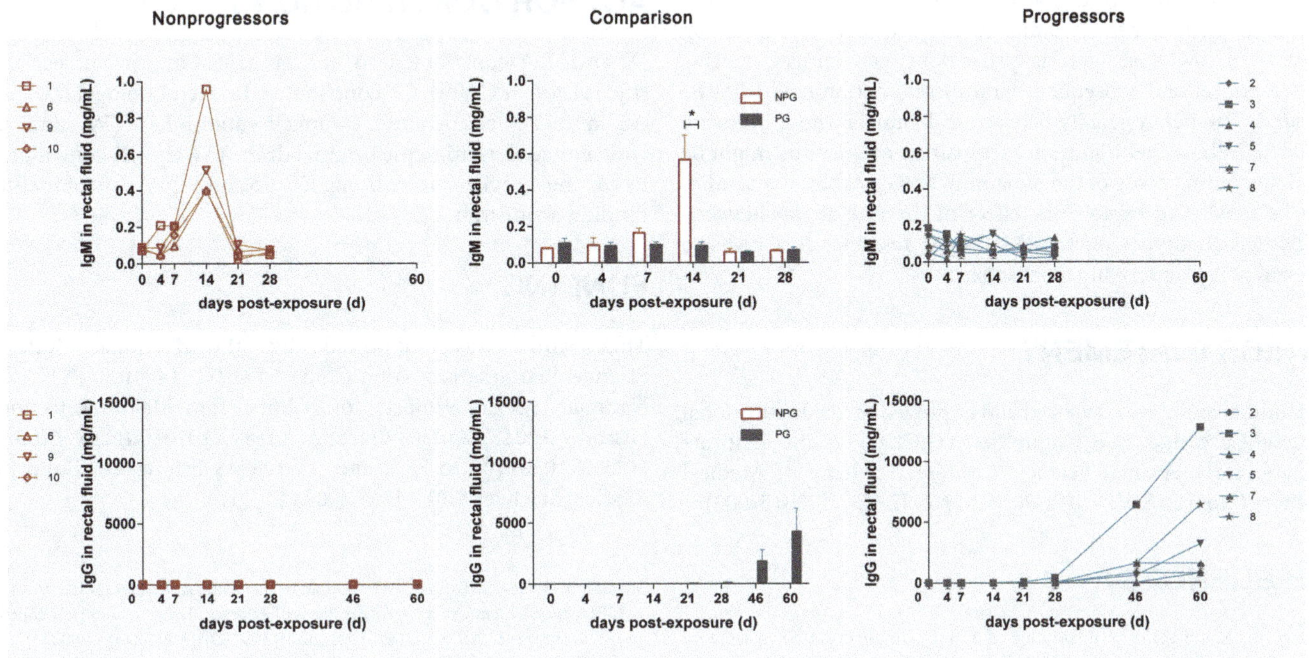

FIGURE 7 | Levels of IgM and IgG in rectal fluid in non-progressive and progressive monkeys. The levels of IgM and IgG were detected after initial exposure. A precipitously elevated IgM level in rectal fluid was found in four non-progressive monkeys during the early stage after initial exposure. In six progressive monkeys, a gradual increase in IgG was observed during the late stage 2 weeks after the first exposure. According to unpaired t test results, the level of IgM in the four non-progressive monkeys was significantly higher than that in the six progressive monkeys, whereas the level of IgG in the six progressive monkeys was significantly higher than that in the four non-progressive monkeys (*$P < 0.01$).

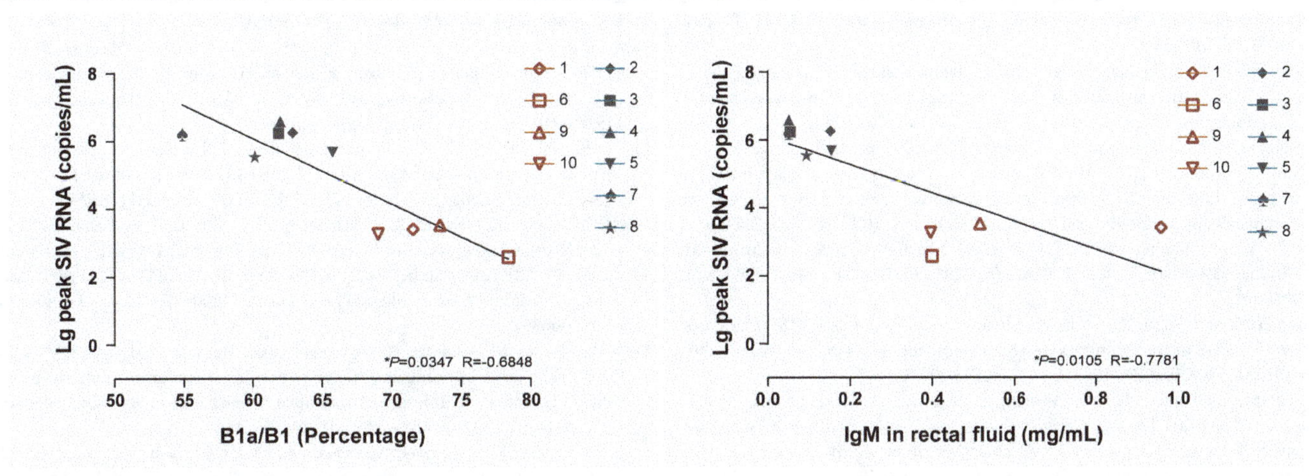

FIGURE 8 | Correlation of the B1a/B1 cell ratio among LPMCs and the IgM level in rectal fluid with peak viremia in 10 ChRhs. The correlations of peak viremia with the B1a/B1 cell ratio among LPMCs detected on day 11 post infection (left panel) and the level of IgM in rectal fluid detected at day 14 post infection (right panel) are shown. Using the Spearman correlation, strong significant linear correlations were observed between the B1a/B1 cell ratio and peak viremia ($R = -0.6848$) and between the level of IgM in rectal fluid and peak viremia ($R = -0.7781$) in 10 ChRhs with mucosal SIV exposure (*$P < 0.05$).

Taken together, our results support the hypothesis that an accumulative mucosal immune response induced by repetitive antigenic stimulation results in a peak IgM response in LPMCs. This mechanism may be the reason that ~30% of ChRhs were protected from dissemination and led to their becoming NPGs. The exposure-dependent immune response was mild yet accumulative and produced a robust non-specific IgM to neutralize insufficient antigens, followed by the blockage of dissemination. We hypothesize that early B1 cell activation along with the IgM peak in LPMCs might exert a "decapacitating effect" to protect ChRhs from progression. The primary cause of this result was the characterized genotypes, which were characterized as central to the PG. On the other hand, susceptible animals who acquired SIV infection, albeit at a low dose, gradually developed an antigen-specific IgG response, and subsequent viral dissemination could not be avoided. The heterogeneity between individuals whose minority could be initiated with minimal acquisition of the virus might be the determining cause of the remaining NPGs. Additional studies will be needed to explore the effect of the interaction between individual genotypes on the GALT-IgM response in ChRhs to determine the underlying mechanism.

ETHICS STATEMENT

The animal study was reviewed and approved by the Institutional Animal Care and Use Committee (IACUC) at the Institute of Laboratory Animal Science, Chinese Academy of Medical Sciences (No. ILAS-VL-2012-002 and No. ILAS-VL-2015-003).

AUTHOR CONTRIBUTIONS

JX and CQ contributed to conceptualization, resources, and supervision. ZC and LT contributed to methodology. ZC, LT, AS, and TC contributed to investigation. LT, YW, and JX contributed to writing the original draft. YW and JX contributed to writing—review and editing. ZC, JX, and QW contributed to funding acquisition.

FUNDING

This work was supported by the National Natural Science Foundation of China (81971944 to JX), the National Mega Projects of China for Major Infectious Diseases (2017ZX10304402 and 2018ZX10101001 to JX and 2018ZX10301103 to ZC), and the CAMS Innovation Fund for Medical Sciences (2017-I2M-1-014 to QW).

REFERENCES

Baumgarth, N. (2011). The double life of a B-1 cell: self-reactivity selects for protective effector functions. *Nat. Rev. Immunol.* 11, 34–46. doi: 10.1038/nri2901

Bendenoun, M., Samri, A., Avettand-Fenoel, V., Cardinaud, S., Descours, B., Carcelain, G., et al. (2018). What is the most important for elite control: genetic background of patient, genetic background of partner, both or neither? Description of complete natural history within a couple of MSM. *EBioMedicine* 27, 51–60. doi: 10.1016/j.ebiom.2017.12.003

Bolton, D. L., Song, K., Wilson, R. L., Kozlowski, P. A., Tomaras, G. D., Keele, B. F., et al. (2012). Comparison of systemic and mucosal vaccination: impact on intravenous and rectal SIV challenge. *Mucosal Immunol.* 5, 41–52. doi: 10.1038/mi.2011.45

Brocca-Cofano, E., Kuhrt, D., Siewe, B., Xu, C., Haret-Richter, G. S., Craigo, J., et al. (2017). Pathogenic correlates of simian immunodeficiency virus-associated B cell dysfunction. *J. Virol.* 91:e1051-17. doi: 10.1128/JVI.01051-17

Cheeseman, H. M., Olejniczak, N. J., Rogers, P. M., Evans, A. B., King, D. F. L., Ziprin, P., et al. (2017). Broadly neutralizing antibodies display potential for prevention of HIV-1 infection of mucosal tissue superior to that of nonneutralizing antibodies. *J. Virol.* 91:e1762-16. doi: 10.1128/JVI.01762-16

Choi, Y. S., and Baumgarth, N. (2008). Dual role for B-1a cells in immunity to influenza virus infection. *J. Exp. Med.* 205, 3053–3064. doi: 10.1084/jem.20080979

Chong, H., Xue, J., Zhu, Y., Cong, Z., Chen, T., Guo, Y., et al. (2018). Design of novel HIV-1/2 fusion inhibitors with high therapeutic efficacy in rhesus monkey models. *J. Virol.* 92:e775-18. doi: 10.1128/JVI.00775-18

Cottrell, M. L., Prince, H. M., Allmon, A., Mollan, K. R., Hudgens, M. G., Sykes, C., et al. (2016). Cervicovaginal and rectal fluid as a surrogate marker of antiretroviral tissue concentration: implications for clinical trial design. *J. Acquir. Immune Defic. Syndr.* 72, 498–506. doi: 10.1097/QAI.0000000000000996

Deng, W., Guan, G., Xiao, C., Qu, G., Xue, J., Qin, C., et al. (2019). Construction of a comprehensive observer-based scale assessing aging-related health and functioning in captive rhesus macaques. *Aging (Albany NY)* 11, 6892–6903. doi: 10.18632/aging.102219

Devito, C., Ellegard, R., Falkeborn, T., Svensson, L., Ohlin, M., Larsson, M., et al. (2018). Human IgM monoclonal antibodies block HIV-transmission to immune cells in cervico-vaginal tissues and across polarized epithelial cells in vitro. *Sci. Rep.* 8:10180. doi: 10.1038/s41598-018-28242-y

Greene, J. M., Weiler, A. M., Reynolds, M. R., Cain, B. T., Pham, N. H., Ericsen, A. J., et al. (2014). Rapid, repeated, low-dose challenges with SIVmac239 infect animals in a condensed challenge window. *Retrovirology* 11:66. doi: 10.1186/s12977-014-0066-z

Gurdasani, D., Iles, L., Dillon, D. G., Young, E. H., Olson, A. D., Naranbhai, V., et al. (2014). A systematic review of definitions of extreme phenotypes of HIV control and progression. *AIDS* 28, 149–162. doi: 10.1097/QAD.0000000000000049

Haase, A. T. (2010). Targeting early infection to prevent HIV-1 mucosal transmission. *Nature* 464, 217–223. doi: 10.1038/nature08757

Hara, A., Furuichi, K., Higuchi, M., Iwata, Y., Sakai, N., Kaneko, S., et al. (2013). Autoantibodies to erythropoietin receptor in patients with immune-mediated diseases: relationship to anaemia with erythroid hypoplasia. *Br. J. Haematol.* 160, 244–250. doi: 10.1111/bjh.12105

Haseltine, W. A. (1989). Silent HIV infections. *N. Engl. J. Med.* 320, 1487–1489. doi: 10.1056/nejm198906013202210

Hladik, F., and McElrath, M. J. (2008). Setting the stage: host invasion by HIV. *Nat. Rev. Immunol.* 8, 447–457. doi: 10.1038/nri2302

Lama, J. R., Karuna, S. T., Grant, S. P., Swann, E. M., Ganoza, C., Segura, P., et al. (2016). Transient peripheral immune activation follows elective sigmoidoscopy or circumcision in a cohort study of MSM at risk of HIV infection. *PLoS One* 11:e0160487. doi: 10.1371/journal.pone.0160487

Li, Q., Skinner, P. J., Ha, S. J., Duan, L., Mattila, T. L., Hage, A., et al. (2009). Visualizing antigen-specific and infected cells in situ predicts outcomes in early viral infection. *Science* 323, 1726–1729. doi: 10.1126/science.1168676

Lim, S. Y., Chan, T., Gelman, R. S., Whitney, J. B., O'Brien, K. L., Barouch, D. H., et al. (2010). Contributions of Mamu-A*01 status and TRIM5 allele expression, but not CCL3L copy number variation, to the control of SIVmac251 replication in Indian-origin rhesus monkeys. *PLoS Genet.* 6:e1000997. doi: 10.1371/journal.pgen.1000997

Ling, B., Mohan, M., Lackner, A. A., Green, L. C., Marx, P. A., Doyle, L. A., et al. (2010). The large intestine as a major reservoir for simian immunodeficiency virus in macaques with long-term, nonprogressing non-progressing infection. *J. Infect. Dis.* 202, 1846–1854. doi: 10.1086/657413

Ling, B., Veazey, R. S., Luckay, A., Penedo, C., Xu, K., Lifson, J. D., et al. (2002). SIV(mac) pathogenesis in rhesus macaques of Chinese and Indian origin compared with primary HIV infections in humans. *AIDS* 16, 1489–1496. doi: 10.1097/00002030-200207260-00005

Loffredo, J. T., Maxwell, J., Qi, Y., Glidden, C. E., Borchardt, G. J., Soma, T., et al. (2007). Mamu-B*08-positive macaques control simian immunodeficiency virus replication. *J. Virol.* 81, 8827–8832. doi: 10.1128/jvi.00895-07

Loffredo, J. T., Sidney, J., Wojewoda, C., Dodds, E., Reynolds, M. R., Napoe, G., et al. (2004). Identification of seventeen new simian immunodeficiency virus-derived CD8 + T cell epitopes restricted by the high frequency molecule, Mamu-A*02, and potential escape from CTL recognition. *J. Immunol.* 173, 5064–5076. doi: 10.4049/jimmunol.173.8.5064

McDermott, A. B., Mitchen, J., Piaskowski, S., De Souza, I., Yant, L. J., Stephany, J., et al. (2004). Repeated low-dose mucosal simian immunodeficiency virus

SIVmac239 challenge results in the same viral and immunological kinetics as high-dose challenge: a model for the evaluation of vaccine efficacy in nonhuman non-human primates. *J. Virol.* 78, 3140–3144. doi: 10.1128/jvi.78.6.3140-3144.2004

McGary, C. S., Alvarez, X., Harrington, S., Cervasi, B., Ryan, E. S., Iriele, R. I., et al. (2017). The loss of CCR6 (+) and CD161 (+) CD4 (+) T-cell homeostasis contributes to disease progression in SIV-infected rhesus macaques. *Mucosal Immunol.* 10, 1082–1096. doi: 10.1038/mi.2016.116

Miller, C. J., Alexander, N. J., Sutjipto, S., Lackner, A. A., Gettie, A., Hendrickx, A. G., et al. (1989). Genital mucosal transmission of simian immunodeficiency virus: animal model for heterosexual transmission of human immunodeficiency virus. *J. Virol.* 63, 4277–4284. doi: 10.1128/jvi.63.10.4277-4284.1989

Miller, C. J., Li, Q., Abel, K., Kim, E. Y., Ma, Z. M., Wietgrefe, S., et al. (2005). Propagation and dissemination of infection after vaginal transmission of simian immunodeficiency virus. *J. Virol.* 79, 9217–9227. doi: 10.1128/jvi.79.14.9217-9227.2005

Nishimura, Y., Gautam, R., Chun, T. W., Sadjadpour, R., Foulds, K. E., Shingai, M., et al. (2017). Early antibody therapy can induce long-lasting immunity to SHIV. *Nature* 543, 559–563. doi: 10.1038/nature21435

Pal, R., Venzon, D., Letvin, N. L., Santra, S., Montefiori, D. C., Miller, N. R., et al. (2002). ALVAC-SIV-gag-pol-env-based vaccination and macaque major histocompatibility complex class I (A*01) delay simian immunodeficiency virus SIVmac-induced immunodeficiency. *J. Virol.* 76, 292–302. doi: 10.1128/jvi.76.1.292-302.2002

Sahu, G. K., Chen, J. J., Huang, J. C., Ramsey, K. M., and Cloyd, M. W. (2001). Transient or occult HIV-1 infection in high-risk adults. *AIDS* 15, 1175–1177. doi: 10.1097/00002030-200106150-00013

Sahu, G. K., McNearney, T., Evans, A., Turner, A., Weaver, S., Huang, J. C., et al. (2005). Transient or occult HIV infections may occur more frequently than progressive infections: changing the paradigm about HIV persistence. *Arch. Virol. Suppl.* 19, 131–145. doi: 10.1007/3-211-299 81-5_11

Shacklett, B. L., and Ferre, A. L. (2011). Mucosal immunity in HIV controllers: the right place at the right time. *Curr. Opin. HIV AIDS* 6, 202–207. doi: 10.1097/COH.0b013e3283453e2b

Silver, Z. A., and Watkins, D. I. (2017). The role of MHC class I gene products in SIV infection of macaques. *Immunogenetics* 69, 511–519. doi: 10.1007/s00251-017-0997-3

Sui, Y., Lewis, G. K., Wang, Y., Berckmueller, K., Frey, B., Dzutsev, A., et al. (2019). Mucosal vaccine efficacy against intrarectal SHIV is independent of anti-Env antibody response. *J. Clin. Invest.* 129, 1314–1328. doi: 10.1172/JCI122110

Sutton, M. S., Burns, C. M., Weiler, A. M., Balgeman, A. J., Braasch, A., Lehrer-Brey, G., et al. (2016). Vaccination with live attenuated simian immunodeficiency virus (SIV) protects from mucosal, but not necessarily intravenous, challenge with a minimally heterologous SIV. *J. Virol.* 90, 5541–5548. doi: 10.1128/JVI.00192-16

Tasca, S., Tsai, L., Trunova, N., Gettie, A., Saifuddin, M., Bohm, R., et al. (2007). Induction of potent local cellular immunity with low dose X4 SHIV(SF33A) vaginal exposure. *Virology* 367, 196–211. doi: 10.1016/j.virol.2007.05.021

Tebit, D. M., Ndembi, N., Weinberg, A., and Quinones-Mateu, M. E. (2012). Mucosal transmission of human immunodeficiency virus. *Curr. HIV Res.* 10, 3–8. doi: 10.2174/157016212799304689

Theze, J., Chakrabarti, L. A., Vingert, B., Porichis, F., and Kaufmann, D. E. (2011). HIV controllers: a multifactorial phenotype of spontaneous viral suppression. *Clin. Immunol.* 141, 15–30. doi: 10.1016/j.clim.2011.07.007

Xiao, P., Patterson, L. J., Kuate, S., Brocca-Cofano, E., Thomas, M. A., Venzon, D., et al. (2012). Replicating adenovirus-simian immunodeficiency virus (SIV) recombinant priming and envelope protein boosting elicits localized, mucosal IgA immunity in rhesus macaques correlated with delayed acquisition following a repeated low-dose rectal SIV (mac251) challenge. *J. Virol.* 86, 4644–4657. doi: 10.1128/JVI.06812-11

Xu, H., Wang, X., and Veazey, R. S. (2013). Mucosal immunology of HIV infection. *Immunol. Rev.* 254, 10–33. doi: 10.1111/imr.12072

Xue, J., Cong, Z., Xiong, J., Wang, W., Jiang, H., Chen, T., et al. (2013). Repressive effect of primary virus replication on superinfection correlated with gut-derived central memory CD4 (+) T cells in SHIV-infected Chinese rhesus macaques. *PLoS One* 8:e72295. doi: 10.1371/journal.pone.0072295

Yant, L. J., Friedrich, T. C., Johnson, R. C., May, G. E., Maness, N. J., Enz, A. M., et al. (2006). The high-frequency major histocompatibility complex class I allele Mamu-B*17 is associated with control of simian immunodeficiency virus SIVmac239 replication. *J. Virol.* 80, 5074–5077. doi: 10.1128/jvi.80.10.5074-5077.2006

3

Vaccines and Therapeutics Against Hantaviruses

Rongrong Liu[1†], Hongwei Ma[1†], Jiayi Shu[2,3], Qiang Zhang[4], Mingwei Han[5], Ziyu Liu[1], Xia Jin[2], Fanglin Zhang[1*] and Xingan Wu[1*]*

[1] Department of Microbiology, School of Basic Medicine, Fourth Military Medical University, Xi'an, China, [2] Scientific Research Center, Shanghai Public Health Clinical Center & Institutes of Biomedical Sciences, Key Laboratory of Medical Molecular Virology of Ministry of Education & Health, Shanghai Medical College, Fudan University, Shanghai, China, [3] Viral Disease and Vaccine Translational Research Unit, Institut Pasteur of Shanghai, Chinese Academy of Sciences, Shanghai, China, [4] School of Biology and Basic Medical Sciences, Soochow University, Suzhou, China, [5] Cadet Brigade, School of Basic Medicine, Fourth Military Medical University, Xi'an, China

***Correspondence:**
Xia Jin
xiajin2012@outlook.com
Fanglin Zhang
flzhang@fmmu.edu.cn
Xingan Wu
wuxingan@fmmu.edu.cn

Hantaviruses (HVs) are rodent-transmitted viruses that can cause hantavirus cardiopulmonary syndrome (HCPS) in the Americas and hemorrhagic fever with renal syndrome (HFRS) in Eurasia. Together, these viruses have annually caused approximately 200,000 human infections worldwide in recent years, with a case fatality rate of 5–15% for HFRS and up to 40% for HCPS. There is currently no effective treatment available for either HFRS or HCPS. Only whole virus inactivated vaccines against HTNV or SEOV are licensed for use in the Republic of Korea and China, but the protective efficacies of these vaccines are uncertain. To a large extent, the immune correlates of protection against hantavirus are not known. In this review, we summarized the epidemiology, virology, and pathogenesis of four HFRS-causing viruses, HTNV, SEOV, PUUV, and DOBV, and two HCPS-causing viruses, ANDV and SNV, and then discussed the existing knowledge on vaccines and therapeutics against these diseases. We think that this information will shed light on the rational development of new vaccines and treatments.

Keywords: hantavirus, vaccine, therapeutic strategies, HFRS, HPCS

INTRODUCTION

In recent years, the repeated outbreak of hantavirus disease has caused a serious threat to human health. The spread of hantavirus from natural hosts to humans is a natural ecological process; however, the outbreak of hantavirus is driven by striped field mouse population cycle dynamics and seasonal climate change (Tian and Stenseth, 2019).

Hantavirus is a virus transmitted mainly by rodent animals, mainly through urine, feces, and saliva and the aerosols produced by them, but rarely by the bites of infected animals (Brocato and Hooper, 2019). In recent years, the infection rate of hantavirus has increased in China and Europe (Dong et al., 2019). Hantavirus disease has turned out to be a newly identified but not a "new" disease in Germany (Kruger et al., 2013). The clinical presentations may vary according to viral strains prevalence in different regions. In Asia, hantavirus infection by Hantan virus (HTNV) and Seoul virus (SEOV) targets mainly the human kidney and causes hemorrhagic fever with renal syndrome (HFRS). In North America, infection by Andes virus (ANDV) and Sin Nombre virus (SNV) manifests in mainly the lung and leads to hantavirus pulmonary syndrome (HPS) or hantavirus cardiopulmonary syndrome (HCPS), with high mortality rates; in Europe, infection by

Puumala virus (PUUV) and Dobrava-Belgrade virus (DOBV) typically causes a milder form of HFRS, nephropathia epidemica (NE) (Echterdiek et al., 2019).

Currently, there is no approved post-exposure therapeutic countermeasure against hantaviral infection, but diversified treatment strategies have been developed and applied to manage HFRS or HCPS. These strategies target viral life cycle, host immunological factors, or patient clinical symptoms. Preventive measures against hantaviral infection, especially vaccine development, are essential for future pandemics. In this paper, we reviewed the epidemiology and pathogenesis of hantavirus, and discuss the existing knowledge on vaccine and therapeutics against these diseases in order to shed light on the development of new vaccines and treatments.

THE RE-EMERGENCE OF HANTAVIRUS

The Epidemiology of HFRS and HCPS

China has the highest incidence and mortality of HFRS in the world, accounting for more than 90% of the total number of HFRS cases in the world (Zheng et al., 2018). In 2004, the Chinese Center for Disease Control and Prevention (China CDC) established the National Notifiable Disease Surveillance System (NNDSS) online, and HFRS cases of the whole country were reported daily through this system (Zhang et al., 2014). From 2006 to 2012, a total of 77,558 cases and 866 deaths were reported with the average annual incidence rate of 0.83 per 100,000, mortality rate of 0.01 per 100,000 and case fatality rate of 1.13% (Zhang et al., 2014), and its main causative pathogens are HTNV and SEOV (Tian and Stenseth, 2019). So far, HFRS cases have been reported in 30 out of 32 provinces in China (excluding Hong Kong, Macao, and Taiwan) (Zhang et al., 2014). In recent years, the incidence is still high in eastern China (Tian et al., 2017). The distribution map of hantavirus cases reported in recent Chinese literatures is summarized in **Figure 1**. More than 90% of the total cases were clustered in nine provinces and mainly reported in spring and autumn–winter seasons. We can observe that the annual average number of cases in Shaanxi Province was higher than 2000, ranking at the top of the list (**Figure 1**). From 2006 to 2017, Shaanxi has gradually become the province with the highest incidence in China, with approximately 4.51 cases/100,000 cases, of which more than 90% are concentrated in the central region (Xi'an, Xianyang, Baoji, and Weinan cities) (Zheng et al., 2018). By November 20 of 2017, 878 people were recorded infected in Shaanxi Province (Dong et al., 2019). We also can observe that the average annual number of cases in the cities of Shannxi, Shandong, and Jiangxi Province rank the top three (**Supplementary Figure 1**). Another place with a high incidence of HFRS is Qingdao city of Shandong Province, where HFRS incidence is three times higher than the national average, reaching 0.83/100,000 (Jiang et al., 2017).

In the US, 34 states have confirmed and recorded HCPS cases since 1993 (Prince and Lieberman, 2013). In 2008, the first locally acquired case of HFRS caused by the SEOV was confirmed. In 2017, the US CDC investigated an outbreak of SEOV infection that has infected 17 rat owners in seven states (Kerins et al., 2018). The number of hantavirus cases by year in different states is summarized in **Figure 2**. In Canada, HCPS is still very rare, but cases are recorded every year and show seasonal patterns, mainly between March and May and between September and November. A total of 64 cases have been confirmed since 2000, of which 12 were reported in 2013, most in western Canadian provinces such as Alberta, Manitoba, British Columbia, and Saskatchewan (Kerins et al., 2018). SNV and ANDV are responsible for the majority of hantavirus cases leading to HCPS.

Outside North America, individual cases and small clusters of HCPS have been reported in Balkans, northern Sweden (Bergstedt Oscarsson et al., 2016), Argentina (Pini et al., 2003), Chile (Toro et al., 1998), Poland (Gut et al., 2018), Bolivia (1998), Brazil (Suzuki et al., 2004; Limongi et al., 2009), Serbia (Stanojevic et al., 2019), United Kingdom (Duggan, 2019), Panama (Bayard et al., 2004), and Germany (Ettinger et al., 2012). Overall, in Europe, the incidence of hantavirus infections has steadily increased in recent years: In 2014, a record number of 3754 infections were registered across Europe (Vaheri et al., 2013). Chile has had an average of 67 cases per year since 1995; the disease occurs mainly in spring and summer. However, between June and October 2011, there was an increase in cases and rodent populations (Toro et al., 1998). In Paraguay, an HCPS case was first found in the Chako region in 1995. A total of 56 cases were reported in 2011, and 18 cases were reported in 2012 (Padula et al., 2007). In Panama, HCPS first appeared in 1999, with an average of 12 patients per year. However, 16 cases were reported in 2012, and 14 cases were confirmed as of 21 August 2013. For the first time since 1997, Uruguay has experienced HCPS cases, with an average of nine cases per year. The first case was recorded in northern Uruguay in 2010. In Poland, the infections are caused by mainly the PUUV and DOBV serotypes. The morbidity is not high; it ranges between 0.02 and 0.14 per 100,000 cases, but some papers suggest that the data concerning Poland is underestimated (Gut et al., 2018), because the number of infections then was higher, and it was most likely the epidemic year. In the following year, 2015, there were 6 infections, and in 2016 and 2017, there were 8 and 14 cases registered, respectively. In Germany, from 2001 to 2010, the incidence increased from 0.09 to 2.47/100,000 (Ettinger et al., 2012). In United Kingdom, the virus was first identified in laboratory rats in Scotland in 1977, and all but 1 of the 15 cases of SEOV caused acute kidney injury, which were diagnosed by the Rare and Imported Pathogens Laboratory (Duggan, 2019).

Hantavirus Virology

Hantaviruses belong to the Family *Hantaviridae* of *Bunyavirales* and are a kind of enveloped single negative chain RNA virus (Abudurexiti et al., 2019). A maximum likelihood phylogenetic tree of the complete amino acid and CDS sequence of the M segment of hantaviruses was made based on the international Committee on Taxonomy of Viruses (ICTV) updated taxonomy of the order *Bunyavirales* in 2019 (see **Figure 3**). This phylogeny shows the modest genetic diversity of the virus family.

The diameter of hantavirus particles is 80–US210 nm, and the structure is spherical or ovoid. They are composed of 20–30%

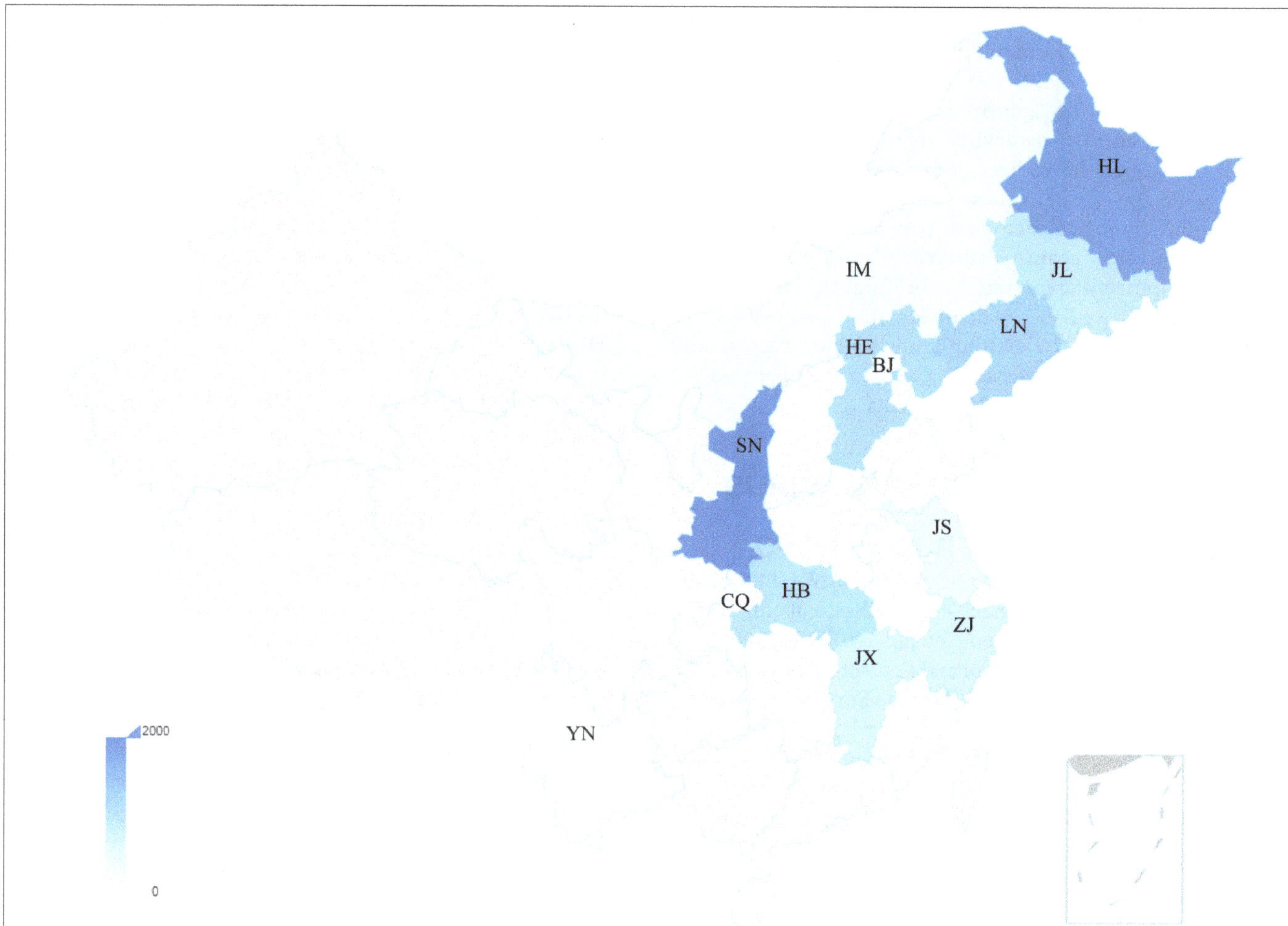

FIGURE 1 | The distribution map of the average hantavirus cases in China of recent years. The main provinces shown in the map were Shaanxi: SN; Heilongjiang: HL; Liaoning: LN; Hebei: HE; Hubei: HB; Jilin: JL; Jiangxi: JX; Zhejiang: ZJ; Jiangsu: JS; Inner Mongoria: IM; Beijing: BJ; Yunnan: YN; Chongqing: CQ. The bar represents the annual average number of cases. These data were published by Chinese literatures.

fat, >50% protein, 7% carbohydrates, and 2% RNA. They are very stable and can survive for more than 18 days at 4°C and −20°C and 10 days at room temperature (Vaheri et al., 2013). The genome comprises three negative sense, single-stranded RNAs that consist the small (S), medium (M), and large (L) segments that encode the nucleoprotein (Np), envelope glycoproteins (Gn and Gc), and viral RNA-dependent RNA polymerase (RdRp), respectively (Graham et al., 2019). The outer membrane of hantavirus is composed of Gn and Gc glycoprotein, which mediates the recognition of and entry into host cells. The crystal structure of HTNV Gn is very similar to that of PUUV Gn, which confirms that hantavirus Gn is conserved in hantavirus (Li et al., 2016; Rissanen et al., 2017).

CLINICAL EVALUATION OF EXISTING VACCINES

Although there have been substantial vaccines, there is no licensed vaccine against hantavirus infection that can be widely used. Despite inactivated hantavirus vaccines being licensed for human use in China and Korea, no such vaccine has been approved in the US or Europe (Tian and Stenseth, 2019). Current clinical studies of inactivated hantavirus vaccine in China or Korea and clinical trials of DNA vaccines in the US are summarized in **Table 1**.

Protective Efficacy of Inactivated Hantavirus Vaccines

The inactivated vaccines comprise entire virions that are inactivated physically (heat) or chemically. In Korea, Lee and An (Cho et al., 2002) first developed an inactivated HTNV vaccine (IHV), which was prepared from the HTNV strain ROK 84/105, which proliferates in the brains of lactating mice. It has been proven that it can induce protein immunization in mice and humans (Yamanishi et al., 1988). In 1990, the Korean HFRS vaccine Hantavax was put into commercial production. The total number of HFRS patients hospitalized in South Korea fell sharply from 1234 in 1991 to 415 in 1997 (Cho et al., 2002). To evaluate

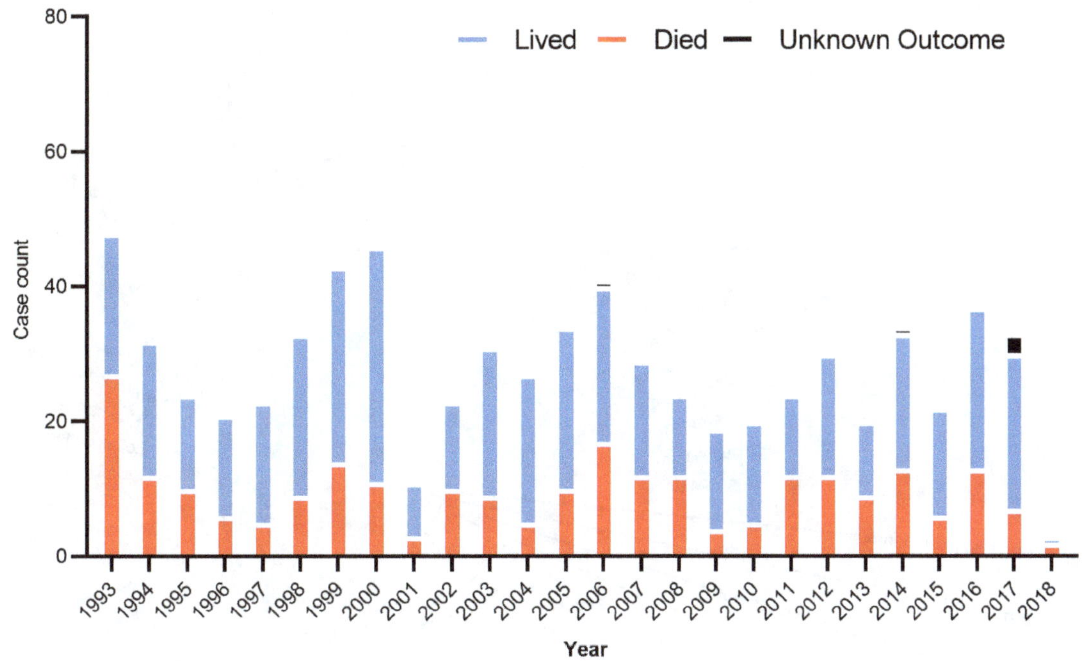

FIGURE 2 | US hantavirus cases from 1993 to 2018. These data were published by the Centers for Disease Control and Prevention, United States.

the immunogenicity and safety of Hantavax™ in healthy adults in multicenter phase III clinical trials, three dose schedules at 0, 1, and 13 months were used. The seroconversion rate was 90.14% by IFA but only 23.24% by PRNT50 after two primary doses. One month after vaccination, the positive rate of serum was 87.32 and 45.07% according to IFA and PRNT50, respectively. The neutralizing antibody response of the two initial doses of Hantavax™ was very poor. Therefore, it is necessary to carry out enhanced immunization within 2–6 months to provide timely protection for high-risk groups (Song et al., 2016).

From January 2011 to February 2017, the South Korean military conducted a case–control study of 100 patients to evaluate the effect of an IHV on HFRS. The vaccine effectiveness (VE) value of the IHV was 59.1%, but the VE value of HFRS high-incidence area was higher (78.7%) (Jung et al., 2018). However, in 2018, the efficacy of iHV on the progression of HFRS did not show a statistically significant protective effect. From 2009 to 2017, 18 patients inoculated with HFRS vaccine and 110 patients not vaccinated with the HFRS vaccine were recruited at Korean Army Hospital to investigate the severity (AKI) and the efficacy of dialysis events in acute renal injury. Overall, 33.3% of the effective vaccination group had three stages of AKI, compared with 54.5% for the non-vaccinated group. The curative effect of IHV on disease progression was 58.1%, but the curative effect of IHV on HFRS progress did not show a statistically significant protective effect (Yi et al., 2018).

In China, bivalent inactivated vaccines against HTNV and SEOV infection were produced in 1994 and approved by the Pharmacopoeia of China in 2005. Since 2008, the Chinese government has implemented an expanded immunization program targeting HFRS. China uses approximately 2 million doses of HFRS vaccine every year (Schmaljohn, 2012). HFRS cases have significantly dropped to less than 20,000 per year. Phase 4 clinical trials of inactivated hantavirus vaccine showed that the median OD values of IgG antibody were 0.005 (0.004–0.016), 0.116 (0.036–0.620), 0.320 (0.065–0.848), and 0.128 (0.011–0.649), and that the positivity rate was 7.7, 40.6, 62.2, and 48.2% at pre-vaccination, 1 month after the two primary doses, at the booster dose and at 18 months after the booster dose, respectively. Although two main doses can help healthy individuals develop immune responses, the three-dose series should be better than the two-dose series (Zheng et al., 2018). Another clinical study in Xian Yang city in northwest China showed that the positive rate of neutralizing antibody in the unvaccinated group was 10.0%, and the positive rate was 80.0, 90.0, 50.0, and 90%, respectively, at 1, 3, 29, and 33 months after immunization with a vaccine consisting of a mixture of inactivated HTNV and SEOV. This finding indicates that the vaccination program can induce effective humoral immunity in northwestern China and can be maintained up to 33 months after vaccination (Li et al., 2017) (**Table 1**).

Clinical Trials of DNA Vaccines for HFRS

At present, DNA vaccines are the most popular method in the research of HFRS and HCPS vaccines, mainly focusing on the use of a hetero-expression system to produce recombinant M protein. DNA vaccines are characterized by safety because they have replication defects, cannot restore the virulence, and cannot spread from person to person or to the environment. A variety of DNA vaccines against the hantavirus envelope glycoprotein gene were developed by Hopper's group (Schmaljohn et al., 2014).

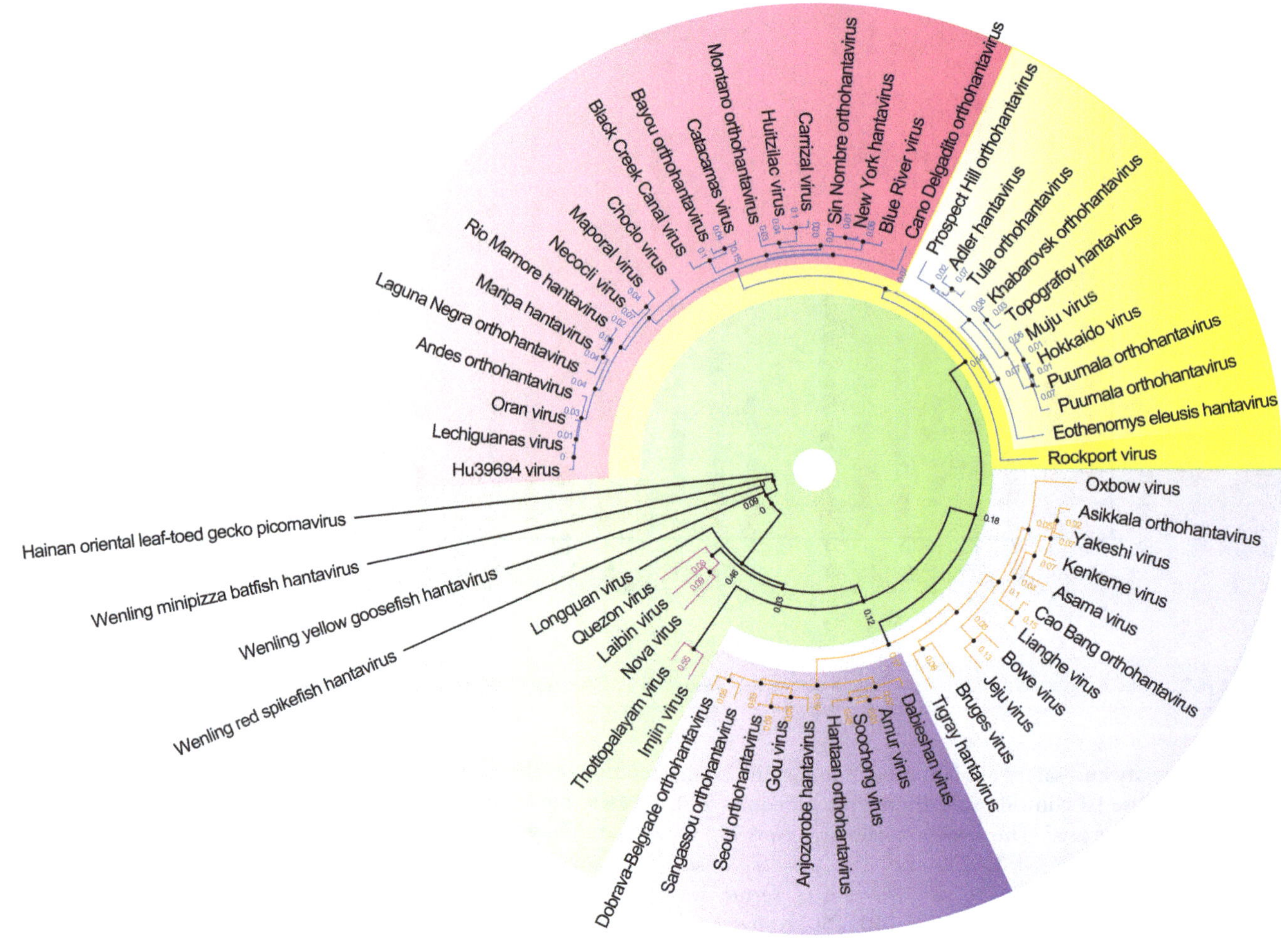

FIGURE 3 | Hantavirus phylogenetic tree on the basis of the M segment sequences. A maximum clade credibility tree of the complete amino acid sequence of the protein encoded by the M segment of viruses belonging to Hantavirus. Different colors represent different clade. These proteins had a high similar signature domain and highly unconserved terminal sequences, which could artificially create similarities between sequences if the alignment was not properly made. Therefore, the phylogenetic tree was made with more robust methods using T-Coffee (default parameter, removed the unconserved sites by filtering the column scores < 4) for multiple sequence alignment and SMS-PhyML (default parameter, bootstrap = 1000, best model = LG +G) for ML (Maximum Likelihood) tree construction.

Their studies have confirmed that these DNA vaccines produce neutralizing antibodies in multiple experimental animal species and protected hamsters from HFRS (Schmaljohn et al., 2014).

Next, they developed HFRS candidate DNA vaccines expressing HTNV or PUUV Gn and GC genes and evaluated them in an open-labeled single-center phase 1 study. The results showed that HTNV and PUUV DNA vaccines prepared by electroporation were safe. When mixed together, the response to PUUV was greater than that to the HTNV DNA vaccine, and both DNA vaccines had immunogenicity (Hooper et al., 2014).

The vaccine entered phase 2a trial in 2014 to compare the immune responses to two different doses, 1.0 and 2.0 mg, and mixed HTNV and PUUV DNA vaccines in healthy participants. All groups also received booster doses 6 months after the first vaccination to determine which doses and vaccination plans will be the best way to advance the vaccine development process. To evaluate the safety, responsiveness and immunogenicity of an ANDV DNA vaccine to prevent HPS, the first phase I clinical trials of the ANDV DNA vaccine began in February 2019[1] (**Table 1**).

PRE-CLINICAL DEVELOPMENT OF NEW VACCINES

DNA Vaccines

Similarly, all DNA vaccines developed against hantavirus target the M gene expressing the envelope GP (Gn and Gc) of hantaviruses (**Table 2**, part 1).

In the United States, a variety of DNA vaccines express the envelope glycoprotein gene of hantaviruses that were developed by Hopper's group (Schmaljohn et al., 2014). In 1999, HFRS candidate naked DNA vaccine was constructed by the subcloning method. The subcloned cDNA represented the medium fragment

[1] www.clinicaltrials.gov

TABLE 1 | Existing vaccines in clinical trials and case–control studies.

Number	Title	Conditions	Interventions	Type	Funder Type	Age	Number Enrolled	Date	Status	References
AFMC-17082-IRB-17-077	Effectiveness of inactivated hantavirus vaccine on the disease severity of hemorrhagic fever with renal syndrome	HFRS	Hantavax®	Case–control study	Korea	20–22	129	March-09 March-17	Completed	Jung et al., 2018
	Protective effectiveness of inactivated hantavirus vaccine against hemorrhagic fever with renal syndrome	HFRS	Hantavax®	Case–control study	Korea	20–30	100	January-11 February-17	Completed	Yi et al., 2018
	Persistence of immune responses to vaccine against hemorrhagic fever with renal syndrome	HFRS	Inactivated hantavirus vaccine	Phase 4	China	16–60	143	June-11 June -13	Completed	Zheng et al., 2018
	The assessment of Hantaan virus-specific antibody responses after the immunization program for hemorrhagic fever with renal syndrome in northwest China	HFRS	HFRS inactivated vaccine [a mixture of HTNV (type I) and SEOV (type II)]	Case–control study	China	16–60	100		Completed	Li et al., 2017
NCT01502345	Study to evaluate the safety, tolerability, and immunogenicity of Hantaan and Puumala virus DNA vaccines	HFRS	HTNV/PUUV DNA vaccine/device combination	Phase 1	U. S. Fed | Industry	18–49	31	January-12 January-13	Completed	Hooper et al., 2014
NCT02116205	Phase 2a immunogenicity study of Hantaan/Puumala virus DNA vaccine for prevention of hemorrhagic fever	HFRS	HTNV/PUUV DNA vaccine	Phase 2a	V. S. Fed | Industry	18–49	132	May-14 July-19	Active, not recruiting	
NCT03682107	Andes virus DNA vaccine for the prevention of hantavirus pulmonary syndrome using the PharmaJetStratis(R) needle-free injection delivery device	HPS	Andes virus DNA vaccine	Phase 1	NIH	18–49	48	February-19 October-19	Recruiting	
NCT03718130	Combination HTNV and PUUV DNA vaccine	HFRS	HTNV vaccine PUUV vaccine HTNV/PUUV virus vaccines	Phase 1	U.S. Fed	18–49	72	May-19 May-21	Not yet recruiting	

TABLE 2 | Pre-clinical development of new vaccines.

DNA vaccine					
Virus	**Antigens**	**Vector**	**Delivery Methodology**	**Animal Model**	**References**
SEOV	M/S	pWRG7077	I.M.	Hamsters	Hooper et al., 1999
PUUV	Npeptide	HuAC/pUC19	I.M.	BALB/c mice	Bucht et al., 2001
HTNV and SEOV	M	pWRG/SEO-M,pWRG/HTN-M	I.M.	Rhesus monkeys	Hooper et al., 2001
ANDV	M	pWRG/AND-M	Gene gun	Rhesus macaques	Custer et al., 2003
HTNV and ANDV	M	pWRG/HA-M	Gene gun	Rhesus macaques	Hooper et al., 2006
ANDV	M	pWRG/AND-M	Twin Injector electroporation device. I.M.	Hamster; rabbits	Hooper et al., 2008
HTNV and PUUV	M	pWRG7077	Gene Gun or I.M. EP	Hamsters	Spik et al., 2008
PUUV	M	pWRG/PUU-M	Gene gun	Hamsters	Brocato et al., 2012
ANDV	M	pWRG/AND-M	I.M.	Hamsters; ducks	Brocato et al., 2012
SNV ANDV and SNV HTNV and PUUV Pan-hantavirus	M	pWRG/SN-M	Muscle electroporation (me)	Female New Zealand white rabbits (*Oryctolagus cuniculus*)	Hooper et al., 2013
SNV ANDV	M	pWRG/SN-M, pWRG/AND-M	DSJI system, IM and ID needle-free devices	Rabbits and NHPs (Syrian hamsters; Rhesus macaques; Cynomolgus macaques)	Kwilas et al., 2014
ANDV and SNV	Gp	pWRG/AND-M;pWRG/SN-M	Needle-free jet injection device	Syrian hamsters	Hooper et al., 2014
ANDV	M	pWRG/AND-M	I.M.	Syrian hamsters	Haese et al., 2015
SEOV, HTNV and PUUV	25 Gp epitopes	pcDNA3.1-SHP pGEX-6p-1-SHP	I.M.	BALB/c mice	Zhao et al., 2012
HTNV	Gn	pVAX-LAMP/Gn	I.M.	BALB/c mice	Jiang et al., 2015
HTNV	Gn	pVAX-Gn, pVAX-LAMP and pVAX-LAMP/Gn;	I.M.	BALB/c mice	Jiang et al., 2017
Subunit Vaccine					
Virus	**Antigens**	**Vector**	**Expression system**	**Results**	**References**
PUUV, TOPV, AMDV and DOBV	NP	pQE-32	*Escherichia coli* cells	Immunization with NP from PUUV, TOPV, ANDV, or DOBV has cross-protection against PUUV	de Carvalho Nicacio et al., 2002
PUUV	NP, G1and G2	pBSK.K27S pWRG7079 K27 G1 pELVS K27 G2 pSC11T7	CV-1 cells COS-7 cells	These recombinant vaccinia viruses were used to detect and clone PUUV-specific CTLs from the PBMC of NE patients. An HLA-A24-restricted CTL line recognizing the G2 protein was isolated and its 9-mer epitope was determined.	Terajima et al., 2002
PUUV, DOBV, and HTNV	NP	pFX7-His6	Yeast *Saccharomyces cerevisiae*	The yield for all nucleocapsid proteins ranged from 0.5 to 1.5 mg per g wet weight of yeast cells	Razanskiene et al., 2004

(Continued)

TABLE 2 | Continued

Subunit Vaccine					
Virus	**Antigens**	**Vector**	**Expression system**	**Results**	**References**
DOBV	NP	pFX7-derived expression plasmids	Yeast *S. cerevisiae*	The antibodies induced by DOBV rN protein were highly cross-reactive to the rN proteins of HTNV and PUUV. In both mice strains, DOBV rN protein induced N-specific antibodies of all IgG sub classes, suggesting a mixed Th1/Th2 immune response.	Geldmacher et al., 2004
PUUV	Gn and Gc	pTrcHis2 Topo® TA vector	COS-1 cells	The diversity between different Puumala virus: N-linked glycosylation occurs at three sites in Gn (N142, N357, and N409), and at one site in Gc (N937). Also, one possible *O*-glycosylation site was identified in Gc (T985).	Johansson et al., 2004
SEOV	NP	pSTBLUE-1/SEOV-N pFX7-His-SEOV-N	Yeast *S. cerevisiae*	The immunization of a rabbit with the recombinant NP resulted in the induction of a high-titered antibody response and was able to detect antibodies in sera of experimentally infected laboratory rats and in human anti-hantavirus-positive sera or serum pools of patients from different geographical origin.	Schmidt et al., 2005
PUUV	NP	pFD3	*S. cerevisiae* FH4C/pFD3-h-N–GFP	The maximal volumetric yield of N protein was 316 mg L^{-1}, the respective yield of h-N protein was 284 mg L^{-1}	Antoniukas et al., 2006
PUUV	NP	pTEXmp18	*E. coli* mutant ICONE 200	P40-Puu118 in particular is a good candidate for a recombinant vaccine against PUUV. All recombinant proteins linked to rP40 induced high antibody responses, indicating that rP40 is a carrier protein with potential for use in other vaccines.	Maes et al., 2008

(Continued)

TABLE 2 | Continued

VLP vaccine					
Virus	**Antigens**	**Vector**	**Expression system**	**Results**	**References**
HTNV	M	pFastBacTM Dual vector	Sf9 insect cells	Chimeric HTNV VLPs containing GPI-anchored GM-CSF or CD40L induced stronger humoral immune responses and cellular immune responses compared to the HTNV VLPs and Chinese commercial inactivated hantavirus vaccine.	Cheng et al., 2016
HTNV	M	pCI-neo	dhfr-deficient CHO cells	*In vitro* stimulation with CD40L or GM-CSF anchored HTNV VLP showed enhanced activation of macrophages and DCs. *In vivo*, it can induce higher level of HTNV specific antibody and neutralizing antibody in mice. Immunized mice splenocytes showed higher ability of secreting IFN-γ and IL-2, as well as enhancing CTL activity.	Ying et al., 2016
HTNV	M	pCI-neo	dhfr-deficient CHO cells	GM-CSF and CD40L VLPs provided stable, long-term protection with a high titer of neutralizing antibody in mice 6 months after immunization. Furthermore, VLPs increased HTNV-specific cellular immune responses via higher expression of IFN-g and CTL responses. HTNV challenge assay results showed long-term protection against HFRS. No significant pathological alteration was observed in the organs of mice after immunization.	Dong et al., 2019

(M; encoding G 1 and G 2 glycoprotein) or small fragment (S; encoding nucleocapsid protein) of SEOV and was cloned into the expression vector WRG 7077. Syrian hamsters were vaccinated with the M or S vaccine with a gene gun, and hantavirus-specific antibodies were found in 5 of 5 hamsters or 4 of 5 hamsters, respectively. Evidence of infection was monitored after challenge with SEOV. Twenty-eight days later, hamsters vaccinated with M were protected hamsters from infection, but those inoculated with S were not protected (Hooper et al., 1999).

Then, HTNV M gene products G 1 and G 2 were expressed in 2001, and non-human primates were evaluated. The HTNV M gene has protective effects against HTNV, SEOV, and DOBV in hamsters. The HTNV and ANDV M genes can induce high level of neutralizing antibodies in rhesus monkeys (Hooper et al., 2001). Next, a DNA vaccine plasmid containing the full-length M genome fragment of ANDV (pWRG/AND-M) was constructed (Hooper et al., 2008). Rhesus monkeys inoculated with pWRG/AND-M with gene guns produced very high levels of neutralizing antibodies that neutralized not only ANDV but also other HCPS-related hantavirus strains, such as SNV. On the 4th or 5th day after injection, monkey serum protected 100% of hamsters from fatal diseases (Custer et al., 2003).

Then the pWRG/HA-M plasmid containing the HTNV and ANDV M gene fragments was constructed. Rhesus monkeys were immunized with the pWRG/HA-M vaccine to produce antibodies binding to M gene products (G 1 and G 2 glycoproteins) and neutralize HTNV and ANDV. Subsequently, 1–2 years after the initial vaccination series, the neutralizing antibody titers induced by the double immunogen pWRG/HA-M or a single immunogen expressing only HTNV or ANDV Gp increased rapidly to a high level. This result is the first time that the hantavirus M gene DNA vaccine has been shown to elicit a strong memory response and stimulate an antibody response to neutralize HFRS and HCPS viruses (Hooper et al., 2006; Kwilas et al., 2014) detected the high-titer neutralizing antibody induced by an SNV/ANDV DNA vaccine encoding viral envelope Gp in laboratory animals and non-human primates (NHCPS). It can be delivered effectively using a disposable syringe injection (DSJI) system (Kwilas et al., 2014). Brocato et al. (2013) cloned codon-optimized PUUV M fragments into DNA vaccine vectors to produce the plasmid pWRG/PUU-M, which can produce high-titer neutralizing antibodies in hamsters and NHCPs. The pWRG/PUU-M vaccine protects hamsters from PUUV infection and is not affected by DOBV infection. Unexpectedly, vaccination could protect hamsters in the absence of ANDV cross-neutralizing antibodies in a lethal ANDV disease model (Brocato et al., 2013). Then, the authors tried to produce the pan-hantavirus vaccine with a mixed plasmid DNA vaccine. A study of ANDV hamster model showed that the neutralizing antibody produced by DNA vaccine technology can be used to resist the challenge of an SNV full-length M gene DNA vaccine to prevent the occurrence of HCPS. Rabbits vaccinated with SNV DNA vaccine with muscle electroporation (mEP) produced increased neutralizing antibody titers. In addition, hamsters vaccinated three times with the SNV DNA vaccine with a gene gun were completely free from SNV infection. Rabbits were vaccinated with HCPS mixture (ANDV and SNV plasmid), HFRS mixed (HTNV and PUUV plasmid), or HCPS/HFRS mixture (all four plasmids) by mEP. The results showed that the HCPS mixture and HFRS mixture produce neutralizing antibodies against ANDV/SNV and HTNV/PUUV, respectively. In addition, a mixture of HCPS/HFRS triggered neutralizing antibodies against all four viruses (Hooper et al., 2013). Spik et al. (2008) reported that PUUV and HTNV DNA vaccines should serve as separate regulators. Both vaccines produced neutralizing antibodies when injected alone, but when they were administered as mixtures, only one of the two hantavirus antibodies could be detected. In contrast, if the DNA was administered to an animal as a separate vaccine, a reaction to both was observed. To improve the use of DNA vaccine, a multihead intradermal electroporation device was developed, which can be used to vaccinate with an increased dose of DNA vaccine to the skin. The device will enable multiplasmid vaccine preparation to provide multiplasmid vaccine preparation without interference (Mackow et al., 2014).

In China, a DNA vaccine targeting hantavirus Gn merges the antigen with lysosome-associated membrane protein 1 (LAMP 1), thereby changing the antigen presentation pathway and activating CD4 T cells. The LAMP 1 targeting strategy successfully enhanced the effectiveness of the HTNV Gn vaccine. Further studies showed that pVAX-LAMP/Gn established a memory response during long-term protection (6 months) in mice. Zhao et al. constructed a multi-epitope chimeric DNA vaccine—named the SHP chimeric gene, which contains 25 glycoprotein epitopes of SEOV, HTNV, and PUUV. The humoral and cellular responses were significantly enhanced in vaccinated BALB/c mice (Zhao et al., 2012).

Subunit Vaccines

Subunit protein vaccines not only are safe and easy to produce but also do not easily cause interference between the components of a multivalent formulation (Sun et al., 2017; Liang et al., 2018; Qu et al., 2018). Because the N protein of hantavirus circulating in different continents can provide high cross-protection in animals, the N protein is considered to be an important part of a wide range of reactive vaccines against hantavirus infection (de Carvalho Nicacio et al., 2002). Research has shown that recombinant nucleocapsid protein (rN) from PUUV, TOPV, ANDV, and DOBV could induce a cross-protective immune response to PUUV. The cross-reaction to PUUV antigen was the highest in the serum of animals immunized with ANDV rN, followed by that to TOPV and DOBV rN. In a proliferation test, T lymphocytes immunized with heterogenic rNs were effectively recalled by PUUV rN *in vitro*, as were animal T lymphocytes immunized with homologous proteins (de Carvalho Nicacio et al., 2002). In addition, recombinant vaccinia virus carrying PUUV N or the first half of the G2 gene was constructed. Detection and cloning of PUUV-specific CTLs from PBMCs of patients with NE by recombinant PUUV vaccinia virus led to the isolation of an HLA-A24-restricted CTL cell line recognizing the G2 protein, and its 9-mer epitope was determined (Terajima et al., 2002). Razanskiene et al. (2004) reported that the stability and high purity of NP of PUUV, DOBV, and HTNV ranged from 0.5 to 1.5 mg/g wet weight of yeast cells. DOBV rN protein is a promising vaccine candidate protein that can induce N-specific antibodies, and its terminal titer is as high as 1:1,000,000 in C57BL/6 mice. The antibody induced by DOBV rN protein has a high cross-reaction with rN protein of PUUV and HTNV (Geldmacher et al., 2004). It was found that there might be RNA fragment exchange between the two PUUV strains. N-linked glycosylation occurred at one site of Gn (N 142, N357, and N409) and GC (N 937), and a possible *O*-glycosylation site was identified in GC (T 985). The study of coding gene products is of great significance for the design of new vaccines (Johansson et al., 2004). Schmidt et al. (2005) reports that NP of SEOV reacts with SEOV-specific monoclonal antibodies and some HTNV- and PUUV cross-reactive monoclonal antibodies. Rabbits immunized with recombinant NP can induce a high-titer antibody response, and NP-specific antibodies were detected in the serum of experimental infected rats and human exposed to hantavirus from different geographical sources. Yeast-expressed SEOV N protein represents a promising antigen for serological epidemiological research and vaccine development (Schmidt et al., 2005). Antoniukas et al. (2006) reported that the biomass and the expression level of recombinant PUUV NP were increased by adding plant extract to YNB medium. The maximum volume yield of the N protein was 316 mg L^{-1} (Antoniukas et al., 2006) (**Table 2**, part 2).

VLP Vaccines

Virus-like particle vaccines are similar to natural virus particles but lack infectious genetic material. They are composed of repetitive viral structural proteins with inherent self-assembly characteristics (Yong et al., 2019). How to improve the immunogenicity of VLPs is very important. It was reported that either CD40L- or GM-CSF-contained HTNV VLP expression in sf9 insect cells (Cheng et al., 2016) or CHO cells (Ying et al., 2016) could enhance the activation of macrophages and dendritic cells. CD40L/GM-CSF incorporation into VLPs induced elevated levels of HTNV-specific antibodies and neutralizing antibodies in mice. The spleen cells of immunized mice had an enhanced ability to secrete IFN-γ and IL-2, increasing CTL activity (Cheng et al., 2016). The GM-CSF and CD40L-containing VLPs expressed in a eukaryotic expression vector had a stable, long-term protective effect, with a high titer of neutralizing antibody, on mice within 6 months after immunization (Dong et al., 2019). These results suggest that CD40L/GM-CSF-containing VLPs can be used as a potential candidate vaccine (**Table 2**, part 3).

THERAPEUTIC STRATEGIES AGAINST HANTAVIRUS INFECTION

Hantaviruses primarily infect host capillary endothelial cells of various organs, especially those of kidneys and lungs, and could spark robust immune response in humans. The basic pathological feature of both old world hantaviruses causing HFRS and new world hantaviruses leading to HCPS is dramatically increased vascular permeability, the pathogenesis of which is highly involved in viral infection and excessive immune responses of the host. Extensive capillary leakage results in multiple clinical manifestations, such as hypotensive shock in HFRS and non-cardiogenic pulmonary edema in HCPS, which might deteriorate into multisystem organ failure. Currently, there are no approved post-exposure therapeutic countermeasures against hantaviral infection, but diversified treatment strategies, which target the viral life cycle, host immunological factors or patient clinical symptoms, have been developed and applied to manage HFRS or HCPS (see **Table 3**). Virus-targeting antivirals, including classical antiviral drugs, antibodies, or novel small molecules, are tested mainly to block hantavirus entry or restrain virus replication. Although several antivirals have been proven to be protective *in vitro* or *in vivo*, there still exist some problems for their clinical application. Host-targeting medicines are designed to improve vascular function or rebuild immune homeostasis, while their curative effects are still under debate. Supportive care is universally applied for HFRS or HCPS, and the specific treatments depend on clinical findings of different disease phases.

Virus-Targeting Antivirals

Blocking Viral Entry

The viral entry process is composed of virus attachment or absorption on susceptible cells, penetration and subsequent uncoating, which is the first step for hantaviral life cycle. Neutralizing antibodies (NAbs) could interact with viral envelope proteins and disturb their binding with receptors on host cells, thus blocking viral attachment. During hantavirus infection, the Gn and Gc glycoproteins, but not nucleocapsid proteins (NP) are considered the major antigens in inducing NAb production (Jiang et al., 2016). High levels of NAbs could be detected in the convalescent phase of HFRS or HCPS patients, and these NAbs could protect the individual from hantaviral infection and have been used as passive immunotherapy (Manigold and Vial, 2014; Jiang et al., 2016). Presently, there are no reported clinical randomized controlled trials using NAbs in immunotherapy for HFRS or HCPS in humans. Most studies measure antibody efficacy through the focus reduction neutralization test (FRNT) and hemagglutination inhibition (HI) test at the cellular level, as well as animal experiments against lethal hantavirus challenge (sucking mice or newborn rat models for HTNV or SEOV infection and hamster models for ANDV or SNV infection) (Zhang et al., 1989; Xu et al., 2002; Manigold and Vial, 2014). For old world hantaviruses, 13 crude Fab preparations directed to the PUUV Gc protein were generated from splenic lymphocytes of a PUUV-immune individual and exhibited type-specific neutralization of PUUV, with a 44–54% reduction in FRNT (de Carvalho Nicacio et al., 2000). Anti-SR-11 (SEOV) rat serum applied 4 h before or 72 h after the challenge could protect against lethal SR-11 (SEOV) infection in newborn rats, and cross-protection effects were also found against KI-262 (SEOV) and 76-118 (HTNV) (Zhang et al., 1989). In China, 18 murine monoclonal antibodies (MAbs) targeting HTNV were prepared in our lab, among which 14 targeted NP, 4 reacted with Gc, and 1 recognized both NP and Gc. The Gc-related MAbs were active in the HI test and displayed high virus-neutralizing activity *in vitro*, and they could be regarded as HTNV NAbs. Consistently, administration of these NAbs within 48 hpi could protect suckling mice from lethal HTNV infection, indicating that NAbs might be a potentially treatment strategy for preexposure prophylaxis and postexposure therapy against HTNV infection (Xu et al., 2002). Phase I clinical pharmacology and toxicity tests for HTNV NAbs in healthy volunteers were performed, and phase II clinical trials to assess the therapeutic efficacy of these NAbs in early stages of HFRS were carried out in endemic settings in China (Xu et al., 2002, 2009). For new world hantaviruses, passive immunization with either patient-derived or vaccine-induced NAbs was capable of protecting against lethal ANDV challenge in hamsters (Manigold and Vial, 2014). A non-randomized multicenter trial using plasma from HCPS convalescent patients for the treatment of acute HCPS has been carried out in Chile, showing that plasma containing high titers of NAbs against ANDV could significantly reduce case fatality rate from 32 to

TABLE 3 | Potential therapeutic strategies for hantaviral infection.

Purpose	Drugs	Type	Known/ Putative target	Virus/Evidence	Diseases	References
Blocking Viral Entry	MAb Fab 4G2 and 1C9	Human MAbs Fab fragments	Gc glycoprotein	PUUV/ Vero E6 cells	HFRS	de Carvalho Nicacio et al., 2000
	Anti-SR rat serum	Rat PAbs	Viral GP	SEOV/ newborn rats		Zhang et al., 1989
	3D8, 3G1, 8G3, 8F8, 8G2	Mice MAbs	Gc, or both NP and Gc	HTNV/Vero E6 cells/suckling mice/phase II clinical trials		Xu et al., 2002, 2009
	Patient-derived or vaccine-induced NAbs	Human PAbs	Viral GP	ANDV/hamsters	HCPS	Manigold and Vial, 2014
	Human immune plasma	Human PAbs	Viral GP	ANDV/clinical trials		Vial et al., 2015
	IgY/IgY ΔFc	Goose PAbs	Viral GP	ANDV/hamsters		Haese et al., 2015
	JL16 and MIB22	Human MAbs	Viral GP	ANDV/hamsters		Garrido et al., 2018
	Lactoferin	Lactoferin	Viral GP/monocyte and NK	SEOV/ Vero E6 cell/suckling mice	HFRS	Murphy et al., 2000, 2001
	Domain III and stem peptides	Peptides	Gc glycoprotein	ANDV, PUUV/Vero E6 cells	HCPS and HFRS	Barriga et al., 2016
	CLVRNLAWC and CQATTARNC	Cyclic nonapeptides	Host receptor	SNV, ANDV/Vero E6 cells	HCPS	Hall et al., 2008
	012-0652, C481-1256 and G319-0078	Peptidomimetic compounds	Host receptor	SNV, ANDV, HTNV/Vero E6 cells	HCPS and HFRS	Hall et al., 2010
	Favipiravir	Pyrazine derivative	RdRp	SNV, ANDV/Vero E6 cells/hamsters	HCPS	Safronetz et al., 2013
Inhibiting Viral Replication	Ribavirin	Nucleoside analogs/ mutagen/ T cell	RdRp	HTNV, PUUV, ANDV/Vero E6 cells/suckling mice (HTNV)/hamsters (ANDV)	HCPS and HFRS	Mertz et al., 2004; Safronetz et al., 2011; Kobayashi et al., 2012; Chung et al., 2013; Ogg et al., 2013; Westover et al., 2016; Malinin and Platonov, 2017
	ETAR	Nucleoside analogs	RdRp	HTNV, ANDV/ Vero E6 cells/suckling mice (HTNV)	HCPS and HFRS	Chung et al., 2008
	K31, K34 and 103772	Small molecules	Viral RNA-NP interaction	SNV, ANDV/ Vero E6 cells	HCPS	Salim et al., 2016
	Arbidol	Small molecules	Unclear	HTNV/Vero E6 cells/suckling mice	HFRS	Deng et al., 2009
	siRNA	Small interfering RNA	S, M, and L segments	ANDV/Vero E6 cells	HCPS	Chiang et al., 2014
	siRNA and 3G1-Cκ-tP	Small interfering RNA and Abs	S, M, and L segments	HTNV/Vero E6 cells/suckling mice	HFRS	Yang et al., 2017
Improving Vascular Function	Pazopanib, dasatinib, PP1, bosutinib, and Src inhibitor 1	VEGFR2 kinase inhibitor or SFK inhibitor	Vascular function/VEGF	ANDV/HUVECs	HCPS	Gorbunova et al., 2011
	Vandetanib	Tyrosine-kinase inhibitor	Vascular function/VEGF	ANDV/HUVECs/ hamsters	HCPS	Bird et al., 2016
	Ang-1 and S1P	Compounds	Vascular function	HTNV, ANDV, NY-1/HUVECs	HCPS and HFRS	Gavrilovskaya et al., 2008
	Icatibant	Small molecules	BK type 2 receptor	PUUV/clinical case report	HFRS	Antonen et al., 2013; Laine et al., 2015
Rebuilding Immune Homeostasis	Clofilium phosphate	Compounds	Alveolar macrophages	ANDV/hamsters	HCPS	Hammerbeck et al., 2016
	Corticoids or methylprednisolone	Hormone	Immunotherapy	HTNV, ANDV/clinical trials	HCPS and HFRS	Vial et al., 2013; Brocato and Hooper, 2019

14% (Vial et al., 2015). Considering the limited availability of convalescent plasma from HCPS survivors, goose polyclonal antibodies were acquired from ANDV DNA vaccine, and the purified IgY/IgY ΔFc from egg yolks could protect hamsters from lethal ANDV infection. Recently, two NAbs, JL16 and MIB22, were developed from the ANDV GP-specific memory B cells of convalescent HCPS patients, both of which reached in a 100% protection rate against lethal ANDV challenge (Garrido et al., 2018). Although NAbs from convalescent patient or immunized animals could obviously restrain hantaviral infection and improve disease outcome, purified human or humanized NAbs against hantaviruses with increased security and efficacy should be developed for clinical experiments. Additionally, research on broadly neutralizing antibodies against hantaviruses is still lacking.

Hantaviral attachment or absorption could also be restrained by lactoferin (LF), an iron-binding glycoprotein that was reported to have broad antibacterial, antifungal, and antiviral activities. LF-pretreated Vero E6 cells showed a reduced number of SR-11 (SEOV) foci, while its antiviral effects were obviously compromised if the LF-pretreated cell monolayer was washed before SEOV infection (Murphy et al., 2000). Further, LF could suppress viral shedding within 24 hpi, the effectiveness of which failed after 48 hpi (Murphy et al., 2001). These results indicated that LF might adhere to cell surface and inhibit SEOV adsorption to host cells. Intriguingly, although LF could not inhibit the expression of NP and Gc, once hantaviral amplification was established in cells, LF contributed to higher survival rates, which might be due to LF-enhanced cytocidal function of natural killer (NK) cells (Murphy et al., 2001). Even so, the specific mechanisms of how LF inhibits SEOV absorption and influences host immune responses, as well as the effects of LF on other species of hantaviruses, remain obscure.

Hantaviral fusion with cell membrane facilitates its entry process. The Hantavirus Gc envelope glycoprotein acts as a viral fusion protein that is essential for viral entry. It has been demonstrated that Gc shares similar features with class II fusion proteins, which means that three domains of viral fusion proteins are connected by a stem region anchoring in the viral envelope (Cifuentes-Munoz et al., 2011). Exogenous protein fragments containing fusion protein domain III (DIII) and the stem region could bind to the core of the fusion protein and interfere with its conformation transition, inhibiting the membrane fusion process. Based on this effect, soluble recombinant peptides that mimic DIII and the stem region were prepared, and were proven to block both ANDV and PUUV infection in Vero E6 cells by blocking membrane fusion (Barriga et al., 2016). The strategy using viral Gc DIII and stem fragments to suppress fusion might be feasible for other hantaviruses, while the protective effects *in vivo* still need further studies to confirm.

Furthermore, antivirals targeting hantaviral receptors have been synthesized. It has been demonstrated that pathogenic hantaviruses attach to the cell surface via host-specific $\alpha_{IIb}\beta_3$ or$\alpha_v\beta_3$integrins while non-pathogenic hantaviruses initiate cellular entry relying on $\alpha_v\beta_1$ integrins (Jiang et al., 2016). Based on the structure of cyclic peptides known to bind the $\alpha_v\beta_3$ receptor, a few of cyclic peptides or small molecules were designed and screened for their antihantaviral function. The cyclic nonapeptides CLVRNLAWC and CQATTARNC could inhibit SNV and ANDV infection *in vitro* (Hall et al., 2008). After two rounds of biological screening, the peptidomimetic compounds 8012-0652, C481-1256, and G319-0078 were screened out with potency in the nanomolar range against infection of a panel of hantaviruses, including SNV, ANDV, and HTNV (Hall et al., 2010). Further studies should be performed to evaluate the safety and efficacy of these small molecules *in vivo*.

Inhibiting Viral Replication

Viral proteins are the working molecules for viral biosynthesis, among which RdRp plays an important role in hantaviral transcription and replication and is considered a desirable drug target. The pyrazine derivative Favipiravir and the nucleoside analogs Ribavirin (RBV) and ETAR have been tested effective antihantaviral drugs that directly or indirectly affect the biological function of RdRp. Favipiravir (Avigan; T-705) was initially discovered in 2002 as an antiviral drug selectively inhibiting the RdRp of influenza virus and then reported to have a high activity against a panel of Bunyaviruses (Gowen et al., 2007; Westover et al., 2016). Favipiravir could attenuate the viral RNA replication level and decrease the progeny virus yield of SNV and ANDV *in vitro*. *In vivo* studies, including non-lethal SNV challenged and lethal ANDV challenged hamster model, demonstrated that oral administration favipiravir at the dosage of 100 mg/kg twice daily could prominently reduce viral load in hamster serum and various organs and resulted in 100% survival in the ANDV lethal infection model (Safronetz et al., 2013). Delayed favipiravir administration after the onset of viremia exerted no protective effects against ANDV infection. Notably, there is no reported clinical trial with favipiravir as an antiviral treatment in HFRS and HCPS.

RBV and ETAR are nucleoside analogs that interfere with viral replication. They can inhibit inosine monophosphate dehydrogenase and reduce the synthesis GTP *de novo*, hence affecting the function of viral RdRp. As a potent mutagen, RBV could induce RNA mutagenesis in subsequent generations of HTNV virions (Chung et al., 2013), while it is not expected that ETAR induces mutation, probably due to the lack of pseudobase pair presence (Chung et al., 2008). Additionally, RBV was reported to modulate host immune responses by suppressing interleukin-10-producing regulatory T cells (Kobayashi et al., 2012), while there is no evidence showing that ETAR could exert immunoregulatory effects (Szabo, 2017). Both *in vitro* and *in vivo* antihantaviral activity of RBV and ETAR have been confirmed by a series of studies. For HFRS therapy, RBV-treated suckling mice had a higher survival rate upon HTNV infection than the placebo control group (Huggins et al., 1986). In China, a double-blind placebo-controlled clinical trial enrolled 242 HFRS patients caused by HTNV infection. The result showed that postexposure administration of RBV could decrease mortality by sevenfold and reduce the risk of entering the oliguric phase, suggesting that RBV is effective against HTNV-induced HFRS (Huggins et al., 1991). However, a clinical trial for HFRS caused by PUUV infection in Russia showed that RBV could not improve patient condition, especially reducing viral load, and that RBV could increase the occurrence of side effects of RBV, including rash, sinus bradycardia, hyperbilirubinemia, and reduced hemoglobin. These data suggested insufficient efficacy and safety of RBV in the treatment of HFRS caused by PUUV (Malinin and Platonov, 2017). For HCPS treatment, two studies confirmed that RBV could protect hamsters from lethally intraperitoneal or intranasal ANDV challenge without toxicity, and even abbreviated treatment regimens from 7 days to 3 days worked if therapy commenced 1 day following virus challenge (Safronetz et al., 2011; Ogg et al., 2013). Unfortunately, two clinical trials for the treatment of HCPS using RBV did not show any improvement in survival rates compared with those for patients during the same time frame or receiving placebo treatment. It is speculated that RBV treatment might be ineffective once HCPS progresses to the cardiopulmonary phase. ETAR showed an EC(50) value of 10 and 4.4 μmol/L for HTNV and ANDV in Vero E6 cells, respectively, which is much lower than its toxic dosage of 880 μmol/L (Chung et al., 2008). Moreover, ETAR administration in sucking mice with a dosage of 12.5 or 25 mg/kg at 10 days post HTNV infection could significantly increase the survival rate from 10 to 25%, an effect equal to that of RBV (Chung et al., 2008). To date, there were no studies on the antiviral activity of ETAR on other hantaviruses.

Hantaviral NP could bind to an evolutionary conserved sequence at the 5′ terminus of hantaviral genomic RNA. The interaction of NP with the viral genome could protect viral RNA from host recognition and degradation, facilitate the N-mediated viral RNA translation process, and help package the viral genome into nucleocapsids. Several compounds, namely, lead inhibitor K31, K34, and 103772, were reported to interrupt the NP-RNA interaction against SNV and ANDV infection. They could abrogate both viral RNA synthesis and translation without affecting the normal biological process of host cells, among which K31 showed antiviral activity similar to that of RBV (Salim et al., 2016). However, K31 failed to affect the replication of HIV or adenovirus, demonstrating its selectivity for hantaviruses. Arbidol, an immunomodulator developed in Russia, was also found to protect against HTNV infection both *in vivo* and *in vitro* (Deng et al., 2009).

Targeting viral RNAs is the most direct and effective way to curb hantaviral replication. Small interfering RNA (siRNA) directed against hantaviral genes could facilitate viral RNA clearance based on the RNA interfering (RNAi) mechanisms and has been tested as a potential antiviral strategy *in vitro* and *in vivo*. It has been demonstrated that siRNAs targeting the S, M, or L segment of ANDV could reduce viral replication in Vero E6 cells or human lung microvascular endothelial cells and that an S-targeted siRNA pool seemed to be more efficient in reducing viral transcription and replication than M- or L-targeted siRNA in Vero E6 cells. Importantly, these siRNAs could inhibit ANDV replication even if given after infection (Chiang et al., 2014). Although siRNAs could effectively suppress hantavirus amplification in host cells most likely through promoting viral RNA clearance, their antiviral activity might be greatly compromised considering their poor biological stability and targeting ability *in vivo*. One strategy is to combine siRNAs targeting encoding sequences of HTNV genome with recombinant antibodies (3G1-Cκ-tP) recognizing HTNV Gc, which were applied by intraperitoneal injection in an HTNV-induced encephalitis mouse model. The result indicated that through combination, siRNAs could be specifically delivered to the HTNV-infected brain cells and protect against HTNV intracranial infection (Yang et al., 2017). On all accounts, novel delivery system should be developed to ensure the stability and selectivity of siRNAs, and the efficacy and safety of these systems remained unclear for the treatment of HFRS or HCPS.

Host-Targeting Medicines

Improving Vascular Function

Increased capillary leakage due to hantaviral infection is the basic pathogenic feature for both HFRS and HCPS. Therefore, treatment strategies improving microvascular endothelial cell function seem to be feasible in mitigating disease severity and reducing mortality (Alkharsah, 2018). Hantavirus-disturbed vascular function is a multifactorial event whose complicated mechanisms still need to be elucidated, and two kinds of hypothesis have been developed. The vascular endothelial growth factor (VEGF) theory was first proposed and studied in depth. VEGF binding to VEGF receptor 2 (VEGFR2) could activate SFK (Src family kinases) signaling, which may result in dissociation, internalization, and degradation of VE-cadherin. Altered expression and localization of VE-cadherin contributed to impaired barrier structure of adherent junctions, which could lead to incremental cellular permeability (Jiang et al., 2016). It has been demonstrated HTNV or ANDV infection could disrupt the interaction of β3 integrin with VEGFR2 and induce VEGFR2 hyper phosphorylation, which may enhance the permeability of infected endothelial cells by sensitizing them to VEGF (Gavrilovskaya et al., 2012; Wang et al., 2012). As increased VEGF content has been noted in the plasma of HFRS and HCPS patients and is closely related to disease severity in the acute phase (Bird et al., 2016; Pal et al., 2018), it is feasible to repurpose those FDA-approved drugs targeting vasoactive mediators for use as hantaviral infection therapy. In line with this strategy, one study reported that the VEGFR2 kinase inhibitor, as well as SFK inhibitors, could obviously stabilize ANDV-induced endovascular permeability, among which the SFK inhibitors dasatinib and pazopanib blocked VE-cadherin dissociation by more 90% (Gorbunova et al., 2011). Another study also indicated that application of vandetanib, a tyrosine-kinase inhibitor preventing VEGFR2 phosphorylation, before ANDV infection could delay animal lethality and increase total survival by 23% in ANDV-challenged hamsters (Bird et al., 2016). In contrast, similar small molecules administered after the onset of viremia failed to protect hamsters from lethal ANDV challenge (Brocato and Hooper, 2019). Moreover, some other small molecules, such as angiopoietin 1 (Ang-1) and sphingosine 1-phosphate (S1P), were found to inhibit hantavirus-directed endothelial cell permeability *in vitro* (Gavrilovskaya et al., 2008), while further research *in vivo* should be performed to confirm their efficacy.

Another promising theory is increased activation of the kinin–kallikrein system (KKS) during hantavirus infection. One study using a model with co-cultured endothelial and vascular smooth muscle cells demonstrated that activation of KKS and subsequent liberation of bradykinin (BK), but not VEGF, were mainly responsible for the dramatic increase in endothelial cell permeability after hantavirus infection (Taylor et al., 2013). BK, a nonapeptide that binds BK type 2 receptor, could induce blood vessel dilatation and vascular permeability increase, resulting in collapsed blood pressure. Icatibant is a peptidomimetic drug that can block the interaction of BK with the BK type 2 receptor by binding to this receptor itself. One case reported that a 37-year-old male who once underwent splenectomy due to congenital spherocytosis manifested with severe capillary leakage syndrome caused by PUUV infection. With a single dose of icatibant, the condition of the patient stabilized, followed by gradual improvement and full recovery (Antonen et al., 2013). Another case report also confirmed the efficient treatment of icatibant in a 67-year-old female HFRS patient (Laine et al., 2015). These clinical data indicated that BK receptor antagonist might be a novel treatment strategy for hantavirus diseases. Nevertheless, it should also be noted that the foresaid two patients had spleen abnormalities, which might be related to the curative effect of icatibant. Clinical trials enrolling a large number of HFRS or HCPS patients should be performed to further identify the remedy effects of bradykinin receptor antagonists.

Rebuilding Immune Homeostasis

It is wildly accepted that HFRS and HCPS are caused by uncontrolled systemic inflammatory responses, in which multiple inflammatory cytokines, especially TNF-α, IL-8, and RANTES, contributed to disease progression (Manigold and Vial, 2014; Schonrich and Raftery, 2017); however, immunoregulation treatment in HFRS or HCPS is undesirable. A recent study with depletion of alveolar macrophages, which are considered the main resource for proinflammatory responses, could not prevent ANDV-caused pathogenesis in hamsters (Hammerbeck et al., 2016). The immunomodulatory treatment of corticoids was firstly performed during the Korean war, but the case fatality rate was not improved (Sayer et al., 1955). In Chile, a retrospective analysis suggested that a high dose of methylprednisolone could reduce mortality in 22 HCPS patients (Brocato and Hooper, 2019). However, a double-blind clinical trial in Chile failed to observe a significantly improved outcome between methylprednisolone recipients and placebo recipients for HCPS. Similarly, another randomized prospective study did not show any benefit from corticosteroid treatment in HFRS patients (Qian et al., 1990).

Supportive Care

The initiation of careful observation and prompt but judicious supportive treatment is crucial to improve patient survival condition for both HFRS and HCPS (Sargianou et al., 2012). It has been demonstrated that admission to the ICU and supportive treatment could greatly reduce the mortality rate of HFRS (Huggins et al., 1991). In general, the treatment principle for HFRS patients is using intravenous hydration and electrolyte therapy to maintain physiological blood pressure. Platelet transfusions can be applied to reduce the mortality in patients with severe thrombocytopenia. Intermittent hemodialysis (IHD) is the first choice to improve uremia condition and rectify kidney dysfunction in patients with acute kidney injury. Continuous renal replacement therapy (CRRT) should be applied for those critical HFRS patients, especially when they have a complication, such as multi-organ injury pulmonary edema, or cerebropathy (Jiang et al., 2016). Treatment of patients with HCPS should also be performed in the ICU with continuous cardiac monitoring and respiratory support. The palliative treatments for HCPS usually include mechanical ventilation, extracorporeal membrane oxygenation, and hemofiltration (Sargianou et al., 2012).

DISCUSSION

HFRS and HCPS caused by hantavirus infection are reemerging infectious diseases that greatly threaten global public health. At present, there are currently no US FDA-approved treatments or vaccines available; only the whole virus-inactivated vaccine against HTNV or SEOV is available in China and Korea. With the implementation of intervention measures, the incidence of hantavirus infections seems to have shown a decline in recent years. In China and Korea, the number of HFRS cases has been drastically reduced. But the vaccines elicit suboptimal immune responses, confer inadequate protection, and may cause safety concerns. In 2017, the recurrence of global outbreak of HFRS has drawn renewed attention to this old disease, which seriously threatens human health. HFRS in China was still a natural focal disease with relatively high morbidity and fatality, and its distribution and epidemic trends had also changed. Surveillance measures, together with prevention and control strategies, should be improved and strengthened to reduce HFRS infection in China. Therefore, the best solution is to develop a functional vaccine to prevent hantavirus infection. Among the three types of vaccines discussed above, only DNA vaccine candidates have progressed to clinical trials. Subunit protein vaccines not only are safe and easy to produce but also do not easily cause interference between the components of a multivalent formulation (Sun et al., 2017; Liang et al., 2018; Qu et al., 2018). To resolve the above problems, we propose to construct a universal genetic engineering novel subunit protein vaccine against HTNV and SEOV by combining bioinformatics methods, viral surface protein structure biology knowledge, and molecular biology tools.

Antiviral treatment only works when applied during the early infection stage, possibly because uncontrolled immune responses occur and predominate the pathogenesis process post-acute infection. Immunomodulatory therapy hardly improves the patient survival rate, possibly because suppressed inflammatory responses inhibit prompt viral clearance and enhance virus-caused injury increase. Therefore, based on rapid supportive care, effectively combining antiviral treatment and immunomodulatory therapy is a potential strategy for HFRS and HPS. 3G1 and 3D8, the mice MAbs against HTNV developed by our team, have been used for HFRS treatment and the result indicated that application of 3G1 and 3D8 at early stage of disease could significantly improve the patient condition and increase survival rates, especially for those severe or critical HFRS patients (data unpublished). Hence, NAbs might be the most promising treatment for HFRS or HPS, and the effective humanized neutralizing antibodies should be further developed.

Moreover, it is universally acknowledged that type I IFN responses are essential for hosts to defend against hantaviral infection. Multiple IFN stimulated genes (ISG) were confirmed to have antihantaviral activity. The interferon-induced MxA protein, a GTPase with extensive antiviral activity, notably against influenza viruses, was reported to inhibit HTNV and PUUV replication in Vero cells (Frese et al., 1996). The interferon-induced IFITM3 protein was able to inhibit HTNV infection in both HUVEC and A549 cells by inhibiting virus entry (Xu-Yang et al., 2016). Several studies have shown that pretreatment with type I IFN could effectively inhibit hantaviral infection. Pretreating endothelial cells (ECs) with IFNα blocks hantavirus replication, and this inhibitory effect is still observed when IFNα is added to ECs within 12 hpi; however, the addition of IFNα 15–24 h after infection had little effect on hantavirus replication. Clinical data indicated that IFN treatment is only effective prophylactically or shortly after hantavirus infection. In fact, during the natural infection process, compared with non-pathogenic hantaviruses, pathogenic hantaviruses could inhibit host IFN production at an early infection stage, but the specific mechanism remains ambiguous. Our team recently found that HTNV could induce complete autophagy at an early phase, which promotes host MAVS degradation and disturbs RIG-I-MAVS signaling-mediated IFN production. The application of autophagy inhibitors, including 3-MA and CQ, could significantly enhance type I IFN responses and inhibit HTNV replication both *in vitro* and *in vivo*. We also demonstrated that lncRNA NEAT1 could positively regulate RIG-I-DDX60-mediated IFN responses during HTNV infection and that overexpression of NEAT1 could restrain HTNV amplification both *in vitro* and *in vivo*. These results suggest that enhancing host IFN responses during the early infection phase may be a novel therapeutic strategy for HFRS and HCPS, while there is still much work to be done to translate basic medicine research to clinical practice.

AUTHOR CONTRIBUTIONS

RL and HM wrote the manuscript. JS, MH, and ZL provided published evidence. QZ made the phylogenetic tree. XJ, FZ, and XW edited, reviewed, and approved its final version.

FUNDING

This work was supported by grants from the National Science Foundation (Nos. 81772167, 81971563, 81602494, and 81671994) and the Key Research and Development Project of Shaanxi Province (No. 2019ZDLSF02-03).

REFERENCES

Abudurexiti, A., Adkins, S., Alioto, D., Alkhovsky, S. V., Avsic-Zupanc, T., Ballinger, M. J., et al. (2019). Taxonomy of the order Bunyavirales: update 2019. *Arch. Virol.* 164, 1949–1965. doi: 10.1007/s00705-019-04253-6

Alkharsah, K. R. (2018). VEGF upregulation in viral infections and its possible therapeutic implications. *Int. J. Mol. Sci.* 19:E1642. doi: 10.3390/ijms1906 1642

Antonen, J., Leppanen, I., Tenhunen, J., Arvola, P., Makela, S., Vaheri, A., et al. (2013). A severe case of *Puumala hantavirus* infection successfully treated with bradykinin receptor antagonist icatibant. *Scand. J. Infect. Dis.* 45, 494–496. doi: 10.3109/00365548.2012.755268

Antoniukas, L., Grammel, H., and Reichl, U. (2006). Production of hantavirus *Puumala nucleocapsid* protein in *Saccharomyces cerevisiae* for vaccine and diagnostics. *J. Biotechnol.* 124, 347–362. doi: 10.1016/j.jbiotec.2005.12.028

Barriga, G. P., Villalon-Letelier, F., Marquez, C. L., Bignon, E. A., Acuna, R., Ross, B. H., et al. (2016). Inhibition of the hantavirus fusion process by predicted domain III and stem peptides from glycoprotein Gc. *PLoS Negl. Trop. Dis.* 10:e0004799. doi: 10.1371/journal.pntd.0004799

Bayard, V., Kitsutani, P. T., Barria, E. O., Ruedas, L. A., Tinnin, D. S., Muñoz, C., et al. (2004). Outbreak of hantavirus pulmonary syndrome, Los Santos, Panama, 1999-2000. *Emerg. Infect. Dis.* 10, 1635–1642. doi: 10.3201/eid1009. 040143

Bergstedt Oscarsson, K., Brorstad, A., Baudin, M., Lindberg, A., Forssen, A., Evander, M., et al. (2016). Human *Puumala hantavirus* infection in northern Sweden; increased seroprevalence and association to risk and health factors. *BMC Infect. Dis.* 16:566. doi: 10.1186/s12879-016-1879-2

Bird, B. H., Shrivastava-Ranjan, P., Dodd, K. A., Erickson, B. R., and Spiropoulou, C. F. (2016). Effect of Vandetanib on *Andes virus* survival in the hamster model of Hantavirus pulmonary syndrome. *Antiviral Res.* 132, 66–69. doi: 10.1016/j. antiviral.2016.05.014

Brocato, R. L., and Hooper, J. W. (2019). Progress on the prevention and treatment of hantavirus disease. *Viruses* 11:E610. doi: 10.3390/v11070610

Brocato, R., Josleyn, M., Ballantyne, J., Vial, P., and Hooper, J. W. (2012). DNA vaccine-generated duck polyclonal antibodies as a postexposure prophylactic to prevent hantavirus pulmonary syndrome (HPS). *PLoS one* 7:e35996. doi: 10.1371/journal.pone.0035996

Brocato, R. L., Josleyn, M. J., Wahl-Jensen, V., Schmaljohn, C. S., and Hooper, J. W. (2013). Construction and nonclinical testing of a puumala virus synthetic M gene-based DNA vaccine.*Clin. Vaccine Immunol.* 20, 218–226. doi: 10.1128/ CVI.00546-12

Bucht, G., Sjolander, K. B., Eriksson, S., Lindgren, L., Lundkvist, A., and Elgh, F. (2001). Modifying the cellular transport of DNA-based vaccines alters the immune response to hantavirus nucleocapsid protein. *Vaccine* 19, 3820–3829. doi: 10.1016/s0264-410x(01)00151-7

Cheng, L. F., Wang, F., Zhang, L., Yu, L., Ye, W., Liu, Z. Y., et al. (2016). Incorporation of GM-CSF or CD40L enhances the immunogenicity of *Hantaan virus*-like particles. *Front. Cell Infect. Microbiol.* 6:185. doi: 10.3389/fcimb.2016. 00185

Chiang, C. F., Albarino, C. G., Lo, M. K., and Spiropoulou, C. F. (2014). Small interfering RNA inhibition of *Andes virus* replication. *PLoS One* 9:e99764. doi: 10.1371/journal.pone.0099764

Cho, H. W., Howard, C. R., and Lee, H. W. (2002). Review of an inactivated vaccine against hantaviruses. *Intervirology* 45, 328–333. doi: 10.1159/000067925

Chung, D. H., Kumarapperuma, S. C., Sun, Y., Li, Q., Chu, Y. K., Arterburn, J. B., et al. (2008). Synthesis of 1-beta-D-ribofuranosyl-3-ethynyl-[1,2,4]triazole and its *in vitro* and *in vivo* efficacy against hantavirus. *Antiviral Res.* 79, 19–27. doi: 10.1016/j.antiviral.2008.02.003

Chung, D. H., Vastermark, A., Camp, J. V., Mcallister, R., Remold, S. K., Chu, Y. K., et al. (2013). The murine model for *Hantaan virus*-induced lethal disease shows two distinct paths in viral evolutionary trajectory with and without ribavirin treatment. *J. Virol.* 87, 10997–11007. doi: 10.1128/JVI.01394-13

Cifuentes-Munoz, N., Barriga, G. P., Valenzuela, P. D., and Tischler, N. D. (2011). Aromatic and polar residues spanning the candidate fusion peptide of the *Andes virus* Gc protein are essential for membrane fusion and infection. *J. Gen. Virol.* 92, 552–563. doi: 10.1099/vir.0.027235-0

Custer, D. M., Thompson, E., Schmaljohn, C. S., Ksiazek, T. G., and Hooper, J. W. (2003). Active and passive vaccination against hantavirus pulmonary syndrome with *Andes virus* M genome segment-based DNA vaccine. *J. Virol.* 77, 9894–9905. doi: 10.1128/jvi.77.18.9894-9905.2003

de Carvalho Nicacio, C., Gonzalez Della Valle, M., Padula, P., Björling, E., Plyusnin, A., and Lundkvist, Å (2002). Cross-protection against challenge with *Puumala virus* after immunization with nucleocapsid proteins from different hantaviruses. *J. Virol.* 76, 6669–6677. doi: 10.1128/jvi.76.13.6669-6677.2002

de Carvalho Nicacio, C., Lundkvist, A., Sjolander, K. B., Plyusnin, A., Salonen, E. M., and Bjorling, E. (2000). A neutralizing recombinant human antibody Fab fragment against *Puumala hantavirus*. *J. Med. Virol.* 60, 446–454. doi: 10.1002/(sici)1096-9071(200004)60:4<446::aid-jmv13>3.0.co;2-v

Deng, H. Y., Luo, F., Shi, L. Q., Zhong, Q., Liu, Y. J., and Yang, Z. Q. (2009). Efficacy of arbidol on lethal *hantaan virus* infections in suckling mice and *in vitro*. *Acta Pharmacol. Sin.* 30, 1015–1024. doi: 10.1038/aps.2009.53

Dong, Y., Ma, T., Zhang, X., Ying, Q., Han, M., Zhang, M., et al. (2019). Incorporation of CD40 ligand or granulocyte-macrophage colony stimulating factor into *Hantaan virus* (HTNV) virus-like particles significantly enhances the long-term immunity potency against HTNV infection. *J. Med. Microbiol.* 68, 480–492. doi: 10.1099/jmm.0.000897

Duggan, J. M. (2019). Prevalence of *Seoul hantavirus* in UK wild rats: an emerging public health problem? *Vet. Rec.* 184, 523–524. doi: 10.1136/vr.l1163

Echterdiek, F., Kitterer, D., Alscher, M. D., Schwenger, V., Ruckenbrod, B., Bald, M., et al. (2019). Clinical course of hantavirus-induced nephropathia epidemica in children compared to adults in Germany—analysis of 317 patients. *Pediatr. Nephrol.* 34, 1247–1252. doi: 10.1007/s00467-019-04215-9

Ettinger, J., Hofmann, J., Enders, M., Tewald, F., Oehme, R. M., Rosenfeld, U. M., et al. (2012). Multiple synchronous outbreaks of *Puumala virus*, Germany, 2010. *Emerg. Infect. Dis.* 18, 1461–1464. doi: 10.3201/eid1809.111447

Frese, M., Kochs, G., Feldmann, H., Hertkorn, C., and Haller, O. (1996). Inhibition of bunyaviruses, phleboviruses, and hantaviruses by human MxA protein. *J. Virol.* 70, 915–923. doi: 10.1128/jvi.70.2.915-923.1996

Garrido, J. L., Prescott, J., Calvo, M., Bravo, F., Alvarez, R., Salas, A., et al. (2018). Two recombinant human monoclonal antibodies that protect against lethal *Andes hantavirus* infection *in vivo*. *Sci. Transl. Med.* 10:eaat6420. doi: 10.1126/scitranslmed.aat6420

Gavrilovskaya, I. N., Gorbunova, E. E., and Mackow, E. R. (2012). *Andes virus* infection of lymphatic endothelial cells causes giant cell and enhanced permeability responses that are rapamycin and vascular endothelial growth factor C sensitive. *J. Virol.* 86, 8765–8772. doi: 10.1128/JVI.00817-12

Gavrilovskaya, I. N., Gorbunova, E. E., Mackow, N. A., and Mackow, E. R. (2008). Hantaviruses direct endothelial cell permeability by sensitizing cells to the vascular permeability factor VEGF, while angiopoietin 1 and sphingosine 1-phosphate inhibit hantavirus-directed permeability. *J. Virol.* 82, 5797–5806. doi: 10.1128/JVI.02397-07

Geldmacher, A., Schmaler, M., Kruger, D. H., and Ulrich, R. (2004). Yeast-expressed hantavirus Dobrava nucleocapsid protein induces a strong, long-lasting, and highly cross-reactive immune response in mice. *Viral. Immunol.* 17, 115–122. doi: 10.1089/088282404322875511

Gorbunova, E. E., Gavrilovskaya, I. N., Pepini, T., and Mackow, E. R. (2011). VEGFR2 and Src kinase inhibitors suppress *Andes virus*-induced endothelial cell permeability. *J. Virol.* 85, 2296–2303. doi: 10.1128/JVI.02319-10

Gowen, B. B., Wong, M. H., Jung, K. H., Sanders, A. B., Mendenhall, M., Bailey, K. W., et al. (2007). In vitro and in vivo activities of T-705 against arenavirus and bunyavirus infections. *Antimicrob. Agents Chemother.* 51, 3168–3176. doi: 10.1128/aac.00356-07

Graham, B. S., Gilman, M. S. A., and Mclellan, J. S. (2019). Structure-based vaccine antigen design. *Annu. Rev. Med.* 70, 91–104. doi: 10.1146/annurev-med-121217-094234

Gut, A. K., Gut, R., Rymarz, A., and Wozniak-Kosek, A. (2018). Hemorrhagic fever with renal syndrome (HFRS) in Poland. *Przegl. Epidemiol.* 72, 477–485. doi: 10.32394/pe.72.4.23

Haese, N., Brocato, R. L., Henderson, T., Nilles, M. L., Kwilas, S. A., Josleyn, M. D., et al. (2015). Antiviral biologic produced in DNA vaccine/goose platform protects hamsters against hantavirus pulmonary syndrome when administered post-exposure. *PLoS Negl. Trop. Dis.* 9:e0003803. doi: 10.1371/journal.pntd.0003803

Hall, P. R., Hjelle, B., Brown, D. C., Ye, C., Bondu-Hawkins, V., Kilpatrick, K. A., et al. (2008). Multivalent presentation of antihantavirus peptides on nanoparticles enhances infection blockade. *Antimicrob. Agents Chemother.* 52, 2079–2088. doi: 10.1128/AAC.01415-07

Hall, P. R., Leitao, A., Ye, C., Kilpatrick, K., Hjelle, B., Oprea, T. I., et al. (2010). Small molecule inhibitors of hantavirus infection. *Bioorg. Med. Chem. Lett.* 20, 7085–7091. doi: 10.1016/j.bmcl.2010.09.092

Hammerbeck, C. D., Brocato, R. L., Bell, T. M., Schellhase, C. W., Mraz, S. R., Queen, L. A., et al. (2016). Depletion of alveolar macrophages does not prevent hantavirus disease pathogenesis in golden syrian hamsters. *J. Virol.* 90, 6200–6215. doi: 10.1128/jvi.00304-16

Hooper, J. W., Custer, D. M., Smith, J., and Wahl-Jensen, V. (2006). Hantaan/*Andes virus* DNA vaccine elicits a broadly cross-reactive neutralizing antibody response in nonhuman primates. *Virology* 347, 208–216. doi: 10.1016/j.virol.2005.11.035

Hooper, J. W., Custer, D. M., Thompson, E., and Schmaljohn, C. S. (2001). DNA vaccination with the *Hantaan virus* M gene protects Hamsters against three of four HFRS hantaviruses and elicits a high-titer neutralizing antibody response in Rhesus monkeys. *J. Virol.* 75, 8469–8477. doi: 10.1128/jvi.75.18.8469-8477.2001

Hooper, J. W., Ferro, A. M., and Wahl-Jensen, V. (2008). Immune serum produced by DNA vaccination protects hamsters against lethal respiratory challenge with *Andes virus*. *J. Virol.* 82, 1332–1338. doi: 10.1128/jvi.01822-07

Hooper, J. W., Josleyn, M., Ballantyne, J., and Brocato, R. (2013). A novel Sin Nombre virus DNA vaccine and its inclusion in a candidate pan-hantavirus vaccine against hantavirus pulmonary syndrome (HPS) and hemorrhagic fever with renal syndrome (HFRS). *Vaccine* 31, 4314–4321. doi: 10.1016/j.vaccine.2013.07.025

Hooper, J. W., Kamrud, K. I., Elgh, F., Custer, D., and Schmaljohn, C. S. (1999). DNA vaccination with hantavirus M segment elicits neutralizing antibodies and protects against *Seoul virus* infection. *Virology* 255, 269–278. doi: 10.1006/viro.1998.9586

Hooper, J. W., Moon, J. E., Paolino, K. M., Newcomer, R., Mclain, D. E., Josleyn, M., et al. (2014). A Phase 1 clinical trial of *Hantaan virus* and *Puumala virus* M-segment DNA vaccines for haemorrhagic fever with renal syndrome delivered by intramuscular electroporation. *Clin. Microbiol. Infect.* 20(Suppl. 5), 110–117. doi: 10.1111/1469-0691.12553

Huggins, J. W., Hsiang, C. M., Cosgriff, T. M., Guang, M. Y., Smith, J. I., Wu, Z. O., et al. (1991). Prospective, double-blind, concurrent, placebo-controlled clinical trial of intravenous ribavirin therapy of hemorrhagic fever with renal syndrome. *J. Infect. Dis.* 164, 1119–1127. doi: 10.1093/infdis/164.6.1119

Huggins, J. W., Kim, G. R., Brand, O. M., and Mckee, K. T. Jr. (1986). Ribavirin therapy for *Hantaan virus* infection in suckling mice. *J. Infect. Dis.* 153, 489–497. doi: 10.1093/infdis/153.3.489

Jiang, H., Du, H., Wang, L. M., Wang, P. Z., and Bai, X. F. (2016). Hemorrhagic fever with renal syndrome: pathogenesis and clinical picture. *Front. Cell Infect. Microbiol.* 6:1. doi: 10.3389/fcimb.2016.00001

Jiang, D., Sun, Y., Cheng, L., Zhang, G., Dong, C., and Jin, B. (2015). Construction and evaluation of DNA vaccine encoding Hantavirus glycoprotein N-terminal fused with lysosome-associated membrane protein. *Vaccine* 33, 3367–3376.doi: 10.1016/j.vaccine.2015.05.007

Jiang, F., Wang, L., Wang, S., Zhu, L., Dong, L., Zhang, Z., et al. (2017). Meteorological factors affect the epidemiology of hemorrhagic fever with renal syndrome via altering the breeding and hantavirus-carrying states of rodents and mites: a 9 years' longitudinal study. *Emerg. Microbes Infect.* 6:e104. doi: 10.1038/emi.2017.92

Johansson, P., Olsson, M., Lindgren, L., Ahlm, C., Elgh, F., Holmstrom, A., et al. (2004). Complete gene sequence of a human *Puumala hantavirus* isolate, *Puumala Umea*/hu: sequence comparison and characterisation of encoded gene products. *Virus Res.* 105, 147–155. doi: 10.1016/j.virusres.2004.05.005

Jung, J., Ko, S. J., Oh, H. S., Moon, S. M., Song, J. W., and Huh, K. (2018). Protective effectiveness of inactivated hantavirus vaccine against hemorrhagic fever with renal syndrome. *J. Infect. Dis.* 217, 1417–1420. doi: 10.1093/infdis/jiy037

Kerins, J. L., Koske, S. E., Kazmierczak, J., Austin, C., Gowdy, K., and Dibernardo, A. (2018). Outbreak of *Seoul virus* among rats and rat owners — United States and Canada, 2017. *Can. Commun. Dis. Rep.* 44, 71–74. doi: 10.14745/ccdr.v44i02a07

Kobayashi, T., Nakatsuka, K., Shimizu, M., Tamura, H., Shinya, E., Atsukawa, M., et al. (2012). Ribavirin modulates the conversion of human CD4(+) CD25(−) T cell to CD4(+) CD25(+) FOXP3(+) T cell via suppressing interleukin-10-producing regulatory T cell. *Immunology* 137, 259–270. doi: 10.1111/imm.12005

Kruger, D. H., Ulrich, R. G., and Hofmann, J. (2013). Hantaviruses as zoonotic pathogens in Germany. *Dtsch. Arztebl. Int.* 110, 461–467. doi: 10.3238/arztebl.2013.0461

Kwilas, S., Kishimori, J. M., Josleyn, M., Jerke, K., Ballantyne, J., Royals, M., et al. (2014). A hantavirus pulmonary syndrome (HPS) DNA vaccine delivered using a spring-powered jet injector elicits a potent neutralizing antibody response in rabbits and nonhuman primates. *Curr. Gene Ther.* 14, 200–210. doi: 10.2174/1566523214666140522122633

Laine, O., Leppanen, I., Koskela, S., Antonen, J., Makela, S., Sinisalo, M., et al. (2015). Severe *Puumala virus* infection in a patient with a lymphoproliferative disease treated with icatibant. *Infect. Dis.* 47, 107–111. doi: 10.3109/00365548.2014.969304

Li, S., Rissanen, I., Zeltina, A., Hepojoki, J., Raghwani, J., Harlos, K., et al. (2016). A molecular-level account of the antigenic hantaviral surface. *Cell Rep.* 15, 959–967. doi: 10.1016/j.celrep.2016.03.082

Li, Z., Zeng, H., Wang, Y., Zhang, Y., Cheng, L., Zhang, F., et al. (2017). The assessment of *Hantaan virus*-specific antibody responses after the immunization program for hemorrhagic fever with renal syndrome in northwest China. *Hum. Vaccin. Immunother.* 13, 802–807. doi: 10.1080/21645515.2016.1253645

Liang, H., Yang, R., Liu, Z., Li, M., Liu, H., and Jin, X. (2018). Recombinant *Zika virus* envelope protein elicited protective immunity against *Zika virus* in immunocompetent mice. *PLoS One* 13:e0194860. doi: 10.1371/journal.pone.0194860

Limongi, J. E., Da Costa, F. C., Pinto, R. M., De Oliveira, R. C., Bragagnolo, C., Lemos, E. R., et al. (2009). Cross-sectional survey of hantavirus infection, Brazil. *Emerg. Infect. Dis.* 15, 1981–1983. doi: 10.3201/eid1512.090229

Mackow, E. R., Dalrymple, N. A., Cimica, V., Matthys, V., Gorbunova, E., and Gavrilovskaya, I. (2014). Hantavirus interferon regulation and virulence determinants. *Virus Res.* 187, 65–71. doi: 10.1016/j.virusres.2013.12.041

Maes, P., Clement, J., Cauwe, B., Bonnet, V., Keyaerts, E., Robert, A., et al. (2008). Truncated recombinant puumala virus nucleocapsid proteins protect mice against challenge *in vivo*. *Viral Immunol.* 21, 49–60. doi: 10.1089/vim.2007.0059

Malinin, O. V., and Platonov, A. E. (2017). Insufficient efficacy and safety of intravenous ribavirin in treatment of haemorrhagic fever with renal syndrome caused by *Puumala virus*. *Infect. Dis.* 49, 514–520. doi: 10.1080/23744235.2017.1293841

Manigold, T., and Vial, P. (2014). Human hantavirus infections: epidemiology, clinical features, pathogenesis and immunology. *Swiss Med. Wkly.* 144:w13937.

Mertz, G. J., Miedzinski, L., Goade, D., Pavia, A. T., Hjelle, B., Hansbarger, C. O., et al. (2004). Placebo-controlled, double-blind trial of intravenous ribavirin for the treatment of hantavirus cardiopulmonary syndrome in North America. *Clin. Infect. Dis.* 39, 1307–1313. doi: 10.1086/425007

Murphy, M. E., Kariwa, H., Mizutani, T., Tanabe, H., Yoshimatsu, K., Arikawa, J., et al. (2001). Characterization of in vitro and in vivo antiviral activity of lactoferrin and ribavirin upon hantavirus. *J. Vet. Med. Sci.* 63, 637–645. doi: 10.1292/jvms.63.637

Murphy, M. E., Kariwa, H., Mizutani, T., Yoshimatsu, K., Arikawa, J., and Takashima, I. (2000). In vitro antiviral activity of lactoferrin and ribavirin upon hantavirus. *Arch. Virol.* 145, 1571–1582. doi: 10.1007/s007050070077

Ogg, M., Jonsson, C. B., Camp, J. V., and Hooper, J. W. (2013). Ribavirin protects Syrian hamsters against lethal hantavirus pulmonary syndrome–after intranasal exposure to *Andes virus*. *Viruses* 5, 2704–2720. doi: 10.3390/v5112704

Padula, P., Martinez, V. P., Bellomo, C., Maidana, S., San Juan, J., Tagliaferri, P., et al. (2007). Pathogenic hantaviruses, northeastern Argentina and eastern Paraguay. *Emerg. Infect. Dis.* 13, 1211–1214. doi: 10.3201/eid1308.061090

Pal, E., Korva, M., Resman Rus, K., Kejzar, N., Bogovic, P., Strle, F., et al. (2018). Relationship between circulating vascular endothelial growth factor and its soluble receptor in patients with hemorrhagic fever with renal syndrome. *Emerg. Microbes Infect.* 7:89. doi: 10.1038/s41426-018-0090-5

Pini, N., Levis, S., Calderón, G., Ramirez, J., Bravo, D., Lozano, E., et al. (2003). Hantavirus infection in humans and rodents, Northwestern Argentina. *Emerg. Infect. Dis.* 9, 1070–1076. doi: 10.3201/eid0909.020768

Prince, H. E., and Lieberman, J. M. (2013). Impact of the Yosemite hantavirus outbreak on hantavirus antibody testing at a national reference laboratory. *Clin. Vaccine Immunol.* 20, 1213–1216. doi: 10.1128/CVI.00326-13

Qian, D. Y., Ding, Y. S., Chen, G. F., Ding, J. J., Chen, Y. X., Lu, T. F., et al. (1990). A placebo-controlled clinical trial of prednisone in the treatment of early hemorrhagic fever. *J. Infect. Dis.* 162, 1213–1214. doi: 10.1093/infdis/162.5.1213

Qu, P., Zhang, W., Li, D., Zhang, C., Liu, Q., Zhang, X., et al. (2018). Insect cell-produced recombinant protein subunit vaccines protect against *Zika virus* infection. *Antivir. Res.* 154, 97–103. doi: 10.1016/j.antiviral.2018.04.010

Razanskiene, A., Schmidt, J., Geldmacher, A., Ritzi, A., Niedrig, M., Lundkvist, Å, et al. (2004). High yields of stable and highly pure nucleocapsid proteins of different hantaviruses can be generated in the yeast *Saccharomyces cerevisiae*. *J. Biotechnol.* 111, 319–333. doi: 10.1016/j.jbiotec.2004.04.010

Rissanen, I., Stass, R., Zeltina, A., Li, S., Hepojoki, J., Harlos, K., et al. (2017). Structural transitions of the conserved and metastable hantaviral glycoprotein envelope. *J. Virol.* 91:e378-17. doi: 10.1128/JVI.00378-17

Safronetz, D., Falzarano, D., Scott, D. P., Furuta, Y., Feldmann, H., and Gowen, B. B. (2013). Antiviral efficacy of favipiravir against two prominent etiological agents of hantavirus pulmonary syndrome. *Antimicrob. Agents Chemother.* 57, 4673–4680. doi: 10.1128/AAC.00886-13

Safronetz, D., Haddock, E., Feldmann, F., Ebihara, H., and Feldmann, H. (2011). In vitro and in vivo activity of ribavirin against *Andes virus* infection. *PLoS One* 6:e23560. doi: 10.1371/journal.pone.0023560

Salim, N. N., Ganaie, S. S., Roy, A., Jeeva, S., and Mir, M. A. (2016). Targeting a novel RNA-protein interaction for therapeutic intervention of Hantavirus disease. *J. Biol. Chem.* 291, 24702–24714. doi: 10.1074/jbc.m116.750729

Sargianou, M., Watson, D. C., Chra, P., Papa, A., Starakis, I., Gogos, C., et al. (2012). Hantavirus infections for the clinician: from case presentation to diagnosis and treatment. *Crit. Rev. Microbiol.* 38, 317–329. doi: 10.3109/1040841X.2012.673553

Sayer, W. J., Entwhisle, G., Uyeno, B., and Bignall, R. C. (1955). Cortisone therapy of early epidemic hemorrhagic fever: a preliminary report. *Ann. Intern. Med.* 42, 839–851.

Schmaljohn, C. S. (2012). Vaccines for hantaviruses: progress and issues. *Expert Rev. Vaccines* 11, 511–513. doi: 10.1586/erv.12.15

Schmaljohn, C. S., Spik, K. W., and Hooper, J. W. (2014). DNA vaccines for HFRS: laboratory and clinical studies. *Virus Res.* 187, 91–96. doi: 10.1016/j.virusres.2013.12.020

Schmidt, J., Jandrig, B., Klempa, B., Yoshimatsu, K., Arikawa, J., Meisel, H., et al. (2005). Nucleocapsid protein of cell culture-adapted *Seoul virus* strain 80-39: analysis of its encoding sequence, expression in yeast and immuno-reactivity. *Virus Genes* 30, 37–48. doi: 10.1007/s11262-004-4580-2

Schonrich, G., and Raftery, M. J. (2017). Exploring the immunopathogenesis of viral hemorrhagic fever in mice with a humanized immune system. *Front. Immunol.* 8:1202. doi: 10.3389/fimmu.2017.01202

Song, J. Y., Woo, H. J., Cheong, H. J., Noh, J. Y., Baek, L. J., and Kim, W. J. (2016). Long-term immunogenicity and safety of inactivated *Hantaan virus* vaccine (Hantavax) in healthy adults. *Vaccine* 34, 1289–1295. doi: 10.1016/j.vaccine.2016.01.031

Spik, K. W., Badger, C., Mathiessen, I., Tjelle, T., Hooper, J. W., and Schmaljohn, C. (2008). Mixing of M segment DNA vaccines to Hantaan virus and Puumala virus reduces their immunogenicity in hamsters. *Vaccine* 26, 5177–5181.doi: 10.1016/j.vaccine.2008.03.097

Stanojevic, M., Cirkovic, V., Siljic, M., Gligic, A., and Stamenkovic, G. (2019). Molecular characterization of Dobrava-Belgrade hantavirus in Serbia, 2007-2011. *J. Infect. Public Health* 12, 645–649. doi: 10.1016/j.jiph.2019.02.021

Sun, J., Li, M., Wang, Y., Hao, P., and Jin, X. (2017). Elaboration of tetravalent antibody responses against dengue viruses using a subunit vaccine comprised of a single consensus dengue envelope sequence. *Vaccine* 35, 6308–6320. doi: 10.1016/j.vaccine.2017.09.063

Suzuki, A., Bisordi, I., Levis, S., Garcia, J., Pereira, L. E., Souza, R. P., et al. (2004). Identifying rodent hantavirus reservoirs, Brazil. *Emerg. Infect. Dis.* 10, 2127–2134. doi: 10.3201/eid1012.040295

Szabo, R. (2017). Antiviral therapy and prevention against hantavirus infections. *Acta Virol.* 61, 3–12. doi: 10.4149/av_2017_01_3

Taylor, S. L., Wahl-Jensen, V., Copeland, A. M., Jahrling, P. B., and Schmaljohn, C. S. (2013). Endothelial cell permeability during hantavirus infection involves factor XII-dependent increased activation of the kallikrein-kinin system. *PLoS Pathog.* 9:e1003470. doi: 10.1371/journal.ppat.1003470

Terajima, M., Van Epps, H. L., Li, D., Leporati, A. M., Juhlin, S. E., Mustonen, J., et al. (2002). Generation of recombinant vaccinia viruses expressing *Puumala virus* proteins and use in isolating cytotoxic T cells specific for *Puumala virus*. *Virus Res.* 84, 67–77. doi: 10.1016/s0168-1702(01)00416-6

Tian, H., and Stenseth, N. C. (2019). The ecological dynamics of hantavirus diseases: from environmental variability to disease prevention largely based on data from China. *PLoS Negl. Trop. Dis.* 13:e0006901. doi: 10.1371/journal.pntd.0006901

Tian, H., Yu, P., Cazelles, B., Xu, L., Tan, H., Yang, J., et al. (2017). Interannual cycles of *Hantaan virus* outbreaks at the human-animal interface in Central China are controlled by temperature and rainfall. *Proc. Natl. Acad. Sci. U.S.A.* 114, 8041–8046. doi: 10.1073/pnas.1701777114

Toro, J., Vega, J. D., Khan, A. S., Mills, J. N., Padula, P., Terry, W., et al. (1998). An outbreak of hantavirus pulmonary syndrome, Chile, 1997. *Emerg. Infect. Dis.* 4, 687–694. doi: 10.3201/eid0404.980425

Vaheri, A., Henttonen, H., Voutilainen, L., Mustonen, J., Sironen, T., and Vapalahti, O. (2013). Hantavirus infections in Europe and their impact on public health. *Rev. Med. Virol.* 23, 35–49. doi: 10.1002/rmv.1722

Vial, P. A., Valdivieso, F., Calvo, M., Rioseco, M. L., Riquelme, R., Araneda, A., et al. (2015). A non-randomized multicentre trial of human immune plasma for treatment of hantavirus cardiopulmonary syndrome caused by *Andes virus*. *Antivir. Ther.* 20, 377–386. doi: 10.3851/IMP2875

Vial, P. A., Valdivieso, F., Ferres, M., Riquelme, R., Rioseco, M. L., Calvo, M., et al. (2013). High-dose intravenous methylprednisolone for hantavirus cardiopulmonary syndrome in Chile: a double-blind, randomized controlled clinical trial. *Clin. Infect. Dis.* 57, 943–951. doi: 10.1093/cid/cit394

Wang, W., Zhang, Y., Li, Y., Pan, L., Bai, L., Zhuang, Y., et al. (2012). Dysregulation of the beta3 integrin-VEGFR2 complex in *Hantaan virus*-directed hyperpermeability upon treatment with VEGF. *Arch. Virol.* 157, 1051–1061. doi: 10.1007/s00705-012-1245-7

Westover, J. B., Sefing, E. J., Bailey, K. W., Van Wettere, A. J., Jung, K. H., Dagley, A., et al. (2016). Low-dose ribavirin potentiates the antiviral activity of favipiravir against hemorrhagic fever viruses. *Antivir. Res.* 126, 62–68. doi: 10.1016/j.antiviral.2015.12.006

Xu, R., Yang, X. Y., Yang, D. F., Zou, C. Y., Gong, P. L., and Zeng, F. D. (2009). Phase I evaluation of the safety and pharmacokinetics of a single-dose intravenous injection of a murine monoclonal antibody against *Hantaan virus* in healthy volunteers. *Antimicrob. Agents Chemother.* 53, 5055–5059. doi: 10.1128/AAC.00728-09

Xu, Z., Wei, L., Wang, L., Wang, H., and Jiang, S. (2002). The *in vitro* and *in vivo* protective activity of monoclonal antibodies directed against *Hantaan virus*: potential application for immunotherapy and passive immunization. *Biochem. Biophys. Res. Commun.* 298, 552–558. doi: 10.1016/s0006-291x(02)02491-9

Xu-Yang, Z., Pei-Yu, B., Chuan-Tao, Y., Wei, Y., Hong-Wei, M., Kang, T., et al. (2016). Interferon-induced transmembrane protein 3 inhibits *Hantaan virus* infection, and its single nucleotide polymorphism rs12252 influences the severity of hemorrhagic fever with renal syndrome. *Front. Immunol.* 7:535. doi: 10.3389/fimmu.2016.00535

Yamanishi, K., Tanishita, O., Tamura, M., Asada, H., Kondo, K., Takagi, M., et al. (1988). Development of inactivated vaccine against virus causing haemorrhagic fever with renal syndrome. *Vaccine* 6, 278–282. doi: 10.1016/0264-410x(88)90224-1

Yang, J., Sun, J. F., Wang, T. T., Guo, X. H., Wei, J. X., Jia, L. T., et al. (2017). Targeted inhibition of hantavirus replication and intracranial pathogenesis by a chimeric protein-delivered siRNA. *Antivir. Res.* 147, 107–115. doi: 10.1016/j.antiviral.2017.10.005

Yi, Y., Park, H., and Jung, J. (2018). Effectiveness of inactivated hantavirus vaccine on the disease severity of hemorrhagic fever with renal syndrome. *Kidney Res. Clin. Pract.* 37, 366–372. doi: 10.23876/j.krcp.18.0044

Ying, Q., Ma, T., Cheng, L., Zhang, X., Truax, A. D., Ma, R., et al. (2016). Construction and immunological characterization of CD40L or GM-CSF incorporated *Hantaan virus* like particle. *Oncotarget* 7, 63488–63503. doi: 10.18632/oncotarget.11329

Yong, C. Y., Ong, H. K., Yeap, S. K., Ho, K. L., and Tan, W. S. (2019). Recent advances in the vaccine development against middle east respiratory syndrome-coronavirus. *Front. Microbiol.* 10:1781. doi: 10.3389/fmicb.2019.01781

Zhang, S., Wang, S., Yin, W., Liang, M., Li, J., Zhang, Q., et al. (2014). Epidemic characteristics of hemorrhagic fever with renal syndrome in China, 2006-2012. *BMC Infect. Dis* 14:384. doi: 10.1186/1471-2334-14-384

Zhang, X. K., Takashima, I., and Hashimoto, N. (1989). Characteristics of passive immunity against hantavirus infection in rats. *Arch. Virol.* 105, 235–246. doi: 10.1007/bf01311360

Zhao, C., Sun, Y., Zhao, Y., Wang, S., Yu, T., Du, F., et al. (2012). Immunogenicity of a multi-epitope DNA vaccine against hantavirus. *Hum. Vaccin. Immunother.* 8, 208–215. doi: 10.4161/hv.18389

Zheng, Y., Zhou, B. Y., Wei, J., Xu, Y., Dong, J. H., Guan, L. Y., et al. (2018). Persistence of immune responses to vaccine against haemorrhagic fever with renal syndrome in healthy adults aged 16-60 years: results from an open-label2-year follow-up study. *Infect. Dis.* 50, 21–26. doi: 10.1080/23744235.2017.1353704

4

The Rationale for a Preventative HCV Virus-Like Particle (VLP) Vaccine

*Joseph Torresi**

Department of Microbiology and Immunology, The Peter Doherty Institute for Infection and Immunity, University of Melbourne, Parkville, VIC, Australia

***Correspondence:**
Joseph Torresi
josepht@unimelb.edu.au

HCV represents a global health problem with ~200 million individuals currently infected, worldwide. With the high cost of antiviral therapies, the global burden of chronic hepatitis C infection (CHCV) infection will be substantially reduced by the development of an effective vaccine for HCV. The field of HCV vaccines is generally divided into proponents of strategies to induce neutralizing antibodies (NAb) and those who propose to elicit cell mediated immunity (CMI). However, for a hepatltis C virus (HCV) vaccine to be effective in preventing infection, it must be capable of generating cross-reactive CD4+, CD8+ T cell, and NAb responses that will cover the major viral genotypes. Simulation models of hepatitis C have predicted that a vaccine of even modest efficacy and coverage will significantly reduce the incidence of hepatitis C. A HCV virus like particle (VLP) based vaccine would fulfill the requirement of delivering critical conformational neutralizing epitopes in addition to providing HCV specific $CD4^+$ and $CD8^+$ epitopes. Several approaches have been reported including insect cell-derived genotype 1b HCV VLPs; a human liver-derived quadrivalent genotype 1a, 1b, 2, and 3a vaccine; a genotype 1a HCV E1 and E2 glycoprotein/MLV Gag pseudotype VLP vaccine; and chimeric HBs-HCV VLP vaccines. All to result in the production of cross-NAb and/or T cell responses against HCV. This paper summarizes the evidence supporting the development of a HCV VLP based vaccine.

Keywords: Hepatitis C, neutralizing antibody, virus like particles, Hepatitis C vaccines

INTRODUCTION

The substantial global health burden posed by hepatitis C infection can only be addressed in part by antiviral therapies, regardless of their success rates. New and reinfection of high risk populations, such as people who inject drugs (PWID) (Sacks-Davis et al., 2013) makes the expectation of controlling hepatitis C infection with antiviral drugs alone unrealistic (Sievert et al., 2014). In Australia, there is an estimated 308,110 persons infected with hepatitis C virus (HCV), with a prevalence of HCV of 1.3%. It is estimated that 80,000 individuals have cleared infection leaving a total number of viraemic cases of 230,000 (prevalence of 1.0%). The problem of hepatitis C in Australia is also compounded by the fact there are an estimated 50,000 individuals who are unaware that they are infected. This means that there is a large residual pool of chronically infected individuals who will contribute to the ongoing transmission of HCV (Sievert et al., 2014). A similar picture exists in the US where there are ~3.9 million infected individuals and an estimated 50% unaware of their diagnosis. The prevalence of HCV in the US is 1.67% (Rosenberg et al., 2017). China, also has a large burden of HCV with an estimated 25–50 million infected individuals and a prevalence of 1.8–3.7% of the populations, accounting for 15–30% of all HCV infected individuals globally (Sievert et al., 2011; Peng et al., 2015; Wu et al., 2017; Zhang et al., 2017).

Limited access to treatment has also hampered the control of HCV. Several modeling studies have shown that for antiviral therapies alone to control HCV the uptake of treatment will need to increase substantially (Hellard et al., 2012; Martin et al., 2013; Sievert et al., 2014). A recent Australian study examined three treatment scenarios based on the availability of directly acting antiviral agents (Sievert et al., 2014). The outcomes of this study could be extrapolated to similar populations in the US and Europe. In the first scenario the effect of more efficacious treatments alone on HCV burden was assessed. This resulted in a fall in the predicted number of chronically infected individuals by 12,300 over the first 18 years of the introduction of these treatments. HCV-related mortality, the prevalence of compensated and decompensated cirrhosis and hepatocellular carcinoma (HCC) were reduced by 4%, respectively. In a second scenario, the impact of both highly effective therapies together with an expanded uptake of these treatments was assessed. This approach was predicted to be far more effective, resulting in a 60% reduction in the predicted number of chronically infected individuals. This was associated with a 43% reduction in mortality associated with HCV and a 52% reduction in both compensated and decompensated cirrhosis. The number of cases of HCC was also predicted to be 45% lower. These reductions were associated with a 24% reduction in the overall cumulative cost of treating CHCV. The last scenario examined the predicted impact of implementing highly effective therapies only in individuals with advanced fibrosis in the first 3 years followed by broadening access to these treatments to all individuals with CHCV. Of the three treatment scenarios this proved to be the most effective, with a 56% reduction in the predicted number of individuals with CHCV. This was associated with a 52% reduction in the mortality associated with CHCV, a 56 and 54% fall in the number of cases of compensated and decompensated cirrhosis, respectively, and halving of the number of cases of HCC. However, these reductions were only associated with a 26% reduction in the cumulative costs of managing CHCV (Sievert et al., 2014).

In another study, the impact of scaling up antiviral treatment was estimated in three cities with increasing HCV prevalence rates in populations of people who inject drugs (PWID), Edinburgh (baseline prevalence 25%), Melbourne (baseline prevalence 50%), and Vancouver (baseline prevalence 65%). Increasing treatment rates from around 5/1,000 PWID annually to 80/1,000 PWID annually over a 15-year period resulted in an estimated 90% reduction in HCV prevalence in Edinburgh and Melbourne but only an approximate 55% reduction in Vancouver (Martin et al., 2013). These findings suggest that especially in a high prevalence population, even a 20-fold increase in treatment rates would be insufficient to eliminate HCV.

Reinfection after treatment also remains a problem in a proportion of individuals. Some studies examining HCV reinfection in PWID who have cleared infection with antiviral therapy have suggested that the rates of reinfection are low. However, the follow-up period in these reports was relatively short and possibly insufficient to determine the true rate of reinfection (Grebely et al., 2010; Grady et al., 2012). In contrast studies that have examined a longer-term follow period up have reported high rates of reinfection, with one study from Australia reporting a high prevalence of late recurrence of viremia and reinfection of 17% (Bate et al., 2010). A study from Norway also examined reinfection after a sustained virological response (SVR) to antiviral therapy and followed patients for over 8 years (Midgard et al., 2016). Of individuals who had a history of injecting drug use 11% became reinfected with HCV. In contrast, in those who returned to injecting drug use 27% became reinfected with HCV. Interestingly the majority of reinfections occurred 5–8 years after having achieved a SVR with antiviral therapy (Midgard et al., 2016). These studies highlight that reinfection with HCV is not an infrequent occurrence, even after successful antiviral therapy.

MODELING THE IMPACT OF HCV VACCINES

Limitations in access to antiviral therapies for HCV for all chronically infected individuals and the limited ability to significantly scale up access to treatment globally along with significant reinfection rates after clearance of HCV will negatively impact on our ability to eliminate hepatitis C infection and disease. An effective vaccine would be a substantial benefit to the overall aim of eradicating HCV globally. By utilizing mathematical models of HCV infection in high risk populations, it has also been possible to demonstrate that the introduction of a preventative HCV vaccine would have a substantial benefit in reducing the incidence of CHCV (Hahn et al., 2009; Scott et al., 2015).

One such study from San Francisco examined three vaccination strategies (Sacks-Davis et al., 2013); no targeting and selecting PWID for vaccination at random; risk targeting which prioritized high-risk PWID; and sero-targeting, which prioritized HCV antibody negative individuals to receive vaccine (Hahn et al., 2009). The investigators also modeled predicted vaccine efficacies of 50, 65, and 80% and vaccination coverage rates of 0.2, 0.6, and 1% PWID per month. In an approach targeting high-risk individuals or by sero-targeting, the incidence of CHCV was predicted to fall 13.5–4.3, 3.2, and 2.3% per person years at 5, 10, and 30 years after the introduction of a vaccine with 80% efficacy and with a high vaccination rate of 15% per month. The predicted reduction in HCV incidence was only marginally lower if the vaccination coverage fell to 0.6% per month, resulting in a fall in the incidence of CHCV to 2.9% after 30 years. Finally, even a vaccine with 50% efficacy and a moderate to high coverage rate targeted to high-risk PWID was predicted to dramatically reduce the incidence of HCV at 30 years (Hahn et al., 2009).

A more recent UK study also showed that a halving chronic HCV prevalence was possible over a period of 40 years by achieving annual vaccination rates of 162 (72%), 77 (56%), and 44 (38%) per 1,000 PWID for low (50% protection for 5 years), moderate (70% protection for 10 years), and high (90% protection for 20 years) vaccine efficacies. The model predicted that HCV prevalence could be halved over 20 years and this required a doubling in vaccination rates, but only for vaccines of moderate and high efficacy (Stone et al., 2016).

Finally, a subsequent simulation study has shown that vaccination after successful treatment with DAAs is also be as effective at reducing HCV prevalence as vaccinating an equivalent number of people who inject drugs (PWID) in the community (Scott et al., 2015). In this study, a vaccine of 60–90% efficacy was predicted to be beneficial in reducing HCV prevalence especially in populations of PWID with high (50%) to very high (75%) initial chronic HCV prevalence (Scott et al., 2015).

THE IMPORTANCE OF NEUTRALIZING ANTIBODY RESPONSES IN PROTECTION AND VIRAL CLEARANCE

The clearance of hepatitis C infection requires strong and broad cross-reactive T cell and neutralizing antibody (NAb) responses.

Although the proportion of individuals is lower and the time to clearance of HCV after reinfection is twice as likely compared to individuals with primary infection (Sacks-Davis et al., 2013) this does not necessarily result in complete protection against reinfection, suggesting that sterilizing immunity against HCV may not occur frequently (Aitken et al., 2008; Osburn et al., 2010; Grebely et al., 2012; Sacks-Davis et al., 2013). However, these findings indicate that the development of a vaccine that is able to produce protective immunity to prevent persistent infection is possible. The development of early and multi-specific class 1 CD8+ and class II CD4+ T cell and NAb responses during acute HCV infection are associated with the spontaneous clearance of infection (Schulze Zur Wiesch et al., 2012). T cell responses to HCV have been reviewed comprehensively elsewhere (Park and Rehermann, 2014; Holz and Rehermann, 2015). However, the clearance of HCV may require substantially more than strong T cell responses alone (Puig et al., 2006). There is strong evidence that cross-NAb responses to epitopes in the E2 glycoproteins are associated with HCV clearance of existing infection and protection against new HCV infection in animal models.

In humans, the early induction of NAb has been associated with control of viraemia and resolution of infection (Pestka et al., 2007). Similarly, immunoglobulin prepared from the serum of anti-HCV positive humans (Yu et al., 2004) protects chimpanzees against viral challenge. In this study, immune globulin samples prepared from the anti-HCV positive donor plasma were first tested for HCV neutralizing activity using an *in vitro* infectious HCV pseudoparticle assay. The IgG showing neutralizing activity in this assay were then mixed with a standardized HCV inoculum prepared from the acute phase plasma of a patient with hepatitis C infection before been administered to chimpanzees. Control chimpanzees were administered the same inoculum mixed with HCV Ab negative IgG. Weekly serum samples were collected from the chimpanzees and tested for the presence of HCV viremia using RT-PCR. The chimpanzees administered with the mixture of HCV neutralizing IgG and inoculum were protected against HCV infection while the control chimpanzees became infected (Yu et al., 2004).

The early appearance of broad NAb is also an important determinant of clearance of HCV and it is the breadth and not just the presence of heterologous NAb alone that has been associated with protection against persistent infection with HCV (Osburn et al., 2014).

Early studies in chimpanzees has provided valuable insight into the importance of NAb to HCV. These studies demonstrated that NAb develops against the hypervariable region 1 (HVR1) of the E2 glycoprotein and that neutralization of HCV with anti-HVR1 antibodies prevents HCV infection in chimpanzees (Farci et al., 1994, 1996). In addition, vaccination of chimpanzees with mammalian cell expressed recombinant E1 and E2 glycoproteins resulted in protection against challenge with HCV (Choo et al., 1994; Rosa et al., 1996). The recombinant E1 and E2 proteins were produced in HeLa or CHO cells and purified by affinity chromatography and ultrafiltration. Chimpanzees were injected recombinant HCV antigens and received several immunizations over a 7–9-month period followed by challenge with HCV-1 isolated from a chronically infected chimpanzee. None of the immunized chimpanzees became viremic following challenge in contrast to the control animals, all of which became infected (Choo et al., 1994). In a subsequent study the ability of antibodies from the immunized chimpanzees to neutralize the binding of recombinant E2 to MOLT-4 cells was assessed (Rosa et al., 1996). In this report, the neutralization of binding of HCV E2 protein to MOLT-4 cells was found to correlate with protection against challenge with HCV-1.

Neutralization of HCV with rabbit hyperimmune serum to a homologous HVR1 sequence prior to injection into chimpanzees has also been demonstrated (Farci et al., 1994). Following on from these studies it was shown that immunoglobulin prepared from the serum of anti-HCV positive humans protected chimpanzees against viral challenge (Yu et al., 2004). In addition, cross-NAb to epitopes in the E1 and E2 glycoproteins of HCV have also been shown to be protective (Owsianka et al., 2008; Broering et al., 2009; Dowd et al., 2009; Raghuraman et al., 2012).

The limited number of suitable animal models has hampered ongoing studies into the nature of protective NAb responses to HCV. However, the development of humanized uPa-SCID liver chimeric mice has enabled significant progress to be made (Meuleman et al., 2008). Using this model it has been possible to demonstrate that human IgG from HCV-infected individuals and human anti-E2 monoclonal antibodies protect uPA-SCID liver chimeric mice against homologous and heterologous HCV challenge (Law et al., 2008; Vanwolleghem et al., 2008; Meuleman et al., 2011). Furthermore, broad NAb are able to cure uPA-SCID liver chimeric mice of HCV infection (de Jong et al., 2014). In a separate model, anti-E2 sero-positive immunocompetent humanized mice were protected against homologous HCV challenge with a recombinant vaccinia-HCV virus encoding the structural proteins of HCV (Dorner et al., 2011). Furthermore, broad neutralizing human monoclonal antibodies that interfere with the binding of HCV E2 to CD81 on the surface of hepatocytes and a second subset of broad NAbs recognizing native E1E2 heterodimers protect liver chimeric mice against heterologous HCV challenge (Giang et al., 2012). These studies all reinforce the important role of NAb in protection against hepatitis C infection (Owsianka et al., 2008; Broering et al., 2009; Dowd et al., 2009; Raghuraman et al., 2012). Although, studies in liver chimeric mice have provided valuable information regarding NAb to HCV they are immunocompromised and therefore limited by the inability to directly assess the immunogenicity of HCV vaccines.

HCV NAB VACCINE APPROACHES

A number of approaches have been developed to induce the production of broad protective NAb responses. It has been possible to prevent persistent infection with both homologous and heterologous HCV challenge in chimpanzees following vaccination with recombinant E1 and E2 glycoproteins produced in mammalian cells. Recombinant HCV E1E2 adjuvanted with MF59C is also safe and immunogenic in humans resulting in the production of NAb and $CD4^{+}$ T cell responses (Frey et al., 2010). Furthermore, immunization of human volunteers with recombinant gpE1/E2 (HCV genotype 1a) resulted in the production of broad cross-NAb responses (Law et al., 2013). Finally, IgG isolated from mice immunized with inactivated cell culture derived HCV has been shown to neutralize HCV pseudo-particles and protect liver chimeric mice against homologous HCV challenge (Akazawa et al., 2013).

Although, a vaccine derived from a single genotype can elicit NAb, the inclusion of antigens of a number of different genotypes is expected to produce a broader cross-NAb response and thereby be more effective than a single antigen. Broad NAbs act by recognizing native E1E2 heterodimers (Giang et al., 2012) and by blocking the interaction of the virus with critical co-receptors like CD81, scavenger receptor class B type 1 (SR-B1) and Claudin-1 (Scarselli et al., 2002; Koutsoudakis et al., 2007; Zeisel et al., 2007; Meuleman et al., 2008; Douam et al., 2014). For a vaccine to be able to produce effective NAb responses it is therefore likely that such a vaccine will need to express native E1E2 structures. The significance of these regions on the viral envelope is further highlighted by the ability of polyclonal and monoclonal antibodies directed to these regions to protect human liver chimeric mice against HCV challenge (Meuleman et al., 2011). These findings are highly significant for HCV vaccine design because they reinforce the need to present both E1 and E2 proteins in the correct structural organization in a vaccine.

HEPATITIS C VIRUS-LIKE PARTICLES (HCV VLPS) AS NEUTRALIZING VACCINE CANDIDATES

A number of HCV vaccines that produce cellular immune responses against the core or non-structural proteins have entered clinical trials. A recent Phase I study reported using chimpanzee Ad3 and MVA encoding the HCV non-structural (NS) proteins in a prime-boost approach (Swadling et al., 2014). The adenoviral and MVA HCV vaccine were safe and resulted in the production of strong cross-genotypic CD4+ and CD8+ T cell responses. However, in a meta-analysis of the efficacy of various vaccine approaches in chimpanzees it was found that protection against HCV was more closely correlated with immune responses against the viral structural proteins rather than the non-structural proteins (Dahari et al., 2010). An effective preventative vaccine will therefore need to include HCV structural in addition to non-structural proteins in order to produce broad T and B cell responses. HCV VLPs have the potential to fulfill these requirements (**Table 1**).

HCV VLPs elicit both NAb and cellular immune responses (Chua et al., 2012; Beaumont et al., 2013; Kumar et al., 2015; Earnest-Silveira et al., 2016a; **Table 1**). Compared to HCV core, E1 and E2 DNA vaccines HCV VLPs produce stronger cytotoxic T cell responses in mice (Murata et al., 2003). This is significant given the important role of HCV core specific T cell responses in clearance of HCV (Smyk-Pearson et al., 2006). HCV VLPs produced in insect cells also produce maturation of dendritic cells (DC) (Barth et al., 2005; Chua et al., 2012; Earnest-Silveira et al., 2016b), another important consideration given the role of DC in directing adaptive immune responses to viruses and vaccines (Li et al., 2006; Yu et al., 2008; Alloatti et al., 2016). These are important findings for the development of HCV VLP vaccine as both the human papilloma virus (HPV) and hepatitis B virus (HBV) VLP vaccines have been shown to result in strong T cell responses in humans (Pinto et al., 2006; Vandepapeliere et al., 2008; Yokomine et al., 2017).

The development of cross-NAb to epitopes on the surface of HCV that develop in the course of natural infection provides further encouragement for the development of a neutralizing HCV VLP vaccine (Mancini et al., 2009). Furthermore, as HCV-specific NAbs recognize tertiary or quaternary structures (Giang et al., 2012) this makes VLPs attractive as a potential vaccine for HCV (Garrone et al., 2011; Chua et al., 2012; Beaumont et al., 2013). HCV VLPs are able to present conformational epitopes in their native state and consequently several approaches have been described. Favorable immune responses, both humoral and cellular, have been shown with an insect cell-derived vaccine based on genotype 1b HCV VLP. This vaccine was also partially protective in chimpanzees (Elmowalid et al., 2007). A HCV genotype 1a E2 glycoprotein/retroviral Gag pseudotype vaccine has also been shown to produce high-titre NAb in both mice and macaques (Garrone et al., 2011). Vaccination of rabbits with chimeric HBV-HCV VLPs produced in CHO cells and containing genotype 1a E1E2 heterodimers has also been shown to result in the production of cross-NAb responses against heterologous HCV genotypes (Beaumont et al., 2013; **Table 1**).

Neutralizing Epitopes in the E2 Protein

The E2 protein contains the major conformational neutralizing antigenic regions organized into a number of important antigenic domains (A–E or the AR3 and AR4 regions; Keck et al., 2004, 2008; Giang et al., 2012; Pierce et al., 2016). Antibodies against these epitopes have been shown to be broadly cross-neutralizing

TABLE 1 | Summary of various HCV VLP approaches and immune responses reported in different animal models.

HCV VLP type	Genotype	*In-vitro* cell line for production	Neutralization HCVcc or HCVpp (Genotype)	Binding of human NAb	DC maturation	Memory B cell responses	HCV specific CD8+ and/or CD4+ T cell responses	Animal models tested	Protection from HCV Challenge	References
Insect cell derived	1b	Sf9	No Strong antibody response in mice. Neutralization of vaccinia virus-HCV with Baboon immune sera. (Poor antibody responses in Chimpanzees)	Yes	Yes (*in-vitro*)	Yes	Yes (CD4+, CD8+, CTL)	(1) BALB/c mice (2) HLA2.1 transgenic mice (3) Baboons (4) Chimpanzee	(1) BALB/c and HLA2.1 transgenic mice vaccinia virus-HCV (2) Protection against persistent infection with homologous HCV in Chimpanzees	Baumert et al., 1998, 1999; Murata et al., 2003; Steinmann et al., 2004
Mammalian cell derived	1a, 1b, 2, 3a	Huh7	Yes (HCVcc 1b and 2)	Yes	Yes (*in-vitro*)	Yes	Yes (CD4+, CD8+, Granzyme B)	(1) C57BL/6 and BALB/c mice, (2) HLA2.1 transgenic mice	No	Chua et al., 2012; Earnest-Silveira et al., 2016b
CHIMERIC HBsAg/HCV LPs										
(1) HBs-HCV E1 and E2 VLPs	1a	CHO	Yes (HCVcc and HCVpp 1a, 1b, 2a, and 3)	No	No	No	No	Rabbits	No	Patient et al., 2009; Beaumont et al., 2013
(2) HBsAg/HCV HVR1	1a and 1b	Huh7	Yes (HCVpp 1a)	No	No	No	No	C57BL/6 and BALB/c mice	No	Netter et al., 2001, 2003; Woo et al., 2006; Haqshenas et al., 2007; Vietheer et al., 2007; Cheong et al., 2009
RETROVIRAL HCV-LIKE PARTICLES										
(1) $RetroVLP^{E1E2}$ (2) $RetroVLP^{NS3}$ (3) Plasmo-$retroVLP^{E1E2}$ (4) rAdE1E2 (Prime-boost strategies)	1a		Yes (1b, 2a, 2b, 4, and 5)	No	No	No	Yes (CD8+, CTL)	(1) C57BL/6 and BALB/c mice (2) Macaques	No	Bartosch et al., 2003; Bellier et al., 2006, 2009; Desjardins et al., 2009; Garrone et al., 2011; Huret et al., 2013

and protective against HCV challenge in human liver chimeric mice (Giang et al., 2012).

Distinct broad neutralizing epitopes in and downstream of hypervariable region 1 (HVR1) of the E2 protein have been described (Keck et al., 2013, 2014), with at least four distinct clusters of overlapping epitopes mediating broad virus neutralization (Keck et al., 2004, 2008, 2011). It has also been possible to define a neutralizing and a non-neutralizing face to the E2 core antigenic surface (Kong et al., 2013; Khan et al., 2014). Together with comprehensive alanine substitution studies it has also been possible to map the binding of human monoclonal antibodies (HuMAbs) to these critical regions of E2, with the most potent binding to domains B and D of E2 the protein (Fauvelle et al., 2016). Several HuMabs also bind to the non-neutralizing face of E2 (Fauvelle et al., 2016; **Figure 1**). In a recent report, a comprehensive analysis of the E2 binding residues of neutralizing HuMabs was described (Pierce et al., 2016). This study identified the critical binding residues for HuMAbs on the neutralizing face of E2 and for which limited epitope mapping was previously described (**Figure 2**) together with the critical residues defining the major antigenic domains A–D of the E2 protein. It also mapped the binding residues for HuMAbs targeting antigenic domains A and C for which there was little or no previous epitope mapping data nor crystal structures available (Pierce et al., 2016; **Figure 1**). This information provides critical data for the design of neutralizing antibody vaccines for HCV.

Neutralizing Epitopes in the E1 Protein

The E2 glycoprotein also contains neutralizing epitopes, although there is less information available characterizing these. A broad cross-neutralizing epitope has been identified between amino acids 313 and 327 (Meunier et al., 2008). Monoclonal antibodies to these epitopes neutralized HCV/retroviral pseudotype particles (HCVpp) of genotypes 1a, 1b, 4a, and 6a and HCVcc of genotype 1a and 2a. By using epitope extraction and mass spectrometry it has also been possible to identify a potentially neutralizing epitope in E1 (aa 313 and 327) that overlaps the cross-neutralizing epitope 313–327 described by Meunier and coworkers (Grollo et al., 2006; Torresi et al., 2007; Meunier et al., 2008). A more recent study using chimeric hepatitis B S envelope protein subviral particles expressing HCV E1 and E2 proteins alone or as E1E2 dimers also demonstrated that anti-E1 antibodies produced following immunization of rabbits were able to neutralize HCVcc *in vitro* and had additive cross neutralizing activity with anti-E2 antibodies against heterologous HCVcc genotypes *in vitro* (Beaumont et al., 2016). This study reinforces the importance of including both E1 and E2 in a neutralizing HCV vaccine.

These studies highlight the complex organization of neutralizing epitopes on the surface of HCV and argue that for a vaccine to be effective it would need to be able to closely reproduce these quaternary structures (Pierce et al., 2016). An HCV VLP based vaccine will fulfill the requirement of delivering critical conformational neutralizing epitopes in addition to providing HCV core specific CD4+ and CD8+ epitopes.

INSECT CELL DERIVED HCV VLPS

Insect cell-derived VLPs produced using a baculovirus system expressing the core, E1 and E2 structural proteins of HCV (genotype 1b) were able to induce broad HCV specific immune responses (Baumert et al., 1998, 1999; Murata et al., 2003; Steinmann et al., 2004). These studies first demonstrated that the HCV structural proteins were able to self-assemble into 40–60 nm VLPs that were representative of HCV (Baumert et al., 1998). The HCV VLPs were shown to be similar structurally and antigenically in composition to putative HCV virions (Baumert et al., 1999). However, the glycosylated forms of E1 and E2 and the size of E2 in the insect cell derived HCV VLPs was different from E1 and E2 expressed in mammalian cells and this was attributed in part to the less efficient cleavage of E2 in insect cells (Baumert et al., 1999). Immunization of mice resulted in antibody responses against the HCV structural proteins and the HCV VLPs were immunoreactive with sera from individuals infected with different HCV genotypes suggesting that the HCV VLPs may have exhibited broad cross-neutralizing epitopes (Baumert et al., 1998). In a follow up study, HLA-A2.1 transgenic mice were immunized with genotype 1b HCV VLPs. Humoral responses were assessed by ELISA while T cell responses were assessed using pools of HCV core and envelope specific peptides in ELISPOT and intracellular cytokine staining assays (Baumert et al., 1998, 1999; Murata et al., 2003; Steinmann et al., 2004). The HCV VLP immunized mice developed strong humoral and HCV core-specific CD4+ and CD8+ T cell responses (Baumert et al., 1998, 1999; Murata et al., 2003; Steinmann et al., 2004). In a surrogate HCV challenge model to assess the importance of these immune responses, BALB/c and HLA-A2.1 mice were immunized with the vaccine and then challenged with recombinant vaccinia virus expressing the HCV structural proteins (vvHCV.S) and compared to unimmunized mice as a negative control followed by harvesting of the mouse ovaries and determining vaccinia virus titres by plaque assay. In contrast to negative control mice, the HCV VLP immunized mice had >5 log10 reductions in viral titres and no detectable viremia. Finally, adoptive transfer of splenocytes from immunized BALB/c mice protected non-immunized mice from vvHCV.S challenge (Baumert et al., 1998, 1999; Murata et al., 2003; Steinmann et al., 2004). In addition, the HCV VLPs were able to stimulate the maturation of human dendritic cells (Barth et al., 2005), an important response for an effective vaccine. The HCV VLPs demonstrated a saturable binding to human hepatoma cells that was efficiently blocked by anti-E2 antibodies (Wellnitz et al., 2002). Antibodies and IgG isolated from the sera of patients with acute and chronic hepatitis C infection also inhibited the binding of HCV VLPs to human hepatoma cells (Steinmann et al., 2004).

Immunization of HLA2.1 transgenic mice with the insect cell-derived HCV VLPs also resulted in the production of strong humoral and HCV-specific T helper and CTL responses (Lechmann et al., 2001). The HCV-specific T cell responses produced in the HLA2.1 transgenic mice were also substantially stronger than responses against recombinant HCV protein and DNA based vaccines (Lechmann et al., 2001; Murata et al., 2003). In a surrogate challenge model, immunized mice (including

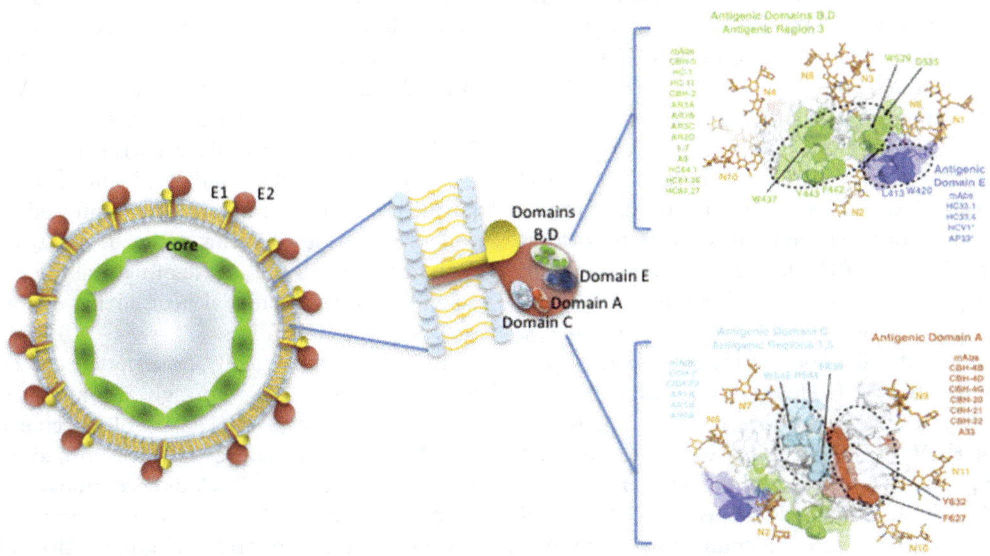

FIGURE 1 | HCV virus like particle showing E1 and E2 protein dimers embedded in a lipid bilayer, surrounding the core nucleocapsid. Major neutralizing regions are situated on the surface of the E2 protein. Antigenic domains and antigenic regions with the key binding sites of key human Mabs are shown on the right, with the neutralizing antibody face (antigenic domains B, D; Antigenic Region 3; antigenic domain E) above and the non-neutralizing face (antigenic domains A,C) of E2 below. Adapted from Fauvelle et al. (2016) and with permission from Prof S Foung.

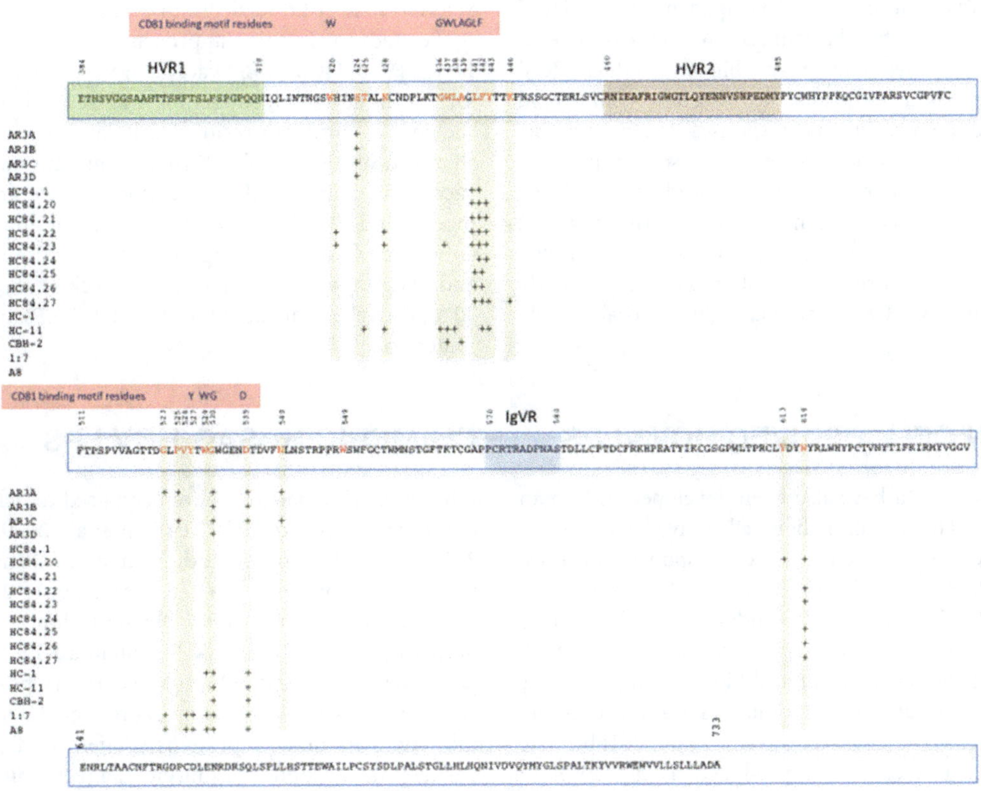

FIGURE 2 | Map of the E2 protein showing the position of amino acid contact residues (red) of HuMabs binding the Domains B and D and Antigenic Region 3 on the neutralizing face of E2 (Pierce et al., 2016). The positions of HVR1, HVR2, IgVR, and the CD81 binding motif residues on E2 are highlighted.

HLA2.1 transgenic mice) were protected from challenge with recombinant vaccinia virus expressing HCV structural proteins (Murata et al., 2003). The significant role of both CD4+ and CD8+ T cells in providing protection against vaccinia-HCV was confirmed with adoptive transfer experiments following lymphocyte depletion (Murata et al., 2003).

The immunogenicity of HCV VLPs and the effects of novel adjuvants were further tested in a nonhuman primate model (Jeong et al., 2004). Baboons were immunized with four doses of HCV VLPs plus adjuvant AS01B alone or the combination of AS01B and CpG oligodeoxynucleotides. All animals developed HCV specific antibody, CD4+ and CD8+ T cell responses. The addition of adjuvants did not significantly increase the immunogenicity of the HCV VLPs (Jeong et al., 2004).

These encouraging results paved the way to evaluate the immunogenicity of HCV VLPs in the chimpanzee (Elmowalid et al., 2007). Chimpanzees were immunized with HCV VLPs alone or with AS01B adjuvant. HCV-specific CD4+ and CD8+ T cell responses developed in all chimpanzees, although antibody responses were generally poor (Elmowalid et al., 2007). The chimpanzees were then challenged with HCV. One chimpanzee developed a transient low-level viremia. Three other chimpanzees developed high level viremia however all went on to clear infection 10 weeks after HCV challenge. The challenge with HCV also resulted in a significantly stronger peripheral and intra-hepatic T cell response. In contrast, 3 of 4 naïve chimpanzees developed persistent HCV infection. Vaccination of the chimpanzees was clearly able to induce immune responses that were able to control HCV and prevent progression to persistent infection (Elmowalid et al., 2007). The poor antibody responses to the vaccine were in contrast to the strong responses observed in mice and may have been a reflection of the production of the VLPs in insect cells. This is perhaps not surprising as E2 protein produced in insect cells has previously been shown to not to result in the production of protective antibody responses in primates (Choo et al., 1994; Rosa et al., 1996).

MAMMALIAN CELL DERIVED HCV VLPS

HCV VLPs of genotype 1a have also been developed in human hepatocyte-derived. These mammalian cell derived HCV VLPs produce NAb and HCV specific T cell responses in mice (Chua et al., 2012; Earnest-Silveira et al., 2016b). Similarly, a genotype 3a HCV VLP vaccine also induced broad humoral and cellular immune responses in mice (Kumar et al., 2015). HCV VLPs possess the biochemical and biophysical properties that are characteristic of HCV virions (Gastaminza et al., 2010; Catanese et al., 2013; Earnest-Silveira et al., 2016b). The envelope proteins E1 and E2 are produced as glycoprotein heterodimers that self-assemble with the HCV core protein into VLPs that are morphologically typical of HCV virions by electron microscopy (EM) and cryo-EM (Earnest-Silveira et al., 2016a,b). The morphology of these hepatocyte-derived HCV VLPs is consistent with the findings of other investigators (Gastaminza et al., 2010; Catanese et al., 2013) who have shown that HCV virions isolated from sera of infected individuals are spherical, heterogeneous, vary in size from 40 to 100 nm (Earnest-Silveira et al., 2016b). Like HCV virions, these HCV VLPs incorporate apolipoproteins C and E (Gastaminza et al., 2010; Catanese et al., 2013; Earnest-Silveira et al., 2016a). The entry of the genotype 1a VLPs into Huh7 cells could also be blocked effectively with IgG purified from the sera of individuals infected with HCV genotype 1a and 3a (Earnest-Silveira et al., 2016b). This shows that cross-NAb generated in the course of natural infection in humans are able to recognize potential neutralizing epitopes present on the surface of the HCV VLPs.

In a subsequent study, a genotype 3a HCV VLP vaccine was also shown to be strongly immunogenic (Kumar et al., 2015). The genotype 3a HCV VLP vaccine resulted in strong T cell and NAb responses in mice. In addition, a prime-boost strategy using a HCV DNA or recombinant adenovirus vaccine encoding genotype 3a HCV core, E1 and E2 proteins resulted in even stronger humoral (including NAb) and cellular immune responses (Kumar et al., 2015).

The mammalian cell derived HCV VLPs also induced the production of HCV-specific CD4+ and CD8+ T cell in mice. This is an important finding as spontaneous clearance of HCV, control of HCV viremia and the development of HCV specific memory B cell and NAb responses are all associated with the development of $CD4^+$ T helper cell responses (Schulze Zur Wiesch et al., 2012; Raziorrouh et al., 2015; Spaan et al., 2015).

To advance this approach, a quadrivalent genotype 1a/1b/2a/3a HCV VLP vaccine was produced and a method for the large-scale production and refined purification of the vaccine to eliminate residual cellular proteins was established (Earnest-Silveira et al., 2016a). The immunogenicity of this vaccine in humanized liver chimeric mice and a large animal model and the binding of neutralizing human monoclonal antibodies (HuMAbs) targeting conserved antigenic domain B and D epitopes of the E2 protein (Keck et al., 2004, 2008, 2011, 2016; Fauvelle et al., 2016) to the HCV VLPs are currently under evaluation.

CHIMERIC HBSAG/HCV LPS

HBsAg subviral particles have been used to deliver the complete envelope proteins of HCV (Patient et al., 2009; Beaumont et al., 2013, 2016; Beaumont and Roingeard, 2015) or specific E2 neutralizing epitopes (Netter et al., 2001, 2003; Woo et al., 2006; Vietheer et al., 2007). By replacing the transmembrane domain (TMD) of the HBV S protein a with the TMD of HCV genotype 1a E1 and E2 proteins it was possible to produce chimeric HBs-HCV particles expressing HBs protein fused to full-length E1 and E2 proteins (Patient et al., 2009). Chimeric particles were produced using either a recombinant Semliki forest virus expression system to transduce CHO cells or by producing stably transfected CHO cells. The chimeric fusion proteins efficiently self-assembled into VLPs containing HCV E1 and E2 glycoproteins (Patient et al., 2009; Beaumont et al., 2013). The immunogenicity of the chimeric HBs-HCV particles was assessed in rabbits and induced strong HCV E1 and E2 specific antibody responses against. Immune sera from rabbits vaccinated with chimeric HBs-HCV E1 or E2 particles neutralized both HCVpp and HCVcc of several genotypes, including 1a, 1b, 2a, and 3 (Beaumont et al., 2013). Antibody responses were also found to be less sustained in E1-S-immunized than in E2-S-immunized rabbits (Beaumont et al., 2013). The immunogenicity of the chimeric vaccine and the strength of the HCV E2 responses was not affected by pre-existing immunity to HBsAg (Beaumont and Roingeard, 2015). In a further follow-up study these investigators compared the immunogenicity and NAb responses of chimeric particles expressing HCV E1 and E2 proteins alone with chimeric particles expressing E1E2 heterodimers (Beaumont et al., 2016). Interestingly the investigators found that immunization of rabbits with the chimeric vaccine expressing the E1E2 dimers resulted in poorer NAb responses compared to the vaccine with E1 and E2 expressed separately. However, an additive effect was found in anti-E1 and anti-E2 responses that was associated with increased cross-neutralization of heterologous HCV genotypes (Beaumont et al., 2016). This finding reinforces the requirement of including both E1 and E2 proteins for an effective vaccine.

In an alternative approach Netter and coworkers modified HBsAg particles by introducing HCV specific B and T cell epitopes into the "a" determinant of the HBs protein (Netter et al., 2001, 2003; Woo et al., 2006; Haqshenas et al., 2007; Vietheer et al., 2007). Sequences from HVR1 of the E2 gene of HCV were inserted into the HBsAg gene so that varying lengths of the HCV HVR1 were expressed on the "a" determinant of the HBsAg protein (Netter et al., 2001). By using this approach it was possible to produce HBsAg subviral particles in Huh7 cells containing inserts of up to 36 aa from the HCV HVR1 in mammalian cells. The particles were secreted as efficiently as wild-type HBsAg particles (Netter et al., 2001). However, the ability to produce secreted particles is influenced by the way in which the "a" determinant is altered by the insertion of foreign sequences and in particular cysteine rich sequences which dramatically reduced particle secretion (Cheong et al., 2009). Also, immunization of mice with HBs/ HCV genotype 1a or 1b particles resulted in the production of specific antibody responses. Immunization with a combination of these particles resulted in a synergistic effect with stronger antibody responses against both the HVR1 epitopes than with the individual particles (Netter et al., 2001). To determine if pre-existing anti-HBs might reduce the antibody response to the HCV HVR1 sequences included in the chimeric particles these investigators also immunized mice with a commercial HBV vaccine followed by the chimeric HBsAg/HVR1 particles. The presence of pre-existing anti-HBs antibody had no effect on anti-HVR1 antibody titres, suggesting the HBsAg/HVR1 particles could be used in HBV vaccinated individuals (Netter et al., 2001). In addition, anti-HVR1 antisera blocked the entry of HCVpps containing homologous or heterologous HVR1 sequences into Huh7 cells, showing that the chimeric particles were able to induce the production of HVR1-specific neutralizing antibody (Vietheer et al., 2007).

RETROVIRAL HCV-LIKE PARTICLES

Retroviral expression vectors have also proven useful in developing produce neutralizing HCV vaccines. Bellier and coworkers have developed a DNA vaccine expressing murine leukemia virus (MLV) Gag and modified MLV Env proteins capable of assembling into "retroVLPs." The aim of these particles was to induce stronger immune responses than DNA vaccines expressing single or multiple monomeric proteins. These investigators also developed "plasmo-retroVLPs," consisting of DNA plasmids that could be used to transform cells to produce retroVLPs carrying foreign epitopes like the E1E2 proteins of HCV (Bartosch et al., 2003; Bellier et al., 2006). RetroVLPs presenting foreign antigens induced stronger immune responses than matching antigens not presented as VLPs (Bellier et al., 2006). RetroVLPs pseudotyped with the Gag protein of MLV and the envelope proteins of Vesicular Stomatitis virus (VSV) or West Nile virus (WNV) were also produced. Antibodies against VSV or WNV were detected earlier and had stronger neutralizing activity than with plasmids not generating VLPs (Bellier et al., 2009). The advantage of this system is that the plasmo-retroVLPs can be combined with the retroVLPs in a prime boost strategy.

These initial studies were followed by a prime-boost immunization series using plasmo-retroVLPs and a recombinant serotype 5 adenovirus (rAd5) expressing HCV-E1/E2 envelope glycoprotein (plasmo-retroVLP^{E1E2}) (Desjardins et al., 2009). Mice were primed with rAdE1E2 followed by boosting with plasmo-retroVLP^{E1E2}. The plasmo-retroVLP^{E1E2} significantly increased E1E2-specific T cell responses and also increased the production of E2-specific antibody. In comparison, plasmids that were unable to form E1E2-pseudotyped retroVLPs did not produce boosted immune (Desjardins et al., 2009). This was a significant finding as it highlighted the importance of including the HCV E1 and E2 proteins as heterodimers in a particle to ensure that critical neutralizing epitopes are presented correctly.

The rAdE1E2 and plasmo-retroVLP^{E1E2} were next tested in a prime-boost strategy in mice and macaques (Garrone et al., 2011). Immunization of mice with E1E2-expressing vectors elicited anti-E2 antibodies, and the response was significantly enhanced after boosting with retroVLP^{E1E2}. A group of four macaques were also primed with rAdE1E2 followed by boosting with retroVLP^{E1E2}. Priming with rAdE1E2 resulted in strong T cell responses, but weak anti-E2 antibody responses. In contrast, strong NAb responses were observed after boosting with retroVLP^{E1E2}. In addition, the prime boost strategy was shown to produce HCV NAb that cross-neutralized five other HCV genotypes (Garrone et al., 2011). These results highlight the importance of delivering E1E2 on a particulate structure.

In a subsequent study, mice were immunized with plasmo-retroVLPs expressing genotype 1a HCV-envelope glycoproteins and cross-reactive HCV immune responses were assessed by restimulating T cells with heterologous E1E2 antigens from genotypes 1b, 2b, 3a, 4c or 5 (Huret et al., 2013). Stronger T cell responses were found after restimulating with HCV genotype 1b, 3a, and 4c E1E2 VLPs than restimulation with homologous

VLPs. To broaden the cross-reactive T cell responses retroVLPs displaying the NS3 polypeptide fused to Gag were produced. Mice were immunized with plasmo-retroVLP^{NS3} and plasmid DNA encoding GagNS3 and the HCV E1E2 proteins. Strong HCV NS3 and E1E2 specific T cell responses were produced. In addition, strong anti-E1 and anti-E2 NAb responses were produced after priming with plasmo-retroVLPs followed by boosting with retroVLP^{E1E2} (Huret et al., 2013).

CONCLUSION

Although the development of protective immune responses against HCV is possible, the major challenge facing researchers is how best to reproduce these responses in a vaccine. A HCV VLP-based vaccine has the potential to fulfill the requirements of an effective vaccine for hepatitis C. Several approaches have shown that HCV VLPs are immunogenic and capable of eliciting robust CD4+, CD8+, and cross reactive NAb responses. The results reported with each of these approaches has provided important preclinical data for the progression to broader studies in HCV challenge models and ultimately to clinical trials for development of an effective preventative vaccine for HCV.

AUTHOR CONTRIBUTIONS

JT wrote the paper in its entirety, created the figures and tables and was responsible for the editing thc final draft.

FUNDING

This work was supported by the National Health and Medical Research Council (NHMRC) of Australia, grant numbers 1060436 and 1126379. JT is supported by an NHMRC Practitioner Fellowship, grant number 106043.

REFERENCES

Aitken, C. K., Lewis, J., Tracy, S. L., Spelman, T., Bowden, D. S., Bharadwaj, M., et al. (2008). High incidence of hepatitis C virus reinfection in a cohort of injecting drug users. *Hepatology* 48, 1746–1752. doi: 10.1002/hep.22534

Akazawa, D., Moriyama, M., Yokokawa, H., Omi, N., Watanabe, N., Date, T., et al. (2013). Neutralizing antibodies induced by cell culture-derived hepatitis C virus protect against infection in mice. *Gastroenterology* 145, 447.e1-4–455.e1-4. doi: 10.1053/j.gastro.2013.05.007

Alloatti, A., Kotsias, F., Magalhaes, J. G., and Amigorena, S. (2016). Dendritic cell maturation and cross-presentation: timing matters! *Immunol. Rev.* 272, 97–108. doi: 10.1111/imr.12432

Barth, H., Ulsenheimer, A., Pape, G. R., Diepolder, H. M., Hoffman, M., Neumann-Haefelin, C., et al. (2005). Uptake and presentation of hepatitis C virus-like particles by human dendritic cells. *Blood* 105, 3605–3614. doi: 10.1182/blood-2004-05-1952

Bartosch, B., Dubuisson, J., and Cosset, F. L. (2003). Infectious hepatitis C virus pseudo-particles containing functional E1-E2 envelope protein complexes. *J. Exp. Med.* 197, 633–642. doi: 10.1084/jem.20021756

Bate, J. P., Colman, A. J., Frost, P. J., Shaw, D. R., and Harley, H. A. (2010). High prevalence of late relapse and reinfection in prisoners treated for chronic hepatitis C. *J. Gastroenterol. Hepatol.* 25, 1276–1280. doi: 10.1111/j.1440-1746.2010.06295.x

Baumert, T. F., Ito, S., Wong, D. T., and Liang, T. J. (1998). Hepatitis C virus structural proteins assemble into viruslike particles in insect cells. *J. Virol.* 72, 3827–3836

Baumert, T. F., Vergalla, J., Satoi, J., Thomson, M., Lechmann, M., Herion, D., et al. (1999). Hepatitis C virus-like particles synthesized in insect cells as a potential vaccine candidate. *Gastroenterology* 117, 1397–1407. doi: 10.1016/S0016-5085(99)70290-8

Beaumont, E., Patient, R., Hourioux, C., Dimier-Poisson, I., and Roingeard, P. (2013). Chimeric hepatitis B virus/hepatitis C virus envelope proteins elicit broadly neutralizing antibodies and constitute a potential bivalent prophylactic vaccine. *Hepatology* 57, 1303–1313. doi: 10.1002/hep.26132

Beaumont, E., Roch, E., Chopin, L., and Roingeard, P. (2016). Hepatitis C Virus E1 and E2 proteins used as separate immunogens induce neutralizing antibodies with additive properties. *PLoS ONE* 11:e0151626. doi: 10.1371/journal.pone.0151626

Beaumont, E., and Roingeard, P. (2015). Chimeric hepatitis B virus (HBV)/hepatitis C virus (HCV) subviral envelope particles induce efficient anti-HCV antibody production in animals pre-immunized with HBV vaccine. *Vaccine* 33, 973–976. doi: 10.1016/j.vaccine.2015.01.007

Bellier, B., Dalba, C., Clerc, B., Desjardins, D., Drury, R., Cosset, F., et al. (2006). DNA vaccines encoding retrovirus-based virus-like particles induce efficient immune responses without adjuvant. *Vaccine* 24, 2643–2655. doi: 10.1016/j.vaccine.2005.11.034

Bellier, B., Huret, C., Miyalou, M., Desjardins, D., Frenkiel, M. P., Despres, P., et al. (2009). DNA vaccines expressing retrovirus-like particles are efficient immunogens to induce neutralizing antibodies. *Vaccine* 27, 5772–5780. doi: 10.1016/j.vaccine.2009.07.059

Broering, T. J., Garrity, K. A., Boatright, N. K., Sloan, S. E., Sandor, F., Thomas, W. D. Jr., et al. (2009). Identification and characterization of broadly neutralizing human monoclonal antibodies directed against the E2 envelope glycoprotein of Hepatitis C virus. *J. Virol.* 83, 12473–12482. doi: 10.1128/JVI.01138-09

Catanese, M. T., Uryu, K., Kopp, M., Edwards, T. J., Andrus, L., Rice, W. J., et al. (2013). Ultrastructural analysis of hepatitis C virus particles. *Proc. Natl. Acad. Sci. U.S.A.* 110, 9505–9510. doi: 10.1073/pnas.1307527110

Cheong, W. S., Drummer, H. E., and Netter, H. J. (2009). Delivery of a foreign epitope by sharing amino acid residues with the carrier matrix. *J. Virol. Methods* 158, 35–40. doi: 10.1016/j.jviromet.2009.01.015

Choo, Q. L., Kuo, G., Ralston, R., Weiner, A., Chien, D., Van Nest, G., et al. (1994). Vaccination of chimpanzees against infection by the hepatitis C virus. *Proc. Natl. Acad. Sci. U.S.A.* 91, 1294–1298. doi: 10.1073/pnas.91.4.1294

Chua, B. Y., Johnson, D., Tan, A., Earnest-Silveira, L., Sekiya, T., Chin, R., et al. (2012). Hepatitis C VLPs delivered to dendritic cells by a TLR2 targeting lipopeptide results in enhanced antibody and cell-mediated responses. *PLoS ONE* 7:e47492. doi: 10.1371/journal.pone.0047492

Dahari, H., Feinstone, S. M., and Major, M. E. (2010). Meta-analysis of hepatitis C virus vaccine efficacy in chimpanzees indicates an importance for structural proteins. *Gastroenterology* 139, 965–974. doi: 10.1053/j.gastro.2010.05.077

de Jong, Y. P., Dorner, M., Mommersteeg, M. C., Xiao, J. W., Balazs, A. B., Robbins, J. B., et al. (2014). Broadly neutralizing antibodies abrogate established hepatitis C virus infection. *Sci. Transl. Med.* 6:254ra129. doi: 10.1126/scitranslmed.3009512

Desjardins, D., Huret, C., Dalba, C., Kreppel, F., Kochanek, S., Cosset, F., et al. (2009). Recombinant retrovirus-like particle forming DNA vaccines in prime-boost immunization and their use for hepatitis C virus vaccine development. *J. Gene Med.* 11, 313–325. doi: 10.1002/jgm.1307

Dorner, M., Horwitz, J. A., Robbins, J. B., Barry, W. T., Feng, Q., Mu, K., et al. (2011). A genetically humanized mouse model for hepatitis C virus infection. *Nature* 474, 208–211. doi: 10.1038/nature10168

Douam, F., Dao Thi, V. L., Maurin, G., Fresquet, J., Mompelat, D., Zeisel, M. B., et al. (2014). Critical interaction between E1 and E2 glycoproteins determines binding and fusion properties of hepatitis C virus during cell entry. *Hepatology* 59, 776–788. doi: 10.1002/hep.26733

Dowd, K. A., Netski, D. M., Wang, X. H., Cox, A. L., and Ray, S. C. (2009). Selection pressure from neutralizing antibodies drives sequence evolution during acute infection with hepatitis C virus. *Gastroenterology* 136, 2377–2386. doi: 10.1053/j.gastro.2009.02.080

Earnest-Silveira, L., Christiansen, D., Herrmann, S., Ralph, S. A., Das, S., Gowans, E. J., et al. (2016a). Large scale production of a mammalian cell derived quadrivalent hepatitis C virus like particle vaccine. *J. Virol. Methods* 236, 87–92. doi: 10.1016/j.jviromet.2016.06.012

Earnest-Silveira, L., Chua, B., Chin, R., Christiansen, D., Johnson, D., Herrmann, S., et al. (2016b). Characterization of a hepatitis C virus-like particle vaccine produced in a human hepatocyte-derived cell line. *J. Gen. Virol.* 97, 1865–1876. doi: 10.1099/jgv.0.000493

Elmowalid, G. A., Qiao, M. S., Jeong, H., Borg, B. B., Baumer, T. F., Sapp, R. K., et al. (2007). Immunization with hepatitis C virus-like particles results in control of hepatitis C virus infection in chimpanzees. *Proc. Natl. Acad. Sci. U.S.A.* 104, 8427–8432. doi: 10.1073/pnas.0702162104

Farci, P., Alter, H. J., Wong, D. C., Miller, R. H., Govindarajan, S., Engle, R., et al. (1994). Prevention of hepatitis C virus infection in chimpanzees after antibody-mediated *in vitro* neutralization. *Proc. Natl. Acad. Sci. U.S.A.* 91, 7792–7796. doi: 10.1073/pnas.91.16.7792

Farci, P., Shimoda, A., Wong, D., Cabezon, T., De Gioannis, D., Strazzera, A., et al. (1996). Prevention of hepatitis C virus infection in chimpanzees by hyperimmune serum against the hypervariable region 1 of the envelope 2 protein. *Proc. Natl. Acad. Sci. U.S.A.* 93, 15394–1539. doi: 10.1073/pnas.93.26.15394

Fauvelle, C., Colpitts, C. C., Keck, Z. Y., Pierce, B. G., Foung, S. K., and Baumert, T. F. (2016). Hepatitis C virus vaccine candidates inducing protective neutralizing antibodies. *Expert Rev. Vaccines* 15, 1535–1544. doi: 10.1080/14760584.2016.1194759

Frey, S. E., Houghton, M., Coates, S., Abrignani, S., Chien, D., Rosa, D., et al. (2010). Safety and immunogenicity of HCV E1E2 vaccine adjuvanted with MF59 administered to healthy adults. *Vaccine* 28, 6367–6373. doi: 10.1016/j.vaccine.2010.06.084

Garrone, P., Fluckiger, A. C., Mangeot, P. E., Gauthier, E., Dupeyrot-Lacas, P., Mancip, J., et al. (2011). A prime-boost strategy using virus-like particles pseudotyped for HCV proteins triggers broadly neutralizing antibodies in macaques. *Sci. Transl. Med.* 3:94ra71. doi: 10.1126/scitranslmed.3002330

Gastaminza, P., Dryden, K. A., Boyd, B., Wood, M. R., Law, M., Yeager, M., et al. (2010). Ultrastructural and biophysical characterization of hepatitis C virus particles produced in cell culture. *J. Virol.* 84, 10999–11009. doi: 10.1128/JVI.00526-10

Giang, E., Dorner, M., Prentoe, J. C., Dreux, M., Evans, M. J., Bukh, J., et al. (2012). Human broadly neutralizing antibodies to the envelope glycoprotein complex of hepatitis C virus. *Proc. Natl. Acad. Sci. U.S.A.* 109, 6205–6210. doi: 10.1073/pnas.1114927109

Grady, B. P., Vanhommerig, J. W., Schinkel, J., Weegink, C. J., Bruisten, S. M., Lindenburg, C. E., et al. (2012). Low incidence of reinfection with the hepatitis C virus following treatment in active drug users in Amsterdam. *Eur. J. Gastroenterol. Hepatol.* 24, 1302–1307. doi: 10.1097/MEG.0b013e32835702a8

Grebely, J., Knight, E., Ngai, T., Genoway, K. A., Raffa, J. D., Storms, M., et al. (2010). Reinfection with hepatitis C virus following sustained virological response in injection drug users. *J. Gastroenterol. Hepatol.* 25, 1281–1284. doi: 10.1111/j.1440-1746.2010.06238.x

Grebely, J., Prins, M., Hellard, M., Cox, A. L., Osburn, W. O., Lauer, G., et al. (2012). Hepatitis C virus clearance, reinfection, and persistence, with insights from studies of injecting drug users: towards a vaccine. *Lancet Infect. Dis.* 12, 408–414. doi: 10.1016/S1473-3099(12)70010-5

Grollo, L., Torresi, J., Drummer, H., Zeng, W., Williamson, N., and Jackson, D. C. (2006). Cross-reactive epitopes of hepatitis C virus induce antibodies that capture virions and inhibit pseudo virus particle cell entry. *Antivir. Ther.* 11, 1005–1014.

Hahn, J. A., Wylie, D., Dill, J., Sanchez, M. S., Lloyd-Smith, J. O., Page-Shafer, K., et al. (2009). Potential impact of vaccination on the hepatitis C virus epidemic in injection drug users. *Epidemics* 1, 47–57. doi: 10.1016/j.epidem.2008.10.002

Haqshenas, G., Dong, X., Netter, H., Torresi, J., and Gowans, E. J. (2007). A chimeric GB virus B encoding the hepatitis C virus hypervariable region 1 is infectious *in vivo*. *J. Gen. Virol.* 88(Pt 3), 895–902. doi: 10.1099/vir.0.82467-0

Hellard, M. E., Jenkinson, R., Higgs, P., Stoove, M. A., Sacks-Davis, R., Gold, J., et al. (2012). Modelling antiviral treatment to prevent hepatitis C infection among people who inject drugs in Victoria, Australia. *Med. J. Aust.* 196, 638–641. doi: 10.5694/mja11.10981

Holz, L., and Rehermann, B. (2015). T cell responses in hepatitis C virus infection: historical overview and goals for future research. *Antiviral Res.* 114, 96–105. doi: 10.1016/j.antiviral.2014.11.009

Huret, C., Desjardins, D., Miyalou, M., Levacher, B., Amadoudji Zin, M., Bonduelle, O., et al. (2013). Recombinant retrovirus-derived virus-like particle-based vaccines induce hepatitis C virus-specific cellular and neutralizing immune responses in mice. *Vaccine* 31, 1540–1547. doi: 10.1016/j.vaccine.2012.05.025

Jeong, S. H., Qiao, M., Nascimbeni, M., Hu, Z., Rehermann, B., Murthy, K., et al. (2004). Immunization with hepatitis C virus-like particles induces humoral and cellular immune responses in nonhuman primates. *J. Virol.* 78, 6995–7003. doi: 10.1128/JVI.78.13.6995-7003.2004

Keck, Z., Op De Beeck, A., Hadlock, K. G., Xia, J., Li, T. K., Dubuisson, J., et al. (2004). Hepatitis C virus E2 has three immunogenic domains containing conformational epitopes with distinct propertires and biological functions. *J. Virol.* 78, 9224–9232. doi: 10.1128/JVI.78.17.9224-9232.2004

Keck, Z., Wang, W., Wang, Y., Lau, P., Carlsen, T. H., Prentoe, J., et al. (2013). Cooperativity in virus neutralization by human monoclonal antibodies to two adjacent regions located at the amino terminus of hepatitis C virus E2 glycoprotein. *J. Virol.* 87, 37–51. doi: 10.1128/JVI.01941-12

Keck, Z. Y., Angus, A. G., Wang, W., Lau, P., Wang, Y., Gatherer, D., et al. (2014). Non-random escape pathways from a broadly neutralizing human monoclonal antibody map to a highly conserved region on the hepatitis C virus E2 glycoprotein encompassing amino acids 412-423. *PLoS Pathog.* 10:e1004297. doi: 10.1371/journal.ppat.1004297

Keck, Z. Y., Li, T. K., Xia, J., Gal-Tanamy, M., Olson, O., Li, SH., et al. (2008). Definition of a conserved immunodominant domain on hepatitis C virus E2 glycoprotein by neutralizing human monoclonal antibodies. *J. Virol.* 82, 6061–6066. doi: 10.1128/JVI.02475-07

Keck, Z. Y., Saha, A., Xia, J., Wang, Y., Lau, P., Krey, T., et al. (2011). Mapping a region of hepatitis C virus E2 that is responsible for escape from neutralizing antibodies and a core CD81-binding region that does not tolerate neutralization escape mutations. *J. Virol.* 85, 10451–10463. doi: 10.1128/JVI.05259-11

Keck, Z. Y., Wang, Y., Lau, P., Lund, G., Rangarajan, S., Fauvelle, C., et al. (2016). Affinity maturation of a broadly neutralizing human monoclonal antibody that prevents acute hepatitis C virus infection in mice. *Hepatology* 64, 1922–1933. doi: 10.1002/hep.28850

Khan, A. G., Whidby, J., Miller, M. T., Scarborough, H., Zatorski, A. V., Cygan, A., et al. (2014). Structure of the core ectodomain of the hepatitis C virus envelope glycoprotein 2. *Nature* 509, 381–384. doi: 10.1038/nature13117

Kong, L., Giang, E., Nieusma, T., Kadam, R. U., Cogburn, K. E., Hua, Y., et al. (2013). Hepatitis C virus E2 envelope glycoprotein core structure. *Science* 342, 1090–1094. doi: 10.1126/science.1243876

Koutsoudakis, G., Herrmann, E., Kallis, S., Bartenschlager, R., and Pietschmann, T. (2007). The level of CD81 cell surface expression is a key determinant for productive entry of hepatitis C virus into host cells. *J. Virol.* 81, 588–598. doi: 10.1128/JVI.01534-06

Kumar, A., Das, S., Mullick, R., Lahiri, P., Tatineni, R., Goswami, D., Bhat, P., et al. (2015). Immune responses against hepatitis C virus genotype 3a virus-like particles in mice: a novel VLP prime-adenovirus boost strategy. *Vaccine* 34, 1115–1125. doi: 10.1016/j.vaccine.2015.11.061

Law, J. L., Chen, C., Wong, J., Hockman, D., Santer, D. M., Frey, S. E., et al. (2013). A hepatitis C virus (HCV) vaccine comprising envelope glycoproteins gpE1/gpE2 derived from a single isolate elicits broad cross-genotype neutralizing antibodies in humans. *PLoS ONE* 8:e59776. doi: 10.1371/journal.pone.0059776

Law, M., Maruyama, T., Lewis, J., Giang, E., Tarr, A. W., Stamataki, Z., et al. (2008). Broadly neutralizing antibodies protect against hepatitis C virus quasispecies challenge. *Nat. Med.* 14, 25–27. doi: 10.1038/nm1698

Lechmann, M., Murata, K., Satoi, J., Vergalla, J., Baumert, T., F., and Liang, T. J. (2001). Hepatitis C virus-like particles induce virus-specific humoral and cellular immune responses in mice. *Hepatology* 34, 417–423. doi: 10.1053/jhep.2001.26523

Li, W., Krishnadas, D. K., Li, J., Tyrrell, D. L., and Agrawal, B. (2006). Induction of primary human T cell responses against hepatitis C virus-derived antigens NS3 or core by autologous dendritic cells expressing hepatitis C virus antigens: potential for vaccine and immunotherapy. *J. Immunol.* 176, 6065–6075. doi: 10.4049/jimmunol.176.10.6065

Mancini, N., Diotti, R. A., Perotti, M., Sautto, G., Clementi, N., Nitti, G., et al. (2009). Hepatitis C virus (HCV) infection may elicit neutralizing antibodies targeting epitopes conserved in all viral genotypes. *PLoS ONE* 4:e8254. doi: 10.1371/journal.pone.0008254

Martin, N. K., Vickerman, P., Grebely, J., Hellard, M., Hutchinson, S. J., Lima, V. D., et al. (2013). Hepatitis C virus treatment for prevention among people who inject drugs: modeling treatment scale-up in the age of direct-acting antivirals. *Hepatology* 58, 1598–1609. doi: 10.1002/hep.26431

Meuleman, P., Bukh, J., Verhoye, L., Farhoudi, A., Vanwolleghem, T., Wang, R., et al. (2011). *In vivo* evaluation of the cross-genotype neutralizing activity of polyclonal antibodies against hepatitis C virus. *Hepatology* 53, 755–762. doi: 10.1002/hep.24171

Meuleman, P., Hesselgesser, J., Paulson, M., Vanwolleghem, T., Desombere, I., Reiser, H., et al. (2008). Anti-CD81 antibodies can prevent a hepatitis C virus infection *in vivo*. *Hepatology* 48, 1761–1768. doi: 10.1002/hep.22547

Meunier, J. C., Russell, R. S., Goossens, V., Priem, S., Walter, H., Depla, E., et al. (2008). Isolation and characterization of broadly neutralizing human monoclonal antibodies to the E1 glycoprotein of hepatitis C virus. *J. Virol.* 82, 966–973. doi: 10.1128/JVI.01872-07

Midgard, H., Bjoro, B., Maeland, A., Konopski, Z., Kileng, H., Damas, J., et al. (2016). Hepatitis C reinfection after sustained virological response. *J. Hepatol.* 64, 1020–1026. doi: 10.1016/j.jhep.2016.01.001

Murata, K., Lechmann, M., Qiao, M., Gunji, T., Alter, H. J., and Liang, T. J. (2003). Immunization with hepatitis C virus-like particles protects mice from recombinant hepatitis C virus-vaccinia infection. *Proc. Natl. Acad. Sci. U.S.A.* 100, 6753–6758. doi: 10.1073/pnas.1131929100

Netter, H. J., Macnaughton, T. B., Woo, W. P., Tindle, R., and Gowans, E. J. (2001). Antigenicity and immunogenicity of novel chimeric hepatitis B surface antigen particles with exposed hepatitis C virus epitopes. *J. Virol.* 75, 2130–241. doi: 10.1128/JVI.75.5.2130-2141.2001

Netter, H. J., Woo, W. P., Tindle, R., Macfarlan, R. I., and Gowans, E. J. (2003). Immunogenicity of recombinant HBsAg/HCV particles in mice pre-immunised with hepatitis B virus-specific vaccine. *Vaccine* 21, 2692–2697. doi: 10.1016/S0264-410X(03)00182-8

Osburn, W. O., Fisher, B. E., Dowd, K. A., Urban, G., Liu, L., Ray, S. C., et al. (2010). Spontaneous control of primary hepatitis C virus infection and immunity against persistent reinfection. *Gastroenterology* 138, 315–324. doi: 10.1053/j.gastro.2009.09.017

Osburn, W. O., Snider, A. E., Wells, B. L., Latanich, R., Bailey, J. R., Thomas, D. L., et al. (2014). Clearance of hepatitis C infection is associated with the early appearance of broad neutralizing antibody responses. *Hepatology* 59, 2140–2151. doi: 10.1002/hep.27013

Owsianka, A. M., Tarr, A. W., Keck, Z. Y., Li, T. K., Witteveldt, J., Adair, R., et al. (2008). Broadly neutralizing human monoclonal antibodies to the hepatitis C virus E2 glycoprotein. *J. Gen. Virol.* 89(Pt 3), 653–659. doi: 10.1099/vir.0.83386-0

Park, S. H., and Rehermann, B. (2014). Immune responses to HCV and other hepatitis viruses. *Immunity* 40, 13–24. doi: 10.1016/j.immuni.2013.12.010

Patient, R., Hourioux, C., Vaudin, P., Pages, J. C., and Roingeard, P. (2009). Chimeric hepatitis B and C viruses envelope proteins can form subviral particles. Implications for the design of new vaccine strategies. *New Biotechnol.* 25, 226–234. doi: 10.1016/j.nbt.2009.01.001

Peng, J., Lu, Y., Liu, W., Zhu, Y., Yan, X., Xu, J., et al. (2015). Genotype distribution and molecular epidemiology of hepatitis C Virus in Hubei, central China. *PLoS ONE* 10:e0137059. doi: 10.1371/journal.pone.0137059

Pestka, J. M., Zeisel, M. B., Blaser, E., Schurmann, P., Bartosch, B., Cosset, F. L., et al. (2007). Rapid induction of virus-neutralizing antibodies and viral clearance in a single-source outbreak of hepatitis C. *Proc. Natl. Acad. Sci. U.S.A.* 104, 6025–6030. doi: 10.1073/pnas.0607026104

Pierce, B. G., Keck, Z.-Y., Lau, P., Fauvelle, C., Gowthaman, R., Baumert, T. F., et al. (2016). Global mapping of antibody recognition of the hepatitis C virus E2 glycoprotein: implications for vaccine design. *Proc. Natl. Acad. Sci. U.S.A.* 113, E6946–E6954. doi: 10.1073/pnas.1614942113

Pinto, L. A., Viscidi, R., Harro, C. D., Kemp, T. J., Garcia-Pineres, A. J., Trivett, M., et al. (2006). Cellular immune responses to HPV-18,−31, and−53 in healthy volunteers immunized with recombinant HPV-16 L1 virus-like particles. *Virology* 353, 451–462. doi: 10.1016/j.virol.2006.06.021

Puig, M., Mihalik, K., Tilton, J. C., Williams, O., Merchlinsky, M., Connors, M., et al. (2006). CD4+ immune escape and subsequent T-cell failure following chimpanzee immunization against hepatitis C virus. *Hepatology* 44, 736–745. doi: 10.1002/hep.21319

Raghuraman, S., Park, H., Osburn, W. O., Winkelstein, E., Edlin, B. R., and Rehermann, B. (2012). Spontaneous clearance of chronic hepatitis C virus infection is associated with appearance of neutralizing antibodies and reversal of T-cell exhaustion. *J. Infect. Dis.* 205, 763–771. doi: 10.1093/infdis/jir835

Raziorrouh, B., Sacher, K., Tawar, R. G., Emmerich, F., Neumann-Haefelin, C., Baumert, T. F., et al. (2015). Virus-specific CD_{4+} T cells have functional and phenotypic characteristics of follicular T-helper cells in patients with acute and chronic HCV infections. *Gastroenterology* 150, 696–706. doi: 10.1053/j.gastro.2015.11.005

Rosa, D., Campagnoli, S., Moretto, C., Guenzi, E., Cousens, L., Chin, M., et al. (1996). A quantitative test to estimate neutralizing antibodies to the hepatitis C virus: cytofluorimetric assessment of envelope glycoprotein 2 binding to target cells. *Proc. Natl. Acad. Sci. U.S.A.* 93, 1759–163. doi: 10.1073/pnas.93.5.1759

Rosenberg, E. S., Hall, E. W., Sullivan, P. S., Sanchez, T. H., Workowski, K. A., Ward, J. W., et al. (2017). Estimation of state-level prevalence of hepatitis C virus infection, US states and district of Columbia, 2010. *Clin. Infect. Dis.* 64, 1573–1581. doi: 10.1093/cid/cix202

Sacks-Davis, R., Aitken, C. K., Higgs, P., Spelman, T., Pedrana, A. E., Bowden, S., et al. (2013). High rates of hepatitis C virus reinfection and spontaneous clearance of reinfection in people who inject drugs: a prospective cohort study. *PLoS ONE* 8:e80216. doi: 10.1371/journal.pone.0080216

Scarselli, E., Ansuini, H., Cerino, R., Roccasecca, R. M., Acali, S., Filocamo, G., et al. (2002). The human scavenger receptor class B type I is a novel candidate receptor for the hepatitis C virus. *EMBO J.* 21, 5017–525. doi: 10.1093/emboj/cdf529

Schulze Zur Wiesch, J., Ciuffreda, D., Lewis-Ximenez, L., Kasprowicz, V., Nolan, B. E., Streeck, H., et al. (2012). Broadly directed virus-specific CD4+ T cell responses are primed during acute hepatitis C infection, but rapidly disappear from human blood with viral persistence. *J. Exp. Med.* 209, 61–75. doi: 10.1084/jem.20100388

Scott, N., McBryde, E., Vickerman, P., Martin, N. K., Stone, J., Drummer, H., et al. (2015). The role of a hepatitis C virus vaccine: modelling the benefits alongside direct-acting antiviral treatments. *BMC Med.* 13:198. doi: 10.1186/s12916-015-0440-2

Sievert, W., Altraif, I., Razavi, H. A., Abdo, A., Ahmed, E. A., Alomair, A., et al. (2011). A systematic review of hepatitis C virus epidemiology in Asia, Australia and Egypt. *Liver Int.* 31(Suppl. 2), 61–80. doi: 10.1111/j.1478-3231.2011.02540.x

Sievert, W., Razavi, H., Estes, C., Thompson, A. J., Zekry, A., Roberts, S. K., et al. (2014). Enhanced antiviral treatment efficacy and uptake in preventing the rising burden of hepatitis C-related liver disease and costs in Australia. *J. Gastroenterol. Hepatol.* 29(Suppl. 1), 1–9. doi: 10.1111/jgh.12677

Smyk-Pearson, S., Tester, I. A., Lezotte, D., Sasaki, A. W., Lewinsohn, D. M., and Rosen, H. R. (2006). Differential antigenic hierarchy associated with spontaneous recovery from hepatitis C virus infection: implications for vaccine design. *J. Infect. Dis.* 194, 454–463. doi: 10.1086/505714

Spaan, M., Kreefft, K., de Graav, G. N., Brouwer, W. P., de Knegt, R. J., ten Kate, F. J., et al. (2015). $CD4^+CXCR5^+$ T cells in chronic HCV infection produce less IL-21, yet are efficient at supporting B cell responses. *J. Hepatol.* 62, 303–310. doi: 10.1016/j.jhep.2014.09.024

Steinmann, D., Barth, H., Gissler, B., Schurmann, P., Adah, M. I., Gerlach, J. T., et al. (2004). Inhibition of hepatitis C virus-like particle binding to target cells by antiviral antibodies in acute and chronic hepatitis. *J. Virol.* 78, 9030–9040. doi: 10.1128/JVI.78.17.9030-9040.2004

Stone, J., Martin, N. K., Hickman, M., Hellard, M., Scott, N., McBryde, E., et al. (2016). The potential impact of a hepatitis C vaccine for people who inject drugs: Is a vaccine needed in the age of direct-acting antivirals? *PLoS ONE* 11:e0156213. doi: 10.1371/journal.pone.0156213

Swadling, L., Capone, S., Antrobus, R. D., Brown, A., Richardson, R., Newell, E. W., et al. (2014). A human vaccine strategy based on chimpanzee adenoviral and MVA vectors that primes, boosts, and sustains functional HCV-specific T cell memory. *Sci. Transl. Med.* 6:261ra153. doi: 10.1126/scitranslmed.3009185

Torresi, J., Fischer, A., Grollo, L., Zeng, W., Drummer, H., and Jackson, D. C. (2007). Induction of neutralizing antibody responses to hepatitis C virus with synthetic peptide constructs incorporating both antibody and T-helper epitopes. *Immunol. Cell Biol.* 85, 169–173. doi: 10.1038/sj.icb.7100021

Vandepapeliere, P., Horsmans, Y., Moris, P., Van Mechelen, M., Janssens, M., Koutsoukos, M., et al. (2008). Vaccine adjuvant systems containing monophosphoryl lipid A and QS21 induce strong and persistent humoral and T cell responses against hepatitis B surface antigen in healthy adult volunteers. *Vaccine* 26, 1375–1386. doi: 10.1016/j.vaccine.2007.12.038

Vanwolleghem, T., Bukh, J., Meuleman, P., Desombere, I., Meunier, J. C., Alter, H., et al. (2008). Polyclonal immunoglobulins from a chronic hepatitis C virus patient protect human liver-chimeric mice from infection with a homologous hepatitis C virus strain. *Hepatology* 47, 1846–1855. doi: 10.1002/hep.22244

Vietheer, P. T., Boo, I., Drummer, H. E., and Netter, H. J. (2007). Immunizations with chimeric hepatitis B virus-like particles to induce potential anti-hepatitis C virus neutralizing antibodies. *Antivir. Ther.* 12, 477–487.

Wellnitz, S., Klumpp, B., Barth, H., Ito, S., Depla, E., Dubuisson, J., et al. (2002). Binding of hepatitis C virus-like particles derived from infectious clone H77C to defined human cell lines. *J. Virol.* 76, 1181–1193. doi: 10.1128/JVI.76.3.1181-1193.2002

Woo, W. P., Doan, T., Herd, K. A., Netter, H. J., and Tindle, R. W. (2006). Hepatitis B surface antigen vector delivers protective cytotoxic T-lymphocyte responses to disease-relevant foreign epitopes. *J. Virol.* 80, 3975–3984. doi: 10.1128/JVI.80.8.3975-3984.2006

Wu, E., Yang, M., Rao, H., Fu, S., Feng, B., Fei, R., et al. (2017). Temporal changes in the modes of hepatitis C virus transmission in the USA and Northern China. *Dig. Dis. Sci.* 62, 2141–2149. doi: 10.1007/s10620-017-4619-6

Yokomine, M., Matsueda, S., Kawano, K., Sasada, T., Fukui, A., Yamashita, T., et al. (2017). Enhancement of humoral and cell mediated immune response to HPV16 L1-derived peptides subsequent to vaccination with prophylactic bivalent HPV L1 virus-like particle vaccine in healthy females. *Exp. Ther. Med.* 13, 1500–1505. doi: 10.3892/etm.2017.4150

Yu, H., Babiuk, L. A., and van Drunen Littel-van den Hurk, S. (2008). Strategies for loading dendritic cells with hepatitis C NS5a antigen and inducing protective immunity. *J. Viral Hepat.* 15, 459–470. doi: 10.1111/j.1365-2893.2008.00959.x

Yu, M., Bartosch, B., Zhang, P., Guo, Z., P., Renzi, P. M., Shen, L. M., et al. (2004). Neutralising antibodies to hepatitis C virus (HCV) in immune globulins derived from anti-HCV-positive plasma. *Proc. Natl. Acad. Sci. U.S.A.* 101, 7705–7710. doi: 10.1073/pnas.0402458101

Zeisel, M. B., Koutsoudakis, G., Schnober, E. K., Haberstroh, A., Blum, H. E., Cosset, F. L., et al. (2007). Scavenger receptor class B type I is a key host factor for hepatitis C virus infection required for an entry step closely linked to CD81. *Hepatology* 46, 1722–1731. doi: 10.1002/hep.21994

Zhang, Y., Chen, L. M., and He, M. (2017). Hepatitis C Virus in mainland China with an emphasis on genotype and subtype distribution. *Virol. J.* 14:41. doi: 10.1186/s12985-017-0710-z

5

Anti-TGEV Miller Strain Infection Effect of *Lactobacillus plantarum* Supernatant Based on the JAK-STAT1 Signaling Pathway

Kai Wang[1†], Ling Ran[1†], Tao Yan[2], Zheng Niu[1], Zifei Kan[1], Yiling Zhang[1], Yang Yang[1], Luyi Xie[1], Shilei Huang[1], Qiuhan Yu[1], Di Wu[1] and Zhenhui Song[1]*

[1] *Department of Microbiology and Immunology, College of Animal Science, Southwest University, Chongqing, China,*
[2] *Department of Preventive Veterinary Medicine, Medical College of Animals, Xinjiang Agricultural University, Ürümqi, China*

***Correspondence:**
Zhenhui Song
szh7678@126.com

Transmissible gastroenteritis (TGE), caused by transmissible gastroenteritis virus (TGEV), is one many gastrointestinal inflections in piglets, characterized by diarrhea, and high mortality. Probiotics are ubiquitous bacteria in animal intestines, which have many functions, such as promoting intestinal peristalsis and maintaining the intestinal balance. We found that the supernatant of the Lp-1 strain of *Lactobacillus plantarum*, isolated in our laboratory, and named Lp-1s had marked anti-TGEV effect on IPEC-J2 cells. Lp-1s could induce large amounts of interferon-β in IPEC-J2 cells in the early stage (6 h) of infection with TGEV, and increased the level of phosphorylated signal transducer and activator of transcription and its nuclear translocation in the late stage (24–48 h) of infection. This resulted in upregulated expression of interferon-stimulated genes, and increased the transcription and protein expression of antiviral proteins, resulting in an anti-TGEV effect.

Keywords: transmissible gastroenteritis virus, *Lactobacillus plantarum*, interferon-beta, STAT1, interferon-stimulating genes

INTRODUCTION

Transmissible gastroenteritis virus (TGEV) is the pathogenic agent of porcine transmissible gastroenteritis (TGE), which causes vomiting, diarrhea, and high mortality in suckling piglets (Masters, 2006), resulting in heavy losses to the pig breeding industry (Zhao et al., 2014). In particular, viral diarrhea diseases are more serious because of limited treatment options. Probiotics comprise microorganisms that have beneficial activities to the host, and mainly comprise *Clostridium butyricum*, *Lactobacillus*, *Bifidobacteria*, Actinomycetes, and yeasts. They usually occupy the human gut and reproductive system, and can improve the balance of the host micro-ecology (Fuller, 1989; Maragkoudakis et al., 2010; da Silva Sabo et al., 2017; Stofilova et al., 2017). There is growing interest in the oral administration of appropriate probiotics to reduce the pressure in the intestines and produce an effective innate immune response (Pollmann et al., 2005; Maragkoudakis et al., 2010). In recent years, probiotic animal feed supplements have been developed as viable alternatives to antibiotics because of the ban on antibiotics in feed (Scharek et al., 2007). The addition of probiotic feed can prevent the infection of pathogens causing intestinal diseases, directly benefiting the animal host (Villena et al., 2014), or can indirectly enhance the host's immune response by balancing the disordered microbiota (Lee et al., 2018). In addition, many basic and clinical studies have confirmed that probiotic strains have antiviral effects (Lee et al., 2011; Yuan et al., 2018). Studies have shown that *Lactobacillus plantarum* can stimulate the body's innate and acquired immunity, and contributes to the production of inflammatory factors that inhibit the replication of the virus in the body. For example, *L. plantarum* strain YU (LpYU) not only has high interleukin (IL)-12-inducing activity mediated by Toll-like receptor (TLR) 2 in mouse peritoneal macrophages, but also communicates with natural killer cells (NK) in the spleen to stimulate the production of IgA to enhance the body's anti-H1N1 virus activity (Kawashima et al., 2011). In addition, *L. plantarum* L-137 can stimulate the production of type I interferon (IFN-1) to effectively inhibit the proliferation of H1N1 (Maeda et al., 2009). TGEV is an important gastrointestinal diarrhea virus; therefore, research and exploration into the antiviral mechanism of probiotics could lead to the development of oral probiotics to prevent and treat TGEV infection.

The body reacts rapidly to viral invasion by synthesizing and secreting type I interferon IFN-1 (IFN-α/β), which plays a key role in the host antiviral response. The binding of IFN-1 to its receptor (interferon α/β receptor, IFNAR) leads to activation of the Janus family kinase (JAK) and subsequent signal transduction and transcriptional activator (STAT) signaling cascade, resulting in the activation and upregulation of interferon-stimulating genes (*ISGs*), ultimately activating IFN to exert its antiviral effects (Zhao et al., 2016; Chen et al., 2017).

A strain of *L. plantarum* was successfully isolated and named Lp-1 (Song Han et al., 2017). We wondered whether the IPEC-J2 cells treated by Lp-1 could induce an antiviral mechanism through the IFN-β/JAKs/STAT/*ISGs* pathway after TGEV infection. In the present study, we found that the supernatant of *L. plantarum* Lp-1 (Lp-1s) could significantly inhibit TGEV infection. By detecting the replication of TGEV N gene in porcine intestinal epithelial cells treated with Lp-1s at different time points, we confirmed that Lp-1s had a preventive effect against TGEV. Then, by detecting the levels of IFN, p-STAT and *ISGs*, we further confirmed that Lp-1s exerts its anti-TGEV role by upregulating the expression of IFN-β.

MATERIALS AND METHODS

Cells, Viruses, and Reagents

Porcine kidney cells (ST) to amplify the virus and the experimental model pig jejunal cells (IPEC-J2 cells) were both cultured in Roswell Park Memorial Institute (RPMI) 1640 medium (Gibco, Grand Island, NY, United States) containing 10% fetal bovine serum (FBS, Gibco), under 37°C and 5% CO_2. IPEC-J2 cells and ST cells were purchased from the Shanghai Sur Biotech Co., Ltd (Shanghai, China). *L. plantarum* LP-1 was isolated and stored in our laboratory. Its 16S ribosomal gene sequence has been submitted to GenBank (MH727586). Lp-1s was isolated from a culture of *L. plantarum* LP-1 after shaking for 14 h at 37°C. The TGEV Miller strain (Yang et al., 2018) was preserved in our laboratory. Viral fluid was collected from ST cells after replication for approximately 72 h when the cells showed obvious cytopathic effects (CPEs).

Primer Design and Synthesis

The GenBank sequences of the TGEV N gene (GQ-374566.1) coding sequence (CDS) conserved region, the porcine MX1 CDS (MX dynamin like GTPase 1; AH015318.2), the MX2 CDS (MX dynamin like GTPase 2; AY897395.1), the ISG15 CDS (interferon-stimulated protein, 15 KDa; NM_214303.2), the OASL CDS (2′-5′-oligoadenylate synthetase like; NM_214303.2), the PKR CDS (double stranded RNA-dependent protein kinase; AB104654.1), the ZAP CDS (zeta-chain associated protein; GU_563332.1), and internal reference pig β-Actin gene (ACTB; XM_003124280.2) were obtained and pairs of specific primers were designed using Primer 5.0 software for quantitative real-time PCR [performed using SYBR Premix EX Taq II (Takara, Shiga, Japan)] as follows: TGEV-N (Forward: 5′-TTCAACCCC ATAACCCTCCAACAA-3′ and Reverse: 5′-GGCCCTTCAC CAT GCGATAGC-3′), MX1 (Forward: 5′-ATCTGTAAGCAGG AGACCATCAACTT G-3′ and Reverse: 5′-CTCGCCACGTCCA CTATCTTGTC-3′), MX2 (Forward: 5′-TTCACTCGCATCCGC ACTTCAG-3′ and Reverse: 5′-AGCTCCTCTGTCGCACTC TGG-3′), ISG15 (Forward: 5′-GGCAGCACAGTCCTGTT GATGG-3′ and Reverse: 5′-TGCGTCAGCCAGACCTCAT AGG-3′), OASL (Forward: 5′-CGTTGGTGGTGG AGACACA TACAG-3′ and Reverse: 5′-TCAGGCGACACCTTCCAGG ATC-3′), PKR (Forward: 5′-ACAGGACCTGCACATAACT TGAGG-3′ and Reverse: 5′-TGCTGTCGGCAGTGATGAAGA AC-3′), ZAP (Forward: 5′-GCTCAGTGCGAAC ACCTGGA TG-3′ and Reverse: 5′-TGACAGATGAAGGCGTGGAG AGG-3′), and ACTB (Forward: 5′-CTCTTCCAGC CCTCCT TCC-3′ and Reverse: 5′-GGTCCTTG CGGATGTCG-3′). The designed primers were synthesized by Shanghai Shenggong Biotechnology Service Co., Ltd. (Shanghai, China).

Assessment of Cellular Toxicity of Lp-1s by the CPE Effect and the MTT Assay

After centrifugation of Lp-1 with an OD_{600} of 1.8 at 4000 rpm/min for 10 min, the obtained supernatant was filtered through a 0.22-μm filter, and then diluted with RPMI 1640 high sugar medium to six gradients at two times ratio, i.e., Lp-1s was diluted to obtain OD_{600} values of 0.9, 0.45, 0.225, 0.113, 0.056, and 0.028, respectively. IPEC-J2 cells were seeded at 1×10^5/mL in 96-well plates and incubated overnight in 5% CO_2 at 37°C. The medium was discarded when the cells reached 90% confluence in the 96-well plate, and then 100 μL of each gradient dilution of Lp-1s was added to each well. The medium in the control group was replaced with RPMI 1640. After incubating for 90 min, the supernatant was discarded, and the cells were washed twice with phosphate-buffered saline (PBS). Culture was continued and the cytopathic effect (CPE) was observed daily. The maximum non-toxic dose of Lp-1s to the cells was detected using the 3-(4,5-dimethylthiazol-2-yl)-2,5-diphenyltetrazolium bromide (MTT) reagent (BBI, Shanghai, China), when 80% of the cells in the negative control group were damaged. MTT assays for each dilution were repeated three times independently.

Optimal Concentration of Lp-1s for Anti-TGEV Activity

Lp-1s was prepared as above and then diluted to an OD_{600} of 0.45, 0.225, 0.113, and 0.056 with RPMI 1640 high-sugar medium. IPEC-J2 cells were seeded at 1.8×10^6/mL in 6-well plates and cultured in 5% CO_2 at 37°C. At 90% confluence, the medium was discarded, the cells were washed three times with PBS, 1 mL of each gradient dilution of Lp-1s was added to each well, and the cells incubated at 37°C in 5% CO_2 for 90 min. The medium in the control group was replaced with RPMI 1640. For the other wells, the supernatant was discarded, TGEV (multiplicity of infection (MOI) = 0.1) in RPMI 1640 medium was added to Lp-1s-treated IPEC-J2, and incubated at 37°C in 5% CO_2 for 1.5 h. The supernatants were discarded and incubation continued in RPMI 1640 high glucose medium. After 48 h of culture, proteins were extracted for western blotting to detect the levels of the TGEV N protein after treatment with different concentrations of Lp-1s.

Median Tissue Culture Infectious Dose (TCID50) Analysis

IPEC-J2 cells treated with Lp-1s for 1.5 h were exposed to TGEV (MOI = 0.1). The IPEC-J2 cells treated with Lp-1s were sampled at 12 h post infection (hpi), 24 hpi, and 48 hpi and then frozen and thawed three times to collect virus particles in the cells and supernatants. Gradient dilution of IPEC-J2 cells was performed from 10^{-1} and 10^{-7}, respectively. TGEV titers of IPEC-J2 cells treated with Lp-1s for different times were detected using ST cells in 96-well plates. Each dilution gradient was assayed in 12 replicate wells. The $TCID_{50}$ of the virus in the different groups was calculated by Reed and Muench methods.

Detection of TGEV-N Gene Copy Number and Protein Expression

IPEC-J2 cells were inoculated into 6-well plates at 1.8×10^6/mL. The IPEC-J2 cells treated with Lp-1s for 1.5 h were exposed to TGEV (MOI = 0.1) for RNA extraction and protein sampling. When the cells reached 90% confluence, RNA was extracted and reverse transcribed into cDNA and quantified at 500 ng/mL. Absolute fluorescence quantitative PCR was performed using fluorescence quantitative PCR. The reaction parameters were as follows: Pre-denaturation at 95°C for 3 min, followed by 40 cycles of denaturation at 94°C for 30 s, annealing at 60°C for 30 s, and prolongation at 72°C for 30 s. The reaction for each sample was repeated three times. The Bio-Rad CFX Manager random matrix method was used to analyze the linear relationship between cycle threshold (CT) value and the copy number to calculate the copy number of the TGEV-N gene. Protein samples were also extracted at the same time point and detected using western blotting. The primary antibody was a mouse monoclonal antibody against TGEV-N, and the secondary antibodies were horseradish peroxidase (HRP)-conjugated goat anti-mouse antibodies (Proteintech,Wuhan,China). The immunoreactive protein bands were visualized using a Vilber fusion FX5 chemiluminescent imager.

Effect of Lp-1s on IFN-β Induction in IPEC Cells

IPEC-J2 cells were inoculated into 6-well plates at 1.8×10^6/mL. When they reached 90% confluence, three experimental groups were established: An Lp-1s optimal concentration treatment group infected TGEV, a TGEV single infection group, and the uninfected control group. Cell samples at 6, 12, 24, and 48 hpi were centrifuged at 4000 rpm for 10 min, and the supernatant subjected to an enzyme linked immunosorbent assay (ELISA) to detect IFN-β.

Western Blotting Analysis

Transmissible gastroenteritis virus (MOI = 0.1) was infected to IPEC-J2 cells that had been treated with Lp-1s for 1.5 h, and then cell samples at 12, 24, and 48 hpi were collected to produce protein lysates. In addition, TGEV (MOI = 0.1) was infected into IPEC-J2 cells cultured in RPMI 1640 for 1.5 h as the TGEV control group and the proteins were extracted at the same time points as the Lp-1s group. The protein concentration was determined using the bicinchoninic acid method and subjected to sodium dodecyl sulfate polyacrylamide gel electrophoresis. The separated proteins were transferred to a nitrocellulose membrane (Bio-Rad). The membranes were blocked using 5% skimmed milk and incubated with the following primary antibodies: Anti-STAT1 rabbit polyclonal antibodies (British Biorbyt Company), anti-phospho-(p)STAT1 (Tyr701) rabbit polyclonal antibodies (Biorbyt), anti-ZAP rabbit polyclonal antibodies (Abcam), anti-PKR rabbit polyclonal antibodies (Abcam), anti-(p)PKR (T446) rabbit polyclonal antibodies (Abcam), and anti-β-tubulin rabbit polyclonal antibodies (Proteintech). Secondary antibodies comprised goat anti-rabbit immunoglobulin (H + L). The immunoreactive protein bands were visualized using the Vilber fusion FX5 imaging system (VILBER), and the grayscale values of each band were analyzed by GraphPad Prism.

Indirect Immunofluorescence Detection of Nuclear Displacement

IPEC-J2 cells were seeded at a density of 1.5×10^6 in cell slides in 24-well culture dishes. These cells were set as three experimental groups comprising an Lp-1s optimal concentration treatment group, a TGEV alone infection group, and a blank (uninfected) control group, when they reached 90% confluence. The cells were sampled at 12, 24, and 48 hpi; washed three times with PBS; fixed with 4% paraformaldehyde at 37°C for 1.5 h; washed three times with PBS; permeated by 0.3% Triton-X-100 for 10 min; washed three times with PBS; and blocked by 1% bovine serum albumin for 30 min at room temperature. Primary antibodies comprising anti-p-STAT1 protein rabbit polyclonal antibodies and anti-TGEV-N mouse monoclonal antibodies were added and incubated overnight in 4°C in a wet box. The cells were then washed three times with PBS, proportionally added CY3-goat anti-rabbit fluorescence and fluorescein isothiocyanate (FITC)-labeled goat anti-mouse fluorescent secondary antibodies were then added, the cells were incubated for 1 h in a dark room at 37°C, incubated with 2-(4-amidinophenyl)-1H-indole-6-carboxamidine (DAPI) for 5 min, rinsed with PBS. Laser confocal microscopy was then used to observe p-STAT1, its nuclear translocation, and the TGEV N protein. The protein levels were analyzed using the ZEN software.

Quantitative Real-Time Reverse Transcription Polymerase Chain Reaction (qRT-PCR)

IPEC-J2 cells were seeded at 1.8 × 10^6/mL in 6-well plates, grown to 90% confluence, and then divided into three groups: Cells treated with Lp-1s for 1.5 h and then infected with TGEV (MOI = 0.1), TGEV infection alone, and the blank control (uninfected cells). The IPEC-J2 cells were sampled at 12, 24, and 48 hpi for qRT-PCR. Total RNA was extracted using the RNAiso plus reagent (Takara), and then single-stranded RNA was isolated using an RNA PCR (AMV) ver 3.0 kit (Takara). cDNA was then synthesized via reverse transcription. Quantitative real-time PCR was then performed using the SYBR premix EX Taq II (Takara) to detect the mRNA levels of ZAP, PKR, OASL, and ISG15 (fluorescent primers were synthesized by Shanghai Shenggong Bioengineering Technology Service Co., Ltd.).

Small Interfering RNA (siRNA) Assays

Small interfering RNA (siRNA) targeting STAT1, 5′-GGAACAGAAATACACCTAT-3′ (produced by RIBO, China). Transfected with the STAT1-specific siRNA using LipofectamineTM 3000 (Invitrogen, United States), according to the manufacturer's instructions, to the TGEV-infected groups treated with Lp-1s and TGEV infection alone groups, respectively, in IPEC-J2 cells. ConsiRNA transfected as control groups. The collected samples were analyzed by Western blotting using a rabbit pAb recognizing STAT1 as the primary antibody and HRP-conjugated goat anti-rabbit IgG as the secondary antibody.

Statistical Analyses

All results were plotted and analyzed using GraphPad Prism 6 software (GraphPad Inc., La Jolla, CA, United States). The data were presented as the mean ± standard deviation (SD) of three independent experiments. Data were statistically compared using the t test. A p value < 0.05 ($^*p < 0.05$ and $^{**}p < 0.01$) was considered statistically significant.

RESULTS

MTT Cytotoxicity Test and Lp-1s Concentration Screening

The MTT assay (**Figure 1**) showed that the higher dilution ratio of Lp-1s, the higher the cell viability. The maximum non-toxic dose toward the cells was greater than 50% OD_{490}; therefore, the maximum non-toxic dose of Lp-1s to IPEC-J2 cells is OD_{600} 0.45 (**Figure 1A**). The TGEV inhibition rate of Lp-1s decreased with increasing dilution factor and was thus concentration dependent. The results showed that amount of TGEV Miller strain (MOI = 0.1) was reduced by 1/4-fold by Lp-1s, i.e., the OD_{600} was 0.45, and the treated IPEC-J2 cells received the highest non-toxic dose of Lp-1s (**Figure 1B**).

Results of $TCID_{50}$ Experiment

The experimental data (**Figure 2**) showed that the TGEV titers at 12, 24, and 48 hpi after TGEV infection of IPEC-J2 cells treated with Lp-1s were $10^{2.5}$ $TCID_{50}$/mL, $10^{2.55}$ $TCID_{50}$/mL, and 103.3 $TCID_{50}$/mL, respectively. Compared with the TGEV control group, the amount of viral of lesions decreased by 1.1, 1.9, and 1.8-fold at 12, 24, and 48 hpi, respectively, in the Lp-1s group and no lesions appeared in the blank control group. Therefore, Lp-1s has a significant anti-TGEV effect ($^{**}p < 0.01$) and is optimal for antiviral activity at 24 hpi.

TGEV-N Gene Copy Number and Protein Expression Levels in Response to Lp-1s

We found that the TGEV N gene copy number in IPEC-J2 cells treated with Lp-1s was lower than that in cells infected with TGEV only ($^*p < 0.05$, $^{**}p < 0.01$). In addition, the viral N gene copy number in the TGEV infection group was positively correlated with the infection duration (**Figure 3A**). Western blotting showed that the level of the TGEV N protein in the Lp-1s group was lower than that in the TGEV group at all three time points. No expression of TGEV N protein was observed in the blank control group (**Figures 3B,C**). These results demonstrated that Lp-1s could inhibit the transcription and protein expression of TGEV N.

Lp-1s Induces IFN-β

The results in **Figure 4** indicate that IFN-β levels gradually increased in IPEC-J2 cells during TGEV infection. However, compared with the TGEV-infected group, the IFN-β level of the TGEV (MOI = 0.1)-infected group treated with Lp-1s increased significantly with infection time ($^{**}p < 0.01$). Therefore, Lp-1s can significantly increase the level of intracellular IFN-β during TGEV infection.

Lp-1s Stimulates the Phosphorylation of STAT1

The results in **Figure 5** show that there was almost no change in the total expression of STAT1 in IPEC-J2 cells under different treatments and at different time points; however, the amount of phosphorylated STAT1 changed significantly. The amount of phosphorylated STAT1 in the Lp-1s group was higher than that in the TGEV group at the different time points ($^*p < 0.05$ and $^{**}p < 0.01$), while only a small amount of phosphorylated STAT1 was detected in the blank control group at the different time points. Therefore, although TGEV infection could significantly increase the amount of phosphorylated STAT1, Lp-1s could further significantly increase the amount of phosphorylated STAT1 in cells after TGEV infection.

Lp-1s Activates Nuclear Translocation of p-STAT1

The results in **Figure 6** show that the amount of p-STAT1 (red fluorescence) in the nuclei of TGEV infected cells treated with Lp-1s at different time points was significantly higher than that in the nuclei of cells in TGEV infected group. At the same time, the amount of p-STAT1 correlated positively with the duration

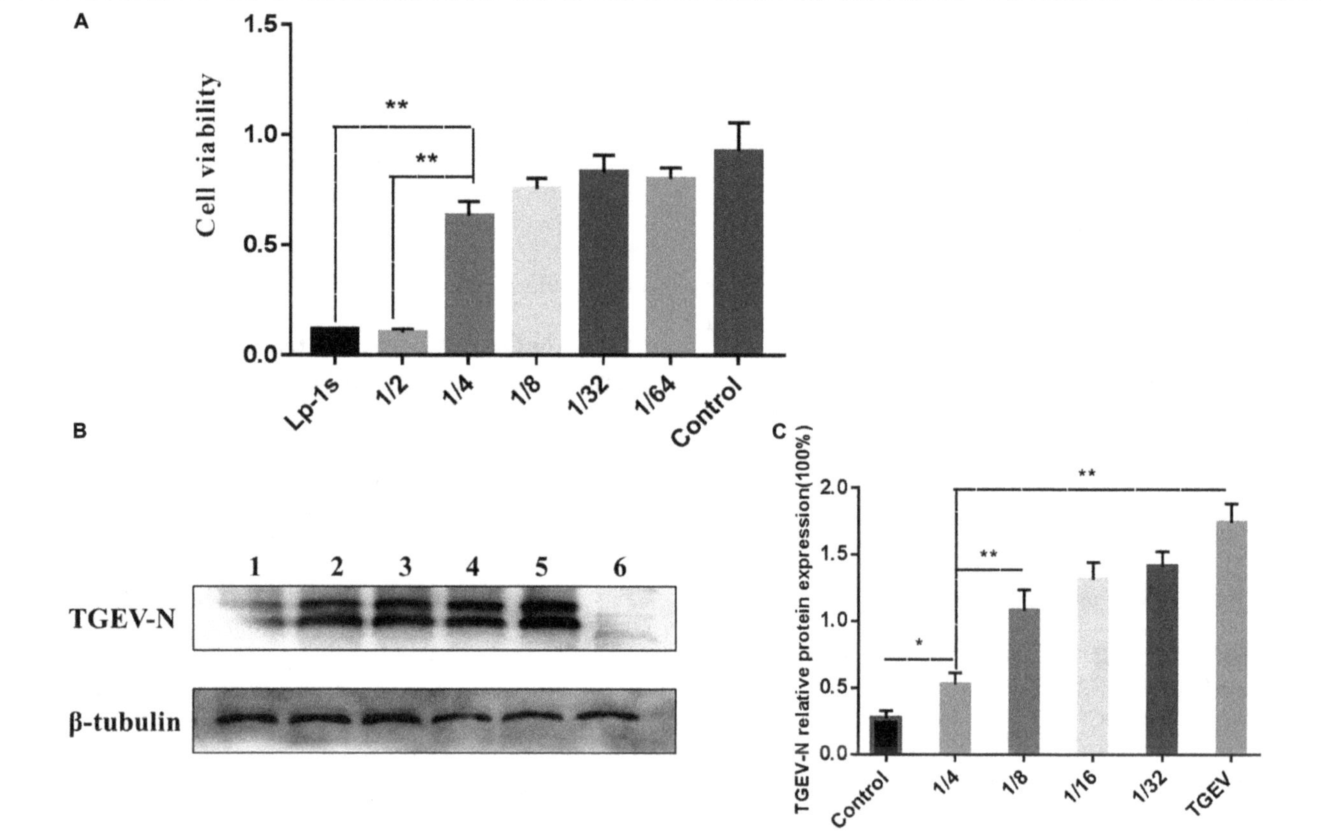

FIGURE 1 | MTT cytotoxicity test and Lp-1s concentration screening. **(A)** Results of Lp-1s cytotoxicity as detected using the MTT method on 1/4, 1/8, 1/32, and 1/64 times dilutions of Lp-1s acting on IPEC-J2 cells. The cell adherence state remained basically unchanged. According to the experimental data, the Lp-1s undiluted group, the 1/2-fold dilution group and the 1/4-fold dilution group showed significantly difference in cytotoxicity (**$P < 0.01$), and the 1/4-fold dilution group showed no significant difference compared with that of the control group ($P > 0.05$). **(B)** The expression of the TGEV N protein in IPEC-J2 cells treated with Lp-1s at different dilutions was detected by western blotting. Lane 1, infected TGEV group after Lp-1s 1/4 dilution pretreatment; Lane 2, infected TGEV group after Lp-1s 1/8 dilution pretreatment; Lane 3, infected TGEV group after Lp-1s 1/16 dilution pretreatment; Lane 4, infected TGEV group after Lp-1s 1/32 dilution pretreatment; Lane 5, TGEV infection group; and Lane 6, uninfected control cells (normal group). **(C)** Grayscale analysis of the relative expression of TGEV N in IPEC-J2 cells infected with Lp-1s at different dilutions showing that TGEV N protein levels were decreased in the 1/4-fold dilution of Lp-1s treatment group after 48 h, compared with the 1/8-fold dilution and TGEV infection group, there was a significant difference (**$P < 0.01$), which was significantly different from the control group (*$P < 0.05$).

of infection after Lp-1s-treatment of IPEC-J2 cells infected with TGEV. However, the amount of red fluorescence emitted by p-STAT1 labeled with Cy3 correlated negatively with the amount of green fluorescence emitted by FITC-labeled TGEV N protein. We found that when TGEV was directly infected into IPEC-J2 cells, the red fluorescence of p-STAT1 was mainly gathered around the cell wall and only a small amount appeared in the nucleus; the green fluorescence and red fluorescence of the blank control group were not obvious. Meanwhile, the signal intensity of p-STAT1 in the nuclei of the Lp-1s treatment group correlated positively with time (**Figure 6**). Therefore, Lp-1s could significantly increase the level of p-STAT1 and promoted its translocation into the nucleus, while simultaneously inhibiting the expression of TGEV N.

Transcriptional Expression of *ISGs*

We found that the mRNA expression levels of *ZAP*, *MX2*, *MX1*, *PKR*, *OASL*, and *ISG15* were significantly higher in the Lp-1s treated group than in the TGEV infected group at various points after infection. The expression levels of *ZAP*, *PKR*, *OASL*, and *ISG15* in each experimental group increased with time. The expression levels of *MX1* and *MX2* peaked at 24 h and then decreased at 48 h (**Figures 7A–F**). The results showed that the best time to STAT1-siRNA targeting gene silencing STAT1 was 48 h (**Figure 7G**), and the best interference fragment was STAT1-siRNA1 (**Figure 7H**). After gene silencing STAT1, we found that the expression of ISGs decreased compared to the groups which no knock down STAT1, and the expression ISGs of Lp-1s-treated TGEV infected group was higher than that of TGEV infected alone group (**Figures 7I–N**). The results showed that TGEV infection of IPEC-J2 cells treated with Lp-1s could stimulate the expression of *ISGs* in cells to inhibit viral replication.

Proteins Levels of ZAP, PKR, and p-PKR

As expected, the protein levels of ZAP, PKR, p-PKR (**Figures 8A–D**) at 24, and 48 hpi in the Lp-1s group were significantly higher than those in negative control group and TGEV group (ZAP, *$P < 0.05$ and PKR, **$P < 0.01$). There was

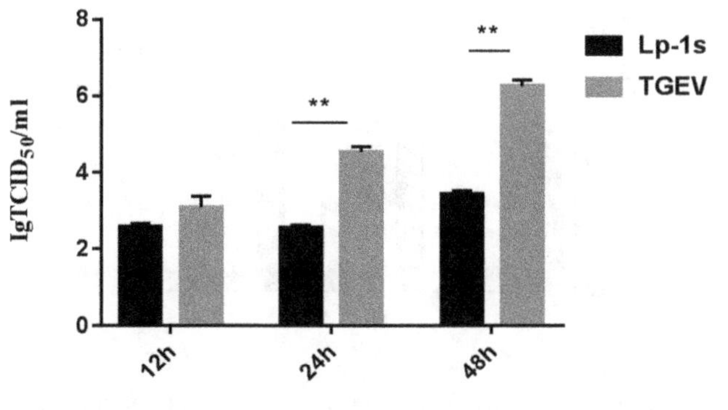

FIGURE 2 | $TCID_{50}$ analysis. The results of statistical analysis showed that the 24 h and 48 h Lp-1s supernatant treatment groups had significantly different $TCID_{50}$ values compared with that of the simultaneous TGEV challenge group ($^{**}P < 0.01$) demonstrating that IPEC-J2 had a reduced viral titer of the TGEV Miller strain after treatment with Lp-1s.

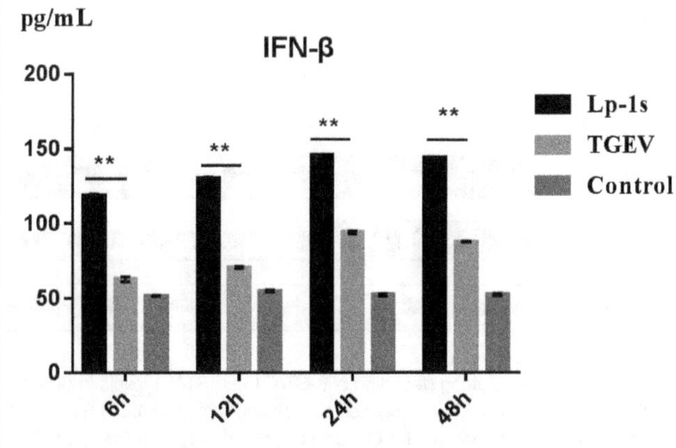

FIGURE 4 | Changes in IFN-β levels induced by cells in different groups. Lp-1s, Lp-1s pretreatment of IPEC-J2 cells infected with TGEV; TGEV, cells directly infected with TGEV; Con, uninfected cells (normal group). There were significant differences in IFN-β levels between the TGEV group and the Lp-1s group at different time points ($^{**}P < 0.01$).

no significant change in the relative expression of p-PKR/PKR, however, the expression level of p-PKR protein varied with the amount of PKR protein. The level of STAT-1 in **Figure 8E** where the expression of this gene was knocked down using siRNA is significantly lower than the level of unknocked down STAT1 in **Figure 5A**. After gene silencing STAT1, the protein levels of STAT1, p-STAT1 ZAP, PKR, p-PKR (**Figures 8E–H**) at 12, 24, and 48 hpi in the Lp-1s group were significantly higher than TGEV group (p-STAT1/STAT1, $^{*}P < 0.05$; ZAP, $^{*}P < 0.05$; and p-PKR/PKR, $^{*}P < 0.05$). The results showed that Lp-1s could

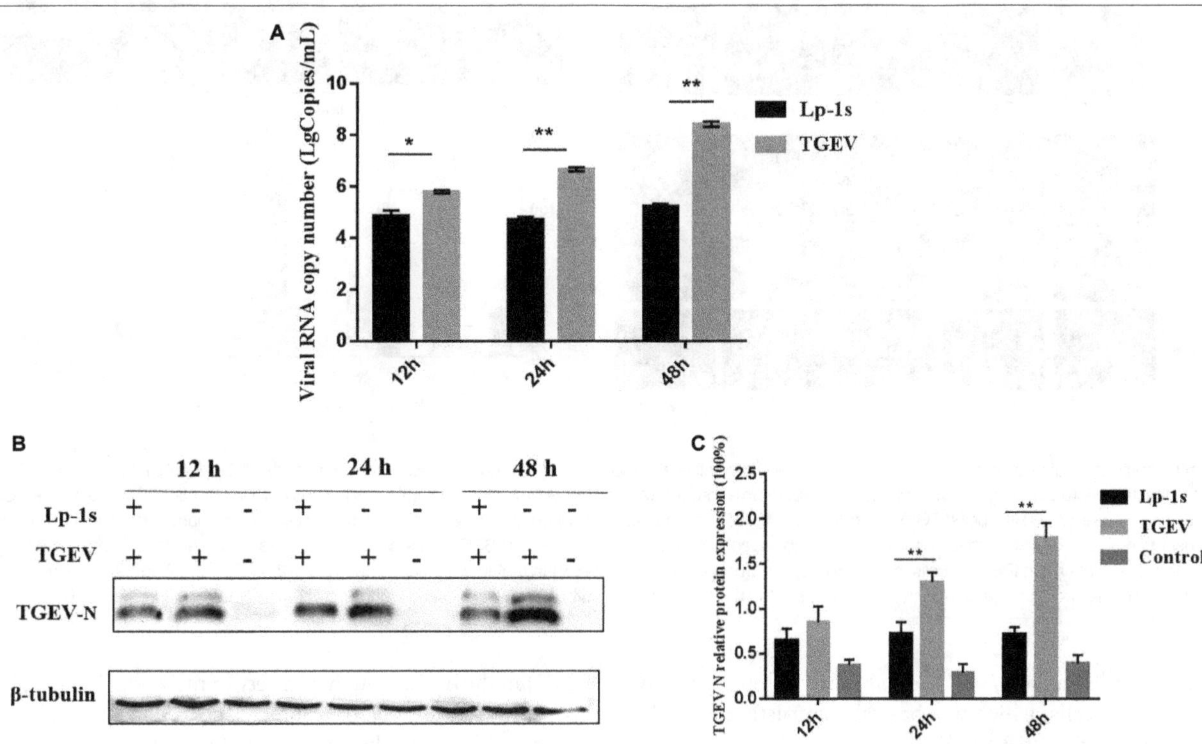

FIGURE 3 | Time course of TGEV N gene and protein expression. **(A)** TGEV N gene copy number in different groups of cells infected with TGEV for 12, 24, and 48 h. The TGEV N gene copy number was significantly different between the TGEV group and the TGEV group after treatment with Lp-1s for 12 h ($^{*}P < 0.05$). The TGEV group and the TGEV group with Lp-1s treatment infected for 24 and 48 h showed a significant difference ($^{**}P < 0.01$). **(B)** Western blotting detection of TGEV N protein levels at different time points after infection of TGEV in Lp-1s-treated cells. **(C)** Grayscale analysis of TGEV N protein levels at different time points after infection of TGEV by Lp-1s treated cells. There was no significant difference between the two groups ($P > 0.05$) at 12 h; however, the difference was extremely significant at 24 and 48 h ($^{**}P < 0.01$). Lp-1s, Lp-1s pretreatment of IPEC-J2 cells infected with TGEV; TGEV, cells directly infected with TGEV.

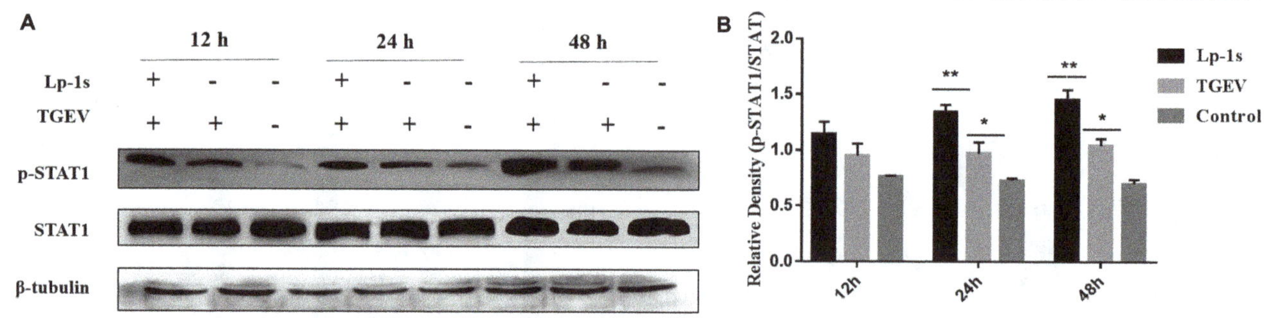

FIGURE 5 | Western blotting detection of p-STAT1 and STAT1 levels in different groups. Lp-1s, Lp-1s pretreatment of IPEC-J2 cells infected with TGEV; TGEV, cells directly infected with TGEV; Con, uninfected cells (normal group). **(A)** STAT1 total protein levels and phosphorylated STAT1 levels at 12–48 h. **(B)** Grayscale analysis of the levels of phosphorylated STAT1 in the different groups. Statistical analysis showed that the level of phosphorylated STAT1 was higher in the Lp-1s group than in the TGEV group after 12 h ($P > 0.05$); after 24 h of Lp-1s treatment, the level of phosphorylated STAT1 in the Lp-1s group was significantly higher than that in the TGEV group ($^{**}P < 0.01$); after 48 h of Lp-1s treatment, the level of phosphorylated STAT1 in the Lp-1s group was significantly higher than that in the TGEV group ($^{*}P < 0.05$). The results showed that treatment of TGEV-infected IPEC-J2 cells with Lp-1s (24–48 h), induced increased of levels of phosphorylated intracellular STAT1.

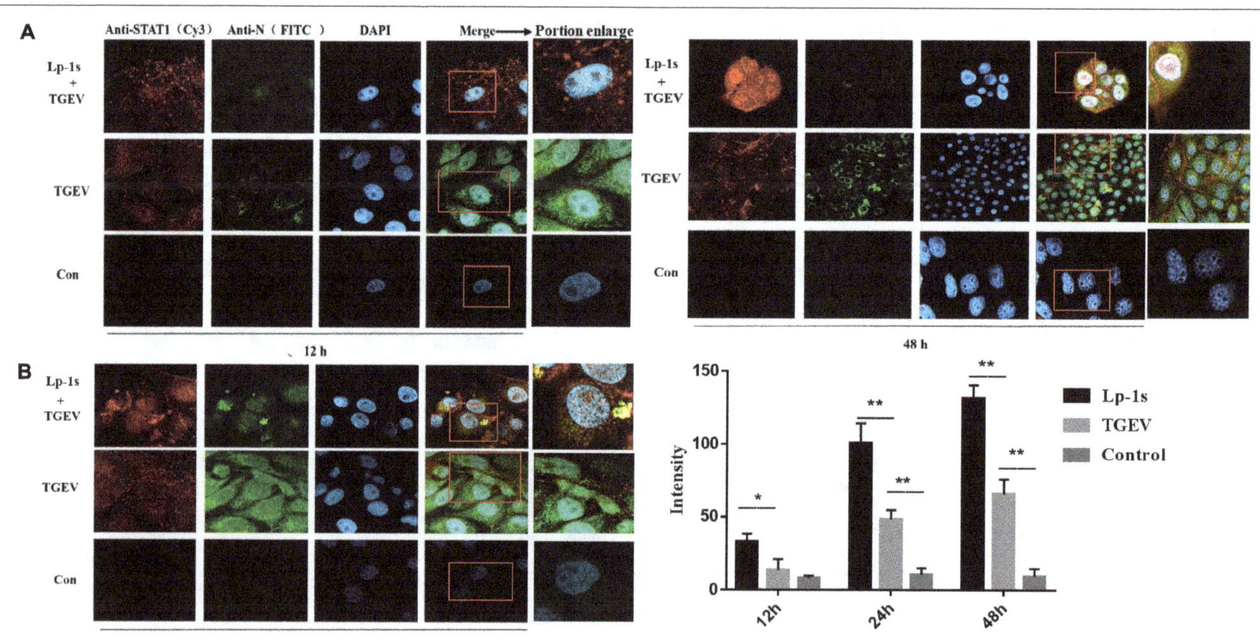

FIGURE 6 | Identification of nuclear translocation in porcine p-STAT by IFA (magnification: 63×). Lp-1s, Lp-1s pretreatment of IPEC-J2 cells infected with TGEV; TGEV, cells directly infected with TGEV; Con, uninfected cells (normal group). **(A)** Anti-pSTAT1 (Cy3), goat anti-rabbit IgG Cy3 labeled p-STAT1 protein; Anti-TGEV N (FITC), goat anti-mouse IgG FITC labeled TGEV N protein; DAPI, DAPI nuclear staining; Merge, fused image of the three fluorescent images. **(B)** The nucleus was identified using Zen blue software and the intensity of red fluorescence emitted by Cy3-labeled p-STAT1 was analyzed. The statistical results showed that the fluorescence intensity of Cy3 in IPEC-J2 cells treated with Lp-1s was significantly higher than that in the TGEV group after 12 h ($^{*}P < 0.05$). In the late stage of TGEV infection (24–48 h), the fluorescence signal intensity of p-STAT1 in the nucleus of this group was significantly higher than that in TGEV group ($^{**}P < 0.01$).

increase the expression of *ISGs* and inhibit the replication of TGEV in IPEC-J2 cells, which was basically consistent with the expression trend of the *PKR* and *ZAP* genes.

DISCUSSION

Previous studies have found that many lactic acid bacteria can inhibit the infection of diarrhea-causing viruses (such as RV and PEDV) in the host through a variety of methods (Hou et al., 2007; Kawakami et al., 2010). Some lactic acid bacteria can be recognized by Toll like receptor (TLR)-2 or TLR-9 to enhance their response to stimulation by the interferon inducer poly (I: C) and induce a large amount of IFN-I (Maeda et al., 2009; Kanmani and Kim, 2018; Lee et al., 2019). At the same time, they can also upregulate the transcription of *IL6* and *TNFA* (Reyes-Diaz et al., 2018). In addition, some lactic acid bacteria can enhance the expression of surface molecules and cytokines in intestinal

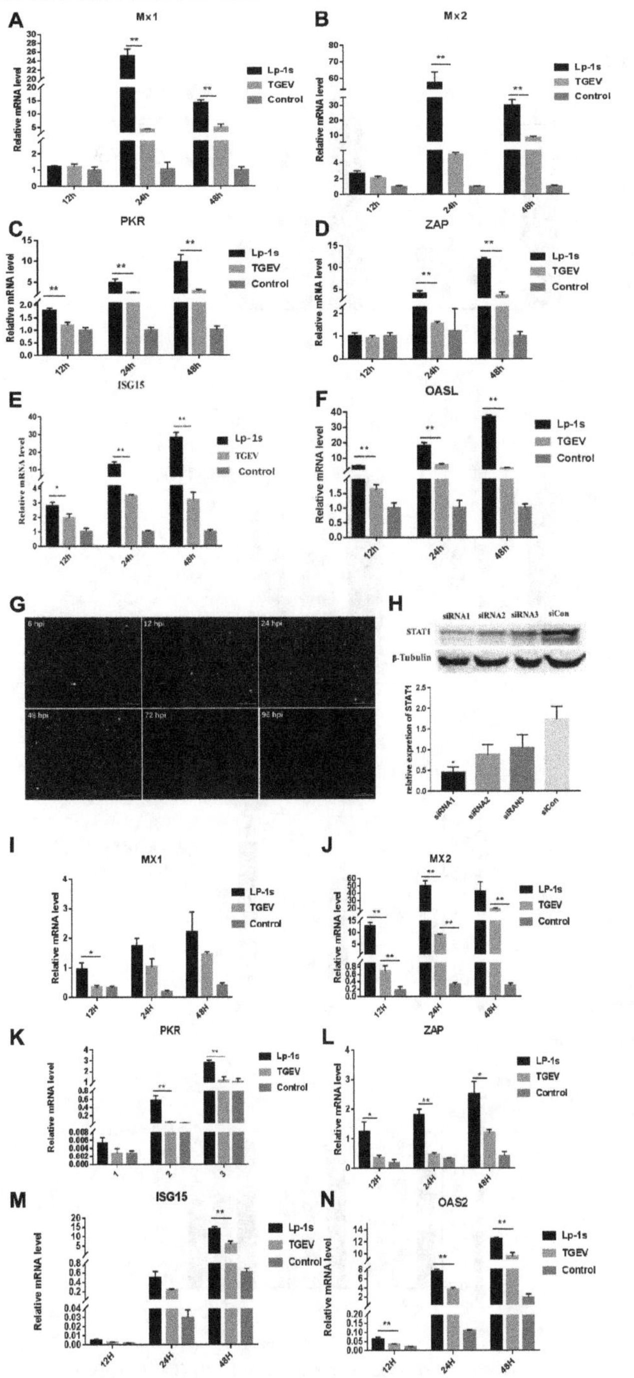

FIGURE 7 | Relative mRNA expression levels of *ISGs* in different experimental groups. Lp-1s, Lp-1s pretreatment of IPEC-J2 cells infected with TGEV; TGEV, cells directly infected with TGEV; Con, uninfected cells (normal group). **(A–F)** Relative mRNA expression levels of *MX1*, *MX2*, *PKR*, *ZAP*, *ISG15*, and *OASL*, respectively. The expression levels of *ZAP*, *MX2*, and *MX1* in Lp-1s group after 12 h were not significantly different from those in the TGEV group ($P > 0.05$). The expression level of *ISG15* was significantly higher in the Lp-1s group than in the TGEV group ($^{*}P < 0.05$). The expression levels of *PKR* and *OASL* were significantly higher in the Lp-1s group than in the TGEV group ($^{**}P < 0.01$). The expression levels of *ZAP*, *MX2*, *MX1*, *PKR*, *OASL*, and *ISG15* in the Lp-1s group after 24 and 48 h were significantly higher than (Continued)

FIGURE 7 | Continued
those in the TGEV group ($^{**}P < 0.01$). **(G,H)** Screening of siRNA targeting STAT1 optimal treatment time and gene silencing efficiency fragment. As shown in the figure, the optimal time for siRNA targeting STAT1 is 48 h, and the best gene silencing siRNA fragment is siRNA1 ($^{*}P < 0.05$). **(I–N)** Relative mRNA expression levels of *MX1*, *MX2*, *PKR*, *ZAP*, *ISG15*, and *OASL*, respectively, after targeting gene silencing STAT1. The expression levels of *PKR* and *OASL* in Lp-1s group after 12 h were not significantly different from those in the TGEV group ($P > 0.05$). The expression level of *MX2*, *PKR*, *ZAP*, *ISG15*, and *OASL* was significantly higher in the Lp-1s group after 24 h than in the TGEV group ($^{*}P < 0.05$ and $^{**}P < 0.01$). The expression levels of *ZAP*, *ISG15* and *OASL* were significantly higher in the Lp-1s group after 48 h than in the TGEV group ($^{*}P < 0.05$ and $^{**}P < 0.01$).

antigen presenting cells (APC), and enhance the molecular expression of MHC-II and IL-1β (Villena et al., 2014). In addition, other lactic acid bacteria can also stimulate the response level of TLR-3 to poly (I: C) (Hosoya et al., 2011). They can also regulate the role of TLR-2, TLR-4, and TLR negative regulators in the immune response, further enhancing the production of IFN-I induced by cells, and upregulate the transcription level of related antiviral factors (such as *MXA* and *OASL*) (Castillo et al., 2011). Other studies have shown that probiotics can inhibit TGEV infection by adsorbing virus particles and stimulating cells to produce innate immunity (Chai et al., 2013).

Recent studies have shown that the main reasons why the body's interferon-beta (IFN-β) cannot fully exert its antiviral effect after TGEV infection are as follows: First, the cells do not respond in time to the immune response because of the level of viral replication and the virus titer of TGEV in the early stage of infection, resulting in lower levels of IFNs, which is the main cause of the short burst of TGEV latency (Zhu et al., 2017). Second, IFN-β does not play a direct antiviral role. Its antiviral function is produced by activating the IFN-mediated JAK-STAT signaling pathway to stimulate downstream interferon-stimulating genes *(ISGs)* (Saha and Pahan, 2006; Li, 2008; Proia et al., 2011). And, activation of the JAK-STAT1 signaling pathway requires Phosphorylated STAT1 (Tyr 701) enters the nucleus to activate interferon-stimulating factors *ISGs* (including MX1, MX2, PKR, OAS, ISG15, and ZAP) (Hovanessian, 1991; Zhu et al., 1997; Shi et al., 2010; Goujon et al., 2013; Amici et al., 2015; Li et al., 2015; Nigg and Pavlovic, 2015). ZAP can bind viral RNA directly and prevent the accumulation of viral RNA in the cytoplasm. It can also recruit RNA exosomes to degrade target viral RNA (Li et al., 2015). PKR-mediated inhibition of viral replication is activated by the formation of dsRNA during the replication of single-stranded RNA after viruses invade cells. The main reason is that the amino terminus of PKR can recognize the dsRNA domain and the carboxyl terminus has the kinase domain. When the viral double-stranded RNA is recognized, the inactive PKR protein located in the cytoplasm is phosphorylated. On the other hand, it can also regulate the cell immune response and autophagy caused by virus invasion to inhibit the virus. At the same time, PKR can activate the nuclear factor kappa B (NF-kB) signaling pathway via phosphorylation and further induce IFN production in cells (Sudhakar et al., 2000; Amici et al., 2015).

In the present study, we found that IPEC-J2 cells still produced IFN-β after infection with TGEV, which increased with time,

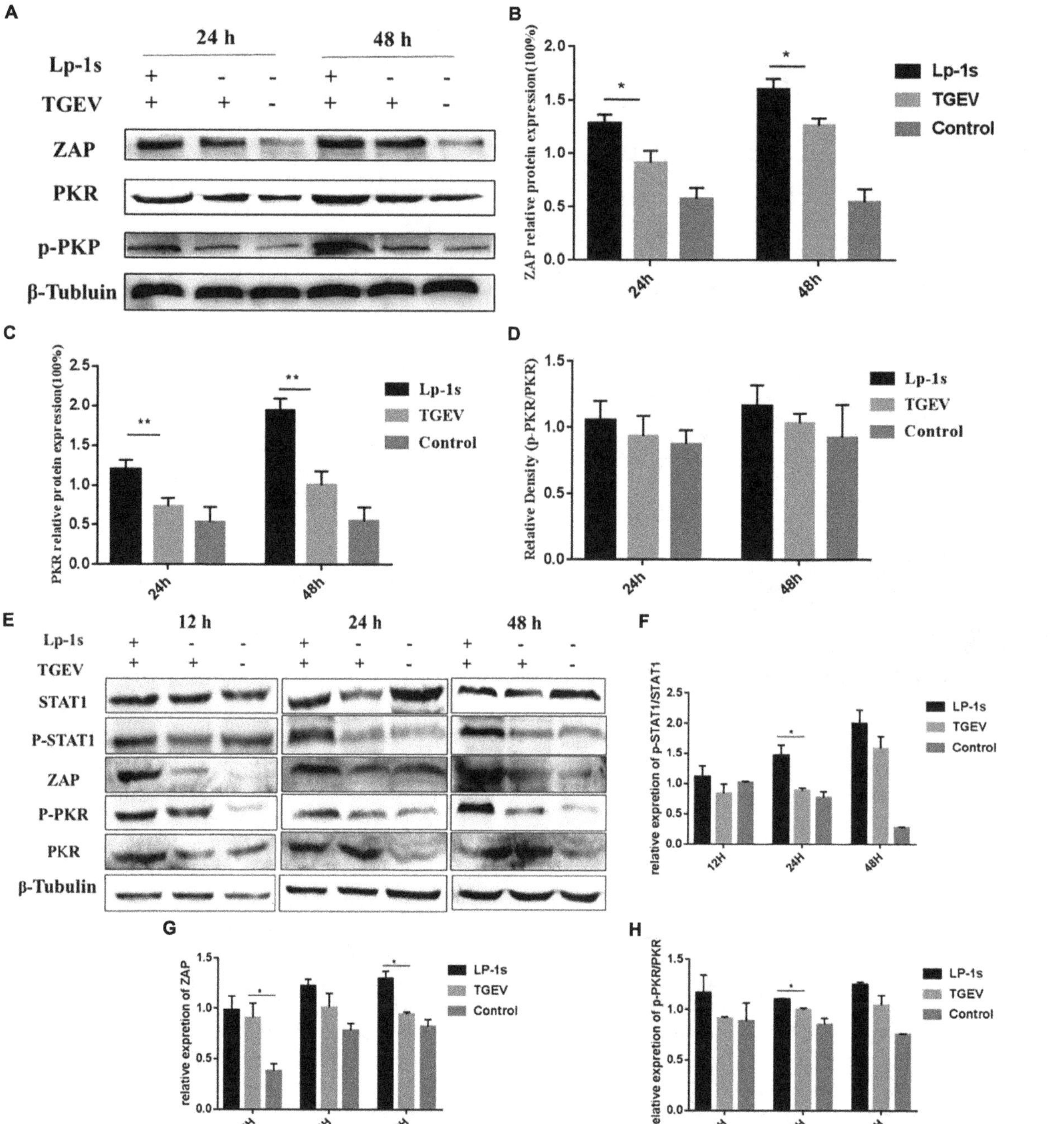

FIGURE 8 | Protein levels of ZAP, PKR and p-PKR in different experimental groups. Lp-1s, Lp-1s pretreatment of IPEC-J2 cells infected with TGEV; TGEV, cells directly infected with TGEV; Con, Uninfected cells (normal group). **(A)** The expression of ZAP, PKR, p-PKR, and β-Tubulin protein. **(B)** Grayscale analysis of the ZAP/β-Tubulin results. The ZAP level of Lp-1s treatment group was significantly higher than TGEV infected alone at 24 and 48 h (*$P < 0.05$). **(C)** Grayscale analysis of the PKR/β-Tubulin ratio. The ratio of PKR/β-Tubulin in the Lp-1s group was significantly higher after 48 h compared with that in the TGEV group (**$P < 0.01$). **(D)** Grayscale analysis of the p-PKR/PKR ratio. There was no significant difference in the p-PKR/PKR ratio at the different time points ($P > 0.05$). **(E–H)** The expression of STAT1, p-STAT1, ZAP, PKR, and p-PKR proteins after silencing STAT1. **(E)** The expression of STAT1, p-STAT1, ZAP, PKR, p-PKR, and β-Tubulin protein. **(F)** Relative expression of p-STAT1/STAT1 in Lp-1s treatment group was significantly higher than TGEV infected alone at 24 h (*$P < 0.05$). **(G)** Relative expression of ZAP in Lp-1s treatment group was significantly higher than TGEV infected alone at 48 h (*$P < 0.05$). **(H)** Relative expression of p-PKR/PKR in Lp-1s treatment group was significantly higher than TGEV infected alone at 24 h (*$P < 0.05$).

reaching a peak at 24 h and no longer increased at 48 h. At the corresponding time points, the level of infection, viral titer, and replication of TGEV on IPEC-J2 cells showed an increasing trend. After Lp-1s treatment, IPEC-J2 cells produced a large amount of IFN-β at the early stage of TGEV infection (6 h), which was significantly higher than that of cells infected with TGEV only.

The induced level of IFN-β in Lp-1s-treated IPEC-J2 cells was significantly different from that in the TGEV infected group at the same time point. The induction level of IFN-β in the Lp-1s treated group was significantly higher than that in TGEV infected group at the different time points. The level of IFN-β induction correlated positively with time, peaking at 24 h before decreasing toward 48 h. The early boost in IFN-β production in IPEC-J2 cells treated with Lp-1s might be one of the reasons for its inhibition of TGEV.

In addition, although TGEV delayed the expression of IFN-β in the early stage of infection, it promoted the expression of IFN-β at the peak of viral replication. The expression of IFN-β was parallel to the increase of viral RNA replication level at 24–48h, which demonstrated that TGEV replication remained high in the late stage of infection when IFN-β was produced in large quantities. This might be caused by the inhibitory effect of TGEV on IFN-β-mediated signaling pathways, resulting in the inability of IFN-β to regulate the transcription and expression of downstream target cytokines and exert an antiviral role.

Although there was no significant difference in the levels of p-STAT1 between the Lp-1s group and the TGEV group at 12 hpi, the level of p-STAT1 in the Lp-1s group was significantly higher than that in the TGEV group at the later stages (24 and 48 h). The level of p-STAT1 in the Lp-1s group correlated positively with time from 12–48 h. The results showed that IPEC-J2 cells treated with Lp-1s could effectively increase STAT1 phosphorylation in the late stage of virus infection. At the same time, the level of p-STAT1 changed slightly from 12–48 h after infection with TGEV. The results were quite different from those reported in previous studies on the infection of ST cells by TGEV. In addition, the level of p-STAT1 in IPEC-J2 cells infected with TGEV from 24–48 h was significantly lower than that in ST cells infected with TGEV from 24–48 h, which might reflect the difference between the cell lines and viruses used.

Further experiments showed that the level p-STAT1 nuclear translocation in the Lp-1s group was significantly higher than that in the TGEV group at the same time points, and p-STAT1 nuclear accumulation correlated positively with time. In TGEV-infected cells, p-STAT1 at the late stage of infection (24–48 h) accumulated in large amounts near the cell membrane and only a few nuclear translocations occurred. We speculated that the reason might be that the intracellular STAT1 protein is activated by IFN-β after IPEC-J2 cells are directly infected with TGEV to form a homologous or heterodimer, and the virus interacts with its receptor IRF9. The interaction resulted in the inability of activated STAT1 to undergo nuclear translocation through receptor-induced endocytosis, and could only dissociate around IFNAR, which reduced the JAK-STAT signaling pathway cascade response and antagonized the antiviral effect of IFN-β. The fluorescence value of activated STAT1 was significantly higher than that of blank control group. This indicated that TGEV could not completely escape the immune mechanism of IFN-β

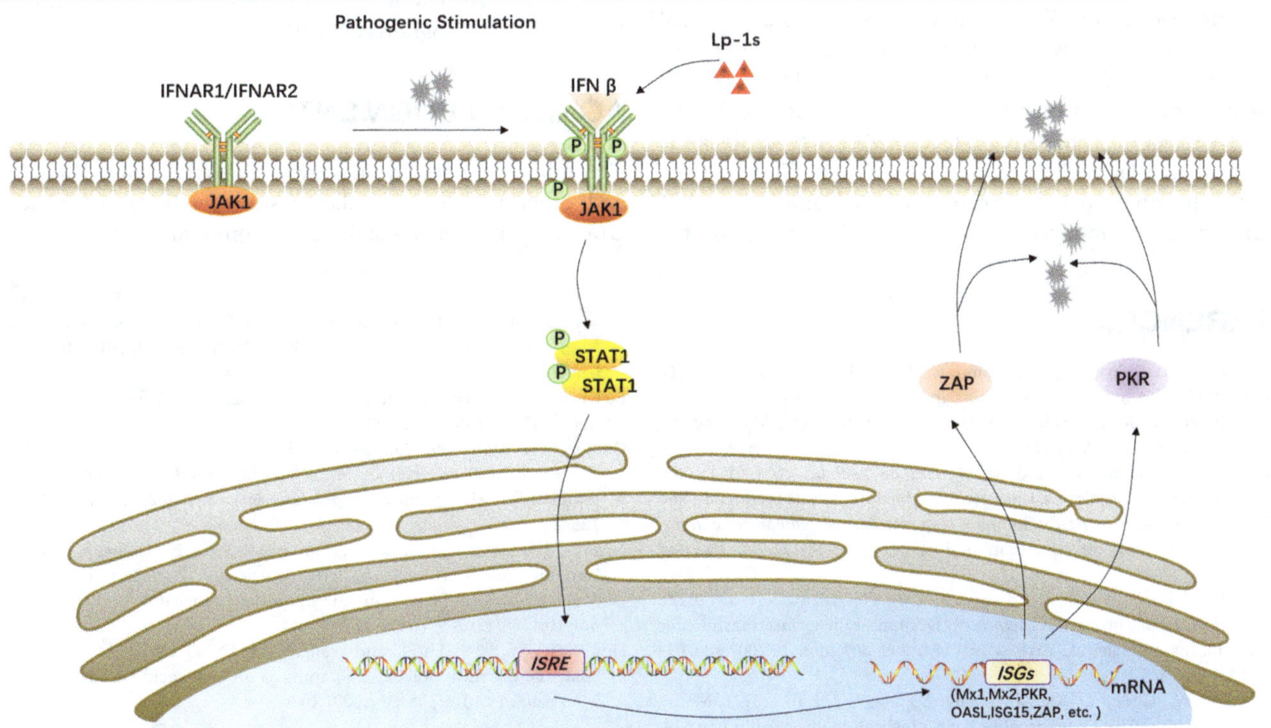

FIGURE 9 | Proposed mechanism of the anti-TGEV effect of Lp-1s. Lp-1s increases IFN-β expression, and the binding of IFN-β to its receptor IFNAR leads to activation of the Janus family kinase (JAK) and subsequent activation of signal transduction and transcriptional activator 1 (STAT1) signaling cascades. These signaling pathways upregulate downstream interferon-stimulated genes (*ISGs*), including *MX1*, *MX2*, *PKR*, *OAS*, *ISG15*, and *ZAP*), which produce the corresponding antiviral proteins, e.g., ZAP and PKR, ultimately activating IFN-β to exert an antiviral effect.

production in IPEC-J2 cells. At the same time, the fluorescence intensity of p-STAT in the nucleus of the cells in the Lp-1s treatment group correlated positively with time, and the intensity of FITC-labeled TGEV N protein was significantly lower than that in the TGEV treatment group at the same time point. These results showed that IPEC-J2 cells treated with Lp-1s could indeed activate the JAK-STAT1 signaling pathway when infected with TGEV, and the intensity of JAK-STAT1 signaling pathway was significantly higher in the Lp-1s-treated cells than in the cells directly infected with TGEV. As the signaling pathway cascade response increased, the replication level of TGEV in IPEC-J2 cells was further inhibited.

Finally, the transcriptional levels of *ISGs* in the Lp-1s treatment group were different at different time points. *MX1* and *MX2* reached their peak at 24 h, while the transcriptional levels of the two *ISGs* decreased at 48 h after TGEV infection. The transcription levels of *PKR*, *ZAP*, OASL and *ISG15* were positively correlated in groups. We speculated that the decrease in *MX1* and *MX2* mRNA transcription levels within 48 h after Lp-1s treatment might be related to the cycle of infected cells. The expression of *ISGs* of gene silenced STAT1 decreased as a whole compared to the groups which no knock down STAT1, indicating that STAT1 could affect downstream *ISGs*. While the *ISGs* of TGEV infected group treated with Lp-1s showed an upward trend, which further confirmed that Lp-1s could activate downstream *ISGs*. To further explore the difference in the intracellular response of Lp-1s treated IPEC-J2 cells to TGEV infection, we detected the changes in ZAP and PKR protein levels. The level of the ZAP protein in the Lp-1s and TGEV groups was consistent with its transcription level at the time point. Although the level of the ZAP protein in Lp-1s treated cells was significantly higher than that in the TGEV infection group, the difference in the transcription level of *ZAP* was significantly lower than that in the TGEV infection group. These results suggested that after Lp-1s treatment, the IFN-β and JAK-STAT1 signaling pathways induced in the cells are enhanced, and the expression of the ZAP protein is still limited, suggesting that other factors have an impact on the transcriptional regulation of ZAP. The protein level of PKR was consistent with its mRNA transcription level. There was no significant difference in the p-PKR/PKR values between the two groups at 24 and 48 h; however, the p-PKR/β-tubulin protein values were in line with our expectations. The results showed that the p-PKR level in the Lp-1s group was significantly higher than that in the TGEV group, and correlated positively with time. Therefore, we believe that the increase in p-PKR is mainly determined by the expression of the PKR protein.

Based on the above results, Lp-1s plays an antiviral role by stimulating the IFN-β-mediated JAK1/STAT pathway, resulting in upregulation interferon-stimulating genes, which induce the synthesis of antiviral proteins such as ZAP and PKR (**Figure 9**).

AUTHOR CONTRIBUTIONS

KW and ZS conceived and designed the experiments. KW, LR, and TY performed the experiments. ZN, ZK, YZ, YY, LX, SH, QY, and DW analyzed the data. LR and ZS wrote the manuscript.

FUNDING

This work was supported by the Fundamental Research Funds for the Central Universities (XDJK2018B023), and the Chongqing Basic Research Program (CYS19137).

ACKNOWLEDGMENTS

The authors gratefully acknowledge Peng Yuan, Zhou Yang, and other veterinary medicine students from the Southwest University for their valuable suggestions and assistance.

REFERENCES

Amici, C., La Frazia, S., Brunelli, C., Balsamo, M., Angelini, M., and Santoro, M. G. (2015). Inhibition of viral protein translation by indomethacin in vesicular stomatitis virus infection: role of eIF2alpha kinase PKR. *Cell Microbiol.* 17, 1391–1404. doi: 10.1111/cmi.12446

Castillo, N. A., Perdigon, G., and de Moreno de Leblanc, A. (2011). Oral administration of a probiotic *Lactobacillus* modulates cytokine production and TLR expression improving the immune response against *Salmonella enterica* serovar Typhimurium infection in mice. *BMC Microbiol.* 11:177. doi: 10.1186/1471-2180-11-177

Chai, W., Burwinkel, M., Wang, Z., Palissa, C., Esch, B., Twardziok, S., et al. (2013). Antiviral effects of a probiotic *Enterococcus* faecium strain against transmissible gastroenteritis coronavirus. *Arch. Virol.* 158, 799–807. doi: 10.1007/s00705-012-1543-0

Chen, J., Xu, W., Chen, Y., Xie, X., Zhang, Y., Ma, C., et al. (2017). Matrix metalloproteinase 9 facilitates hepatitis B virus replication through binding with type I interferon (IFN) receptor 1 to repress IFN/JAK/STAT signaling. *J. Virol.* 91:e1824-16. doi: 10.1128/JVI.01824-16

da Silva Sabo, S., Perez-Rodriguez, N., Dominguez, J. M., and de Souza Oliveira, R. P. (2017). Inhibitory substances production by *Lactobacillus plantarum* ST16Pa cultured in hydrolyzed cheese whey supplemented with soybean flour and their antimicrobial efficiency as biopreservatives on fresh chicken meat. *Food Res. Int.* 99, 762–769. doi: 10.1016/j.foodres.2017.05.026

Fuller, R. (1989). Probiotics in man and animals. *J. Appl. Bacteriol.* 66, 365–378. doi: 10.1111/j.1365-2672.1989.tb05105.x

Goujon, C., Moncorge, O., Bauby, H., Doyle, T., Ward, C. C., Schaller, T., et al. (2013). Human MX2 is an interferon-induced post-entry inhibitor of HIV-1 infection. *Nature* 502, 559–562. doi: 10.1038/nature12542

Hosoya, S., Villena, J., Shimazu, T., Tohno, M., Fujie, H., Chiba, E., et al. (2011). Immunobiotic lactic acid bacteria beneficially regulate immune response triggered by poly(I:C) in porcine intestinal epithelial cells. *Vet Res.* 42, 111. doi: 10.1186/1297-9716-42-111

Hou, X. L., Yu, L. Y., Liu, J., and Wang, G. H. (2007). Surface-displayed porcine epidemic diarrhea viral (PEDV) antigens on lactic acid bacteria. *Vaccine.* 26, 24–31. doi: 10.1016/j.vaccine.2007.10.065

Hovanessian, A. G. (1991). Interferon-induced and double-stranded RNA-activated enzymes: a specific protein kinase and 2′,5′-oligoadenylate synthetases. *J. Interferon Res.* 11, 199–205. doi: 10.1089/jir.1991.11.199

Kanmani, P., and Kim, H. (2018). Protective effects of lactic acid bacteria against TLR4 induced inflammatory response in hepatoma HepG2 cells through modulation of toll-like receptor negative regulators of mitogen-activated protein Kinase and NF-kappaB signaling. *Front. Immunol.* 9:1537. doi: 10.3389/fimmu.2018.01537

Kawakami, S. I., Yamada, T., Nakanishi, N., and Cai, Y. M. (2010). Feeding of lactic acid bacteria and yeast on growth and diarrhea of Holstein Calves. *J. Anim. Vet. Adv.* 9, 1112–1114. doi: 10.3923/javaa.2010.1112.1114

Kawashima, T., Hayashi, K., Kosaka, A., Kawashima, M., Igarashi, T., Tsutsui, H., et al. (2011). *Lactobacillus plantarum* strain YU from fermented foods activates Th1 and protective immune responses. *Int. Immunopharmacol.* 11, 2017–2024. doi: 10.1016/j.intimp.2011.08.013

Lee, B. M., Han, Y. W., Kim, S. B., Rahman, M. M., Uyangaa, E., Kim, J. H., et al. (2011). Enhanced protection against infection with transmissible gastroenteritis virus in piglets by oral co-administration of live attenuated *Salmonella enterica* serovar Typhimurium expressing swine interferon-alpha and interleukin-18. *Comp. Immunol. Microbiol. Infect Dis.* 34, 369–380. doi: 10.1016/j.cimid.2011.05.001

Lee, E. S., Song, E. J., Nam, Y. D., and Lee, S. Y. (2018). Probiotics in human health and disease: from nutribiotics to pharmabiotics. *J. Microbiol.* 56, 773–782. doi: 10.1007/s12275-018-8293-y

Lee, J., Jung, I., Choi, J. W., Lee, C. W., Cho, S., Choi, T. G., et al. (2019). Micronized and heat-treated *Lactobacillus plantarum* LM1004 stimulates host immune responses Via the TLR-2/MAPK/NF-kappaB signalling pathway in vitro and in vivo. *J. Microbiol. Biotechnol.* 29, 704–712. doi: 10.4014/jmb.1812.12059

Li, M., Yan, K., Wei, L., Yang, J., Lu, C., Xiong, F., et al. (2015). Zinc finger antiviral protein inhibits coxsackievirus B3 virus replication and protects against viral myocarditis. *Antiviral. Res.* 123, 50–61. doi: 10.1016/j.antiviral.2015.09.001

Li, W. X. (2008). Canonical and non-canonical JAK-STAT signaling. *Trends Cell Biol.* 18, 545–551. doi: 10.1016/j.tcb.2008.08.008

Maeda, N., Nakamura, R., Hirose, Y., Murosaki, S., Yamamoto, Y., Kase, T., et al. (2009). Oral administration of heat-killed *Lactobacillus plantarum* L-137 enhances protection against influenza virus infection by stimulation of type I interferon production in mice. *Int. Immunopharmacol.* 9, 1122–1125. doi: 10.1016/j.intimp.2009.04.015

Maragkoudakis, P. A., Chingwaru, W., Gradisnik, L., Tsakalidou, E., and Cencic, A. (2010). Lactic acid bacteria efficiently protect human and animal intestinal epithelial and immune cells from enteric virus infection. *Int. J. Food Microbiol.* 141(Suppl. 1), S91–S97. doi: 10.1016/j.ijfoodmicro.2009.12.024

Masters, P. S. (2006). The molecular biology of coronaviruses. *Adv. Virus Res.* 66, 193–292. doi: 10.1016/S0065-3527(06)66005-3

Nigg, P. E., and Pavlovic, J. (2015). Oligomerization and GTP-binding requirements of MxA for viral target recognition and antiviral activity against influenza a virus. *J. Biol. Chem.* 290, 29893–29906. doi: 10.1074/jbc.M115.681494

Pollmann, M., Nordhoff, M., Pospischil, A., Tedin, K., and Wieler, L. H. (2005). Effects of a probiotic strain of *Enterococcus* faecium on the rate of natural chlamydia infection in swine. *Infect Immun.* 73, 4346–4353. doi: 10.1128/IAI.73.7.4346-4353.2005

Proia, D. A., Foley, K. P., Korbut, T., Sang, J., Smith, D., Bates, R. C., et al. (2011). Multifaceted intervention by the Hsp90 inhibitor ganetespib (STA-9090) in cancer cells with activated JAK/STAT signaling. *PLoS One.* 6:e18552. doi: 10.1371/journal.pone.0018552

Reyes-Diaz, A., Mata-Haro, V., Hernandez, J., Gonzalez-Cordova, A. F., Hernandez-Mendoza, A., Reyes-Diaz, R., et al. (2018). Milk fermented by specific *Lactobacillus* strains regulates the serum levels of IL-6, TNF-alpha and IL-10 cytokines in a LPS-stimulated murine model. *Nutrients* 10, E691. doi: 10.3390/nu10060691

Saha, R. N., and Pahan, K. (2006). Regulation of inducible nitric oxide synthase gene in glial cells. *Antioxid Redox Signal.* 8, 929–947. doi: 10.1089/ars.2006.8.929

Scharek, L., Guth, J., Filter, M., and Schmidt, M. F. (2007). Impact of the probiotic bacteria *Enterococcus* faecium NCIMB 10415 (SF68) and Bacillus cereus var. toyoi NCIMB 40112 on the development of serum IgG and faecal IgA of sows and their piglets. *Arch. Anim. Nutr.* 61, 223–234. doi: 10.1080/17450390701431540

Shi, H. X., Yang, K., Liu, X., Liu, X. Y., Wei, B., Shan, Y. F., et al. (2010). Positive regulation of interferon regulatory factor 3 activation by Herc5 via ISG15 modification. *Mol. Cell Biol.* 30, 2424–2436. doi: 10.1128/MCB.01466-09

Song Han, T. L., Li, W., Wei, D., Peng, Y., Zhou, Y., and Zhenhui, S. (2017). Identification of a intestinal probiotic strain from piglets and preliminary study on the strain against the proliferation of TGEV in vitro. *Heilongjiang Animal Husbandry and Veterinary* 17, 178–181.

Stofilova, J., Langerholc, T., Botta, C., Treven, P., Gradisnik, L., Salaj, R., et al. (2017). Cytokine production in vitro and in rat model of colitis in response to *Lactobacillus plantarum* LS/07. *Biomed Pharmacother.* 94, 1176–1185. doi: 10.1016/j.biopha.2017.07.138

Sudhakar, A., Ramachandran, A., Ghosh, S., Hasnain, S. E., Kaufman, R. J., and Ramaiah, K. V. A. (2000). Phosphorylation of serine 51 in initiation factor 2 alpha (eIF2 alpha) promotes complex formation between eIF2 alpha(P) and eIF2B and causes inhibition in the guanine nucleotide exchange activity of eIF2B. *Biochemistry.* 39, 12929–12938. doi: 10.1021/bi0008682

Villena, J., Chiba, E., Vizoso-Pinto, M. G., Tomosada, Y., Takahashi, T., Ishizuka, T., et al. (2014). Immunobiotic *Lactobacillus* rhamnosus strains differentially modulate antiviral immune response in porcine intestinal epithelial and antigen presenting cells. *BMC Microbiol.* 14:126. doi: 10.1186/1471-2180-14-126

Yang, Z., Ran, L., Yuan, P., Yang, Y., Wang, K., Xie, L., et al. (2018). EGFR as a negative regulatory protein adjusts the activity and mobility of NHE3 in the cell membrane of IPEC-J2 cells With TGEV infection. *Front. Microbiol.* 9:2734. doi: 10.3389/fmicb.2018.02734

Yuan, L., Zhang, S., Wang, Y., Li, Y., Wang, X., and Yang, Q. (2018). Surfactin inhibits membrane fusion during invasion of epithelial cells by enveloped viruses. *J. Virol.* 92, e809–e818. doi: 10.1128/JVI.00809-18

Zhao, S., Gao, Q., Qin, T., Yin, Y., Lin, J., Yu, Q., et al. (2014). Effects of virulent and attenuated transmissible gastroenteritis virus on the ability of porcine dendritic cells to sample and present antigen. *Vet. Microbiol.* 171, 74–86. doi: 10.1016/j.vetmic.2014.03.017

Zhao, Y., Valbuena, G., Walker, D. H., Gazi, M., Hidalgo, M., DeSousa, R., et al. (2016). Endothelial cell proteomic response to rickettsia conorii infection reveals activation of the janus kinase (JAK)-signal transducer and activator of transcription (STAT)-interferon stimulated gene (ISG)15 pathway and reprogramming plasma membrane integrin/cadherin signaling. *Mol. Cell Proteomics.* 15, 289–304. doi: 10.1074/mcp.M115.054361

Zhu, L., Yang, X., Mou, C., and Yang, Q. (2017). Transmissible gastroenteritis virus does not suppress IFN-beta induction but is sensitive to IFN in IPEC-J2 cells. *Vet. Microbiol.* 199, 128–134. doi: 10.1016/j.vetmic.2016.12.031

Zhu, X., Wen, Z., Xu, L. Z., and Darnell, J. E. Jr. (1997). Stat1 serine phosphorylation occurs independently of tyrosine phosphorylation and requires an activated Jak2 kinase. *Mol. Cell Biol.* 17, 6618–6623. doi: 10.1128/mcb.17.11.6618

6

Defeat Dengue and Zika Viruses with a One-Two Punch of Vaccine and Vector Blockade

Jin Sun[1], Senyan Du[2], Zhihang Zheng[1,3], Gong Cheng[2] and Xia Jin[1,4*]

[1] Viral Disease and Vaccine Translational Research Unit, CAS Key Laboratory of Molecular Virology and Immunology, Institut Pasteur of Shanghai, Chinese Academy of Sciences, Shanghai, China, [2] Tsinghua-Peking Center for Life Sciences, School of Medicine, Tsinghua University, Beijing, China, [3] Institut Pasteur of Shanghai, Chinese Academy of Sciences, University of Chinese Academy of Sciences, Shanghai, China, [4] Shanghai Public Health Clinical Center, Fudan University, Shanghai, China

***Correspondence:**
Xia Jin
xjin@ips.ac.cn;
jinxia@shphc.org.cn

Dengue virus (DENV) and Zika virus (ZIKV) are two mosquito-borne flaviviruses afflicting nearly half of the world population. Human infection by these viruses can either be asymptomatic or manifest as clinical diseases from mild to severe. Despite more cases are presented as self-limiting febrile illness, severe dengue disease can be manifested as hemorrhagic fever and hemorrhagic shock syndrome, and ZIKV infection has been linked to increased incidence of peripheral neuropathy Guillain-Barre syndrome and central neural disease such as microcephaly. The current prevention and treatment of these infectious diseases are either non-satisfactory or entirely lacking. Because DENV and ZIKV have much similarities in genomic and structural features, almost identical mode of mosquito-mediated transmission, and probably the same pattern of host innate and adaptive immunity toward them, it is reasonable and often desirable to investigate these two viruses side-by-side, and thereby devise common countermeasures against both. Here, we review the existing knowledge on DENV and ZIKV regarding epidemiology, molecular virology, protective immunity and vaccine development, discuss recent new discoveries on the functions of flavivirus NS1 protein in viral pathogenesis and transmission, and propose a one-two punch strategy using vaccine and vector blockade to overcome antibody-dependent enhancement and defeat Dengue and Zika viruses.

Keywords: dengue virus, Zika virus, epidemiology, virology, protective immunity, vaccine, mosquitoes

EPIDEMIOLOGY OF DENGUE VIRUS AND ZIKA VIRUS

Dengue virus (DENV) is the most prevalent mosquito-borne flavivirus that affects over half of the world population in 128 countries and regions (Brady et al., 2012). Zika virus (ZIKV) is another virus that has caught public attention while sweeping across 60 countries and infecting several million people during 2014–2016 (Baud et al., 2017). The transmitting vectors of DENV and ZIKV are *Aedes* mosquitoes, mainly *A. aegypti* and *A. albopictus* (Guzman et al., 2010; Weaver et al., 2016). These viruses cause human diseases that share some similar clinical manifestations but also have features that are distinct from each other.

Dengue viruses are antigenically classified into four serotypes that originate from one ancestor phylogenetically and cause common pathologies in human. Infection by any serotype of dengue virus can be either symptomatic (~25%) or not (Bhatt et al., 2013; St John and Rathore, 2019). The majority of symptomatic infection only develop self-limited febrile illness with manifestations of high fever, facial flushing, rash, myalgia, arthralgia, headache, retro-orbital pain, vomiting, epistaxis, or gum bleeding. Febrile phase lasts 2–7 days, during which viremia and plasma NS1 can be detected in the initial 1–4 days. Only a small percentage of the symptomatic patients (mostly children) progress to more severe forms of dengue disease, Dengue Hemorrhagic Fever (DHF) and Dengue Shock Syndrome (DSS), in which plasma leakage and hemorrhagic manifestations occur; meanwhile, leukopenia, hemoconcentration, and thrombocytopenia can be detected by laboratory tests. Severe plasma leakage that leads to metabolic acidosis and shock with occasional organ impairment is fetal without proper treatment (World Health Organization [WHO], 2009). Immune responses induced during infection by one serotype of dengue virus can confer life-long protection against homotypic viruses and provide cross-protection toward heterotypic viruses for short-term. Strikingly, such cross-reactivities have the potential to enhance disease severity of a secondary heterotypic infection, probably through a mechanism called Antibody Dependent Enhancement (ADE). Consistently, increased risk of DHF/DSS has been observed for secondary dengue virus infections in some epidemiological studies (Sangkawibha et al., 1984; Guzman et al., 2013; Katzelnick et al., 2017). Dengue like disease has been a public health problem for over two centuries. In 1780, Benjamin Rush recorded in Philadelphia an epidemic of bilious remitting fever, which is now considered as one of the earliest descriptions of dengue like diseases in America (Rush, 1951; Packard, 2016). In the following decades, such outbreaks appeared throughout Atlantic World. The name "dengue virus" appeared in the Caribbean in 1820s, it might have derived from Swahili "*Ka-dinga-pepo*" or Spanish "*denguero,*" meaning seizures caused by an evil spirit or referring to the special gait, to describe the agonizing status after infection (Barnett, 2017). Nevertheless, whether all of these early epidemics were caused by dengue virus rather than another clinically similar arbovirus, chikungunya virus, was uncertain, as disease of these outbreaks was often named as "break bone fever" and some were described as rheumatic diseases (Carey, 1971). Although it is unclear when dengue virus was first introduced to Asia, as sylvatic strains of DENV-1 (strain P72-1244), -2 (strain P8-1407), -4 (strain P73-1120 and P75-514, P75-215) were isolated from sentinel monkeys or *A. niveus* mosquitoes in the rainforest of Malaysia, and the existence of sylvatic DENV-3 is supported indirectly by monkey seroconversion against DENV-3 in Malaysia, it is suggested that the four serotype viruses evolved independently in the rainforests of southeast Asia based on the phylogenic analysis (Wang et al., 2000; Holmes and Twiddy, 2003). The huge troop deployments during the Second World War might have also exacerbated the spread of dengue viruses in Asia (Clarke, 2002). Since the beginning of twentieth century, due to the increased urbanization and lacking control of *Aedes* mosquitoes, all four serotypes of dengue viruses have been found in South Asia, causing endemics each year. Similarly, multiple serotypes of dengue virus were circulating in tropical and sub-tropical regions of America after 1950s, leading to regular outbreaks in these regions (Gubler, 1987). Coincide with this, increased DHF and DSS cases were reported in different outbreaks after World War II (Halstead, 1966; World Health Organization [WHO], 1966). Now, the four serotype viruses are co-circulating in all endemic regions (Mackenzie et al., 2004), and estimated to infect 390 million people, causing 10,000 death, and 96 million symptomatic infections in 128 countries each year (Guzman et al., 2010; Brady et al., 2012; Bhatt et al., 2013). Roughly, the world population live under the threat of dengue disease is recently predicted to increase to over 60% by 2080 (Messina et al., 2019). Although modern era of dengue research has begun since Sabin and his colleagues first isolated the virus in 1944 (Sabin, 1952), the dissemination of dengue viruses are still continuing, as no antiviral drugs are available and the only licensed vaccine is far from satisfactory.

In comparison, Zika virus emerged more recently as a public health concern. The historical documents of Zika virus started as its first isolation from a monkey in Zika forest of Uganda in 1947 (Dick et al., 1952). In the following decades, only a few sporadic outbreaks were reported in Africa and South Asia, the number of cases during each outbreak never exceeded a few dozen before 2007 (Duffy et al., 2009; Grard et al., 2014). Symptoms of ZIKV infection including fever, arthralgia, rash and conjunctivitis were presented in patients during the early outbreaks, although 50–80% infections were asymptomatic (Weaver et al., 2016). Fundamental epidemic and clinical changes of the disease first appeared in an outbreak in French Polynesia in 2013, when 28,000 people were infected, and Guillain-Barre syndrome was observed for the first time to be associated with Zika virus infection, implicating the neurotropic feature of Zika virus (Musso et al., 2018); additionally, detection of viral RNA in semen and urine were also documented during this outbreak. Nevertheless, the threat of Zika virus was not recognized until 2015–2016 when it caused much larger outbreaks in South America, most pronounced in Brazil (Campos et al., 2015). In this outbreak, 40% notified Brazilian cases were from northeast region of Brazil (Faria et al., 2017), where Zika virus infected 63% peoples in Salvador. The virus spread to most countries in Americas (Netto et al., 2017), and then further expanded into a pandemic with several outbreaks in South Asia and pacific islands (Baud et al., 2017). In Europe, travel-associated ZIKV cases were reported in most EU (European Union) countries during 2015–2016, with the largest number of cases in France, and largest percentage related to the Caribbean (Spiteri et al., 2017). During the Brazil outbreak, ZIKV has been suspected to persistently replicate in multiple organs for months, and confirmed to be capable of sexual and vertical transmission; and found to be associated with increased ratios of microcephaly and congenital diseases in newborn babies (Weaver et al., 2016). Soon after, the association between Zika virus infection and microcephaly was confirmed by extensive studies in mice (Li et al., 2016; Yockey et al., 2016; Vermillion et al., 2017; Szaba et al., 2018). Furthermore, *in vivo* replication of ZIKV in neuron, placenta and fetus was also verified by using autopsy samples (Martines et al., 2016; Mlakar et al., 2016). Since early 2016, WHO has declared Zika virus disease as a public health emergency of global concern.

It should be noted that ZIKV and DENV spread through the same *Aedes* mosquito vectors in overlapping epidemic areas, and cross-reactivity of their adaptive immune responses are also often observed, therefore, inspecting their similarity in viral and genomic structures should be of value.

VIROLOGICAL FEATURES OF DENGUE VIRUS AND ZIKA VIRUS

Both Dengue virus and Zika virus belong to the genus of *flavivirus* in the *flaviviridae* family, and they have similar genome organization and virion morphology. They both have one single-stranded positive RNA as genome, which contain an open reading frame (ORF) of ~11,000 nucleotides, flanked by 100 nucleotides at the 5′UTR and 400–500 nucleotides at the 3′UTR. The single ORF encodes a polyprotein of 3000-amino acid that is translationally or post-translationally processed into three structural proteins (C, prM, E) and seven non-structural proteins (NS1, NS2A, NS2B, NS3, NS4A, NS5). Generally, the sequence homology between DENV and ZIKV polyprotein is 55–56%, whereas the homology among four serotype dengue virus polyproteins is 69–72%. The three structural proteins and phospholipid bilayers derived from ER of infected cells form the major architecture of viral particles of ZIKV and DENV, whereas the non-structural proteins (except for NS1) mainly retain intracellular location and participate in viral RNA replication and viral polyprotein processing: NS5 is RNA dependent RNA polymerase and methyltransferase, NS3 is helicase, NS2B/NS3 complex is a serine protease that processes polyprotein at C/pr, NS2A/NS2B, NS2B/NS3, NS3/NS4A, NS4A/2K, and NS4B/NS5 junctions. The NS proteins also interact with host immunity: NS2B/NS3, NS4A, NS4B, and NS5 can be antagonists of innate immune responses; NS1 can directly or indirectly cause pathology (Lindenbach et al., 2007; Ngono and Shresta, 2018). On the surface of the mature virus particles, 90 copies of E homodimers lie flat on the virus membrane, packed in a herringbone array; each E dimer is comprised of two antiparallel monomers whose c-terminal helixes are anchored into the lipid bilayer of virus envelope. As envelope protein directly mediates receptor binding and post-entry membrane fusion, it is mostly outwardly exposed and thus contains most neutralization epitopes. Underneath each dimeric E ectodomains are a pair of M proteins buried in the pockets and holes formed between two E subunits on the viral membrane. Similarly, M proteins are anchored to membrane through c-terminal tans-membrane helixes, complexed with each E protein and modulating conformational change of E to initiate membrane fusion at post-entry stage in a pH dependent manner (Zhang et al., 2013; Sirohi et al., 2016). Inside the envelope, the capsids interact with genomic RNA, forming a spherical nucleocapsid, in which ordered structure of capsid surrounding RNA has never been observed in dengue viruses; but a recent study at 9 Å resolution showed structure of immature Zika virus and demonstrated that there was a regular but broken shell of capsid inside the membrane, implying a dynamical morphological alteration during Zika virus maturation (Prasad et al., 2017). Despite minor differences, the structures of DENV and ZIKV are generally similar. A noted difference exists in a region surrounding glycosylation site at Asn^{154} of ZIKV envelope protein and Asn^{153} of DENV envelope protein, these sites may influence virus transmission and pathology through affecting receptor binding and cell tropism (Sirohi et al., 2016).

The precursor of M protein, prM, shields fusion peptide of E protein from acidic environment in trans-Golgi apparatus through its globular "pr" domain when newly budded virus particles transit through exocytosis pathway and thus prevents virus from fusing with Golgi apparatus prematurely. After that, the "pr" peptide is cleaved by a proprotein convertase, Furin, in Golgi apparatus and it dissociates from virus surface once particle reaches extracellular space (Gaucher et al., 2008; Yu et al., 2008, 2009). However, not only fully mature viral particles are produced during viral culture, partially mature or immature virions can also be detected in the supernatant. The immature viruses are those whose pr peptides were not fully proteolytic cleaved from all M proteins on surface. Functionally, in contrast to the mature virus, the immature DENV and ZIKV are non-infectious, however, such immature virus particle can also infect FcγR bearing cells after being bound by antibodies specific for "pr" peptides (Rodenhuis-Zybert et al., 2010; Wirawan et al., 2019), and the uptake of immature virion/antibody complexes creates mature, infectious viruses (Rodenhuis-Zybert et al., 2010).

Besides structural proteins incorporated into viral particles, another membrane associated glycoprotein NS1 can also be secreted extracellularly as hexamers, and detected in blood during acute infection. The NS1 protein can cause pathology in humans through either altering endothelial permeability or inducing antibodies that cross-react with host endothelial proteins; it can also facilitate viral transmission in mosquitoes through antagonizing mosquito innate immunity via suppressing the expression of immune-related genes involved in ROS and JAK/STAT pathways (Liu et al., 2011; Liu J. et al., 2016; Puerta-Guardo et al., 2019). Consistently, antibodies to NS1 can protect mice from lethal diseases in experimental models (Wan et al., 2017; Bailey et al., 2018).

CELL TROPISM OF DENGUE VIRUS AND ZIKA VIRUS

Transmission of DENV and ZIKV are mainly mediated by *Aedes* mosquitoes. When human is bitten by infected mosquitoes, viruses are inoculated directly into the blood vessels or epidermis where keratinocytes, skin dendritic cells (DC) (Limon-Flores et al., 2005), monocytes and myeloid DC are probably infected and become the first virus carriers for further dissemination (Khaiboullina S. F. et al., 2019). An earlier investigation on dengue virus has indicated that immature skin DC, Langerhans cells were infected by dengue virus and then emigrated from the skin to transmit the virus to other organs (Wu et al., 2000). Our studies have demonstrated that monocyte was the principle target cell among PBMCs for both DENV and ZIKV infection, as well as the main mediators for ADE of both viruses in PBMCs (Kou et al., 2008; Li et al., 2018). Consistently, two other studies also provided evidences that circulating CD14 + monocytes were the primary cellular targets of ZIKV infection in PBMCs (Foo et al., 2017; Michlmayr et al., 2017).

As they disseminate through the circulatory and lymphatic system, dengue virus and Zika virus spread to different tissues and organs. Dengue virus infects primary vascular endothelial cells, splenic macrophage and Kupffer cells in *ex vivo* infection assay and immunohistochemistry of autopsy specimens (Marianneau et al., 1999; Jessie et al., 2004; Blackley et al., 2007; Dalrymple and Mackow, 2012). In contrast, besides these tissues, Zika virus also replicates in uterus and many immune privileged organs, including placenta, brain and testicles (Govero et al., 2016; Quicke et al., 2016; Sanchez-San Martin et al., 2018; Khaiboullina S. F. et al., 2019), causing neuropathology, congenital disorders, and damages to reproductive organs. So far, Zika virus has been found to infect a wide range of cell types, including neural progenitor cells, mature neurons and astrocytes in brain, Sertoli cells, Leydig cells, stem-like testicular peritubular cells, primary spermatocytes and spermatogonia in testicles, vaginal epithelium and uterine fibroblast in uterus, and trophoblasts, Hofbauer cells and endothelial cells in placenta (Ma et al., 2016; Miner and Diamond, 2017; Qian et al., 2017). Several investigations indicated Zika virus infects endothelial cells, the key component of blood tissue barriers, a fact that may help to explain how Zika virus crosses blood brain barrier and placental barrier (Liu S. et al., 2016; Papa et al., 2017). However, it is still controversial as to whether Zika virus infection alters endothelial barrier integrity. A recent study showed that ZIKV infection of human umbilical vein endothelial cells (HUVECs) increased endothelial permeability (Khaiboullina S. et al., 2019), whereas some other studies have demonstrated that Zika virus directionally infected polarized epithelial cells from apical side and egressed at basolateral side without a disruption of cell monolayer integrity (Tamhankar and Patterson, 2019).

Understanding of ZIKV cell tropism and dissemination across blood tissue barriers will help to better elucidate Zika pathology, and provide opportunity for the development of efficient treatment or prevention strategy. Meanwhile, pathogenic characteristics and tissue tropism should also been considered during development of prophylactic ZIKV vaccine. Its criteria for protective efficacies need to include not only reduced viral load and neuropathology, but also inhibited vertical transmission, and decreased damages to reproductive systems in animal models (Griffin et al., 2017; Shan et al., 2017; Zou et al., 2018). Different from DENV vaccine candidates, ZIKV vaccine might have to elicit higher level of immune responses (Shan et al., 2019) to overcome the special immune status (such as immune tolerance) of recipients during pregnancy (Nancy et al., 2012), and follow-up studies of the incidence of fetal microcephaly in women received ZIKV vaccine are also necessary in clinical trials.

THE BENEFITS AND LIMITATIONS OF THE ONLY LICENSED DENGUE VACCINE

With effort that lasted two decades, the first licensed vaccine *Dengvaxia* (called CYD-TDV before licensure) has been developed by Sanofi Pasteur. It is a live attenuated vaccine comprised of four Dengue-Yellow Fever virus chimeras in one dose at 1:1:1:1 ratios, and it has been approved to use in over 20 dengue endemic countries and European Union and USA (World Health Organization [WHO], 2017; Halstead and Dans, 2019). Each component of this vaccine was developed on the backbone of Yellow Fever 17D vaccine by replacing prM and E genes with those from each serotype of dengue viruses (Guirakhoo et al., 2000; Guirakhoo et al., 2001). Through such a strategy, CYD-TDV was developed and showed to elicit neutralizing antibodies to four serotype of dengue viruses; moreover, this vaccines has high genetic stability, with limited mosquito transmission, and it is less hepatotropic (one major adverse effect of YF vaccine) (Guirakhoo et al., 2002; Brandler et al., 2005; Higgs et al., 2006; McGee et al., 2008; Mantel et al., 2011). In the large multicenter phase III trials, this vaccine had showed protective efficacies against symptomatic virologically confirmed dengue (VCD) of 54.8% in Asian, and 64.7% in Latin America; the general efficacies against hospitalization and severe dengue cases reached 80.3 and 95.5%, respectively, in Latin America (Capeding et al., 2014; Villar et al., 2015). Though not completely satisfactory, in light of the urgency and significant global demand of a dengue vaccine, CYD-TDV vaccine (*Dengvaxia*) was licensed at the end of 2015, accompanied by the WHO Strategic Advisory Group of Experts (SAGE) recommendation that this vaccine be used in all dengue-endemic counties (World Health Organization [WHO], 2017).

Despite filling in the void of dengue vaccine, its phase II and phase III trials revealed concerns regarding the vaccine's safety. First, the immunogenicity and efficacy of this vaccine varied by age and prior dengue-infections: vaccinees of seronegative and children younger than 9 years' old had increased risk of diseases (Hadinegoro et al., 2015). Vaccination of flavivirus seronegative individuals induced significant lower level of neutralizing antibodies comparing to those having pre-existing flavivirus immunity, specifically, the Geometric Mean Titer (GMTs) of seronegative groups were 47.4–90.8% lower than those of seropositive ones (Guirakhoo et al., 2006; Lanata et al., 2012; Dayan et al., 2013a; Hss et al., 2013). Notably, during long-term follow-up of participants of the two Phase III trials and one Phase IIb trial, vaccinated Asians between ages 2 and 5 years old have had an increased risk of hospitalization in the first year, with a relative risk of 7.5; and vaccinated Thai children between ages 4 and 5 had a relative risk of 2.44 in the 3rd year after vaccination. The vaccine efficacies in children younger than 9 years of age were significantly lower than those of 9 years or older according to a number of criteria (VCD:44.6% vs. 67.8%; hospitalization: 56.1% vs. 86.1%; DHF: 66.7% vs. 90.9%). Further analysis indicated that the lowest vaccine efficacy of 14.4% was in dengue seronegative children younger than 9 years of age (Hadinegoro et al., 2015). It is postulated that vaccination in dengue seronegative recipients had mimicked a course of asymptomatic primary dengue infection, which induced antibodies that enhance subsequent natural dengue infection. Consistently, after the large scale vaccination in Philippines, several vaccinated children and adults have died from lethal dengue diseases. By the time Sanofi Pasteur and WHO modified the instruction for *Dengvaxia* vaccination after those long-term follow-up studies, limiting its use to people who has a previous dengue infection (Vannice et al., 2018), 800,000 Philippine children had already been vaccinated, among them only 100,000 were seropositive, the rest were thus placed at the increased risk of severe DHF/DSS (Fatima and Syed, 2018). Second, *Dengvaxia* has a low protective efficacy against dengue-2 viruses that are endemic in Asia. In a Phase IIb trial, *Dengvaxia* showed poor protection against dengue-2 virus, reached an efficacy of merely 9%, despite having generated decent neutralization antibodies to DENV-2, with similar GMT (Geometric Mean Titer) as those specific for other serotypes when tested at 28 days after the final immunization (Sabchareon et al., 2012). Similarly, in a Phase III trial in Latin America, the GMTs of neutralization antibodies to DENV-1,-2,-3,-4 were 395, 574, 508, and 241, respectively, at 28 days after the 3rd injection; but the corresponding protective efficacy during the 1st year were 50.3, 42.3, 74, and 77.7% for each of the four serotypes (Villar et al., 2015). Based on these large scale clinical studies, an expected correlation between efficacies and neutralizing antibody titer PRNT (Plaque Reduction Neutralizing Test) values were not found for all four serotypes. It should be noted that a waning of cross-genotype neutralization was observed for monovalent CYD-2 vaccine induced antibodies at 6 months post immunization in a Phase I trial; specifically, GMT of neutralizing antibody specific for dengue-2 clinical isolates of heterologous genotype dropped as much as 10-fold compared with those that were specific for laboratory strain 16681 of autologous genotype (Guirakhoo et al., 2006). All these may indicate that high serotype-2 specific neutralization antibodies had been elicited by CYD-TDV, but it only sustained for a short time and was restricted to a limited number of genotypes. Such unsatisfied efficacy and lower neutralizing titers toward one serotype will also increase the risk of infection by that serotype, especially in those who are seronegative at the baseline. Third, although the highest level of protection was supposed to be achieved after the 3rd vaccination, its efficacy was found to be similar with that in peoples only received the 1st dose. How to modify the immunization schedule of this live attenuated vaccine to boost immune responses is still unclear, but it will probably be helpful to improve the efficacy of vaccine itself. Last but not the least, whether the emergence of Zika virus in DENV endemic regions and prior ZIKV immunity in vaccine recipients will affect the efficacy of *Dengvaxia* is unknown, and whether vaccination by *Dengvaxia* will enhance or prevent Zika virus infection is also uncertain. As co-circulation of two viruses and complicated interference between Dengue and Zika virus-specific immunity have already been observed (Bardina et al., 2017; Fowler et al., 2018; Li et al., 2018; Leborgne et al., 2019), it is worthwhile taking the probable influence of ZIKV into consideration during dengue vaccine development. Therefore, either the currently licensed dengue vaccine *Dengvaxia* or other new vaccines must be applied judiciously in epidemic regions.

OTHER DENGUE AND ZIKA VACCINES CURRENTLY IN CLINICAL TRIALS

Other Dengue Vaccines in Clinical Trials

Besides the approved dengue vaccine *Dengvaxia*, several other dengue vaccine candidates have been advanced into clinical trials, these include two recombinant live attenuated vaccines, one subunit protein vaccine, and one DNA vaccine (**Table 1**).

The live attenuated dengue vaccine TAK-003 (DENVax or TDV) is developed by Takeda Vaccine Incorporated. It is comprised of one attenuated dengue-2 viruses, and three other chimeras that contain prM and E genes of other three serotypes built on the backbone of attenuated DENV-2 (Osorio et al., 2015). Here, the backbone DENV-2 in TAK-003 is derived from dengue-2 attenuated virus strain PDK-53, which was obtained through serially passaging of DENV-2 16681 in primary dog kidney cells for 53 times (Bhamarapravati et al., 1987). This tetravalent vaccine has non-structural proteins of DENV-2, and it is capable of activating DENV-2 NS1 specific T cell responses and antibodies (Sharma et al., 2019), both of which *Dengvaxia* is incapable of inducing. But among tetravalent immune responses elicited by the chimeric TDV, the immunity to DENV-4 was the lowest when testing in Phase I and Phase II studies of tetravalent TDV formulations (Osorio et al., 2014; George et al., 2015; Sirivichayakul et al., 2016). Moreover, in the released data from part 1 of its ongoing phase III study, the efficacy of TAK-003 to DENV-4 was still unclear for the insufficient case numbers of DENV-4 infection during study (Biswal et al., 2019). Irrespective of this shortfall, the merits of this vaccine warrants its further testing in several Phase III trials in endemic regions.

A second tetravalent live attenuated dengue vaccine candidate is LAVDelta30 (TV003/TV005), invented by US NIAID and under co-development with Butantan Institute. This vaccine is comprised of attenuated DENV-1, DENV-3, and DENV-4 viruses that contain a 30-nucleotide deletion or additional 31-nucleotide

TABLE 1 | Dengue vaccines in clinical trials.

Name	Vaccine type	Immunogen	Developer	Current status
DENVax (TAK-003)	Live attenuated chimeric vaccine	Attenuated DENV-2; Substitution with DENV-1,3,4 prM and E genes on DENV-2 backbone;	Takeda Vaccine Inc.	Phase III
LAV Delta 30 (TV003/TV005)	Live attenuated chimeric vaccine	Attenuated DENV-1,3 and 4, through deletion in 3′UTR, DENV-2 prME on the backbone of attenuated DENV-4	NIAID/Butantan Institute	Phase III
DENV subunit V180	Subunit protein	Ectodomain (N-terminal 80%) of envelope protein, expressed in S2 cell line	Hawaii Biotech Inc./Merk	Phase I
D1ME100	DNA	prM and E genes	US Naval Research Center	Phase I

deletion in 3′ UTR regions (rDEN1delta30, rDEN3delta30/31, rDEN4delta30) (Blaney et al., 2001, 2008; Whitehead et al., 2003a). Because the same deletion of 30 nucleotides in DENV-2 failed to attenuate it sufficiently, a chimeric virus was obtained by replacing prM and E genes of rDEN4delta30 with DENV-2 prM/E and used instead (Whitehead et al., 2003b). In completed trials and released results, this vaccine was reported to produce neutralizing antibodies and multi-type specific T cell responses in both seronegative and seropositive recipients, although GMTs of neutralizing antibody in seropositive recipients are always higher than those in seronegatives (Weiskopf et al., 2015a; Kirkpatrick et al., 2016). Generally safe, but the vaccine has induced adverse effects such as rash, neutropenia and short-time viremia (Durbin et al., 2005, 2006, 2011, 2013). Its first Phase III trial has been initiated in Brazil.

In contrast to the more rapid progress of live attenuated vaccines into Phase III clinical trials, protein and DNA vaccines are lagging behind in Phase I trials. A subunit dengue vaccine V180 is developed by Hawaii Biotech Inc., and then bought by Merk & Co., Incorporated. This vaccine is comprised of four *Drosophila* S2 cell expressed N-terminal 395aa of envelope proteins (E80) representing four serotype of dengue viruses, and it has been demonstrated to produce neutralizing antibody and provide protection against challenge with multiple serotypes of DENV in murine and non-human primate models (Clements et al., 2010; Govindarajan et al., 2015). In a recent Phase I clinical trial, tetravalent E80 vaccines formulated with different adjuvants were shown to be well tolerated in seronegative recipients in Australia, and they elicited tetravalent neutralizing antibodies, albeit of short duration (Manoff et al., 2019). Use this protein vaccine in adults who previously received attenuated vaccines, TV003 or TV005, has also been tested in clinical trial, the results of which are pending (ID: NCT02450838).

A DNA vaccine under clinical development is developed by US Naval Medical Research Center, and it contains prM and E genes. Monovalent DENV-1 prM and E DNA (D1ME) vaccines showed immunogenicity in Phase I clinical trial after being demonstrated conferring protection in a monkey model (Beckett et al., 2011). The neutralizing antibody was detectable only in the vaccine group receiving higher dose of DNA, and its titer was low. Therefore, tetravalent formulations of this vaccine were tested with combination of Vaxfectin® adjuvant to improve its immunogenicity in further clinical trials (Porter et al., 2012), much of its results have not been published.

Zika Vaccines in Clinical Trials

In contrast to Dengue vaccines, Zika vaccines have only been developed recently since the large ZIKV outbreaks in 2015–2016. Multiple candidates are under development simultaneously, including traditional inactivated vaccine, live attenuated vaccine, and genetically engineered subunit protein vaccine, DNA vaccine, and novel mRNA vaccines; among them, only the seven candidate vaccines that are in Phase I or II clinical trials will be discussed (**Table 2**).

The most advanced Zika vaccine candidates is a DNA vaccine containing Zika virus prM and E genes (VRC5283) that is being developed by NIAID and tested in Phase II clinical trial. The vaccine plasmid expresses prM and E proteins and forms non-infectious but highly antigenic virus like particles (VLP) *in vivo*. Recipients of this vaccine by needle-free injection on both arms with split-dose showed 100% seroconversion, and generated neutralizing antibody with higher GMT values than those received a single-full dose injection on one arm and those administered the vaccine via needle and syringe injection. It is probably because the needle-free injection has enhanced dispersion field and increases the contact area between antigens and dermal APC (Mitragotri, 2006). The split-dose vaccination group also elicited best CD4 + and CD8 + T cell immune responses across all groups (Gaudinski et al., 2018). Another DNA vaccine GLS-5700 (developed by GeneOne/Inovio) containing consensus sequences of ZIKV prM and E genes, delivered via intradermal injection followed by electroporation, produced neutralizing antibodies in 62% participants as measured by the Plaque Reduction Neutralizing Test (PRNT). In addition, adoptive transfer of sera from vaccine recipients protected 92% immune deficient mice from lethal ZIKV challenge (Tebas et al., 2017).

The development of inactivated Zika vaccine was started soon after the ZIKV outbreaks. There are currently two purified inactivated Zika vaccine candidates in Phase I clinical trials, they were developed by WRAIR/NIAID/Harvard University/Sanofi Pasteur (ZPIV) and Valneva Australia GmbH (VLA1601) separately. Inactivated vaccine has the advantages of easy manufacture, established platforms based on many other vaccines, such as those for Japanese Encephalitis (JE) and Polio viruses, have been developed. According to preliminary results of the WRAIR/NIAID vaccine (ZPIV) in three Phase I trials, the formalin-inactivated virus vaccine induced 95% seroconversion, had a peak neutralization antibody GMT of 286, with only moderate adverse effect. Adoptive transfer of human IgG from vaccine recipients to mice prior to challenge with ZIKV led to reduced viremia in mice, indicating its potential for protection in humans (Modjarrad et al., 2018).

Using a similar strategy for DENV-2 vaccine TV003/TV005, recombinant live attenuated Zika vaccine has been constructed with the backbone of attenuated DENV-4 of TV003 (rZIKV/D4delta30), by NIAID, wherein prM and E genes of DEN4delta30 were substituted by the corresponding genes from ZIKV. This vaccine is now in Phase I clinical trial, and might be tested in combination with DENV vaccine TV005 in the future (ID: NCT03611946) (Durbin and Wilder-Smith, 2017; Wilder-Smith et al., 2018). Other viral vectors such as Measles vaccine virus has also been adapted to construct chimeric ZIKV vaccine. One of such vaccine, MV-ZIKA, has been developed by Themis Bioscience GmbH and advanced into Phase I clinical trial (ID: NCT02996890).

Novel vaccine strategy such as lipid nanoparticle-encapsulated modified mRNA has also been used to develop Zika vaccine. An mRNA that contains prM-E genes of ZIKV and optimized 5′ and 3′ untranslated sequences with type-1 cap was obtained through enzymatically synthesis using modified nucleoside, and packaged into lipid nanoparticles (LNP). Such mRNA-LNP vaccine could efficiently produce virus like particle in cells. After intramuscular delivery, two doses of mRNA-LNP vaccine were able to elicit

TABLE 2 | Zika vaccines in clinical trials.

Name	Vaccine type	Immunogen	Developers	Current status
VRC5283	DNA	Wild type prM and E genes, needle-free injection	NIAID	Phase II
GLS-5700	DNA	Consensus prM and E genes, injection & electroporation	GeneOne life science Inc./Inovio Pharmaceuticals	Phase I
ZIKV purified inactivated vaccine (ZPIV)	Inactivated vaccine	Formalin-inactivated whole virus	WRAIR/NIAID/Harvard University/Sanofi Pasteur	Phase I
VLA1601	Inactivated vaccine	Formalin-inactivated whole virus	Valneva Australia GmbH	Phase I
rZIKV/D4delta30	Chimeric live attenuated vaccine	ZIKV prM and E genes inserted to DEN4delta30	NIAID	Phase I
MV-ZIKA	Viral vector	ZIKV prM and E genges inserted to measles virus vector	Themis Bioscience GmbH	Phase I
mRNA-1325	mRNA	Lipid nanoparticle encapsulated modified mRNA of prM and E	ModernaTX, Inc.	Phase I

high titers (~1/100,000) of neutralizing antibodies, and conferred protection against ZIKV challenge in mice (Richner et al., 2017a). An mRNA-based vaccine is now in Phase I clinical trial (ID: NCT03014089).

Besides, other forms of ZIKV vaccine, such as protein based subunit vaccine (Medina et al., 2018; Metz et al., 2019; Slon-Campos et al., 2019) and live attenuated Zika vaccines (Richner et al., 2017b; Xie et al., 2018; Shan et al., 2019) are also under development at the pre-clinical stage. Considering the cross-reactivity and ADE between ZIKV and DENV, newly developed ZIKV vaccine should also be tested for DENV enhancement activity. This additional requirement will likely to be a huge obstacle for both ZIKV and DENV vaccines.

PROTECTIVE IMMUNITY AGAINST DENGUE AND ZIKA VIRUSES

Protective Antibody Response

Although various antibodies targeting different viral proteins are induced after flavivirus infection, only two types of antibodies have been documented to provide significant protection: neutralizing antibodies to viral surface E protein (Crill and Chang, 2004; Dejnirattisai et al., 2015; Stettler et al., 2016; Robbiani et al., 2017) and non-neutralizing antibodies specific for NS1 protein (Henchal et al., 1988; Beatty et al., 2015; Wan et al., 2017; Bailey et al., 2018).

The ectodomain of flavivirus envelope protein can be structurally divided into three sub-domains: Domain II is a long finger-like area lying parallel to virus surface and it contains a fusion peptide on its tip; Domain III is an immunoglobulin-like folded structure projecting slightly away from virus surface, and it is linked to the C-terminal stem region and thought to be involved in virus binding; Domain I is an eight-stranded β-barrel that connects domain II and domain III. Previous study with dengue specific mouse monoclonal antibodies indicated that E domain III was the predominant targets for DENV neutralizing antibodies, and antibodies to this region are mainly serotype specific (Lok et al., 2008); whereas antibodies specific for fusion loop epitopes (FLE) are usually highly cross-reactive with modest neutralization activities (Crill and Chang, 2004). However, in convalescent dengue patient, anti-E Domain III specific neutralizing antibodies only constitute a small proportion of DENV antibody repertoire. Mapping antibody epitope using recombinant envelope proteins, it was found that neutralizing antibody epitopes in human distributed widely across both domain III and domain I/II regions (Beltramello et al., 2010; Stettler et al., 2016), and the depletion of EDIII specific antibodies did not affect the neutralization activity of human immune sera significantly (Williams et al., 2012). Subsequent studies with human samples revealed another class of antibodies that target quaternary epitopes on virus surface, and that these antibodies do not bind to recombinant envelope proteins, but recognize epitopes spanning one dimer or two adjacent dimers of E proteins on the intact virus surface. One group of such antibodies, also called envelope dimer epitope (EDE) antibodies, usually have broad neutralizing activities to all four serotype dengue viruses (Dejnirattisai et al., 2015; Rouvinski et al., 2015).

On the contrary, the importance of ZIKV EDIII specific antibodies has been shown directly in some human studies. In one study with a panel of human mAb isolated from four convalescent patients, antibodies to E domain III and quaternary epitopes were found to be the most potent at neutralization (Stettler et al., 2016). Additionally, using two cohorts of ZIKV infected individuals from Mexico and Brazil, it was revealed that the levels of antibodies specific for the lateral ridge of ZIKV E domain III were positively correlated with sera neutralization antibody titers (Robbiani et al., 2017). Moreover, antibodies to quaternary epitopes formed between E domains II and III of Zika virus were demonstrated to be both protective and therapeutic in murine models (Sapparapu et al., 2016; Hasan et al., 2017; Collins et al., 2019).

DENV and ZIKV show high level of structure homology between their envelope proteins, and share 35, 51, and 29% amino acid identity in EDI, EDII, and EDIII, respectively. Thereby, cross-reactivities are frequently observed between antibodies targeting E domain I/II of two viruses, but less so for domain III antibodies (Stettler et al., 2016). The broadly neutralizing

EDE1 antibodies, one subset of EDE antibodies originally isolated from DENV patients, has been shown to potently neutralize Zika virus *in vitro* and provides protection against lethal challenge of Zika virus in mice. These antibodies recognize a conserved conformational region on the E dimer which prM interacts with during virus maturation. Another subset is EDE2 antibodies that have broader footprints covering N153 glycosylation site of DENV E proteins, these antibodies can also cross-neutralize ZIKV at high concentrations (Fernandez et al., 2017; Abbink et al., 2018; **Figure 1A**). In contrast, ZIKV neutralization antibodies targeting quaternary epitopes identified so far, such as ZIKV-117, A9E, and G9E, are mainly type-specific (Sapparapu et al., 2016; Hasan et al., 2017; Collins et al., 2019). Notably, cross-reactive antibodies EDE1 and EDE2 were isolated mainly from patients of acute secondary DENV infection, whereas A9E and G9E were isolated from DENV naïve ZIKV patients at 6 months after the onset of illness. Whether such cross-complex neutralizing B cell responses can sustain long time after recovery from infection is unclear, and whether its frequency increases after a heterotypic secondary infection is also unknown.

Collectively, neutralization antibodies to dengue or Zika viruses are mainly constituted of type specific EDIII antibodies, cross-reactive EDI/II antibodies, and potently neutralizing quaternary epitope antibodies that often neutralize four serotypes of dengue viruses simultaneously.

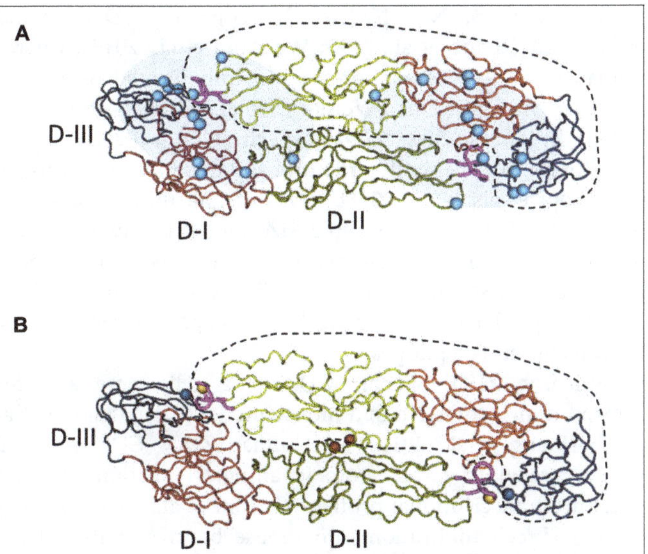

FIGURE 1 | Quaternary epitopes on dengue virus dimeric envelope proteins and stabilizing dimeric structure of E proteins through the addition of disulfate bonds between two monomers. Based on the published structure of DENV-2 E dimer (PDB access NO:1OAN), three domains of E monomer were denoted with different colors on backbones (D-I, red; D-II, yellow; D-III, blue). One of the E monomers in the dimeric structure was circled with dash line. On the tip of domain II, the fusion loop was labeled in pink. The structural image presented the top view, distal from virus membrane. **(A)** Epitopes distribution of EDE epitopes, the residues (cyan spheres) critical for EDE antibody binding were determined by Dejnirattisai et al. Fab binding regions of EDE antibodies were mapped to either end of the dimer (cyan shadow), covering the interface of two monomers. Figure adapted from Dejnirattisai et al. (2015) and Rouvinski et al. (2015). **(B)** Stabilization of dimeric E proteins was achieved through adding disulfate bonds, after introducing mutations into domain II, L107C (yellow spheres) A259C (red spheres) and domain III, A313C (blue spheres). Figure adapted from Rouvinski et al. (2017).

Other than antibodies to envelope proteins, there are abundant prM specific antibodies in human sera after dengue virus infection (Dejnirattisai et al., 2010). However, such antibodies are poorly neutralizing with high cross-reactivity, and induces ADE in a wide range of concentrations, probably because prM antibodies facilitate non-infectious immature virus to become mature and infectious (Rodenhuis-Zybert et al., 2010). In experimental models, immature viral particles may achieve infectivity with the help of antibody against "pr" upon entering the acidic endosome, where the "pr" peptide is cleaved together with the antibody by Furin. Even partially mature viruses that keeping pr peptides in some region on viral surface, can also obtain enhanced infection in Fcγ receptor bearing cells with the help of anti-pr antibodies (Rodenhuis-Zybert et al., 2010; Wirawan et al., 2019). Because of these reasons, prM antibody is now thought to be undesirable among vaccine induced immune responses.

Antibody Dependent Enhancement

One adverse characteristic of flavivirus prM or E antibodies is their ability to induce ADE. When the concentration or affinity of antibodies is too low to neutralize virus infection, the immune complexes formed by virus and antibodies tend to interact with Fcγ receptors on myeloid cell surface through Fc domains of antibodies, they do not induce Fcγ-mediated viral clearance, but aid virus infection by directly increasing virus uptake through Fcγ receptor, or boosting virus replication intracellularly via activating downstream pathway to antagonize the innate immunity (Halstead, 1988; Kliks, 1990). In the latter case, it is hypothesized that legation of Fcγ receptor transmits signals through spleen tyrosine kinase (SYK) to activate extracellular signal-regulated kinase (ERK), and subsequently enhances the transcription of genes including IL-10, which antagonizes type-I IFN pathway through stimulating members of the suppressor of cytokine signaling (SOCs) (Halstead et al., 2010). A number of *in vitro* studies have already demonstrated that most antibodies to DENV or ZIKV prM and E proteins have the potential to enhance viral infections at sub-neutralizing concentrations, irrespective of their neutralization potency (Pierson et al., 2007; Dejnirattisai et al., 2015, 2016). Two classes of antibodies are thought to induce mainly ADE effect rather than neutralization, these are antibodies to fusion-loop and antibodies specific for "pr" peptide, both of which are abundant in patient sera (Beltramello et al., 2010; Dejnirattisai et al., 2010). They are generally highly cross-reactive and marginally neutralizing (Rodenhuis-Zybert et al., 2010; de Alwis et al., 2014). Further investigation on Zika and dengue monoclonal antibodies indicates that antibody concentrations that induce peak ADE are usually negatively correlated with antibodies' neutralizing capacity (Li et al., 2017).

In addition to *in vitro* studies using human samples, ADE of heterotypic DENV infection has been more stringently demonstrated in mouse models. Administering heterotypic DENV immune sera or viral-specific monoclonal antibodies to

AG129 immune deficient mice prior to infection with non-lethal dose of DENV-2 increased viral replication and enhanced disease severity; and increased infection of liver sinusoidal endothelial cells were observed for all four serotypes of clinical isolates (Zellweger et al., 2010). Consistently, clinical evidence of ADE in DENV infection has been reported previously. Infants born to dengue immune mother had elevated risk of DHF/DSS at 6–9 months of age, due to the decay of maternal-derived DENV antibodies (Halstead, 2003). Further, the increased risk of hospitalization in younger children vaccinated with CYD-TDV in Phase III clinical trials are also suspected to have been caused by ADE, as a result of vaccine-induced poorly neutralizing antibodies. More recently, a long-term study on a Nicaragua pediatric cohort showed that the risk of severe dengue diseases was highest within a narrow range of preexisting anti-DENV antibody titers, affirming antibody concentration is a critical determinant of ADE (Katzelnick et al., 2017).

More significantly, a cross-serocomplex ADE between ZIKV and DENV has also been reproduced in mouse model. DENV and WNV immune sera were both found to enhance Zika virus infection in mice (Bardina et al., 2017). Also, the presence of DENV-specific antibodies in ZIKV-infected pregnant mice significantly enhanced viral replication in placenta, and increased placenta damage, reduced fetal growth, and accelerated fetal resorption (Leborgne et al., 2019). Reciprocally, maternally acquired Zika virus antibodies also enhanced dengue disease severity in mice (Fowler et al., 2018). In non-human primate models, the results are not as clear. Two studies did not show enhanced Zika virus infection in macaques that were infected by DENV either 420 days or 2.8 years before experiments (McCracken et al., 2017; Pantoja et al., 2017). However, it should be noted that the interval between primary and secondary DENV infections is critical for disease severity, and DENV ADE in human has only occurred within a relatively narrow range of pre-existing DENV antibody concentration (Katzelnick et al., 2017). In dengue infected patients, this interval was usually 12 months or longer, but unknown for enhancement of Zika virus infection. Limited data from a long-term cohort study in Brazil before and after the 2015 ZIKV outbreak have found that the pre-existing DENV NS1 specific IgG3 antibody within 4–6 months of infection was positively associated with the risk of subsequent ZIKV infection, but high titer of total IgG to DENV was associated with protection against the acquisition of ZIKV infection (Rodriguez-Barraquer et al., 2019). Our previous study using sera of convalescent dengue patients also revealed that stronger cross-serocomplex ADE of ZIKV infection in PBMC appeared more often in sera obtained within 3 months of DENV infection (Li et al., 2018). These results are supportive of the idea that concentrations of cross-reactive antibodies or intervals between two infections are important factors for determining cross-serocomplex enhancement between ZIKV and DENV.

Collectively, ADE is now considered to be the underlying mechanism for enhanced risk of DHF/DSS in secondary dengue virus infection, and it highlights the necessity of avoiding the induction of inadequate immune response toward any serotypes during vaccine development. Despite the impact of prior cross-serocomplex immunity for subsequent ZIKV or DENV infections are clinically unknown, candidate vaccines that provide protection and avoid ADE should be prioritized for development.

T Cell Responses

Aside from the double-edged antibody responses, DENV and ZIKV infections also elicit strong T cell responses of dubious functions. For a long time, T cells activated during dengue virus infection was postulated to cause pathology through producing cytokines such as IFN-γ and TNF-α, which in some models directly increases vascular permeability (Rothman et al., 2014). However, in clinical studies, the appearance of T cell responses was found after the occurrence of hemoconcentration or thrombocytopenia in DHF patients (Jin, 2008; Dung et al., 2010). In mouse models, DENV-specific CD8 + T cell responses were protective and essential for virus clearance during primary infection; and CD4 + T cell responses elicited after peptide vaccination also contributed to protection, although they seemed to be dispensable for virus clearance in primary infection (Yauch et al., 2009; Yauch et al., 2010). A subsequent human cohort study further illustrated that DENV specific CD8 + T cell responses played protective roles against DENV infection in an HLA-linked manner (Weiskopf et al., 2013). DENV-1, -2, -4 specific human CD8 + T cell epitopes are distributed predominantly on NS3, NS4B and NS5 proteins (Duangchinda et al., 2010; Rivino et al., 2013; Weiskopf et al., 2013), whereas human CD4 + T cell epitopes are mainly located on C, NS3, and NS5 viral proteins (Weiskopf et al., 2016; Grifoni et al., 2017a). In some studies, DENV-3 specific CD8 + T cell responses were found to target both structural and non-structural proteins (Weiskopf et al., 2014, 2015b). Of note, all these observations were based on limited sample size and HLA types, and of unknown sequences of heterotypic infections when the subjects had experience secondary infections. These uncertainty in clinical studies might have not revealed the full scope of T cell responses toward conserved epitopes.

Similarly, ZIKV specific CD8 + T cells were also first showed to be protective in a mouse model (Elong Ngono et al., 2017; Huang et al., 2017), and human ZIKV CD8 + T cells were revealed to have cytotoxic antiviral function and bear signature transcriptional profiles (Grifoni et al., 2018). Though, CD8 + T cell infiltration into mouse brain and its antiviral cytotoxicity might be associated with neurological pathology in ZIKV infection, the pre-existence of specific CD8 + T cells did protect mice from CNS disease (Huang et al., 2017; Jurado et al., 2018). Whether ZIKV CD4 + T cell responses are necessary for virus clearance in primary infection is still controversial, but memory CD4 + T cells elicited by infection or peptide immunization have been demonstrated to protect host from subsequent ZIKV infection (Hassert et al., 2018; Elong Ngono et al., 2019). In one cohort study conducted in dengue endemic countries, ZIKV specific CD8 + T cell epitopes were found to be located mainly on C, prM, and E proteins in dengue naïve patients, but targeted broadly across the proteome, especially those conserved regions, in dengue experienced patients (Grifoni et al., 2017b). This is in accord with observations made in human HLA-transgenic mice (Wen et al., 2017b).

Cross-reactive T cell responses were often observed between DENV and ZIKV, because of their homology at amino acid level. DENV specific memory CD8 + T cells could cross-react with Zika virus and protected mice from subsequent lethal ZIKV challenge (Wen et al., 2017a). Adoptive transfer of DENV CD8 + T cells to pregnant mice inhibited Zika virus replication in placenta and increased the survival of fetus (Regla-Nava et al., 2018). In DENV convalescent patients, memory CD4 + and CD8 + T cells could be activated by peptides derived from ZIKV capsid and NS3 proteins, and the activated CD8 + T cells could kill ZIKV infected cells *in vitro* (Lim et al., 2018). Nevertheless, studies on the cross-reactive CD4 + T cells are few, evidence for ZIKV specific memory T cells cross-react with DENV antigens is still lacking.

All above demonstrate that T cell response is an important element of adaptive immunity toward dengue and Zika virus, and T cell component should be considered in the development of protective vaccines.

B AND T CELL VACCINES OF THE NEXT-GENERATION

Based on the existing knowledge of vaccine immunology and protective immunity to DENV and ZIKV, it is predicted that an ideal dengue or Zika vaccine should induce both humoral and cellular immune response to ensure full protection.

Universal B Cell Vaccines for DENV and ZIKV

Previous investigation on dengue and Zika vaccine mainly focused on the B cell immunity, aiming to elicit enough neutralizing antibodies for *in vivo* protection. Because of the complex interaction among antibody responses to four DENV serotypes and ZIKV, an ideal dengue vaccine should elicit long-lasting, serotype-specific neutralizing antibodies to each serotype of virus or broadly neutralizing antibodies that cross-react with all serotypes of viruses. Zika vaccines developed independently need to be able to trigger autologous neutralizing antibodies but minimal cross-reactivity with dengue viruses. Alternatively, pentavalent vaccines would be necessary, if ADE cross sero-complex is verified in epidemiological studies in the future. However, to induce long-term B cell memory response that sustains potent neutralization is not easy, and to produce adequate and relatively balanced neutralizing antibodies against each of these viruses is also difficult. The following approaches may be considered.

First, epitope selection is necessary to design vaccines that produce strong neutralizing antibody responses and minimal ADE effect. Traditional live attenuated vaccines have the advantages of strong immunogenicity and mimicry of wildtype virus. However, the antibody responses elicited by intact or recombinant dengue or Zika viruses still maintain the dual functions of neutralization and enhancement. One prominent source of antigens that induce enhancing antibodies is the immature or partially mature viral particles within the vaccine produced *in vitro* or viruses replicated *in vivo*, and the percentages of which are difficult to determine due to variability in cell cultures for different virus strains. Epitopes on "pr" peptides are probably exposed on immature ZIKV virus surface and elicit abundant ADE inducing antibodies, similar to what happened in DENV infected patients. The same issue must be dealt with for DNA or RNA vaccines that incorporate prM and E genes in order to make virus like particles *in vivo* (Beckett et al., 2011; Porter et al., 2012; Richner et al., 2017a). Similarly, *in vitro* produced virus like particle vaccines will not be ideal unless the immature virus-like particle can be eliminated through procedures such as exogenous Furin cleavage, but how to produce enough immunogens is another problem even more complicated to deal with (Urakami et al., 2017). Therefore, the exact effect and ratio of "pr" antibodies elicited by these vaccines have to be determined during development. In comparison, subunit proteins are easier for epitope selection and quality control. In most subunit candidate vaccines of DENV and ZIKV, soluble EDIII or E80 as antigens were chosen (Block et al., 2010; Liang et al., 2018; Manoff et al., 2019) to induce neutralizing antibodies that block virus attachment or/and inhibit post-entry membrane fusion. Nevertheless, fusion-loop epitope antibodies can still be induced by E80 due to the probable re-exposure of fusion-loop under acidic environment even for an envelope dimer immunogen. One study has attempted to abolish fusion loop through site-directed mutation in mRNA vaccine (Richner et al., 2017a), but both neutralization and enhancement activities were attenuated, indicating this region was probably essential for E dimeric structure on VLP surface. Alternatively, cross-linking of two E80 proteins through additional disulfate bonds in domain II and domain III could stabilize the anti-parallel structure of the soluble E80 dimer, limiting the exposure of fusion-loop, but enabling the presentation of cross-serocomplex broadly neutralizing EDE epitopes (Rouvinski et al., 2017; **Figure 1B**). Consistently, in a recent study, the covalently stabilized ZIKV E dimer has successfully elicited protective antibody responses against ZIKV infection in mice, without causing cross-reactivity to dengue viruses or ADE of DENV (Slon-Campos et al., 2019). Currently, both Zika EDIII and Dengue tetravalent EDIII vaccines are under development. The EDIII component theoretically has more serotype/complex specificity and produce less ADE effect. Whether these type-specific neutralization antibodies induced are strong enough to provide *in vivo* protection toward multiple viruses is to be determined.

Second, relatively balanced neutralization against each of the viruses is required for an ideal tetravalent dengue vaccine or pentavalent Dengue/Zika vaccine. The majority of dengue vaccine candidates are comprised of mixed antigens representing four serotypes, and they are administered to recipients simultaneously to elicit a tetravalent response. When using attenuated viruses, however, different replicative capacity of each virus may produce interference among them, leading to imbalanced neutralizing antibody responses (Dayan et al., 2013b). As for tetravalent protein or DNA vaccines, the immune dominance of specific antigens also affected the balance of neutralizing activities elicited by the vaccines (Block et al., 2010). Thus, modulation of dosage of each serotype of virus or antigen is always needed to improve the relative balance of antibody responses induced. Because the correlation between neutralizing titers and *in vivo* protection varies among four serotypes of dengue viruses or Zika virus, to adjust the balance among immune responses in order to achieve broad protection becomes even more difficult. An alternative strategy is to elicit broadly neutralizing antibodies through a single antigen presenting conserved neutralizing epitopes. To this end, we obtained a consensus E80 sequence that contains epitopes conserved across all four serotype viruses through *in silicon* calculation with a dataset composed of 3,127 published sequences of dengue viruses, and found this single consensus E80 protein was immunogenic and capable of inducing neutralizing antibodies toward all four serotypes of DENV, with less bias than conventional tetravalent E80 vaccine (Sun et al., 2017). When administered in a DNA prime and protein boost regimen, this vaccine conferred protections against all four serotypes of viruses in a mouse model (Wang et al., 2019). This vaccine design strategy uniformly enriched all conserved epitopes on a single E80, further incorporation of consensus E80 monomers derived from both DENV and ZIKV to a stabilized dimer might help to present most cross-neutralizing epitopes on surface.

Moreover, to elicit long-term neutralizing B cell memory response is another essential aim for dengue or Zika vaccine. In clinical trial of CYD-TDV, GMT of antibody to each serotype of viruses was measured at 28 days after each immunization, significant increase of GMT level was only observed after the 1st and 2nd immunization, and protection efficacy in recipients accepted all three doses (per protocol analysis) showed no differences with those only vaccinated for the first dose (intention-to-treat analysis) (Capeding et al., 2014; Villar et al., 2015). Whether B cell memory response elicited by multiple and single doses of CYD-TDV both waned to the same level in the first year is uncertain. For obvious reasons, dengue experienced vaccine recipients have higher GMT than dengue naïve ones, and the formers were better protected from subsequent dengue infections. In an earlier Phase I clinical trial with monovalent CYD-2 vaccine, dramatic decrease of neutralizing antibodies was observed in YF naïve group from 1st to 12th month, whereas YF-immune subjects maintained higher GMTs of antibody responses to dengue virus-2 and heterotypic viruses throughout the first year after immunization, despite the vaccine specific GMT were initially similar for the two groups in the 1st month (Guirakhoo et al., 2006). More followed-up studies are needed for confirmation, but it inferred that boosting with heterologous antigens (i.e., vaccinate recipients having prior flavivirus infection) have helped host immunity to focus on a few conserved epitopes to produce stronger and longer cross-reactive broadly neutralization responses, but repetition of immunization with same antigens (i.e., various antibody responses primed in the first immunization were equally boosted in the following two repeated immunization) only elicited various antibodies of weak cross-neutralization and sustained these responses only for a short-term. In fact, this hypothesis is in line with the theory of "original antigenic sin" (Halstead et al., 1983; Kuno et al., 1993; Zompi and Harris, 2013). Therefore, to achieve long-term antibody responses by B cells toward selected epitopes corresponding to stronger and broader neutralization, heterologous prime-boost immunization to highlight conserved epitopes might be a useful approach.

In summary, through enriching conserved epitopes and selectively presenting broadly neutralizing epitopes, we should be able to construct a universal dengue and Zika B cell vaccine. Furthermore, with suitable heterologous vaccines in prime-and-boost regimens, we might have a chance to achieve the induction of potent, broadly reactive, and protective B cell immune responses that have limited ADE effect.

T Cell Vaccines for DENV and ZIKV

In contrast to the extensive attention on B cell responses, T cell immunity produced by flavivirus vaccine had never been carefully examined until a recent retrospective study that investigated why there was a higher efficacy of CYD-TDV in dengue experienced than dengue naïve vaccine recipients. As a chimera of Dengue virus and YF-17D vaccine, CYD-TDV mainly elicited YFV specific T cell responses through YFV non-structural proteins, of which reactivity to dengue virus was limited. One hypothesis is that, with prior dengue virus infection, dengue specific memory T cell responses were boosted by YFV cross-reactive epitopes in seropositive recipients and contributed to protection. Indeed, the cross-serotype and cross-complex protection of dengue virus specific T cells has already been reported in mouse models. Specifically, memory T cells can relieve mice from lethal disease in an adoptive transfer model, avoiding ADE effect successfully (Wen et al., 2017a). Therefore, T cell vaccine is complementary to traditional B cell vaccines for defense against DENV and ZIKV.

Distinct from B cell epitopes, T cell epitopes are linear, continuous and major histocompatibility complex (MHC) antigen (human leukocyte antigen, HLA, in humans) restricted. Some HLA-linked protective epitopes have already been identified for DENV and ZIKV, it is worthwhile to study epitope distribution for more HLA allotypes. This can be initiated through predictive computational algorithms according to parameters such as MHC affinity, and followed by experimental verification (Elong Ngono et al., 2017, 2019). Viral proteins that contain most epitopes for common HLA allotypes could be included as antigens for T cell vaccines (**Figure 2**). Such an approach had been tested in a study of immunogenicity and protection efficacy of multiepitope DENV NS3 DNA vaccine in Balb/c mice, and it demonstrated that *in vivo* expression of NS3 epitopes elicited T cell responses and protective immunity against DENV-2 infection (Costa et al., 2011). Dominant epitopes from different proteins of different viruses presented by various HLA allotypes can also be integrated into a polypeptide string, which can be made into immunogens to elicit protective T cell immunity in a large population, just as what has been done for HIV CD4 + T cell vaccine (Liu H. et al., 2017).

Live attenuated vaccine has an advantage on eliciting T cell responses. TAK-003 and TV003 containing non-structural proteins of DENV have been shown to elicit both antibody responses and T cell responses. However, to avoid ADE, a flavivirus T cell vaccine without cell surface epitopes is obviously more suitable for the proof-of-concept study. To accomplish

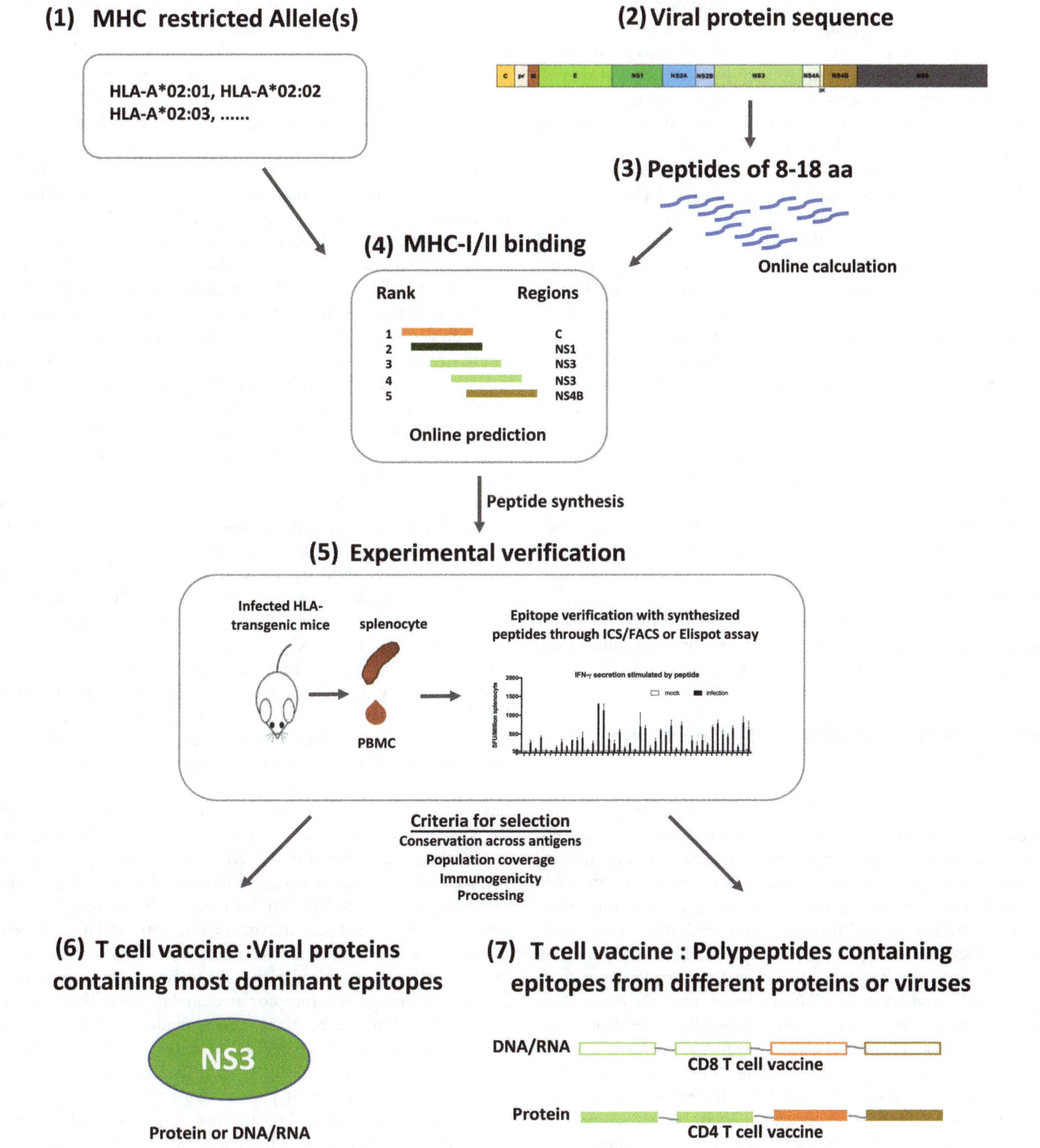

FIGURE 2 | Designing strategy for flavivirus T cell vaccines. Development of T cell vaccine could be initiated from the prediction of T cell epitopes on Immune Epitope Database (IEDB) (1–4). With selected HLA molecules (1) and protein sequences (2), both CD4 + and CD8 + T cell epitopes can be predicted according to the sequences of linear peptides derived from a protein (3), and the affinity of peptides to selected MHC molecules (4). Predicted epitopes were verified in HLA-transgenic mice with synthesized peptides through Elispot or Intracellular cytokine staining assay (5). Verified epitopes were further selected based on their conservation across different strains of viruses (HLA-allotype), population coverage, immunogenicity and processing efficiency, all of which could be calculated online. Some can be tested experimentally. Using these selected epitopes, T cell vaccine can be prepared with two different strategies, one is using antigens which contain most dominant epitopes and have reliable population coverage and sequence conservation (6); the other is to make immunogens with a string of peptides containing epitopes from different genes or strains, thus having higher population and antigen coverage (7). Both kinds of vaccines can be either DNA/RNA or proteins, depending on the T cell subset to be activated.

this goal, many factors affecting the immunogenicity of T cell antigens should be considered. First, immunogens activating two main subsets of T cells have to be delivered in different ways. CD4 + T cell epitopes are mainly presented through an exogenous antigen presentation pathway, whereas CD8 + T cell epitopes are presented more efficiently through an endogenous antigen presentation pathway (Cresswell et al., 2005; Roche and Furuta, 2015; Sadegh-Nasseri and Kim, 2019). Therefore, CD4 + T cell antigens should be administered either directly to extracellular space or secreted to extracellular space after *in vivo* expression. On the other hand, CD8 + T cell antigens are best delivered as DNA or RNA vaccines that have better antigen expression and retention intracellularly. Second, immune dominance of T cell epitopes might be affected by epitope composition of vaccines, and will also be influenced by prior flavivirus infection. How to induce protective T cell immunity toward four serotypes of DENV and ZIKV simultaneously, and whether cross-reactive T cell responses could be induced through heterologous prime-boost vaccination strategy, are all questions that have to be addressed during flavivirus T cell vaccine development. Finally, to achieve sterilizing immunity against viruses is extremely hard through T cell vaccine alone, as the effector T cells are only activated by processed immunogens and only target infected cells bearing linear epitopes on surface, both of which happen after cells were infected.

In summary, we propose an improvement of the strategy for dengue and Zika virus vaccine development by inclusion of T cell epitopes in order to overcome the ADE effect *in vivo*.

VECTOR BLOCKADE THROUGH NS1 ANTIBODIES

As both DENV and ZIKV are transmitted through *Aedes* mosquitoes, countermeasures that block the transmission steps of these vectors are important adjuncts to vaccines or antiviral drugs for controlling their infections. In urban areas, through spraying insecticides and clearing up standing water in containers such as discarded tires and plant pots, adult mosquitoes and mosquito larvae can be effectively removed. These approaches had helped to eliminate dengue fever from southern United States in 1920s. However, absolute elimination of mosquitoes from cities was impossible, reintroduction occurred when global travel became frequent and the new vector, *A. albopictus,* was imported from Asia. Nowadays, investigators are trying to sterilize mosquitoes through genetically engineered endosymbiotic bacteria *Wolbachia* (Zheng et al., 2019), but debate on its long-term ecological influence is continuing.

Leaving the eco-system intact, our investigations on NS1 provided an alternative strategy to block flavivirus-mosquito transmission which is more specific and environmentally friendly. Soluble NS1 hexamers are secreted during virus infection, and a high concentration of plasma NS1 coexists with viremia during the acute phase of disease. We demonstrated that blood meal from infected mice that have NS1 antigenemia can suppress the expression of immune genes (JAK-STAT, ROS) in midgut of mosquitoes, facilitating flavivirus acquisition by mosquitoes. Although transferring NS1 antibody to AG6 mice did not affect the viremia in mice directly, it significantly inhibited DENV-2 transmission from AG6 mice to mosquitoes (Liu J. et al., 2016). Immunization generated NS1 antibodies might competitively bind to soluble NS1 in blood and prevent NS1 from suppressing the expression of immune genes in midgut of mosquitoes after a blood meal. Furthermore, we demonstrated that NS1 antigenemia also determined ZIKV infectivity in mosquitoes. Specifically, comparing with ZIKV Asian strains that were isolated before recent outbreaks, contemporary strains causing recent epidemics have an alanine-to-valine substitution at the 188th residue in NS1. This mutation results in higher level of NS1 secretion, which subsequently dampens the expression of immune genes in mosquito and is responsible for the enhanced infectivity in mosquitoes. This mechanism helps to explain how ZIKV of Asian lineage acquired the ability to rapidly spread from Asia to America (Liu Y. et al., 2017).

Besides blockade of viral transmission, NS1 antibodies have been identified to have multiple other roles in immunity and host pathology, some of which are completely opposite. Previously, soluble DENV NS1 was found to contribute directly to vascular leakage through increasing endothelial permeability and degradation of endothelial glycocalyx components, or indirectly through inducing vasoactive cytokines (TNF-α, IL-1β, and IL-6) via TLR-4 activation (Beatty et al., 2015; Modhiran et al., 2015; Glasner et al., 2017). Further study on DENV, WNV, YFV, JEV, and ZIKV revealed that the effect of NS1 on cell permeability was probably universal in flavivirus but had tissue-specificity and thus there are different disease patterns for different viruses (Puerta-Guardo et al., 2019). In addition, DENV NS1 also facilitates viral immune evasion through inhibiting complement cascade in mammals (Avirutnan et al., 2010). Therefore, blocking NS1 through specific antibodies has been shown to attenuate plasma leakage and mortality in dengue infected mice (Henchal et al., 1988; Wan et al., 2017). Because a fraction of NS1 dimer also presents on the surface of infected cells, antibodies also probably target Fcγ-receptors to mediate viral clearance by phagocytosis or initiate complement dependent cytotoxicity (CDC). Recent investigations show that transferring ZIKV NS1 antibodies from human or vaccinated mice to IFN deficient mice provided protection through Fcγ-receptor mediated pathway (Bailey et al., 2018, 2019). On the contrary, much evidence also indicated NS1 antibodies being capable of cross-react with coagulation factors and adhesin molecules on platelets and endothelial cells, causing disruption of platelet aggregation and apoptosis of endothelial cells, and thus leading to pathology in DENV infections (Falconar, 1997; Lin et al., 2005; Cheng et al., 2009; Liu et al., 2011).

Based on these evidence, we had constructed a modified DENV2 sNS1 with deletion of epitopes mimicking autoantigens (ΔNS1), and found that prior immunization with either ΔNS1 or full-length NS1 in AG6 mice significantly helped to neutralize NS1 antigenemia and block the transmission of virus to mosquitoes. Notably, unlike antibodies elicited to full-length NS1, antibodies generated against ΔNS1 did not cross-react with human endothelial cells or human primary platelets. And after infection, viremia in mice immunized with modified-NS1 (ΔNS1) was significantly lower than those of mock or full-length NS1 immunized mice (Liu J. et al., 2016). In agreement with these results, mice immunized with ΔNS1 showed less vascular leakage and higher survival rate in AG6 mice after DENV-2 challenge, compared to mice that were immunized with full-length NS1 or PBS. Collectively, through antibodies specific to NS1 proteins that have been removed cross-reactive epitopes to autoantigens, we had successfully overcome the adverse effect of NS1 antibodies, blocked virus transmission, inhibited virus replication and protected mice from lethal diseases. Importantly, antibodies to NS1 do not have any risk of inducing ADE.

All above suggest that NS1 is an important target for blocking DENV/ZIKV human-mosquito transmission, and the modified NS1 elicits protective immunity toward ZIKV/DENV infection. Inclusion of suitable form of NS1 in human vaccine might offer a better chance for defeating DENV and ZIKV epidemics.

SPECIAL CONCERNS IN THE DEVELOPMENT OF ZIKV AND DENV VACCINES

Because ZIKV and DENV have different pathogenic characteristics and tropism, special issues should be considered during the development of vaccines to these viruses, especially for prophylactic ZIKV vaccines which are currently under development by several research groups (Richner et al., 2017b; Tebas et al., 2017; Medina et al., 2018; Modjarrad et al., 2018; Zou et al., 2018).

At the early stage of vaccine development for these two viruses, the primary aims are to inhibit virus replication in vaccinated animals, and to reduce mortality in lethal infection murine models. However, ZIKV has the ability to infect and replicate in reproductive systems, it can disseminate through sexual and vertical transmission, and it is associated with increased incidence of microcephaly in fetus. It is still unclear what level of viral load is enough to cause vertical or sexual transmission, or induce inflammation in these tissues and placenta, or damage testicle, or contribute to fetal microcephaly. According to the literature, viral clearance might be more difficult in these organs comparing to others (Barzon et al., 2016; Govero et al., 2016; Mansuy et al., 2016; Prisant et al., 2016; Miner and Diamond, 2017). Therefore, during ZIKV vaccine development, specified criteria for protective efficacies should include reduced neuropathology in adult mice, inhibited vertical transmission to fetus in pregnant animals, and decreased damages to reproductive systems. In contrast, evaluation of DENV vaccine in disease models mainly includes blockage of vascular leakage or hemorrhagic manifestations in mouse model.

Correspondingly, in clinical trial, severe dengue (DHS/DSS), virologically confirmed dengue, and hospitalization were the three major parameters to evaluate DENV vaccine candidates (Hadinegoro et al., 2015; Biswal et al., 2019). In addition to these three parameters, for the evaluation of ZIKV vaccine, other parameters might have to be included, such as neurological diseases (Guillain-Barre syndrome, fetal brain development abnormality).

To fulfill the criteria above, ZIKV vaccine strategy should also be modified, since the characteristics and type of protective immune responses in different organs are not the same. For example, the access of T cells to maternal-fetal interface was limited during pregnancy (Nancy et al., 2012). It has been found that weaker T cell responses were elicited by a live attenuated ZIKV vaccine during pregnancy, comparing to that in non-pregnant mice. In addition, higher neutralizing antibody titers were required to protect pregnant mice and block vertical transmission of ZIKV (Shan et al., 2019). Such evidence warrants a vaccine with higher potency in eliciting T cell and B cell immunity. In another study, it is observed that CD4 + T cell mediated antibody response, but not CD8 + T cells, was essential for viral clearance in intravaginal infection model. Though further investigations are necessary, this might imply the importance of CD4 + T cell immunity in blocking sexual transmission, which should also be considered during vaccine design (Elong Ngono et al., 2019).

A ONE-TWO PUNCH STRATEGY

After it is discovered for 70 years, we are still searching for better approaches to defeat dengue viruses. The sudden outbreaks of Zika virus has brought additional difficulties to solve the dengue problem, because the pre-existing ZIKV antibodies have the potential to enhance DENV infection, and antibodies elicited by dengue vaccines also have the potential to augment ZIKV infection. However, as for any other scientific challenges before, the large global outbreak of ZIKV has brought in extensive investigations on flavivirus virology, immunology, vaccinology, vector biology, and new tools to counteract the diseases. To combat mosquito-borne viruses, a one-two punch strategy that combines human preventive vaccine and vector blockade to cut transmission cycles at multiple steps may be necessary (as **Figure 3** shows). Compared with other approaches for vector blockade, active immunization with NS1/ΔNS1 in human, is more feasible and has less spillover effect on ecology. Application of B cell vaccines producing broadly neutralizing antibodies may efficiently block virus infection in human and inhibit both vertical and sexual transmission of ZIKV. In addition, T cell vaccine can act in synergy with B cell vaccine to elicit functional T cell responses that inhibit virus replication in human, aiding to protect human from severe disease. At a minimal, incorporating NS1 within both B cell and T cell vaccines will likely to help overcoming the effect of ADE in human, blocking transmission to mosquitos, and providing opportunities for total disease control. However, further experimental evaluation on the feasibility, efficiency and safety of these approaches are necessary.

SUMMARY

We have reviewed the existing knowledge on epidemiology, molecular virology, and vaccine development of DENV and ZIKV; and updated our understanding on

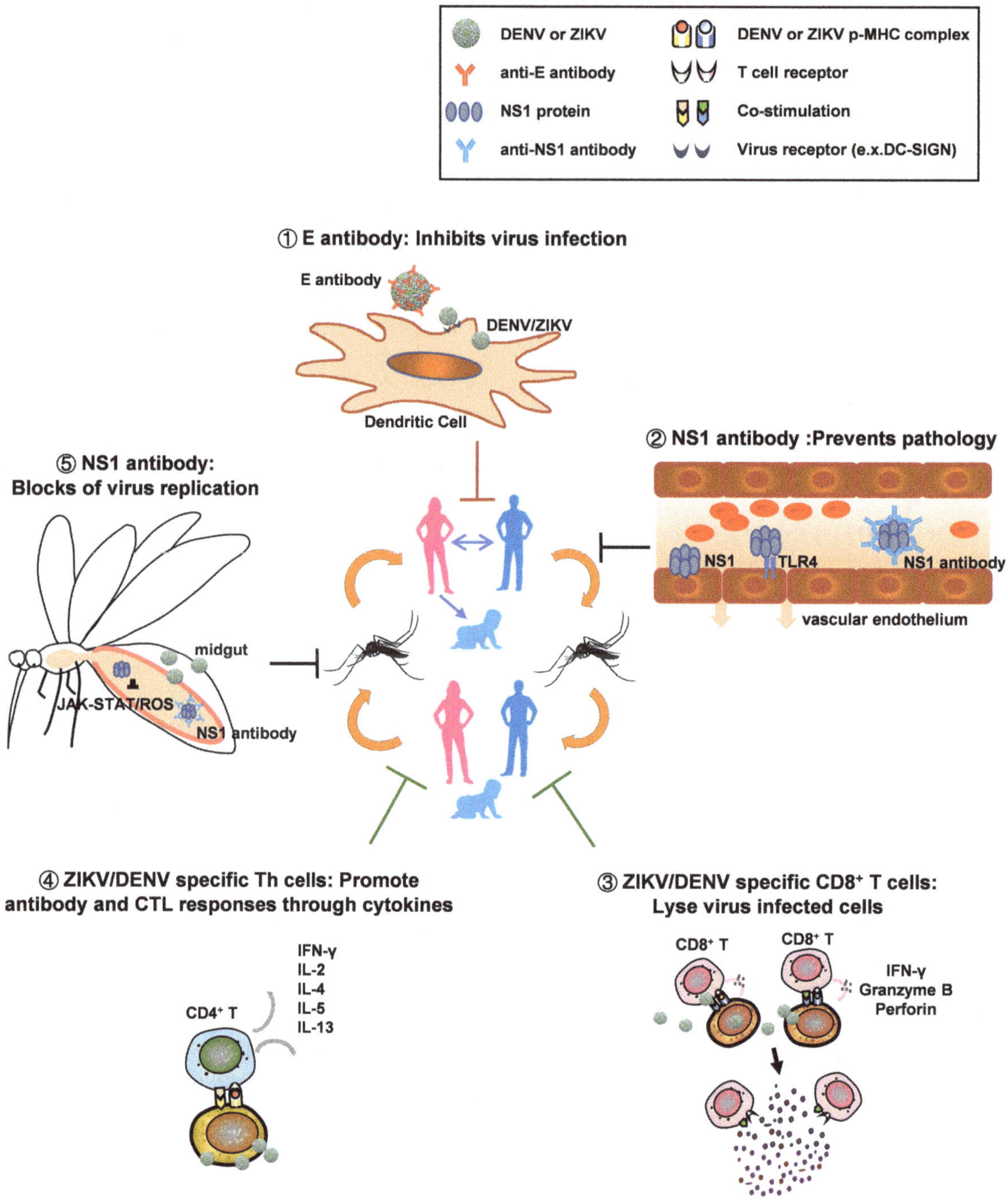

FIGURE 3 | Urban cycle of dengue and Zika virus transmission can be blocked at multiple steps by vaccine elicited immune responses. Both dengue and Zika viruses are transmitted between human through mosquitoes in urban areas, where prevention measures can be applied. By human immunization with universal or pentavalent vaccines that elicit both T cell and B cell responses, especially those that also target NS1antigens, viral transmission in the urban cycle may be blocked and viral diseases can be controlled at multiple steps: (1) Virus transmission to humans and virus replication *in vivo* are inhibited by broadly neutralizing antibodies specific for envelope proteins; these antibodies block virus attachment and virus entry in dendritic cells or other target cells such as monocytes and macrophages; (2) Antibodies specific for NS1 proteins; these can reduce virus induced pathology in human through preventing NS1 hexamers attachment to endothelial cells, because the attachment may trigger the degradation of endothelial glycocalyx components or activate TLR4 pathway to produce vasoactive cytokines, both of which will increase endothelium permeability; (3) Virus replication in human is inhibited by functional CD8 + T cells. Vaccine induced memory CD8 + T cells can be activated by infected cells that present DENV or ZIKV peptides in the context of MHC-I molecules, and activated CD8 + T cells directly lyse infected cells by secreting granzyme B and perforin; (4) Both CD8 + T cell and antibody-producing B cell responses are facilitated by activated CD4 + T helper (Th) cells that secret cytokines such as IFN-γ, IL-2,IL-4, IL-5, or IL-13; (5) Viral transmission to mosquitoes is inhibited by NS1 antibodies. Mosquitoes acquire both NS1 protein and virus particles during a blood meal from acutely infected patients. The NS1 antigenemia could help virus to replicate in the midgut of mosquitoes, by antagonizing mosquito immunity such as JAK-STAT and ROS pathways. The abundant NS1 antibodies in human plasma of vaccine recipients may bind to NS1 protein and thus neutralize the antagonistic effect of NS1 to mosquito immunity, resulting in restriction of virus propagation in the midgut of mosquitoes.

protective immunity against DENV and ZIKV. We have also discussed recent discoveries on the functions of flavivirus NS1 in viral pathogenesis and transmission. Based on such knowledge, we proposed a potential one-two punch strategy that overcomes ADE and defeats Dengue and Zika viruses through a combination of vaccines and vector blockade.

AUTHOR CONTRIBUTIONS

XJ conceived, drafted, and wrote the manuscript. JS drafted and wrote the manuscript. ZZ assisted to make the tables and drew the figure. SD and GC modified the manuscript, assisted to write, and amended the sections on NS1.

FUNDING

This work was supported by the grant: National Natural Science Foundation of China, 31670941; Ministry of Science and Technology of People's Republic of China, 2016YFC1201000; Strategic Priority Research Program of the Chinese Academy of Sciences, XDB29040000; and Science and Technology Commission of Shanghai Municipality, 19ZR1462900.

REFERENCES

Abbink, P., Larocca, R. A., Dejnirattisai, W., Peterson, R., Nkolola, J. P., Borducchi, E. N., et al. (2018). Therapeutic and protective efficacy of a dengue antibody against Zika infection in rhesus monkeys. *Nat. Med.* 24, 721–723. doi: 10.1038/s41591-018-0056-0

Avirutnan, P., Fuchs, A., Hauhart, R. E., Somnuke, P., Youn, S., Diamond, M. S., et al. (2010). Antagonism of the complement component C4 by flavivirus nonstructural protein NS1. *J. Exp. Med.* 207, 793–806. doi: 10.1084/jem.20092545

Bailey, M. J., Broecker, F., Duehr, J., Arumemi, F., Krammer, F., Palese, P., et al. (2019). Antibodies elicited by an ns1-based vaccine protect mice against Zika Virus. *MBio* 10, e2861–e2818. doi: 10.1128/mBio.02861-18

Bailey, M. J., Duehr, J., Dulin, H., Broecker, F., Brown, J. A., Arumemi, F. O., et al. (2018). Human antibodies targeting Zika virus NS1 provide protection against disease in a mouse model. *Nat. Commun.* 9:4560. doi: 10.1038/s41467-018-07008-0

Bardina, S. V., Bunduc, P., Tripathi, S., Duehr, J., Frere, J. J., Brown, J. A., et al. (2017). Enhancement of Zika virus pathogenesis by preexisting antiflavivirus immunity. *Science* 356, 175–180. doi: 10.1126/science.aal4365

Barnett, R. (2017). Dengue. *Lancet* 390:1941. doi: 10.1016/S0140-6736(17)32651-X

Barzon, L., Pacenti, M., Franchin, E., Lavezzo, E., Trevisan, M., Sgarabotto, D., et al. (2016). Infection dynamics in a traveller with persistent shedding of Zika virus RNA in semen for six months after returning from Haiti to Italy, January 2016. *Euro Surveill* 21:30316. doi: 10.2807/1560-7917.ES.2016.21.32.30316

Baud, D., Gubler, D. J., Schaub, B., Lanteri, M. C., and Musso, D. (2017). An update on Zika virus infection. *Lancet* 390, 2099–2109. doi: 10.1016/S0140-6736(17)31450-2

Beatty, P. R., Puerta-Guardo, H., Killingbeck, S. S., Glasner, D. R., Hopkins, K., and Harris, E. (2015). Dengue virus NS1 triggers endothelial permeability and vascular leak that is prevented by NS1 vaccination. *Sci. Transl. Med/.* 7:304ra141. doi: 10.1126/scitranslmed.aaa3787

Beckett, C. G., Tjaden, J., Burgess, T., Danko, J. R., Tamminga, C., Simmons, M., et al. (2011). Evaluation of a prototype dengue-1 DNA vaccine in a Phase 1 clinical trial. *Vaccine* 29, 960–968. doi: 10.1016/j.vaccine.2010.11.050

Beltramello, M., Williams, K. L., Simmons, C. P., Macagno, A., Simonelli, L., Quyen, N. T., et al. (2010). The human immune response to Dengue virus is dominated by highly cross-reactive antibodies endowed with neutralizing and enhancing activity. *Cell Host Microbe* 8, 271–283. doi: 10.1016/j.chom.2010.08.007

Bhamarapravati, N., Yoksan, S., Chayaniyayothin, T., Angsubphakorn, S., and Bunyaratvej, A. (1987). Immunization with a live attenuated dengue-2-virus candidate vaccine (16681-PDK 53): clinical, immunological and biological responses in adult volunteers. *Bull World Health Organ.* 65, 189–195.

Bhatt, S., Gething, P. W., Brady, O. J., Messina, J. P., Farlow, A. W., Moyes, C. L., et al. (2013). The global distribution and burden of dengue. *Nature* 496, 504–507. doi: 10.1038/nature12060

Biswal, S., Reynales, H., Saez-Llorens, X., Lopez, P., Borja-Tabora, C., Kosalaraksa, P., et al. (2019). Efficacy of a tetravalent dengue vaccine in healthy children and adolescents. *N. Engl. J. Med.* 381, 2009–2019. doi: 10.1056/NEJMoa1903869

Blackley, S., Kou, Z., Chen, H., Quinn, M., Rose, R. C., Schlesinger, J. J., et al. (2007). Primary human splenic macrophages, but not T or B cells, are the principal target cells for dengue virus infection in vitro. *J. Virol.* 81, 13325–13334. doi: 10.1128/JVI.01568-07

Blaney, JE Jr, Johnson, D. H., Firestone, C. Y., Hanson, C. T., Murphy, B. R., and Whitehead, S. S. (2001). Chemical mutagenesis of dengue virus type 4 yields mutant viruses which are temperature sensitive in vero cells or human liver cells and attenuated in mice. *J. Virol.* 75, 9731–9740. doi: 10.1128/JVI.75.20.9731-9740.2001

Blaney, JE Jr, Sathe, N. S., Goddard, L., Hanson, C. T., Romero, T. A., Hanley, K. A., et al. (2008). Dengue virus type 3 vaccine candidates generated by introduction of deletions in the 3′ untranslated region (3′-UTR) or by exchange of the DENV-3 3'-UTR with that of DENV-4. *Vaccine* 26, 817–828. doi: 10.1016/j.vaccine.2007.11.082

Block, O. K., Rodrigo, W. W., Quinn, M., Jin, X., Rose, R. C., and Schlesinger, J. J. (2010). A tetravalent recombinant dengue domain III protein vaccine stimulates neutralizing and enhancing antibodies in mice. *Vaccine* 28, 8085–8094. doi: 10.1016/j.vaccine.2010.10.004

Brady, O. J., Gething, P. W., Bhatt, S., Messina, J. P., Brownstein, J. S., Hoen, A. G., et al. (2012). Refining the global spatial limits of dengue virus transmission by evidence-based consensus. *PLoS Negl. Trop. Dis.* 6:e1760. doi: 10.1371/journal.pntd.0001760

Brandler, S., Brown, N., Ermak, T. H., Mitchell, F., Parsons, M., Zhang, Z., et al. (2005). Replication of chimeric yellow fever virus-dengue serotype 1-4 virus vaccine strains in dendritic and hepatic cells. *Am. J. Trop. Med. Hyg.* 72, 74–81. doi: 10.4269/ajtmh.2005.72.74

Campos, G. S., Bandeira, A. C., and Sardi, S. I. (2015). Zika virus outbreak. Bahia, Brazil. *Emerg. Infect. Dis.* 21, 1885–1886. doi: 10.3201/eid2110.150847

Capeding, M. R., Tran, N. H., Hadinegoro, S. R., Ismail, H. I., Chotpitayasunondh, T., Chua, M. N., et al. (2014). Clinical efficacy and safety of a novel tetravalent dengue vaccine in healthy children in Asia: a phase 3, randomised, observer-masked, placebo-controlled trial. *Lancet* 384, 1358–1365. doi: 10.1016/S0140-6736(14)61060-6

Carey, D. E. (1971). Chikungunya and dengue: a case of mistaken identity? *J. Hist. Med. Allied Sci.* 26, 243–262. doi: 10.1093/jhmas/xxvi.3.243

Cheng, H. J., Lei, H. Y., Lin, C. F., Luo, Y. H., Wan, S. W., Liu, H. S., et al. (2009). Anti-dengue virus nonstructural protein 1 antibodies recognize protein disulfide isomerase on platelets and inhibit platelet aggregation. *Mol. Immunol.* 47, 398–406. doi: 10.1016/j.molimm.2009.08.033

Clarke, T. (2002). Dengue virus: break-bone fever. *Nature* 416, 672–674. doi: 10.1038/416672a

Clements, D. E., Coller, B. A., Lieberman, M. M., Ogata, S., Wang, G., Harada, K. E., et al. (2010). Development of a recombinant tetravalent dengue virus vaccine: immunogenicity and efficacy studies in mice and monkeys. *Vaccine* 28, 2705–2715. doi: 10.1016/j.vaccine.2010.01.022

Collins, M. H., Tu, H. A., Gimblet-Ochieng, C., Liou, G. A., Jadi, R. S., Metz, S. W., et al. (2019). Human antibody response to Zika targets type-specific quaternary structure epitopes. *JCI Insight* 4:e123588. doi: 10.1172/jci.insight.124588

Costa, S. M., Yorio, A. P., Goncalves, A. J., Vidale, M. M., Costa, E. C., Mohana-Borges, R., et al. (2011). Induction of a protective response in mice by the dengue virus NS3 protein using DNA vaccines. *PLoS One* 6:e25685. doi: 10.1371/journal.pone.0025685

Cresswell, P., Ackerman, A. L., Giodini, A., Peaper, D. R., and Wearsch, P. A. (2005). Mechanisms of MHC class I-restricted antigen processing and cross-presentation. *Immunol. Rev.* 207, 145–157. doi: 10.1111/j.0105-2896.2005.00316.x

Crill, W. D., and Chang, G. J. (2004). Localization and characterization of flavivirus envelope glycoprotein cross-reactive epitopes. *J. Virol.* 78, 13975–13986. doi: 10.1128/JVI.78.24.13975-13986.2004

Dalrymple, N. A., and Mackow, E. R. (2012). Endothelial cells elicit immune-enhancing responses to dengue virus infection. *J. Virol.* 86, 6408–6415. doi: 10.1128/JVI.00213-12

Dayan, G. H., Garbes, P., Noriega, F., Izoton, de Sadovsky, A. D., Rodrigues, P. M., et al. (2013a). Immunogenicity and safety of a recombinant tetravalent dengue vaccine in children and adolescents ages 9-16 years in Brazil. *Am. J. Trop. Med. Hyg.* 89, 1058–1065. doi: 10.4269/ajtmh.13-0304

Dayan, G. H., Thakur, M., Boaz, M., and Johnson, C. (2013b). Safety and immunogenicity of three tetravalent dengue vaccine formulations in healthy adults in the USA. *Vaccine* 31, 5047–5054. doi: 10.1016/j.vaccine.2013.08.088

de Alwis, R., Williams, K. L., Schmid, M. A., Lai, C. Y., Patel, B., Smith, S. A., et al. (2014). Dengue viruses are enhanced by distinct populations of serotype cross-reactive antibodies in human immune sera. *PLoS Pathog.* 10:e1004386. doi: 10.1371/journal.ppat.1004386

Dejnirattisai, W., Jumnainsong, A., Onsirisakul, N., Fitton, P., Vasanawathana, S., Limpitikul, W., et al. (2010). Cross-reacting antibodies enhance dengue virus infection in humans. *Science* 328, 745–748. doi: 10.1126/science.1185181

Dejnirattisai, W., Supasa, P., Wongwiwat, W., Rouvinski, A., Barba-Spaeth, G., Duangchinda, T., et al. (2016). Dengue virus sero-cross-reactivity drives antibody-dependent enhancement of infection with zika virus. *Nat. Immunol.* 17, 1102–1108. doi: 10.1038/ni.3515

Dejnirattisai, W., Wongwiwat, W., Supasa, S., Zhang, X., Dai, X., Rouvinski, A., et al. (2015). A new class of highly potent, broadly neutralizing antibodies isolated from viremic patients infected with dengue virus. *Nat. Immunol.* 16, 170–177. doi: 10.1038/ni.3058

Dick, G. W., Kitchen, S. F., and Haddow, A. J. (1952). Zika virus. I. Isolations and serological specificity. *Trans. R Soc. Trop. Med. Hyg.* 46, 509–520. doi: 10.1016/0035-9203(52)90042-4

Duangchinda, T., Dejnirattisai, W., Vasanawathana, S., Limpitikul, W., Tangthawornchaikul, N., Malasit, P., et al. (2010). Immunodominant T-cell responses to dengue virus NS3 are associated with DHF. *Proc. Natl. Acad. Sci. U.S.A.* 107, 16922–16927. doi: 10.1073/pnas.1010867107

Duffy, M. R., Chen, T. H., Hancock, W. T., Powers, A. M., Kool, J. L., Lanciotti, R. S., et al. (2009). Zika virus outbreak on Yap Island. Federated States of Micronesia. *N. Engl. J. Med.* 360, 2536–2543. doi: 10.1056/NEJMoa0805715

Dung, N. T., Duyen, H. T., Thuy, N. T., Ngoc, T. V., Chau, N. V., Hien, T. T., et al. (2010). Timing of CD8+ T cell responses in relation to commencement of capillary leakage in children with dengue. *J. Immunol.* 184, 7281–7287. doi: 10.4049/jimmunol.0903262

Durbin, A., and Wilder-Smith, A. (2017). An update on Zika vaccine developments. *Expert Rev. Vaccines* 16, 781–787. doi: 10.1080/14760584.2017.1345309

Durbin, A. P., Kirkpatrick, B. D., Pierce, K. K., Elwood, D., Larsson, C. J., Lindow, J. C., et al. (2013). A single dose of any of four different live attenuated tetravalent dengue vaccines is safe and immunogenic in flavivirus-naive adults: a randomized, double-blind clinical trial. *J. Infect. Dis.* 207, 957–965. doi: 10.1093/infdis/jis936

Durbin, A. P., McArthur, J. H., Marron, J. A., Blaney, J. E., Thumar, B., Wanionek, K., et al. (2006). rDEN2/4Delta30(ME), a live attenuated chimeric dengue serotype 2 vaccine is safe and highly immunogenic in healthy dengue-naive adults. *Hum. Vaccin* 2, 255–260. doi: 10.4161/hv.2.6.3494

Durbin, A. P., Whitehead, S. S., McArthur, J., Perreault, J. R., Blaney, JE Jr, Thumar, B., et al. (2005). rDEN4delta30, a live attenuated dengue virus type 4 vaccine candidate, is safe, immunogenic, and highly infectious in healthy adult volunteers. *J. Infect. Dis.* 191, 710–718. doi: 10.1086/427780

Durbin, A. P., Whitehead, S. S., Shaffer, D., Elwood, D., Wanionek, K., Thumar, B., et al. (2011). A single dose of the DENV-1 candidate vaccine rDEN1Delta30 is strongly immunogenic and induces resistance to a second dose in a randomized trial. *PLoS Negl. Trop. Dis.* 5:e1267. doi: 10.1371/journal.pntd.0001267

Elong Ngono, A., Vizcarra, E. A., Tang, W. W., Sheets, N., Joo, Y., Kim, K., et al. (2017). Mapping and role of the CD8(+) T cell response during primary Zika Virus Infection in Mice. *Cell Host Microbe* 21, 35–46. doi: 10.1016/j.chom.2016.12.010

Elong Ngono, A., Young, M. P., Bunz, M., Xu, Z., Hattakam, S., Vizcarra, E., et al. (2019). CD4+ T cells promote humoral immunity and viral control during Zika virus infection. *PLoS Pathog.* 15:e1007474. doi: 10.1371/journal.ppat.1007474

Falconar, A. K. (1997). The dengue virus nonstructural-1 protein (NS1) generates antibodies to common epitopes on human blood clotting, integrin/adhesin proteins and binds to human endothelial cells: potential implications in haemorrhagic fever pathogenesis. *Arch. Virol.* 142, 897–916. doi: 10.1007/s007050050127

Faria, N. R., Quick, J., Claro, I. M., Theze, J., de Jesus, J. G., Giovanetti, M., et al. (2017). Establishment and cryptic transmission of Zika virus in Brazil and the Americas. *Nature* 546, 406–410. doi: 10.1038/nature22401

Fatima, K., and Syed, N. I. (2018). Dengvaxia controversy: impact on vaccine hesitancy. *J. Glob. Health* 8:010312. doi: 10.7189/jogh.08-020312

Fernandez, E., Dejnirattisai, W., Cao, B., Scheaffer, S. M., Supasa, P., Wongwiwat, W., et al. (2017). Human antibodies to the dengue virus E-dimer epitope have therapeutic activity against Zika virus infection. *Nat. Immunol.* 18, 1261–1269. doi: 10.1038/ni.3849

Foo, S. S., Chen, W., Chan, Y., Bowman, J. W., Chang, L. C., Choi, Y., et al. (2017). Asian Zika virus strains target CD14(+) blood monocytes and induce M2-skewed immunosuppression during pregnancy. *Nat. Microbiol.* 2, 1558–1570. doi: 10.1038/s41564-017-0016-3

Fowler, A. M., Tang, W. W., Young, M. P., Mamidi, A., Viramontes, K. M., McCauley, M. D., et al. (2018). Maternally acquired zika antibodies enhance dengue disease severity in mice. *Cell Host Microbe* 24, 743.E5–750.e5. doi: 10.1016/j.chom.2018.09.015

Gaucher, D., Therrien, R., Kettaf, N., Angermann, B. R., Boucher, G., Filali-Mouhim, A., et al. (2008). Yellow fever vaccine induces integrated multilineage and polyfunctional immune responses. *J. Exp. Med.* 205, 3119–3131. doi: 10.1084/jem.20082292

Gaudinski, M. R., Houser, K. V., Morabito, K. M., Hu, Z., Yamshchikov, G., Rothwell, R. S., et al. (2018). Safety, tolerability, and immunogenicity of two Zika virus DNA vaccine candidates in healthy adults: randomised, open-label, phase 1 clinical trials. *Lancet* 391, 552–562. doi: 10.1016/S0140-6736(17)33105-7

George, S. L., Wong, M. A., Dube, T. J., Boroughs, K. L., Stovall, J. L., Luy, B. E., et al. (2015). Safety and immunogenicity of a live attenuated tetravalent dengue vaccine candidate in flavivirus-naive adults: a Randomized, double-blinded phase 1 Clinical Trial. *J. Infect. Dis.* 212, 1032–1041. doi: 10.1093/infdis/jiv179

Glasner, D. R., Ratnasiri, K., Puerta-Guardo, H., Espinosa, D. A., Beatty, P. R., and Harris, E. (2017). Dengue virus NS1 cytokine-independent vascular leak is dependent on endothelial glycocalyx components. *PLoS Pathog.* 13:e1006673. doi: 10.1371/journal.ppat.1006673

Govero, J., Esakky, P., Scheaffer, S. M., Fernandez, E., Drury, A., Platt, D. J., et al. (2016). Zika virus infection damages the testes in mice. *Nature* 540, 438–442. doi: 10.1038/nature20556

Govindarajan, D., Meschino, S., Guan, L., Clements, D. E., ter Meulen, J. H., Casimiro, D. R., et al. (2015). Preclinical development of a dengue tetravalent recombinant subunit vaccine: Immunogenicity and protective efficacy in nonhuman primates. *Vaccine* 33, 4105–4116. doi: 10.1016/j.vaccine.2015.06.067

Grard, G., Caron, M., Mombo, I. M., Nkoghe, D., Mboui Ondo, S., Jiolle, D., et al. (2014). Zika virus in Gabon (Central Africa)–2007: a new threat from Aedes albopictus? *PLoS Negl. Trop. Dis.* 8:e2681. doi: 10.1371/journal.pntd.0002681

Griffin, B. D., Muthumani, K., Warner, B. M., Majer, A., Hagan, M., Audet, J., et al. (2017). DNA vaccination protects mice against Zika virus-induced damage to the testes. *Nat. Commun.* 8:15743. doi: 10.1038/ncomms15743

Grifoni, A., Angelo, M. A., Lopez, B., O'Rourke, P. H., Sidney, J., Cerpas, C., et al. (2017a). Global assessment of dengue virus-specific CD4(+) T cell responses in dengue-endemic areas. *Front. Immunol.* 8:1309. doi: 10.3389/fimmu.2017.01309

Grifoni, A., Pham, J., Sidney, J., O'Rourke, P. H., Paul, S., Peters, B., et al. (2017b). Prior dengue virus exposure shapes T Cell Immunity to Zika Virus in Humans. *J. Virol.* 91:e01469-17. doi: 10.1128/JVI.01469-17

Grifoni, A., Costa-Ramos, P., Pham, J., Tian, Y., Rosales, S. L., Seumois, G., et al. (2018). Cutting edge: transcriptional profiling reveals multifunctional and cytotoxic antiviral responses of Zika Virus-Specific CD8(+) T Cells. *J. Immunol.* 201, 3487–3491. doi: 10.4049/jimmunol.1801090

Gubler, D. J. (1987). Dengue and dengue hemorrhagic fever in the Americas. *P R Health Sci. J.* 6, 107–111.

Guirakhoo, F., Arroyo, J., Pugachev, K. V., Miller, C., Zhang, Z. X., Weltzin, R., et al. (2001). Construction, safety, and immunogenicity in nonhuman primates of a chimeric yellow fever-dengue virus tetravalent vaccine. *J. Virol.* 75, 7290–7304. doi: 10.1128/JVI.75.16.7290-7304.2001

Guirakhoo, F., Kitchener, S., Morrison, D., Forrat, R., McCarthy, K., Nichols, R., et al. (2006). Live attenuated chimeric yellow fever dengue type 2 (ChimeriVax-DEN2) vaccine: phase I clinical trial for safety and immunogenicity: effect of yellow fever pre-immunity in induction of cross neutralizing antibody responses to all 4 dengue serotypes. *Hum. Vaccin* 2, 60–67. doi: 10.4161/hv.2.2.2555

Guirakhoo, F., Pugachev, K., Arroyo, J., Miller, C., Zhang, Z. X., Weltzin, R., et al. (2002). Viremia and immunogenicity in nonhuman primates of a tetravalent yellow fever-dengue chimeric vaccine: genetic reconstructions, dose adjustment, and antibody responses against wild-type dengue virus isolates. *Virology* 298, 146–159. doi: 10.1006/viro.2002.1462

Guirakhoo, F., Weltzin, R., Chambers, T. J., Zhang, Z. X., Soike, K., Ratterree, M., et al. (2000). Recombinant chimeric yellow fever-dengue type 2 virus is immunogenic and protective in nonhuman primates. *J. Virol.* 74, 5477–5485. doi: 10.1128/jvi.74.12.5477-5485.2000

Guzman, M. G., Alvarez, M., and Halstead, S. B. (2013). Secondary infection as a risk factor for dengue hemorrhagic fever/dengue shock syndrome: an historical perspective and role of antibody-dependent enhancement of infection. *Arch. Virol.* 158, 1445–1459. doi: 10.1007/s00705-013-1645-3

Guzman, M. G., Halstead, S. B., Artsob, H., Buchy, P., Farrar, J., Gubler, D. J., et al. (2010). Dengue: a continuing global threat. *Nat. Rev,. Microbiol.* 8(Suppl.), S7–S16. doi: 10.1038/nrmicro2460

Hadinegoro, S. R., Arredondo-Garcia, J. L., Capeding, M. R., Deseda, C., Chotpitayasunondh, T., Dietze, R., et al. (2015). Efficacy and long-term safety of a dengue vaccine in regions of endemic disease. *N. Engl. J. Med.* 373, 1195–1206. doi: 10.1056/NEJMoa1506223

Halstead, S. B. (1966). Mosquito-borne haemorrhagic fevers of South and South-East Asia. *Bull. World Health Organ.* 35, 3–15.

Halstead, S. B. (1988). Pathogenesis of dengue: challenges to molecular biology. *Science* 239, 476–481. doi: 10.1126/science.3277268

Halstead, S. B. (2003). Neutralization and antibody-dependent enhancement of dengue viruses. *Adv. Virus Res.* 60, 421–467. doi: 10.1016/s0065-3527(03) 60011-4

Halstead, S. B., and Dans, L. F. (2019). Dengue infection and advances in dengue vaccines for children. *Lancet Child Adolesc. Health* 3, 734–741. doi: 10.1016/S2352-4642(19)30205-6

Halstead, S. B., Mahalingam, S., Marovich, M. A., Ubol, S., and Mosser, D. M. (2010). Intrinsic antibody-dependent enhancement of microbial infection in macrophages: disease regulation by immune complexes. *Lancet Infect. Dis.* 10, 712–722. doi: 10.1016/S1473-3099(10)70166-3

Halstead, S. B., Rojanasuphot, S., and Sangkawibha, N. (1983). Original antigenic sin in dengue. *Am. J. Trop. Med. Hyg.* 32, 154–156. doi: 10.4269/ajtmh.1983.32.154

Hasan, S. S., Miller, A., Sapparapu, G., Fernandez, E., Klose, T., Long, F., et al. (2017). A human antibody against Zika virus crosslinks the E protein to prevent infection. *Nat. Commun.* 8:14722. doi: 10.1038/ncomms14722

Hassert, M., Wolf, K. J., Schwetye, K. E., DiPaolo, R. J., Brien, J. D., and Pinto, A. K. (2018). CD4+T cells mediate protection against Zika associated severe disease in a mouse model of infection. *PLoS Pathog.* 14:e1007237. doi: 10.1371/journal.ppat.1007237

Henchal, E. A., Henchal, L. S., and Schlesinger, J. J. (1988). Synergistic interactions of anti-NS1 monoclonal antibodies protect passively immunized mice from lethal challenge with dengue 2 virus. *J. Gen. Virol.* 69(Pt 8), 2101–2107. doi: 10.1099/0022-1317-69-8-2101

Higgs, S., Vanlandingham, D. L., Klingler, K. A., McElroy, K. L., McGee, C. E., Harrington, L., et al. (2006). Growth characteristics of ChimeriVax-Den vaccine viruses in Aedes aegypti and Aedes albopictus from Thailand. *Am. J. Trop. Med. Hyg.* 75, 986–993. doi: 10.4269/ajtmh.2006.75.986

Holmes, E. C., and Twiddy, S. S. (2003). The origin, emergence and evolutionary genetics of dengue virus. *Infect. Genet. Evol.* 3, 19–28. doi: 10.1016/s1567-1348(03)00004-2

Hss, A. S., Koh, M. T., Tan, K. K., Chan, L. G., Zhou, L., Bouckenooghe, A., et al. (2013). Safety and immunogenicity of a tetravalent dengue vaccine in healthy children aged 2-11 years in Malaysia: a randomized, placebo-controlled. Phase III study. *Vaccine* 31, 5814–5821. doi: 10.1016/j.vaccine.2013.10.013

Huang, H., Li, S., Zhang, Y., Han, X., Jia, B., Liu, H., et al. (2017). CD8(+) T Cell Immune Response in Immunocompetent Mice during Zika Virus Infection. *J. Virol.* 91, e900–e917. doi: 10.1128/JVI.00900-17

Jessie, K., Fong, M. Y., Devi, S., Lam, S. K., and Wong, K. T. (2004). Localization of dengue virus in naturally infected human tissues, by immunohistochemistry and in situ hybridization. *J. Infect. Dis.* 189, 1411–1418. doi: 10.1086/383043

Jin, X. (2008). Cellular and molecular basis of antibody-dependent enhancement in human dengue pathogenesis. *Future Virol.* 3, 343–361. doi: 10.2217/17460794.3.4.343

Jurado, K. A., Yockey, L. J., Wong, P. W., Lee, S., Huttner, A. J., and Iwasaki, A. (2018). Antiviral CD8 T cells induce Zika-virus-associated paralysis in mice. *Nat. Microbiol.* 3, 141–147. doi: 10.1038/s41564-017-0060-z

Katzelnick, L. C., Gresh, L., Halloran, M. E., Mercado, J. C., Kuan, G., Gordon, A., et al. (2017). Antibody-dependent enhancement of severe dengue disease in humans. *Science* 358, 929–932. doi: 10.1126/science.aan6836

Khaiboullina, S., Uppal, T., Kletenkov, K., St Jeor, S. C., Garanina, E., Rizvanov, A., et al. (2019). Transcriptome profiling reveals Pro-Inflammatory cytokines and matrix metalloproteinase activation in Zika Virus infected human umbilical vein endothelial cells. *Front. Pharmacol.* 10:642. doi: 10.3389/fphar.2019.00642

Khaiboullina, S. F., Ribeiro, F. M., Uppal, T., Martynova, E. V., Rizvanov, A. A., and Verma, S. C. (2019). Zika virus transmission through blood tissue barriers. *Front. Microbiol.* 10:1465. doi: 10.3389/fmicb.2019.01465

Kirkpatrick, B. D., Whitehead, S. S., Pierce, K. K., Tibery, C. M., Grier, P. L., Hynes, N. A., et al. (2016). The live attenuated dengue vaccine TV003 elicits complete protection against dengue in a human challenge model. *Sci Transl Med 8(330), 330ra336.* doi: 119710.1126/scitranslmed.aaf1517

Kliks, S. (1990). Antibody-enhanced infection of monocytes as the pathogenetic mechanism for severe dengue illness. *AIDS Res. Hum. Retroviruses* 6, 993–998. doi: 10.1089/aid.1990.6.993

Kou, Z., Quinn, M., Chen, H., Rodrigo, W. W., Rose, R. C., Schlesinger, J. J., et al. (2008). Monocytes, but not T or B cells, are the principal target cells for dengue virus (DV) infection among human peripheral blood mononuclear cells. *J. Med. Virol.* 80, 134–146. doi: 10.1002/jmv.21051

Kuno, G., Gubler, D. J., and Oliver, A. (1993). Use of 'original antigenic sin' theory to determine the serotypes of previous dengue infections. *Trans. R Soc. Trop. Med. Hyg.* 87, 103–105. doi: 10.1016/0035-9203(93)90444-u

Lanata, C. F., Andrade, T., Gil, A. I., Terrones, C., Valladolid, O., Zambrano, B., et al. (2012). Immunogenicity and safety of tetravalent dengue vaccine in 2-11 year-olds previously vaccinated against yellow fever: randomized, controlled, phase II study in Piura. *Peru. Vaccine* 30, 5935–5941. doi: 10.1016/j.vaccine.2012.07.043

Leborgne, C., Latournerie, V., Boutin, S., Desgue, D., Quere, A., Pignot, E., et al. (2019). Prevalence and long-term monitoring of humoral immunity against adeno-associated virus in duchenne muscular dystrophy patients. *Cell Immunol.* 342:103780. doi: 10.1016/j.cellimm.2018.03.004

Li, C., Xu, D., Ye, Q., Hong, S., Jiang, Y., Liu, X., et al. (2016). Zika virus disrupts neural progenitor development and leads to microcephaly in mice. *Cell Stem Cell* 19, 120–126. doi: 10.1016/j.stem.2016.04.017

Li, M., Wang, X., Wang, Q., Yu, L., Wang, L., Yan, J., et al. (2017). Both structure and function of human monoclonal antibodies contribute to enhancement of Zika virus infectivity in vitro. *Sci. China Life Sci.* 60, 1396–1398. doi: 10.1007/s11427-017-9192-0

Li, M., Zhao, L., Zhang, C., Wang, X., Hong, W., Sun, J., et al. (2018). Dengue immune sera enhance Zika virus infection in human peripheral blood monocytes through Fc gamma receptors. *PLoS One* 13:e0200478. doi: 10.1371/journal.pone.0200478

Liang, H., Yang, R., Liu, Z., Li, M., Liu, H., and Jin, X. (2018). Recombinant Zika virus envelope protein elicited protective immunity against Zika virus in immunocompetent mice. *PLoS One* 13:e0194860. doi: 10.1371/journal.pone.0194860

Lim, M. Q., Kumaran, E. A. P., Tan, H. C., Lye, D. C., Leo, Y. S., Ooi, E. E., et al. (2018). Cross-reactivity and anti-viral function of dengue capsid and NS3-specific memory T Cells Toward Zika Virus. *Front. Immunol.* 9:2225. doi: 10.3389/fimmu.2018.02225

Limon-Flores, A. Y., Perez-Tapia, M., Estrada-Garcia, I., Vaughan, G., Escobar-Gutierrez, A., Calderon-Amador, J., et al. (2005). Dengue virus inoculation to human skin explants: an effective approach to assess in situ the early infection and the effects on cutaneous dendritic cells. *Int. J. Exp. Pathol.* 86, 323–334. doi: 10.1111/j.0959-9673.2005.00445.x

Lin, C. F., Chiu, S. C., Hsiao, Y. L., Wan, S. W., Lei, H. Y., Shiau, A. L., et al. (2005). Expression of cytokine, chemokine, and adhesion molecules during endothelial cell activation induced by antibodies against dengue virus nonstructural protein 1. *J. Immunol.* 174, 395–403. doi: 10.4049/jimmunol.174.1.395

Lindenbach, B. D., Thiel, H. J., and Rice, C. M. (2007). "Flaviviridae:the Viruses and Their replication," in *Fields Virology*, ed. P. M. H. D. M. Knipe (Philadelphia: Wolters Kluwer Health/Lippincott Williams & Wilkins), 1101–1152.

Liu, H., Shen, W., Shu, J., Kou, Z., and Jin, X. (2017). A novel polyepitope vaccine elicited HIV peptide specific CD4+ T cell responses in HLA-A2/DRB1 transgenic mice. *PLoS One* 12:e0184207. doi: 10.1371/journal.pone.0184207

Liu, Y., Liu, J., Du, S., Shan, C., Nie, K., Zhang, R., et al. (2017). Evolutionary enhancement of Zika virus infectivity in Aedes aegypti mosquitoes. *Nature* 545, 482–486. doi: 10.1038/nature22365

Liu, I. J., Chiu, C. Y., Chen, Y. C., and Wu, H. C. (2011). Molecular mimicry of human endothelial cell antigen by autoantibodies to nonstructural protein 1 of dengue virus. *J. Biol. Chem.* 286, 9726–9736. doi: 10.1074/jbc.M110.170993

Liu, J., Liu, Y., Nie, K., Du, S., Qiu, J., Pang, X., et al. (2016). Flavivirus NS1 protein in infected host sera enhances viral acquisition by mosquitoes. *Nat. Microbiol.* 1:16087. doi: 10.1038/nmicrobiol.2016.87

Liu, S., DeLalio, L. J., Isakson, B. E., and Wang, T. T. (2016). AXL-Mediated Productive Infection of Human Endothelial Cells by Zika Virus. *Circ. Res.* 119, 1183–1189. doi: 10.1161/CIRCRESAHA.116.309866

Lok, S. M., Kostyuchenko, V., Nybakken, G. E., Holdaway, H. A., Battisti, A. J., Sukupolvi-Petty, S., et al. (2008). Binding of a neutralizing antibody to dengue virus alters the arrangement of surface glycoproteins. *Nat. Struct. Mol. Biol.* 15, 312–317. doi: 10.1038/nsmb.1382

Ma, W., Li, S., Ma, S., Jia, L., Zhang, F., Zhang, Y., et al. (2016). Zika virus causes testis damage and leads to male infertility in mice. *Cell* 167, 1511.e10–1524.e10 doi: 10.1016/j.cell.2016.11.016

Mackenzie, J. S., Gubler, D. J., and Petersen, L. R. (2004). Emerging flaviviruses: the spread and resurgence of Japanese encephalitis, West Nile and dengue viruses. *Nat. Med.* 10(Suppl.), S98–S109. doi: 10.1038/nm1144

Manoff, S. B., Sausser, M., Falk Russell, A., Martin, J., Radley, D., Hyatt, D., et al. (2019). Immunogenicity and safety of an investigational tetravalent recombinant subunit vaccine for dengue: results of a Phase I randomized clinical trial in flavivirus-naive adults. *Hum. Vaccin Immunother.* 15, 2195–2204. doi: 10.1080/21645515.2018.1546523

Mansuy, J. M., Dutertre, M., Mengelle, C., Fourcade, C., Marchou, B., Delobel, P., et al. (2016). Zika virus: high infectious viral load in semen, a new sexually transmitted pathogen? *Lancet Infect Dis.* 16:405. doi: 10.1016/S1473-3099(16)00138-9

Mantel, N., Girerd, Y., Geny, C., Bernard, I., Pontvianne, J., Lang, J., et al. (2011). Genetic stability of a dengue vaccine based on chimeric yellow fever/dengue viruses. *Vaccine* 29, 6629–6635. doi: 10.1016/j.vaccine.2011.06.101

Marianneau, P., Steffan, A. M., Royer, C., Drouet, M. T., Jaeck, D., Kirn, A., et al. (1999). Infection of primary cultures of human Kupffer cells by Dengue virus: no viral progeny synthesis, but cytokine production is evident. *J. Virol.* 73, 5201–5206. doi: 10.1128/jvi.73.6.5201-5206.1999

Martines, R. B., Bhatnagar, J., de Oliveira Ramos, A. M., Davi, H. P., Iglezias, S. D., Kanamura, C. T., et al. (2016). Pathology of congenital Zika syndrome in Brazil: a case series. *Lancet* 388, 898–904. doi: 10.1016/S0140-6736(16)30883-2

McCracken, M. K., Gromowski, G. D., Friberg, H. L., Lin, X., Abbink, P., De La Barrera, R., et al. (2017). Impact of prior flavivirus immunity on Zika virus infection in rhesus macaques. *PLoS Pathog.* 13:e1006487. doi: 10.1371/journal.ppat.1006487

McGee, C. E., Tsetsarkin, K., Vanlandingham, D. L., McElroy, K. L., Lang, J., Guy, B., et al. (2008). Substitution of wild-type yellow fever Asibi sequences for 17D vaccine sequences in ChimeriVax-dengue 4 does not enhance infection of Aedes aegypti mosquitoes. *J. Infect. Dis.* 197, 686–692. doi: 10.1086/527328

Medina, L. O., To, A., Lieberman, M. M., Wong, T. A. S., Namekar, M., Nakano, E., et al. (2018). A recombinant subunit based zika virus vaccine is efficacious in Non-human primates. *Front. Immunol.* 9:2464. doi: 10.3389/fimmu.2018.02464

Messina, J. P., Brady, O. J., Golding, N., Kraemer, M. U. G., Wint, G. R. W., Ray, S. E., et al. (2019). The current and future global distribution and population at risk of dengue. *Nat. Microbiol.* 4, 1508–1515. doi: 10.1038/s41564-019-0476-8

Metz, S. W., Thomas, A., Brackbill, A., Forsberg, J., Miley, M. J., Lopez, C. A., et al. (2019). Oligomeric state of the ZIKV E protein defines protective immune responses. *Nat. Commun.* 10:4606. doi: 10.1038/s41467-019-12677-6

Michlmayr, D., Andrade, P., Gonzalez, K., Balmaseda, A., and Harris, E. (2017). CD14(+)CD16(+) monocytes are the main target of Zika virus infection in peripheral blood mononuclear cells in a paediatric study in Nicaragua. *Nat. Microbiol.* 2, 1462–1470. doi: 10.1038/s41564-017-0035-0

Miner, J. J., and Diamond, M. S. (2017). Zika virus pathogenesis and tissue tropism. *Cell Host Microbe* 21, 134–142. doi: 10.1016/j.chom.2017.01.004

Mitragotri, S. (2006). Current status and future prospects of needle-free liquid jet injectors. *Nat. Rev. Drug Discov.* 5, 543–548. doi: 10.1038/nrd2076

Mlakar, J., Korva, M., Tul, N., Popovic, M., Poljsak-Prijatelj, M., Mraz, J., et al. (2016). Zika virus associated with microcephaly. *N. Engl. J. Med* 374, 951–958. doi: 10.1056/NEJMoa1600651

Modhiran, N., Watterson, D., Muller, D. A., Panetta, A. K., Sester, D. P., Liu, L., et al. (2015). Dengue virus NS1 protein activates cells via Toll-like receptor 4 and disrupts endothelial cell monolayer integrity. *Sci. Transl. Med.* 7:304ra142. doi: 10.1126/scitranslmed.aaa3863

Modjarrad, K., Lin, L., George, S. L., Stephenson, K. E., Eckels, K. H., De La Barrera, R. A., et al. (2018). Preliminary aggregate safety and immunogenicity results from three trials of a purified inactivated Zika virus vaccine candidate: phase 1, randomised, double-blind, placebo-controlled clinical trials. *Lancet* 391, 563–571. doi: 10.1016/S0140-6736(17)33106-9

Musso, D., Bossin, H., Mallet, H. P., Besnard, M., Broult, J., Baudouin, L., et al. (2018). Zika virus in French Polynesia 2013-14: anatomy of a completed outbreak. *Lancet Infect Dis.* 18, e172–e182. doi: 10.1016/S1473-3099(17)30446-2

Nancy, P., Tagliani, E., Tay, C. S., Asp, P., Levy, D. E., and Erlebacher, A. (2012). Chemokine gene silencing in decidual stromal cells limits T cell access to the maternal-fetal interface. *Science* 336, 1317–1321. doi: 10.1126/science.1220030

Netto, E. M., Moreira-Soto, A., Pedroso, C., Hoser, C., Funk, S., Kucharski, A. J., et al. (2017). High Zika virus seroprevalence in salvador, northeastern brazil limits the potential for further outbreaks. *MBio* 8:01390-17. doi: 10.1128/mBio.01390-17

Ngono, A. E., and Shresta, S. (2018). Immune response to dengue and zika. *Annu. Rev. Immunol.* 36, 279–308. doi: 10.1146/annurev-immunol-042617-053142

Osorio, J. E., Partidos, C. D., Wallace, D., and Stinchcomb, D. T. (2015). Development of a recombinant, chimeric tetravalent dengue vaccine candidate. *Vaccine* 33, 7112–7120. doi: 10.1016/j.vaccine.2015.11.022

Osorio, J. E., Velez, I. D., Thomson, C., Lopez, L., Jimenez, A., Haller, A. A., et al. (2014). Safety and immunogenicity of a recombinant live attenuated tetravalent dengue vaccine (DENVax) in flavivirus-naive healthy adults in Colombia: a randomised, placebo-controlled, phase 1 study. *Lancet Infect Dis.* 14, 830–838. doi: 10.1016/S1473-3099(14)70811-4

Packard, R. M. (2016). The Fielding H. Garrison Lecture: "Break-Bone" Fever in Philadelphia, 1780: Reflections on the History of Disease. *Bull. Hist Med.* 90, 193–221. doi: 10.1353/bhm.2016.0041

Pantoja, P., Perez-Guzman, E. X., Rodriguez, I. V., White, L. J., Gonzalez, O., Serrano, C., et al. (2017). Zika virus pathogenesis in rhesus macaques is unaffected by pre-existing immunity to dengue virus. *Nat. Commun.* 8:15674. doi: 10.1038/ncomms15674

Papa, M. P., Meuren, L. M., Coelho, S. V. A., Lucas, C. G. O., Mustafa, Y. M., Lemos Matassoli, F., et al. (2017). Zika Virus infects, activates, and crosses brain microvascular endothelial cells, without barrier disruption. *Front. Microbiol.* 8:2557. doi: 10.3389/fmicb.2017.02557

Pierson, T. C., Xu, Q., Nelson, S., Oliphant, T., Nybakken, G. E., Fremont, D. H., et al. (2007). The stoichiometry of antibody-mediated neutralization and enhancement of West Nile virus infection. *Cell Host Microbe* 1, 135–145. doi: 10.1016/j.chom.2007.03.002

Porter, K. R., Ewing, D., Chen, L., Wu, S. J., Hayes, C. G., Ferrari, M., et al. (2012). Immunogenicity and protective efficacy of a vaxfectin-adjuvanted tetravalent dengue DNA vaccine. *Vaccine* 30, 336–341. doi: 10.1016/j.vaccine.2011.10.085

Prasad, V. M., Miller, A. S., Klose, T., Sirohi, D., Buda, G., Jiang, W., et al. (2017). Structure of the immature Zika virus at 9 A resolution. *Nat. Struct. Mol. Biol.* 24, 184–186. doi: 10.1038/nsmb.3352

Prisant, N., Bujan, L., Benichou, H., Hayot, P. H., Pavili, L., Lurel, S., et al. (2016). Zika virus in the female genital tract. *Lancet Infect Dis.* 16, 1000–1001. doi: 10.1016/S1473-3099(16)30193-1

Puerta-Guardo, H., Glasner, D. R., Espinosa, D. A., Biering, S. B., Patana, M., Ratnasiri, K., et al. (2019). Flavivirus NS1 triggers tissue-specific vascular endothelial dysfunction reflecting disease tropism. *Cell Rep.* 26, 1598.e8–1613.e8. doi: 10.1016/j.celrep.2019.01.036

Qian, X., Nguyen, H. N., Jacob, F., Song, H., and Ming, G. L. (2017). Using brain organoids to understand Zika virus-induced microcephaly. *Development* 144, 952–957. doi: 10.1242/dev.140707

Quicke, K. M., Bowen, J. R., Johnson, E. L., McDonald, C. E., Ma, H., O'Neal, J. T., et al. (2016). Zika Virus Infects Human Placental Macrophages. *Cell Host Microbe* 20, 83–90. doi: 10.1016/j.chom.2016.05.015

Regla-Nava, J. A., Elong Ngono, A., Viramontes, K. M., Huynh, A. T., Wang, Y. T., Nguyen, A. T., et al. (2018). Cross-reactive Dengue virus-specific CD8(+) T cells protect against Zika virus during pregnancy. *Nat. Commun.* 9:3042. doi: 10.1038/s41467-018-05458-0

Richner, J. M., Himansu, S., Dowd, K. A., Butler, S. L., Salazar, V., Fox, J. M., et al. (2017a). Modified mRNA vaccines protect against Zika Virus Infection. *Cell* 169:176. doi: 10.1016/j.cell.2017.03.016

Richner, J. M., Jagger, B. W., Shan, C., Fontes, C. R., Dowd, K. A., Cao, B., et al. (2017b). Vaccine mediated protection against Zika virus-induced congenital disease. *Cell* 170, 273.e12–283.e12. doi: 10.1016/j.cell.2017.06.040

Rivino, L., Tan, A. T., Chia, A., Kumaran, E. A., Grotenbreg, G. M., MacAry, P. A., et al. (2013). Defining CD8+ T cell determinants during human viral infection in populations of Asian ethnicity. *J. Immunol.* 191, 4010–4019. doi: 10.4049/jimmunol.1301507

Robbiani, D. F., Bozzacco, L., Keeffe, J. R., Khouri, R., Olsen, P. C., Gazumyan, A., et al. (2017). Recurrent potent human neutralizing antibodies to zika virus in brazil and mexico. *Cell* 169, 597.e11–609.e11. doi: 10.1016/j.cell.2017.04.024

Roche, P. A., and Furuta, K. (2015). The ins and outs of MHC class II-mediated antigen processing and presentation. *Nat. Rev. Immunol.* 15, 203–216. doi: 10.1038/nri3818

Rodenhuis-Zybert, I. A., van der Schaar, H. M., da Silva, Voorham, J. M., van der Ende-Metselaar, H., Lei, H. Y., et al. (2010). Immature dengue virus: a veiled pathogen? *PLoS Pathog.* 6:e1000718. doi: 10.1371/journal.ppat.1000718

Rodriguez-Barraquer, I., Costa, F., Nascimento, E. J. M., Nery, N. J., Castanha, P. M. S., Sacramento, G. A., et al. (2019). Impact of preexisting dengue immunity on Zika virus emergence in a dengue endemic region. *Science* 363, 607–610. doi: 10.1126/science.aav6618

Rothman, A. L., Medin, C. L., Friberg, H., and Currier, J. R. (2014). Immunopathogenesis versus protection in dengue virus infections. *Curr. Trop. Med. Rep.* 1, 13–20. doi: 10.1007/s40475-013-0009-0

Rouvinski, A., Dejnirattisai, W., Guardado-Calvo, P., Vaney, M. C., Sharma, A., Duquerroy, S., et al. (2017). Covalently linked dengue virus envelope glycoprotein dimers reduce exposure of the immunodominant fusion loop epitope. *Nat. Commun.* 8:15411. doi: 10.1038/ncomms15411

Rouvinski, A., Guardado-Calvo, P., Barba-Spaeth, G., Duquerroy, S., Vaney, M. C., Kikuti, C. M., et al. (2015). Recognition determinants of broadly neutralizing human antibodies against dengue viruses. *Nature* 520, 109–113. doi: 10.1038/nature14130

Rush, B. (1951). An account of the bilious remitting fever: as it appeared in philadelphia, in the summer and autumn of the year 1780. *Am. J. Med.* 11, 546–550. doi: 10.1016/0002-9343(51)90035-6

Sabchareon, A., Wallace, D., Sirivichayakul, C., Limkittikul, K., Chanthavanich, P., Suvannadabba, S., et al. (2012). Protective efficacy of the recombinant, live-attenuated, CYD tetravalent dengue vaccine in Thai schoolchildren: a randomised, controlled phase 2b trial. *Lancet* 380, 1559–1567. doi: 10.1016/S0140-6736(12)61428-7

Sabin, A. B. (1952). Research on dengue during World War II. *Am. J. Trop. Med. Hyg.* 1, 30–50. doi: 10.4269/ajtmh.1952.1.30

Sadegh-Nasseri, S., and Kim, A. (2019). Selection of immunodominant epitopes during antigen processing is hierarchical. *Mol. Immunol.* 113, 115–119. doi: 10.1016/j.molimm.2018.08.011

Sanchez-San Martin, C., Li, T., Bouquet, J., Streithorst, J., Yu, G., Paranjpe, A., et al. (2018). Differentiation enhances Zika virus infection of neuronal brain cells. *Sci. Rep.* 8:14543. doi: 10.1038/s41598-018-32400-7

Sangkawibha, N., Rojanasuphot, S., Ahandrik, S., Viriyapongse, S., Jatanasen, S., Salitul, V., et al. (1984). Risk factors in dengue shock syndrome: a prospective epidemiologic study in Rayong. Thailand. I. The 1980 outbreak. *Am. .J Epidemiol.* 120, 653–669. doi: 10.1093/oxfordjournals.aje.a113932

Sapparapu, G., Fernandez, E., Kose, N., Bin, C., Fox, J. M., Bombardi, R. G., et al. (2016). Neutralizing human antibodies prevent Zika virus replication and fetal disease in mice. *Nature* 540, 443–447. doi: 10.1038/nature20564

Shan, C., Muruato, A. E., Jagger, B. W., Richner, J., Nunes, B. T. D., Medeiros, D. B. A., et al. (2017). A single-dose live-attenuated vaccine prevents Zika virus pregnancy transmission and testis damage. *Nat. Commun.* 8:676. doi: 10.1038/s41467-017-00737-8

Shan, C., Xie, X., Luo, H., Muruato, A. E., Liu, Y., Wakamiya, M., et al. (2019). Maternal vaccination and protective immunity against Zika virus vertical transmission. *Nat. Commun.* 10:5677. doi: 10.1038/s41467-019-13589-1

Sharma, M., Glasner, D. R., Watkins, H., Puerta-Guardo, H., Kassa, Y., Egan, M. A., et al. (2019). Magnitude and functionality of the ns1-specific antibody response elicited by a live-attenuated tetravalent dengue vaccine candidate. *J. Infect. Dis.* 221, 867–877. doi: 10.1093/infdis/jiz081

Sirivichayakul, C., Barranco-Santana, E. A., Esquilin-Rivera, I., Oh, H. M., Raanan, M., Sariol, C. A., et al. (2016). Safety and immunogenicity of a tetravalent dengue vaccine candidate in healthy children and adults in dengue-endemic regions: a randomized, placebo-controlled phase 2 Study. *J. Infect. Dis.* 213, 1562–1572. doi: 10.1093/infdis/jiv762

Sirohi, D., Chen, Z., Sun, L., Klose, T., Pierson, T. C., Rossmann, M. G., et al. (2016). The 3.8 A resolution cryo-EM structure of Zika virus. *Science* 352, 467–470. doi: 10.1126/science.aaf5316

Slon-Campos, J. L., Dejnirattisai, W., Jagger, B. W., Lopez-Camacho, C., Wongwiwat, W., Durnell, L. A., et al. (2019). A protective Zika virus E-dimer-based subunit vaccine engineered to abrogate antibody-dependent enhancement of dengue infection. *Nat. Immunol.* 20, 1291–1298. doi: 10.1038/s41590-019-0477-z

Spiteri, G., Sudre, B., Septfons, A., Beaute, J., The European, Zika Surveillance, et al. (2017). Surveillance of Zika virus infection in the EU/EEA, June 2015 to January 2017. *Euro. Surveill* 22, 17–00254. doi: 10.2807/1560-7917.ES.2017.22.41.17-00254

St John, A. L., and Rathore, A. P. S. (2019). Adaptive immune responses to primary and secondary dengue virus infections. *Nat. Rev. Immunol.* 19, 218–230. doi: 10.1038/s41577-019-0123-x

Stettler, K., Beltramello, M., Espinosa, D. A., Graham, V., Cassotta, A., Bianchi, S., et al. (2016). Specificity, cross-reactivity, and function of antibodies elicited by Zika virus infection. *Science* 353, 823–826. doi: 10.1126/science.aaf8505

Sun, J., Li, M., Wang, Y., Hao, P., and Jin, X. (2017). Elaboration of tetravalent antibody responses against dengue viruses using a subunit vaccine comprised of a single consensus dengue envelope sequence. *Vaccine* 35, 6308–6320. doi: 10.1016/j.vaccine.2017.09.063

Szaba, F. M., Tighe, M., Kummer, L. W., Lanzer, K. G., Ward, J. M., Lanthier, P., et al. (2018). Zika virus infection in immunocompetent pregnant mice causes fetal damage and placental pathology in the absence of fetal infection. *PLoS Pathog.* 14:e1006994. doi: 10.1371/journal.ppat.1006994

Tamhankar, M., and Patterson, J. L. (2019). Directional entry and release of Zika virus from polarized epithelial cells. *Virol. J.* 16:99. doi: 10.1186/s12985-019-1200-2

Tebas, P., Roberts, C. C., Muthumani, K., Reuschel, E. L., Kudchodkar, S. B., Zaidi, F. I., et al. (2017). Safety and Immunogenicity of an Anti-Zika Virus DNA Vaccine - Preliminary Report. *N. Engl. J. Med.* doi: 10.1056/NEJMoa1708120

Urakami, A., Ngwe Tun, M. M., Moi, M. L., Sakurai, A., Ishikawa, M., Kuno, S., et al. (2017). An envelope-modified tetravalent dengue virus-like-particle vaccine has implications for flavivirus vaccine design. *J. Virol.* 91:e01181-17. doi: 10.1128/JVI.01181-17

Vannice, K. S., Wilder-Smith, A., Barrett, A. D. T., Carrijo, K., Cavaleri, M., de Silva, A., et al. (2018). Clinical development and regulatory points for consideration for second-generation live attenuated dengue vaccines. *Vaccine* 36, 3411–3417. doi: 10.1016/j.vaccine.2018.02.062

Vermillion, M. S., Lei, J., Shabi, Y., Baxter, V. K., Crilly, N. P., McLane, M., et al. (2017). Intrauterine Zika virus infection of pregnant immunocompetent mice models transplacental transmission and adverse perinatal outcomes. *Nat. Commun.* 8:14575. doi: 10.1038/ncomms14575

Villar, L., Dayan, G. H., Arredondo-Garcia, J. L., Rivera, D. M., Cunha, R., Deseda, C., et al. (2015). Efficacy of a tetravalent dengue vaccine in children in Latin America. *N. Engl. J. Med.* 372, 113–123. doi: 10.1056/NEJMoa1411037

Wan, S. W., Chen, P. W., Chen, C. Y., Lai, Y. C., Chu, Y. T., Hung, C. Y., et al. (2017). Therapeutic effects of monoclonal antibody against dengue Virus NS1 in a STAT1 knockout mouse model of dengue infection. *J. Immunol.* 199, 2834–2844. doi: 10.4049/jimmunol.1601523

Wang, E., Ni, H., Xu, R., Barrett, A. D., Watowich, S. J., Gubler, D. J., et al. (2000). Evolutionary relationships of endemic/epidemic and sylvatic dengue viruses. *J. Virol.* 74, 3227–3234. doi: 10.1128/jvi.74.7.3227-3234.2000

Wang, R., Zheng, X., Sun, J., Feng, K., Gao, N., Fan, D., et al. (2019). Vaccination with a single consensus envelope protein ectodomain sequence administered in a heterologous regimen induces tetravalent immune responses and protection against dengue viruses in mice. *Front. Microbiol.* 10:1113. doi: 10.3389/fmicb.2019.01113

Weaver, S. C., Costa, F., Garcia-Blanco, M. A., Ko, A. I., Ribeiro, G. S., Saade, G., et al. (2016). Zika virus: History, emergence, biology, and prospects for control. *Antiviral. Res.* 130, 69–80. doi: 10.1016/j.antiviral.2016.03.010

Weiskopf, D., Angelo, M. A., Bangs, D. J., Sidney, J., Paul, S., Peters, B., et al. (2015a). The human CD8+ T cell responses induced by a live attenuated tetravalent dengue vaccine are directed against highly conserved epitopes. *J. Virol.* 89, 120–128. doi: 10.1128/JVI.02129-14

Weiskopf, D., Cerpas, C., Angelo, M. A., Bangs, D. J., Sidney, J., Paul, S., et al. (2015b). Human CD8+ T-Cell responses against the 4 dengue virus serotypes are associated with distinct patterns of protein targets. *J. Infect. Dis.* 212, 1743–1751. doi: 10.1093/infdis/jiv289

Weiskopf, D., Angelo, M. A., de Azeredo, E. L., Sidney, J., Greenbaum, J. A., Fernando, A. N., et al. (2013). Comprehensive analysis of dengue virus-specific responses supports an HLA-linked protective role for CD8+ T cells. *Proc. Natl. Acad. Sci. U.S.A.* 110, E2046–E2053. doi: 10.1073/pnas.1305227110

Weiskopf, D., Angelo, M. A., Grifoni, A., O'Rourke, P. H., Sidney, J., Paul, S., et al. (2016). HLA-DRB1 alleles are associated with different magnitudes of dengue virus-specific CD4+ T-Cell Responses. *J. Infect. Dis.* 214, 1117–1124. doi: 10.1093/infdis/jiw309

Weiskopf, D., Angelo, M. A., Sidney, J., Peters, B., Shresta, S., and Sette, A. (2014). Immunodominance changes as a function of the infecting dengue virus serotype and primary versus secondary infection. *J. Virol.* 88, 11383–11394. doi: 10.1128/JVI.01108-14

Wen, J., Elong Ngono, A., Regla-Nava, J. A., Kim, K., Gorman, M. J., Diamond, M. S., et al. (2017a). Dengue virus-reactive CD8(+) T cells mediate cross-protection against subsequent Zika virus challenge. *Nat. Commun.* 8:1459. doi: 10.1038/s41467-017-01669-z

Wen, J., Tang, W. W., Sheets, N., Ellison, J., Sette, A., Kim, K., et al. (2017b). Identification of Zika virus epitopes reveals immunodominant and protective roles for dengue virus cross-reactive CD8(+) T cells. *Nat. Microbiol,.* 2:17036. doi: 10.1038/nmicrobiol.2017.36

Whitehead, S. S., Falgout, B., Hanley, K. A., Blaney, JE Jr, Markoff, L., and Murphy, B. R. (2003a). A live, attenuated dengue virus type 1 vaccine candidate with a 30-nucleotide deletion in the 3' untranslated region is highly attenuated and immunogenic in monkeys. *J. Virol.* 77, 1653–1657. doi: 10.1128/jvi.77.2.1653-1657.2003

Whitehead, S. S., Hanley, K. A., Blaney, JE Jr, Gilmore, L. E., Elkins, W. R., and Murphy, B. R. (2003b). Substitution of the structural genes of dengue virus type 4 with those of type 2 results in chimeric vaccine candidates which are attenuated for mosquitoes, mice, and rhesus monkeys. *Vaccine* 21, 4307–4316. doi: 10.1016/s0264-410x(03)00488-2

Wilder-Smith, A., Vannice, K., Durbin, A., Hombach, J., Thomas, S. J., Thevarjan, I., et al. (2018). Zika vaccines and therapeutics: landscape analysis and challenges ahead. *BMC Med.* 16:84. doi: 10.1186/s12916-018-1067-x

Williams, K. L., Wahala, W. M., Orozco, S., de Silva, A. M., and Harris, E. (2012). Antibodies targeting dengue virus envelope domain III are not required for serotype-specific protection or prevention of enhancement in vivo. *Virology* 429, 12–20. doi: 10.1016/j.virol.2012.03.003

Wirawan, M., Fibriansah, G., Marzinek, J. K., Lim, X. X., Ng, T. S., Sim, A. Y. L., et al. (2019). Mechanism of enhanced immature dengue virus attachment to endosomal membrane induced by prm antibody. *Structure* 27, 253.e8–267.e8. doi: 10.1016/j.str.2018.10.009

World Health Organization [WHO] (1966). Mosquito-borne hemorrhagic fevers of South-East Asia and the Western Pacific. *Bull World Health Organ.* 35, 17–33.

World Health Organization [WHO] (2009). *Dengue: Guidelines for Diagnosis, Treatment, Prevention and Control: New Edition.* Geneva: WHO.

World Health Organization [WHO] (2017). Dengue vaccine: WHO position paper, July 2016 - recommendations. *Vaccine* 35, 1200–1201. doi: 10.1016/j.vaccine.2016.10.070

Wu, S. J., Grouard-Vogel, G., Sun, W., Mascola, J. R., Brachtel, E., Putvatana, R., et al. (2000). Human skin Langerhans cells are targets of dengue virus infection. *Nat. Med.* 6, 816–820. doi: 10.1038/77553

Xie, X., Kum, D. B., Xia, H., Luo, H., Shan, C., Zou, J., et al. (2018). A single-dose live-attenuated zika virus vaccine with controlled infection rounds that protects against vertical transmission. *Cell Host Microbe* 24, 487.e5–499.e5. doi: 10.1016/j.chom.2018.09.008

Yauch, L. E., Prestwood, T. R., May, M. M., Morar, M. M., Zellweger, R. M., Peters, B., et al. (2010). CD4+ T cells are not required for the induction of dengue virus-specific CD8+ T cell or antibody responses but contribute to protection after vaccination. *J. Immunol.* 185, 5405–5416. doi: 10.4049/jimmunol.1001709

Yauch, L. E., Zellweger, R. M., Kotturi, M. F., Qutubuddin, A., Sidney, J., Peters, B., et al. (2009). A protective role for dengue virus-specific CD8+ T cells. *J. Immunol.* 182, 4865–4873. doi: 10.4049/jimmunol.0801974

Yockey, L. J., Varela, L., Rakib, T., Khoury-Hanold, W., Fink, S. L., Stutz, B., et al. (2016). Vaginal exposure to zika virus during pregnancy leads to fetal brain infection. *Cell* 166, 1247.e4–1256.e4 doi: 10.1016/j.cell.2016.08.004

Yu, I. M., Holdaway, H. A., Chipman, P. R., Kuhn, R. J., Rossmann, M. G., and Chen, J. (2009). Association of the pr peptides with dengue virus at acidic pH blocks membrane fusion. *J. Virol.* 83, 12101–12107. doi: 10.1128/JVI.01637-09

Yu, I. M., Zhang, W., Holdaway, H. A., Li, L., Kostyuchenko, V. A., Chipman, P. R., et al. (2008). Structure of the immature dengue virus at low pH primes proteolytic maturation. *Science* 319, 1834–1837. doi: 10.1126/science.1153264

Zellweger, R. M., Prestwood, T. R., and Shresta, S. (2010). Enhanced infection of liver sinusoidal endothelial cells in a mouse model of antibody-induced severe dengue disease. *Cell Host Microbe* 7, 128–139. doi: 10.1016/j.chom.2010.01.004

Zhang, X., Ge, P., Yu, X., Brannan, J. M., Bi, G., Zhang, Q., et al. (2013). Cryo-EM structure of the mature dengue virus at 3.5-*A resolution. Nat. Struct. Mol. Biol.* 20, 105–110. doi: 10.1038/nsmb.2463

Zheng, X., Zhang, D., Li, Y., Yang, C., Wu, Y., Liang, X., et al. (2019). Incompatible and sterile insect techniques combined eliminate mosquitoes. *Nature* 572, 56–61. doi: 10.1038/s41586-019-1407-9

Zompi, S., and Harris, E. (2013). Original antigenic sin in dengue revisited. *Proc. Natl. Acad. Sci. U.S.A.* 110, 8761–8762. doi: 10.1073/pnas.1306333110

Zou, J., Xie, X., Luo, H., Shan, C., Muruato, A. E., Weaver, S. C., et al. (2018). A single-dose plasmid-launched live-attenuated Zika vaccine induces protective immunity. *EBioMedicine* 36, 92–102. doi: 10.1016/j.ebiom.2018.08.056

7

Nasal IgA Provides Protection Against Human Influenza Challenge in Volunteers with Low Serum Influenza Antibody Titre

Victoria M. W. Gould[1†], James N. Francis[2†], Katie J. Anderson[2], Bertrand Georges[2], Alethea V. Cope[1†] and John S. Tregoning[1]*

[1] *Mucosal Infection and Immunity, Section of Virology, Imperial College London, London, United Kingdom,* [2] *Altimmune, London BioScience Innovation Centre, London, United Kingdom*

Correspondence:
John S. Tregoning
john.tregoning@imperial.ac.uk

In spite of there being a number of vaccines, influenza remains a significant global cause of morbidity and mortality. Understanding more about natural and vaccine induced immune protection against influenza infection would help to develop better vaccines. Virus specific IgG is a known correlate of protection, but other factors may help to reduce viral load or disease severity, for example IgA. In the current study we measured influenza specific responses in a controlled human infection model using influenza A/California/2009 (H1N1) as the challenge agent. Volunteers were pre-selected with low haemagglutination inhibition (HAI) titres in order to ensure a higher proportion of infection; this allowed us to explore the role of other immune correlates. In spite of HAI being uniformly low, there were variable levels of H1N1 specific IgG and IgA prior to infection. There was also a range of disease severity in volunteers allowing us to compare whether differences in systemic and local H1N1 specific IgG and IgA prior to infection affected disease outcome. H1N1 specific IgG level before challenge did not correlate with protection, probably due to the pre-screening for individuals with low HAI. However, the length of time infectious virus was recovered from the nose was reduced in patients with higher pre-existing H1N1 influenza specific nasal IgA or serum IgA. Therefore, IgA contributes to protection against influenza and should be targeted in vaccines.

Keywords: influenza, IgA, nasal, vaccine, Human Infection Challenge study

INTRODUCTION

Better understanding about how individuals are protected against influenza infection will aid vaccine development, by identifying effector mechanisms, and vaccine implementation, by identifying easily measurable correlates of protection (Reber and Katz, 2013). Serum antibodies that bind haemagglutinin and prevent haemagglutination are used as a correlate of protection against influenza: a titre greater than 1:40 in the haemagglutination inhibition (HAI) assay is widely used as a protective value. There are, however, other potentially protective, vaccine-inducible components of the adaptive immune response including mucosal T cells and local IgA (Sridhar et al., 2015).

A range of study types can be used to define correlates of protection. Prospective population surveillance studies can be used as a tool to investigate the correlates of protection (Black et al., 2011), but they are large and expensive and because of the size of the studies, the number of potential correlates measurable may be restricted. An alternative is to use mouse models of influenza infection, which are powerful because all tissues can be sampled, a wide variety of immunological tools are available and more severe infections can be used. But there are differences in the immune response between mouse and man, some of the restriction factors for example MX1 are missing in inbred mouse strains (Pillai et al., 2016) and some strains of virus, for example the current H3N2 strains do not infect mice. An alternative is to use human infection challenge studies: whilst smaller in participant number they allow for an increased strike rate of infection, more intensive sampling and a known start point of infection (Carrat et al., 2008). The HAI titre that is currently used as a correlate of influenza protection was defined in the 1970s in a series of human influenza challenge studies (Hobson et al., 1972).

In the current study, local and systemic antibody correlates of protection were investigated in two human challenge studies. Volunteers were pre-screened for low H1N1 HAI titres and then infected with a virus isolated during the 2009 'swine-flu' pandemic – influenza A/California/2009 (H1N1). Infection was determined by PCR and culture and serum and nasal wash H1N1 specific IgG and IgA measured by ELISA. Serum IgG level prior to infection did not correlate with protection from infection, however, there was a weak but significant correlation between time of virus shedding and serum or local IgA. These results support a protective role for IgA, suggesting that vaccines that can induce it would be protective and that there could be a definable value for IgA that could be used as a correlate of protection.

MATERIALS AND METHODS

Volunteers

The subjects were healthy adults aged 18 to 45 and serologically negative to the challenge virus (serum HAI titres $\leq$1:10). Detailed inclusion/exclusion criteria are described in clinicaltrials.gov under identifier NCT02014870 and NCT02071329. All subjects gave written informed consent to participate in the trial. The protocol and informed consent were approved by an independent ethics committee, Institutional Review Board, ZNA/OCMW, Antwerp, Belgium. The study was conducted in accordance with EU Directive 2001/20/EC and ICH GCP.

Clinical Trial

Data from two studies are included here. Clinical challenge volunteers were inoculated with influenza A/California/2009 (H1N1). The first study was a dose escalation study (NCT02014870) and details of this study have been reported elsewhere (Watson et al., 2015): three cohorts were employed: the low cohort were inoculated with 3.5×10^4 $TCID_{50}$, the medium cohort received 3.5×10^5 $TCID_{50}$ and the high cohort received 3.5×10^6 $TCID_{50}$. Subjects entered the quarantine unit 24 h prior to virus challenge and remained for an additional 7 days. The second study is comprised of placebo subjects from a vaccine study (NCT02071329) who were infected with the 3.5×10^6 $TCID_{50}$ of virus. Data from the first study is used to assess sera responses at day 29 after infection, which was not collected in study 2. For the evaluation of protection, data from the high infection cohort and study 2 are pooled for comparable infection dose.

Immediately before challenge, frozen virus was thawed rapidly in a 37°C water bath before dilution in pre-warmed (37°C) phosphate-buffered saline (PBS, Mediatech) to appropriate challenge dose. Subjects were placed in a semi-recumbent position, with the head tipped slightly back and were asked to close their palate. A total of 0.5 ml of diluted virus stock was administered intranasally to each subject (0.25 ml per nostril) using a pipette.

Symptoms were captured twice daily by self-reporting on 16 events associated with influenza illness (headache, nasal stuffiness, runny nose, sore throat, sneezing, hoarseness, earache, facial or eye pain, cough, wheezy chest, breathing difficulty, musculoskeletal ache, nausea/vomiting, feeling/hot/feverish/chills/rigor, fatigue and diarrhea) and classified as absent, mild, moderate or severe. Classifications were defined as follows: mild: the event causes a minor discomfort, does not interfere with daily activity of the subject or does not lead to establishment of a correcting treatment; moderate: the event perturbs the usual activity of the subject and is of a sufficient severity to make the subject uncomfortable; severe: the event prevents any usual routine activity of the patient and causes severe discomfort. In addition, a more objective targeted physical exam was performed twice daily by the study physician which assessed 6 clinical parameters (nasal discharge, otitis, pharyngitis, sinus tenderness, new wheezes, crackles or rhonchi on lung auscultation and percussion) using the same classification system. Vital signs and safety laboratory tests were performed daily. Temperature was measured twice daily. Nasal washes were performed daily by instilling 5 ml of pre-warmed (37°C) sterile phosphate-buffered saline into each nostril and the effluent was collected, diluted 1:1 in virus transport medium and stored at ≤ -65°C. Daily nasal-discharge weights were determined by the collection of pre-weighed tissues in pre-weighed plastic bags assigned to each subject during each 24-h period. On the day of discharge from the quarantine unit subjects were required to have negative result from a negative rapid influenza test (Directigen™ EZ Flu A+B, BD).

Laboratory Analysis

The haemagglutination-inhibition (HAI) assay at Day-1 and 29 (VisMederi srl, Siena, Italy) for all cohorts. Serum was pre-treated with receptor-destroying enzyme (RDE) II (Denka Seiken, Japan) and twofold serially diluted starting from a dilution of 1:10 to 1:2,560 in physiological saline. Virus (A/H1N1/California/04/2009, NIBSC) or (A/Victoria/361/2011) was added to each well at 4 haemagglutination units (HAU)/50 μl for 1 h at room temperature, followed by 0.35% turkey red blood cells for 1 h at room temperature. Reference sheep hyperimmune antisera were provided by NIBSC.

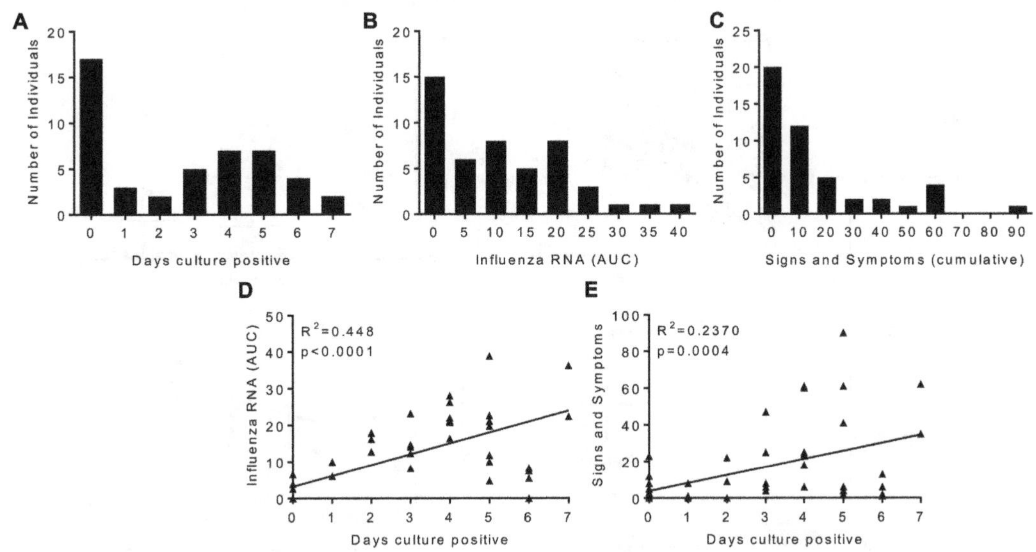

FIGURE 1 | Human influenza infection in clinical volunteers. Patients were inoculated intranasally with 3.5 × 10^6 $TCID_{50}$ influenza A/California/2009 (H1N1). Samples were collected daily and assessed for influenza by culture or rtPCR, and disease signs and symptoms. Cultured virus presented as days virus positive **(A)**, influenza RNA rtPCR data presented as area under the curve plotted over the time course of infection **(B)**, signs and symptoms are presented as cumulative total **(C)**. Correlation plots of days virus positive against detectable Influenza RNA **(D)** or signs and symptoms **(E)**. **(A–C)** Are presented as binned frequencies. Data presented are combined from two studies, n = 47 volunteers.

For real-time RT-PCR (rRT-PCR), the WHO protocol "CDC protocol of real-time RT-PCR for swine influenza A (H1N1)" was followed by VisMederi srl using but only the InfA primer designed for the universal detection influenza A viruses. A specimen was considered positive for influenza A if cycle threshold (Ct) values were within Ct values of 40. A virtual quantification tool was applied to the Ct values to allow the conversion of CDC rRT-PCR Ct values to virus RNA copy number, in the absence of a standard curve run in parallel to the samples (Piralla et al., 2013).

Semi-quantitative Antigen-Specific ELISA

Antibodies specific to influenza were measured using a standardized ELISA (Russell et al., 2016). IgG responses were measured in sera and IgA responses in sera and nasal wash. To detect antigen specific responses, MaxiSorp 96-well plates (Nunc) were coated with 1 μg/ml H1N1 (A/California/09) or H3N2 (A/Texas/50/2012) surface antigens (GSK Vaccines, Sienna, Italy) and incubated overnight at 4°C. Plates were blocked with 1% BSA in PBS. Bound IgG was detected using biotinylated goat anti-human IgG (Sigma) and bound IgA was detected using a biotinylated anti-IgA (AbD Serotec) followed by Poly-HRP40 (Fitzgerald biotech). To quantify the concentration of antigen specific antibody, control wells were coated with a combination of anti-human lambda and kappa light chain specific antibodies (AbDSerotec, Oxford, United Kingdom) and a dilution series of control non-specific human IgG (Sigma) or IgA (Sigma) used as a standard in these wells. TMB with H_2SO_4 as stop solution was used to detect the response and optical densities read at 450 nm.

Statistical Analysis

Correlation of data was performed using Pearson r-test. Comparison between 2 values was performed using t-tests, comparison of 3 variables was performed using ANOVA and Tukey's multiple comparison test. All statistical analyses were performed using GraphPad prism 7.

RESULTS

Variability in Response to Challenge Infection in Individuals with Low HAI

The aim of the study was to define the antibody correlates of protection against influenza, focusing on IgA. To assess this we measured serum and local antibody responses in volunteers challenged intranasally with 3.5 × 10^6 $TCID_{50}$ influenza A/California/2009 (H1N1). Clinical challenge volunteers from two studies were used for this study, the first study was a dose escalation and the second study was a vaccine and challenge study; the high dose challenge group from study one was combined with placebo patients from study two (all data is available in **Supplementary Table S1**). Patients were pre-screened for low H1N1 HAI titres (≤10) to increase the likelihood of infection because of the well-established correlation between HAI titre and protection against infection (Hobson et al., 1972).

There was a range of outcomes to viral challenge, with 14 out of 47 volunteers having no detectable virus by either PCR or culture. The number of days infected patients had culture positive samples recovered from the nose was normally distributed with the median being 4 days (**Figure 1A**). There was influenza RNA detectable in 33 volunteers (**Figure 1B**). Twenty volunteers

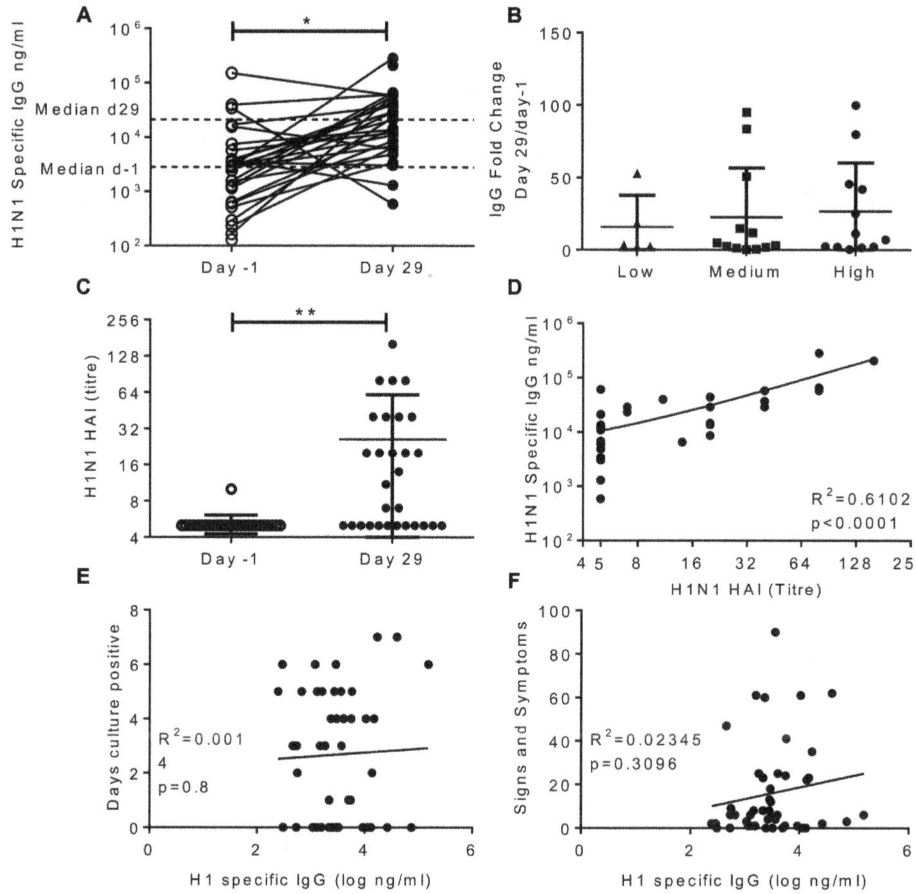

FIGURE 2 | Infection with influenza increases H1 serum IgG antibody responses, but IgG does not correlate with protection. Healthy adult human volunteers were infected intranasally with different doses of H1N1 influenza (low dose: 3.5×10^4 $TCID_{50}$, Medium dose: 3.5×10^5 $TCID_{50}$ and high dose: 3.5×10^6 $TCID_{50}$). H1 specific IgG responses were measured by ELISA in serum on day-1 and day 29 of infection and presented as absolute values **(A)**, fold change based on the infecting dose **(B)**. HAI was assessed at day-1 and day 29 **(C)** and compared with IgG titre on day 29 **(D)**. IgG ELISA titre was compared to days culture positive **(E)** and cumulative signs and symptoms **(F)**. **(A–D)** Represent data from a single study n = 29 volunteers, **(E,F)** Represent data from two studies combined n = 47.

showed no signs and symptoms of clinical illness and the median was for a mild response (**Figure 1C**). When plotted as the area under the curve of the RNA detected over the time course of the study, influenza RNA strongly correlated ($r = 0.4428, p < 0.0001$) with days virus was detectable (**Figure 1D**). Disease signs and symptoms also correlated with days culture positive (**Figure 1E**). Of the virus negative volunteers, 6 were also asymptomatic, interestingly there were virus positive - asymptomatic patients and virus negative - symptomatic patients. Since all the patients had low HAI titres, the variability in responses points to other host factors contributing to protection against infection.

Serum IgG Is Poorly Predictive of Protection

HAI assays measure one facet of antibody immunity, we wished to determine whether H1N1 binding IgG was an independent correlate of protection. Serum was collected 1 day prior to infection and on day 29 after infection in study one only; responses in all three cohorts in this study were compared. There was a significant increase in the H1N1 specific IgG titre in the serum after infection; the median moved from 2,830 to 21,189 ng/ml (**Figure 2A**). The majority of volunteers increased in IgG titre after infection (26 out of 29) and there was no difference in the fold increase in antibody titre between individuals infected with different doses of influenza (**Figure 2B**). Whilst there was detectable IgG in the nose, there was very little H1N1 specific IgG (data not shown). The volunteers all had undetectable HAI prior to challenge, but this significantly increased after challenge (**Figure 2C**), and as seen with IgG challenge dose did not alter the change in HAI. Even though there was a spread of IgG ELISA values, HAI and ELISA IgG did not correlate prior to challenge, presumably as a consequence of pre-screening, but there was a significant correlation between HAI and IgG at day 29 after infection (**Figure 2D**, $R^2 = 0.61$, $p < 0.0001$).

In order to assess possible correlations between IgG and infection, data from the high dose group from the first cohort was combined with subjects from the second study. There was no significant correlation between H1N1 specific IgG and days culture positive ($R^2 = 0.0014$, $p = 0.8$; **Figure 2E**), viral RNA

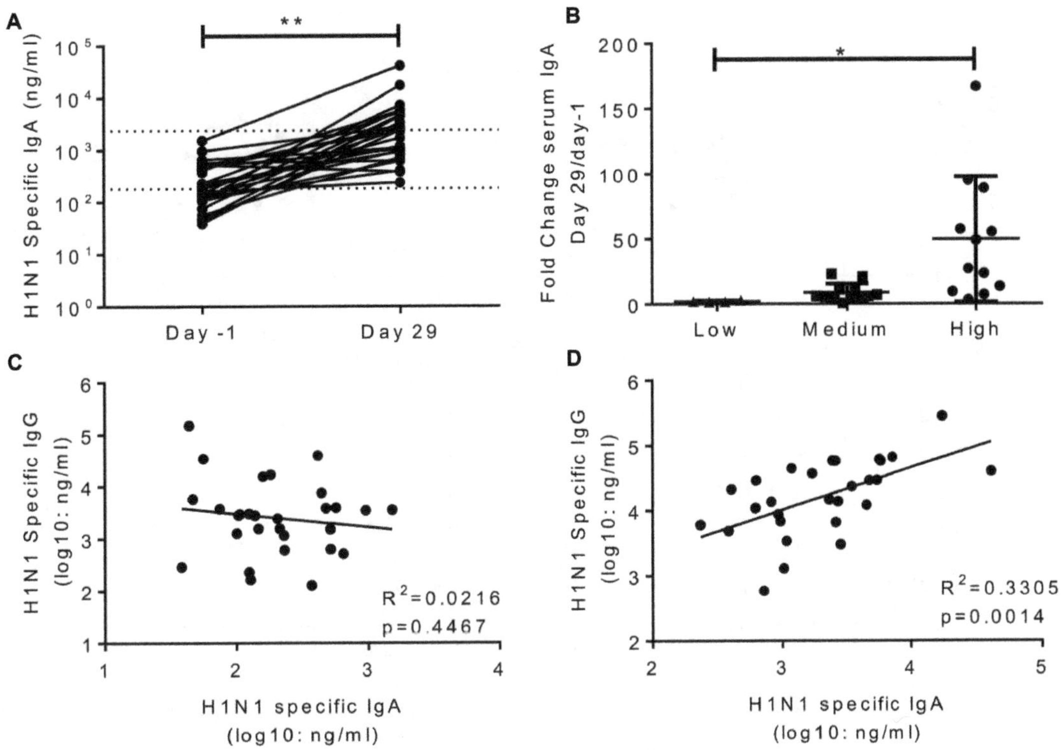

FIGURE 3 | Infection with influenza increases H1 serum IgA antibody responses. Healthy adult human volunteers were infected intranasally with different doses of H1N1 influenza. H1 specific IgA responses were measured by ELISA in serum on day-1 and day 29 of infection and presented as absolute values **(A)** and fold change based on the infecting dose **(B)**. Serum IgA and IgG were compared at day-1 **(C)** and day 29 **(D)**. Data from a single study *n* = 29 volunteers.

copies detected by PCR (data not shown) or cumulative signs and symptoms ($R^2 = 0.023$, $p = 0.31$; **Figure 2F**) infection. This suggests that individuals pre-screened for low HAI also had low serum IgG titres which were also sub-protective, and the two measures do not independently segregate as correlates of protection.

IgA Is Increased by Infection and Weakly Correlates with Protection

A number of studies have indicated that IgA is an independent correlate of protection to IgG (Rossen et al., 1970; Clements et al., 1986; Belshe et al., 2000; Ambrose et al., 2012). H1N1 specific IgA was measured in the serum of volunteers in study 1 on day-1 and day 29. H1N1 specific IgA in the serum significantly increased after infection (**Figure 3A**), the average fold change was 24. Interestingly, challenge dose had a significant effect on the increase in IgA titre, with the IgA increasing more in recipients of higher titre virus than those receiving a low dose (**Figure 3B**). Prior to infection, there was no correlation between serum IgA and IgG (**Figure 3C**). However, IgA and IgG did correlate on day 29 after infection (**Figure 3D**). There was no correlation between HAI and IgA ($R^2 = 0.03$, $p = 0.384$, data not shown).

The main aim of the study was to determine whether systemic or local IgA correlated with protection. H1 specific IgA was measured in nasal lavage; to compensate for dilution effects we normalized the values against total IgA recovered (**Figure 4A**). Prior to infection, H1N1 specific IgA in nasal wash and serum did not correlate (**Figure 4B**). Levels of serum and nasal IgA were compared with the same measures of infection tested for IgG. For both serum IgA ($R^2 = 0.09293$, $p < 0.05$; **Figure 4C**) and nasal IgA ($R^2 = 0.08655$, $p < 0.05$; **Figure 4D**) there was a weak but significant inverse correlation with the number of days detectable virus was shed, measured by culture. There was a similar, but not significant pattern when comparing IgA with either total RNA detection or symptoms. Therefore, IgA provides a separate correlate of protection to IgG against influenza.

Protection Is Independent of the H3 Specific Response

To see if the effects we saw were virus serotype specific, we also measured responses against a recently circulating H3N2 virus (A/Texas/50/2012). After infection, there was a significant increase in H3N2 specific IgG in the sera (**Figure 5A**), but this was significantly lower than the H1 fold change (mean of 4 compared to 23 for H1, **Figure 5B**). This slight increase may reflect overlapping antigen similarity between H1 and H3, though there was no correlation between the individuals in terms of their increase in H1 and H3 titres. There was no increase in H3 HAI titre (**Figure 5C**) or H3 IgA in the sera (**Figure 5D**). There was no correlation between H3 IgA in the serum ($R^2 = 0.0016$, $p = 0.79$; **Figure 5E**) or the nasal lavage ($R^2 = 0.0167$, $p = 0.37$; **Figure 5F**) and protection against infection.

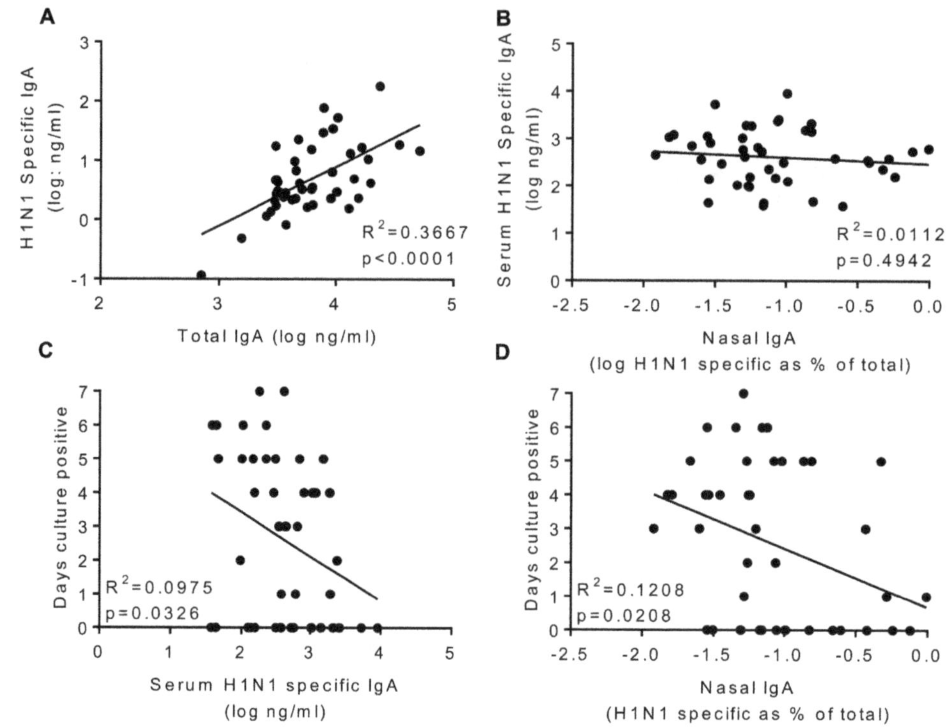

FIGURE 4 | H1N1 specific IgA in nasal wash and serum correlate weakly with protection. H1N1 specific IgA and total IgA were measured in the nasal wash samples collected on day-1 prior to infection **(A)**. H1N1 specific IgA responses were compared between nasal wash and serum **(B)**. Days culture positive virus was recoverable compared to serum IgA **(C)** and nasal IgA **(D)**. Data pooled from two studies, n = 47 volunteers.

DISCUSSION

The aim of the study was to define antibody correlates of protection in a human influenza challenge model. We were able to evaluate the role of IgA in the absence of serum inhibitory antibody because volunteers were pre-screened for low HAI titres. In individuals with low baseline HAI titres, H1N1 strain specific serum IgG measured by ELISA did not correlate with protection against challenge. IgA has previously been proposed as one of the correlates of protection against influenza infection (Rossen et al., 1970; Clements et al., 1986; Belshe et al., 2000; Ambrose et al., 2012). This is supported by murine studies, transfer of nasal IgA from immunized to naïve mice leads to protection against infection (Tamura et al., 1991) and polymeric Ig receptor knockout mice have increased viral load on challenge after intranasal vaccination, with matched virus strains (Asahi et al., 2002). One suggested protective function of influenza specific IgA has been to limit the spread of budding virus from the cell, rather than classical entry inhibiting neutralization (Mazanec et al., 1995), this is supported by studies in guinea pig models demonstrating that IgA prevents influenza transmission (Seibert et al., 2013). In the current study, there was a weak but significant correlation between both nasal lavage and serum IgA and days shedding influenza.

IgA is not the sole protective factor, for example in high dose challenge studies IgA deficient mice had a similar profile on infection as wild type (Mbawuike et al., 1999). Protection also comes from serum IgG transudate into the lungs, which has been observed in both mice (Renegar et al., 2004) and men (Wagner et al., 1987). Serum HAI is a clear correlate of protection against influenza infection (Hobson et al., 1972), though whether the conventional titre of 1:40 is the correct value for all individuals has recently been challenged, especially in more susceptible age groups, for example children (Black et al., 2011). In mouse models the location of the infection determines the functional correlate; IgA is more effective in the upper airway, whilst IgG is more effective in the lower airway (Renegar et al., 2004). The route of antigen exposure affects the type of response, intranasal exposure is more likely to induce IgA, whilst systemic immunization will induce IgG (Clements and Murphy, 1986); in turn, the type of immunity induced has an effect on the correlate of protection –systemic immunization induced protective IgG whilst intranasal immunization induced protective IgA (Clements et al., 1986). In our study we saw that infection boosted influenza specific IgA, as seen in other studies (Wright et al., 1983; Brown et al., 1985), and also IgG. Interestingly, prior to infection IgA and IgG did not correlate, indicating that the different antibody classes can be induced independently. These data suggest IgG and IgA work together to prevent infection.

There are also likely to be factors other than antibody that protect against infection. Of the 47 volunteers challenged in the two studies, 14 had no evidence of infection. These

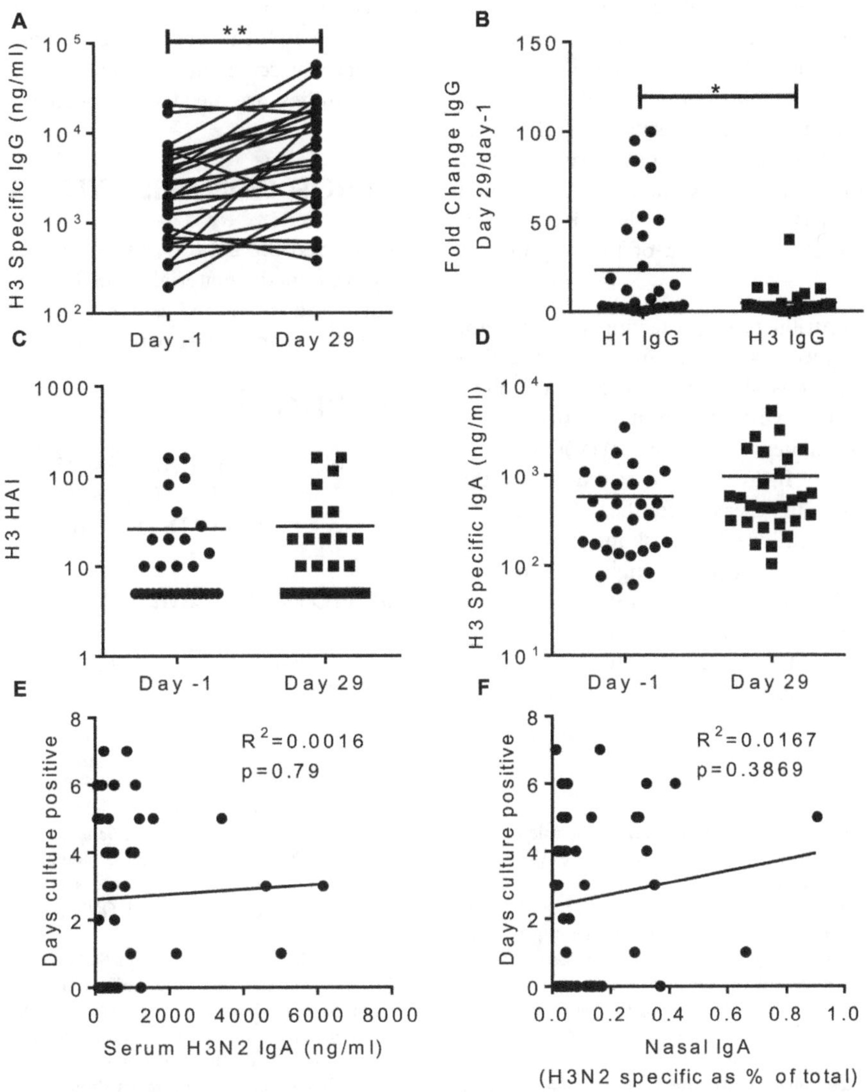

FIGURE 5 | H3N2 specific antibody does not correlate with protection. H3N2 specific IgG **(A)**, HAI **(C)** and IgA **(D)** were measured in serum on day-1 and day 29, fold change in IgG response compared between H1N1 and H3N2 IgG **(B)**. Days culture positive virus was recoverable compared to H3N2 specific serum IgA **(E)** and nasal IgA **(F)**. Data pooled from two studies, $n = 47$ volunteers.

individuals did not have a different distribution of IgA or IgG titres prior to infection to the infected individuals. This suggests that there is not an absolute cut off value of protection, rather that there is a diminishing likelihood of infection as antibody levels increase, this is also seen with HAI (Black et al., 2011). A similar distribution of protective values was seen for IgA in respiratory syncytial virus challenge (Habibi et al., 2015). The data also suggest that there may be other factors that contribute to protection at an individual level. This could include cell intrinsic factors that affect the ability of the virus to replicate in the host cells such as IFITM3 (Everitt et al., 2012; Everitt et al., 2013). It will also reflect the cellular response to infection; T cells will also play a role in protection and clearance of infection (Sridhar et al., 2013), we have previously observed a role for T cell immunity as an additional layer of protection if antibody mediated immunity is circumvented by the virus (Lambert et al., 2016). Most likely all components of the immune response work in concert to prevent infection; cell intrinsic immunity, antibody and T cells.

There are some limitations to the study. There was only a small number of patient samples and in order to define a specific correlate of protection, more individuals would be necessary. Whilst beneficial for dissection of the immune response, the deliberate selection of low HAI individuals will remove the protective role of IgG and conclusions about the relative importance of IgA vs IgG cannot be drawn from this. The nasal wash sampling technique can lead to a degree of variability in recovery of material, we normalized this against the total IgA, but there may be more effective methods of recovering nasal IgA for example nasosorption (Bergin et al., 2016). In some ways the human challenge model is not completely reflective of human infection, for example natural infection probably occurs with a much lower dose of infection (Frise et al., 2016). There is striking variability compared to the mouse model, which are given a similar dose of virus (Mastelic Gavillet et al., 2015; Russell et al., 2015; Lambert et al., 2016), but mice are more homogenous and also infection naïve. Combining the human and animal challenge models with natural infection data is most likely to give us the clearest picture of the response to infection.

Understanding what contributes to protection is important to develop and optimize vaccines against influenza infection and to make informed decisions about the vaccination policy. For example, it is not clear what the best practice is for the use of live attenuated influenza vaccine (LAIV); in 2016, the Advisory Committee on Immunization voted down the use of LAIV for the 2016–2017 season in the US due to a lack of protective efficacy in children (Grohskopf et al., 2016). It had been assumed that LAIV works through IgA not IgG (Barría et al., 2013), though recent studies performed in adults, in which LAIV may have reduced efficacy, indicated no clear correlate of protection (Wright et al., 2016). There is also not a simple value of IgA comparable to HAI >1:40 that could be measured in efficacy studies. Our studies suggest that nasal and serum IgA can contribute to protection against influenza and that a vaccine that can induce IgA will be protective but larger studies are needed to determine a specific protective value.

AUTHOR CONTRIBUTIONS

VG analyzed the data. JF, BG, and KA coordinated the clinical study and made material available for analysis. AC analyzed the data and developed assays. JT designed study, collated and analyzed data and wrote paper.

FUNDING

This work was supported by an NIHR BRC grant to Imperial College London and the European Community's European 7th Framework Program ADITEC (HEALTH-F4-2011-18 280873).

ACKNOWLEDGMENT

Professor Stephen Riley (Imperial College) for productive discussions.

REFERENCES

Ambrose, C. S., Wu, X., Jones, T., and Mallory, R. M. (2012). The role of nasal IgA in children vaccinated with live attenuated influenza vaccine. *Vaccine* 30, 6794–6801. doi: 10.1016/j.vaccine.2012.09.018

Asahi, Y., Yoshikawa, T., Watanabe, I., Iwasaki, T., Hasegawa, H., Sato, Y., et al. (2002). Protection against influenza virus infection in polymeric ig receptor knockout mice immunized intranasally with adjuvant-combined vaccines. *J. Immunol.* 168, 2930–2938. doi: 10.4049/jimmunol.168.6.2930

Barría, M. I., Garrido, J. L., Stein, C., Scher, E., Ge, Y., Engel, S. M., et al. (2013). Localized mucosal response to intranasal live attenuated influenza vaccine in adults. *J. Infect. Dis.* 207, 115–124. doi: 10.1093/infdis/jis641

Belshe, R. B., Gruber, W. C., Mendelman, P. M., Mehta, H. B., Mahmood, K., Reisinger, K., et al. (2000). Correlates of immune protection induced by live, attenuated, cold-adapted, trivalent, intranasal influenza virus vaccine. *J. Infect. Dis.* 181, 1133–1137. doi: 10.1086/315323

Bergin, P., Langat, R., Omosa-Manyonyi, G., Farah, B., Ouattara, G., Park, H., et al. (2016). Assessment of anti-HIV-1 antibodies in oral and nasal compartments of volunteers from three different populations. *J. Acquir. Immune Defic. Syndr.* 73, 130–137. doi: 10.1097/QAI.0000000000001094

Black, S., Nicolay, U., Vesikari, T., Knuf, M., Del Giudice, G., Della Cioppa, G., et al. (2011). Hemagglutination inhibition antibody titers as a correlate of protection for inactivated influenza vaccines in children. *Pediatr. Infect. Dis. J.* 30, 1081–1085. doi: 10.1097/INF.0b013e3182367662

Brown, T. A., Murphy, B. R., Radl, J., Haaijman, J. J., and Mestecky, J. (1985). Subclass distribution and molecular form of immunoglobulin A hemagglutinin antibodies in sera and nasal secretions after experimental secondary infection with influenza A virus in humans. *J. Clin. Microbiol.* 22, 259–264.

Carrat, F., Vergu, E., Ferguson, N. M., Lemaitre, M., Cauchemez, S., Leach, S., et al. (2008). Time lines of infection and disease in human influenza: a review of volunteer challenge studies. *Am. J. Epidemiol.* 167, 775–785. doi: 10.1093/aje/kwm375

Clements, M. L., Betts, R. F., Tierney, E. L., and Murphy, B. R. (1986). Serum and nasal wash antibodies associated with resistance to experimental challenge with influenza A wild-type virus. *J. Clin. Microbiol.* 24, 157–160.

Clements, M. L., and Murphy, B. R. (1986). Development and persistence of local and systemic antibody responses in adults given live attenuated or inactivated influenza A virus vaccine. *J. Clin. Microbiol.* 23, 66–72.

Everitt, A. R., Clare, S., Mcdonald, J. U., Kane, L., Harcourt, K., Ahras, M., et al. (2013). Defining the range of pathogens susceptible to Ifitm3 restriction using a knockout mouse model. *PLoS ONE* 8:e80723. doi: 10.1371/journal.pone.0080723

Everitt, A. R., Clare, S., Pertel, T., John, S. P., Wash, R. S., Smith, S. E., et al. (2012). IFITM3 restricts the morbidity and mortality associated with influenza. *Nature (London)* 484, 519–523. doi: 10.1038/nature10921

Frise, R., Bradley, K., Van Doremalen, N., Galiano, M., Elderfield, R. A., Stilwell, P., et al. (2016). Contact transmission of influenza virus between ferrets imposes a looser bottleneck than respiratory droplet transmission allowing propagation of antiviral resistance. *Sci. Rep.* 6:29793. doi: 10.1038/srep29793

Grohskopf, L. A., Sokolow, L. Z., Broder, K. R., Olsen, S. J., Karron, R. A., Jernigan, D. B., et al. (2016). Prevention and control of seasonal influenza with vaccines. *MMWR Recomm. Rep.* 65, 1–54. doi: 10.15585/mmwr.rr6505a1

Habibi, M. S., Jozwik, A., Makris, S., Dunning, J., Paras, A., Devincenzo, J. P., et al. (2015). Impaired antibody-mediated protection and defective IgA B-cell memory in experimental infection of adults with respiratory syncytial virus. *Am. J. Respir. Crit. Care Med.* 191, 1040–1049. doi: 10.1164/rccm.201412-2256OC

Hobson, D., Curry, R. L., Beare, A. S., and Ward-Gardner, A. (1972). The role of serum haemagglutination-inhibiting antibody in protection against challenge infection with influenza A2 and B viruses. *J. Hyg.* 70, 767–777. doi: 10.1017/S0022172400022610

Lambert, L., Kinnear, E., Mcdonald, J. U., Grodeland, G., Bogen, B., Stubsrud, E., et al. (2016). DNA vaccines encoding antigen targeted to MHC Class II induce influenza-specific CD8+ T cell responses, enabling faster resolution of influenza disease. *Front. Immunol.* 7:321. doi: 10.3389/fimmu.2016.00321

Mastelic Gavillet, B., Eberhardt, C. S., Auderset, F., Castellino, F., Seubert, A., Tregoning, J. S., et al. (2015). MF59 Mediates Its B cell adjuvanticity by promoting T follicular helper cells and thus germinal center responses in adult and early life. *J. Immunol.* 194, 4836–4845. doi: 10.4049/jimmunol.1402071

Mazanec, M. B., Coudret, C. L., and Fletcher, D. R. (1995). Intracellular neutralization of influenza virus by immunoglobulin A anti-hemagglutinin monoclonal antibodies. *J. Virol.* 69, 1339–1343.

Mbawuike, I. N., Pacheco, S., Acuna, C. L., Switzer, K. C., Zhang, Y., and Harriman, G. R. (1999). Mucosal immunity to influenza without IgA: an IgA knockout mouse model. *J. Immunol.* 162, 2530–2537.

Pillai, P. S., Molony, R. D., Martinod, K., Dong, H., Pang, I. K., Tal, M. C., et al. (2016). Mx1 reveals innate pathways to antiviral resistance and lethal influenza disease. *Science* 352, 463–466. doi: 10.1126/science.aaf3926

Piralla, A., Daleno, C., Pariani, E., Conaldi, P., Esposito, S., Zanetti, A., et al. (2013). Virtual quantification of influenza A virus load by real-time RT-PCR. *J. Clin. Virol.* 56, 65–68. doi: 10.1016/j.jcv.2012.09.011

Reber, A., and Katz, J. (2013). Immunological assessment of influenza vaccines and immune correlates of protection. *Expert Rev. Vaccines* 12, 519–536. doi: 10.1586/erv.13.35

Renegar, K. B., Small, P. A. Jr., Boykins, L. G., and Wright, P. F. (2004). Role of IgA versus IgG in the control of influenza viral infection in the murine respiratory tract. *J. Immunol.* 173, 1978–1986. doi: 10.4049/jimmunol.173.3.1978

Rossen, R. D., Butler, W. T., Waldman, R. H., Alford, R. H., Hornick, R. B., Togo, Y., et al. (1970). The proteins in nasal secretion. II. A longitudinal study of IgA and neutralizing antibody levels in nasal washings from men infected with influenza virus. *JAMA* 211, 1157–1161. doi: 10.1001/jama.1970.03170070027005

Russell, R. F., Mcdonald, J. U., Ivanova, M., Zhong, Z., Bukreyev, A., and Tregoning, J. S. (2015). Partial attenuation of respiratory syncytial virus with a deletion of a small hydrophobic gene is associated with elevated interleukin-1beta responses. *J. Virol.* 89, 8974–8981. doi: 10.1128/JVI.01070-15

Russell, R. F., Mcdonald, J. U., Lambert, L., and Tregoning, J. S. (2016). Use of the microparticle NanoSiO2 as an adjuvant to boost vaccine immune responses in neonatal mice against influenza. *J. Virol.* 90, 4735–4744. doi: 10.1128/JVI.03159-15

Seibert, C. W., Rahmat, S., Krause, J. C., Eggink, D., Albrecht, R. A., Goff, P. H., et al. (2013). Recombinant IgA is sufficient to prevent influenza virus transmission in guinea pigs. *J. Virol.* 87, 7793–7804. doi: 10.1128/JVI.00979-13

Sridhar, S., Begom, S., Bermingham, A., Hoschler, K., Adamson, W., Carman, W., et al. (2013). Cellular immune correlates of protection against symptomatic pandemic influenza. *Nat. Med.* 19, 1305–1312. doi: 10.1038/nm.3350

Sridhar, S., Brokstad, K. A., and Cox, R. J. (2015). Influenza vaccination strategies: comparing inactivated and live attenuated influenza vaccines. *Vaccines (Basel)* 3, 373–389. doi: 10.3390/vaccines3020373

Tamura, S., Funato, H., Hirabayashi, Y., Suzuki, Y., Nagamine, T., Aizawa, C., et al. (1991). Cross-protection against influenza A virus infection by passively transferred respiratory tract IgA antibodies to different hemagglutinin molecules. *Eur. J. Immunol.* 21, 1337–1344. doi: 10.1002/eji.1830210602

Wagner, D. K., Clements, M. L., Reimer, C. B., Snyder, M., Nelson, D. L., and Murphy, B. R. (1987). Analysis of immunoglobulin G antibody responses after administration of live and inactivated influenza A vaccine indicates that nasal wash immunoglobulin G is a transudate from serum. *J. Clin. Microbiol.* 25, 559–562.

Watson, J. M., Francis, J. N., Mesens, S., Faiman, G. A., Makin, J., Patriarca, P., et al. (2015). Characterisation of a wild-type influenza (A/H1N1) virus strain as an experimental challenge agent in humans. *Virol. J.* 12, 13. doi: 10.1186/s12985-015-0240-5

Wright, P. F., Hoen, A. G., Ilyushina, N. A., Brown, E. P., Ackerman, M. E., Wieland-Alter, W., et al. (2016). Correlates of immunity to influenza as determined by challenge of children with live, attenuated influenza vaccine. *Open Forum Infect. Dis.* 3:ofw108. doi: 10.1093/ofid/ofw108

Wright, P. F., Murphy, B. R., Kervina, M., Lawrence, E. M., Phelan, M. A., and Karzon, D. T. (1983). Secretory immunological response after intranasal inactivated influenza A virus vaccinations: evidence for immunoglobulin A memory. *Infect. Immun.* 40, 1092–1095.

8

Recent Progress in Vaccine Development Against Chikungunya Virus

Shan Gao[1], *Siqi Song*[1,2] *and Leiliang Zhang*[1]*

[1] *Institute of Basic Medicine, Shandong First Medical University & Shandong Academy of Medical Sciences, Jinan, China,*
[2] *School of Basic Medicine, Qingdao University, Qingdao, China*

***Correspondence:**
Leiliang Zhang
armzhang@hotmail.com

Chikungunya fever (CHIKF) is an acute infectious disease that is mediated by the mosquito-transmitted chikungunya virus (CHIKV). People infected with CHIKV may experience high fever, severe joint pain, skin rash, and headache. In recent years, this disease has become a global public health problem. However, there is no licensed vaccine available for CHIKV. Accumulating research data have provided novel approaches and new directions for the development of CHIKV vaccines. Our review focuses on recent progress in CHIKV vaccine studies. The potential vaccine candidates are classified into seven types: inactivated vaccine, subunit vaccine, live-attenuated vaccine, recombinant virus-vectored vaccine, virus-like particle vaccine, chimeric vaccine, and nucleic acid vaccine. These studies will provide important insights into the future development of CHIKV vaccines.

Keywords: chikungunya fever, CHIKV, live-attenuated vaccine, VLP, chimeric vaccine

INTRODUCTION

Chikungunya fever (CHIKF) is a recurrent infectious disease caused by the chikungunya virus (CHIKV). The main clinical symptoms are arthritis and fever. Patients may also suffer from headache, myalgia, and rash. The mortality of CHIKF is below 0.5%, lower than dengue fever, which has similar clinical symptoms. For infants under 1 year old and people over 60 years old, the mortality will significantly increase (Langsjoen et al., 2018). The acute symptoms usually disappear within about 1–2 weeks, but patients may endure long-lasting joint pain and fatigue (Elsinga et al., 2017). Since CHIKV was first isolated in 1952 from Tanzania, it has induced several outbreaks, mainly in Africa and Asia. However, after re-emerging in 2004 in Kenya, the epidemic area expanded from the tropical zone to even Europe and America (Enserink, 2007). The unprecedentedly rapid and wide spread of this disease calls for efficient preventive measures.

Belonging to the genus Alphavirus of the *Togaviridae* family, CHIKV is an enveloped arthropod-borne virus (arbovirus) with *Aedes aegypti* and *Aedes albopictus* as its primary vectors. The genome of CHIKV consists of a positive-sense RNA approximately 11.5 kb in length. The CHIKV genome comprises two open reading frames (ORFs) that encode four non-structural proteins (nsPs) and one structural polyprotein (**Figure 1**). The nsPs function as a replicase complex, which not only replicates genomic RNA for progeny but also transcribes subgenomic RNA to express structural proteins (Ljungberg and Liljestrom, 2015). As for the structural polyprotein, it will be further cleaved to capsid and E3-E2-6K/TF-E1 (**Figure 1**). The latter is important for virion assembly and virus entry. E1/E2 glycoprotein in the envelope was reported to mediate cell binding at the early stage of infection (Strauss and Strauss, 1994).

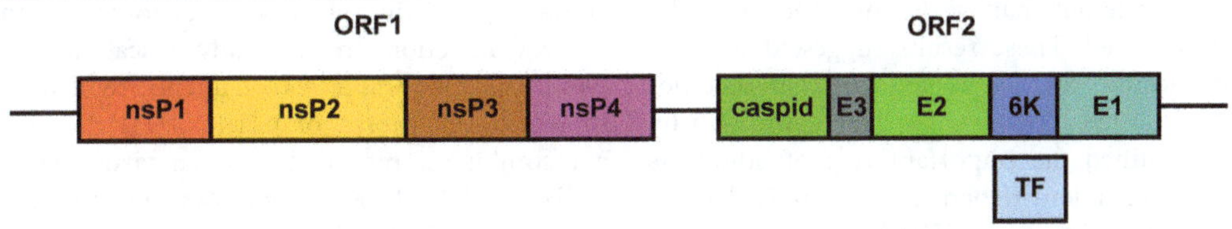

FIGURE 1 | Schematic diagram of the CHIKV genome. The genome of CHIKV is a single-strand RNA compromising two ORFs. ORF1 encodes four nsPs. Translation and further processing of ORF2 produce structural proteins capsid, E3, E2, 6K, and E1. During translation, ribosome shifts to −1 reading frame in 6K, leading to the production of TF protein.

The large-scale resurgence of CHIKV is, to some extent, due to social and economic developments, such as the increased number of overseas tourists, the high population density brought about by urbanization, and the changes in mosquito distribution caused by global warming. A lot of antiviral compounds have shown valuable therapeutic efficacies, especially during CHIKF outbreak. Since it is one of the most cost-benefit public strategies to prevent infectious disease, vaccine is an indispensable means for preventing CHIKF. Considering that the CHIKV antigen variety is limited and infection may lead to lifelong immunity, the advantage of vaccination is particularly prominent.

The attempt to develop a CHIKV vaccine started from the 1960s, not long after the virus was isolated. Since then, researchers have continued to develop CHIKV vaccine candidates that balance immunogenicity and safety. However, there is no licensed CHIKV vaccine available for use. Researchers have taken advantage of progress in biochemical and molecular methods and have utilized various strategies to develop vaccines, which can be classified as inactivated viral vaccine, subunit vaccine, live-attenuated virus (LAV) vaccine, recombinant virus-vectored vaccine, chimeric vaccine, virus-like particle (VLP) vaccine, and nucleic acid vaccine. In the majority of this review, we focus on novel CHIKV vaccine development and progress in the evaluation of vaccine candidates since 2016.

INACTIVATED VACCINE

The first attempts to develop a CHIKV vaccine emerged shortly after the first CHIKF outbreak in the 1960s. Early studies adopted inactivated vaccine as the preferred strategy. By inactivating the virus via heating or chemical treatment (formalin), researchers generated vaccines that could stimulate the immune response without risk of infection, which conferred inactivated vaccine with high safety.

Researchers first infected mouse brains with an African genotype strain of CHIKV and successfully collected neutralizing antibodies 15 days post infection (Kitaoka, 1967). The most prominent achievements in early CHIKV vaccine development were made at the Walter Reed Army Institute of Research, based on a series of platforms including chicken embryos, suckling-mouse brains, and African green monkey kidney cells. The first evaluation of inactivated vaccine in humans was reported in 1971 (Harrison et al., 1971). Two groups of healthy volunteers were vaccinated twice (day 0 and 28) with 0.5 or 1 mL, respectively. Both groups developed neutralizing antibodies within 2 weeks without adverse effects.

In the following 40 years, many vaccine candidates based on inactivation have been developed and have entered the clinical phase. One inactivated vaccine, which was produced in Vero cells, stimulated both cellular and humoral immune responses, with the peak titer of neutralizing antibodies appearing at 6–8 weeks post-vaccination (Tiwari et al., 2009). Kumar et al. (2012) evaluated the protective efficacy of an E2 protein-based recombinant vaccine and whole-virus inactivated vaccine. When measuring the virus load in serum and tissues, both vaccines were verified to protect mice from CHIKV infection. Recently, the means of inoculation has also been improved. Rudd et al. (2015) introduced Foroderm for the delivery of inactivated CHIKV vaccine using cylindrical silica microparticles. This needle-free strategy greatly improves the convenience of vaccination.

The stability and safety of inactivated vaccine come at the expense of efficacy and production cost, which, to a certain extent, impedes its accessibility. The development of inactivated vaccines shows a less prosperous trend than vaccines based on other strategies.

SUBUNIT VACCINE

Subunit vaccine, like inactivated vaccine, is an early mature strategy for vaccine preparation. The viral envelope or capsid is obtained through chemolysis or proteolysis to prepare the vaccine. By using individual viral proteins, subunit vaccines elicit an immune response without inducing the production of antibodies against unrelated antigens or infectious viral particles. This method not only ensures the safety of the vaccine but also makes large-scale manufacturing possible.

The CHIKV envelope glycoproteins E1 and E2 have been selected to develop CHIKV subunit vaccines in different expression systems. Metz et al. (2011) first expressed E1 and E2 in insect cells. Both proteins were N-glycosylated and membrane-targeting, consistent with the maturation of E1 and E2 in whole CHIKV virion. E2 antibody generated by this baculovirus expression system was able to neutralize CHIKV in rabbits. Next, they compared the immunogenicity of three recombinant baculoviruses: E1, E2, and CHIKV VLPs. Although all three baculoviruses induced neutralizing antibodies, the titers of the subunits were not as high as that of VLP. When challenging AG129 mice with infectious CHIKV, VLP protected all animals, while only half of the mice vaccinated by the subunits finally survived. These results suggested that the efficacy of subunit vaccine was not as good as that of other strategies (Metz et al., 2013). This was partially confirmed by other studies that identified the important role of adjuvants in subunit vaccine application (Khan et al., 2012; Kumar et al., 2012). Also, subunits based on CHIKV E1 and E2 were alternatively generated in bacterial expression systems. E1 and E2 proteins from bacteria successfully neutralized CHIKV and completely protected BALB/c mice from disease induced by CHIKV. However, the efficacies varied with different adjuvants, indicating that the immune response to subunit vaccine largely depended on adjuvants.

LAV

Live-attenuated virus is generated by modifying the structure of a virus to significantly weaken its virulence while retaining its immunogenicity. Compared with inactive vaccine, which is a fully inactive pathogen, LAV can stimulate a stronger and long-term immune response. However, higher immunogenic ability is a trade-off for lower safety. In this regard, the safety of LAV should be cautiously evaluated during animal model and clinical trials (Plante et al., 2015). Owing to its high immunogenic potency, LAV is the platform with the best prospects. It can also be combined with other strategies such as vector vaccine, which further extends its application.

After CHIKV enters cells, early immune response is activated by nsPs. Thus, several LAVs have been designed that target nsPs. By the use of the concept well established in the Semliki Forest virus (SFV), Chan et al. (2019) introduced point mutation to generate three CHIKV mutants. The specific mutation sites and corresponding vaccine candidates were as follows: RH-CHIKV, with R532H substitution in the cleavage region between nsP1 and nsP2; EV-CHIKV, with E515V substitution in nsP2; RHEV-CHIKV, with combinational double mutations of R532H and E515V. Researchers characterized the activity of the three mutants *in vitro* and found that the viral RNA titers of both RH-CHIKV and RHEV-CHIKV were lower than that of WT-CHIKV. Consistent with this result, RH-CHIKV and RHEV-CHIKV induced high levels of IFN-α and IFN-γ. To clarify whether the reduced activity exhibited in mouse tail fibroblasts affected symptoms *in vivo*, WT and mutant CHIKV were injected into adult mice. Acute viremia was largely alleviated in RH-CHIKV and RHEV-CHIKV infected mice. Mutant CHIKV also changed the cytokine pathway toward anti-inflammatory response. When challenged by the closely related O'nyong-nyong virus, no obvious viremia was detected in nsP-mutant-infected mice, indicating broad cross-protection by the vaccines.

Another LAV targeting nsP was Δ5nsP3, in which 180 nucleotides in the replicase region of nsP3 were deleted. Single-dose immunization with Δ5nsP3 generated high titers of neutralizing antibodies that lasted until the day of virus challenge (LR2006-OPY1 strain, day 123). It also induced IFN-γ T-cell responses. By determining the viral load in plasma and measuring hematological parameters, Δ5nsP3 vaccination showed protective efficacy in cynomolgus macaques against CHIKV infection. In this study, researchers evaluated another two LAVs. One was a DNA-launched replicon vaccine, DREP-E, in which the capsid of CHIKV was deleted. The other was a recombinant modified vaccinia virus that encoded the full CHIKV C-E3-E2-6K-E1. Both vaccine candidates showed similar results as Δ5nsP3, indicating good prospects for the future application of LAV (Roques et al., 2017).

Capsid was another potential target for LAV development. Recently, a novel vaccine candidate against CHIKV was generated in which the capsid was completely deleted (Zhang et al., 2019). Researchers found that capsid was dispensable for ΔC-CHIKV virion assembly. Consistent with this, ΔC-CHIKV successfully propagated in BHK-21 cells and had similar antigenic activity to WT-CHIKV. Single-dose vaccination (10^4 PFU) of C57BL/6 mice and immunocompromised $IFNAR^{-/-}$ mice protected them from subsequent CHIKV (ECSA strain) challenge. ΔC-CHIKV efficiently induced neutralizing antibodies, comparably with WT CHIKV. No footpad swelling was observed in ΔC-CHIKV immunized mice. The attenuated infection in $IFNAR^{-/-}$ mice indicated that ΔC-CHIKV could be a potential vaccine. The researchers specially assessed the stability of ΔC-CHIKV, since it was an important concern for all LAVs. After five passages, no detectable genomic change was reported. The efficacy and safety of ΔC-CHIKV suggested that it is a promising vaccine candidate.

Taylor et al. (2017) found a nuclear localization sequence (NoLS) in the N-terminal region of capsid protein that was important for virus replication and developed a vaccine candidate by site-directed mutagenesis. Mechanistically, they discovered that the attenuated replication resulted from reduced nuclear import of capsid protein. Attenuation was confirmed by measuring the virus copy number in the supernatants of cultured BHK-21 and C6/36 cells. Mice administered a subcutaneous injection of CHIKV-NoLS showed no disease symptoms. Cross-protection was monitored when CHIKV-NoLS-immunized mice were challenged by another alphavirus, Ross River virus (RRV). The attenuation and stability of CHIKV-NoLS were further evaluated by histological and flow cytometric analysis (Abeyratne et al., 2018). Mice inoculated with CHIKV-NoLS exhibited minimal inflammation in the footpad compared with a CHIKV-WT infected group. When stored at −20°C and −80°C for up to 56 days, the titer of CHIKV-NoLS remained stable. Besides, CHIKV-NoLS showed no loss of infectivity after freeze and thaw. These results confirmed the preclinical safety and stability of CHIKV-NoLS.

Recently, a novel genomic rationale was adopted by Carrau et al. (2019). Multiple replacements of synonymous codons were made in the CHIKV genome to reduce the mutational robustness of the virus and led to a deleterious evolutionary direction (Carrau et al., 2019). Synonymous codons that had the highest likelihood of becoming stop codons ("1-to-Stop," one mutation away from stop) were examined. They constructed two candidates. Specifically, the STOP virus had 151 "1-to-Stop" synonymous codons for all Leu and Ser, while the SuperStop virus had 285 "1-to-Stop" synonymous codons for leucine, serine, arginine, and glycine in the structural-protein-coding region of the CHIKV genome. In experiments on mice, attenuated virus infectivity and diminished disease symptoms were observed. One prominent advantage of this approach was its safety. Since hundreds of synonymous mutations were generated, the reversion risk was greatly reduced.

RECOMBINANT VIRUS-VECTORED VACCINE

Recombinant virus-vectored vaccine is obtained by inserting genes encoding exogenous protective antigen into the vector virus genome. Recombinant vector vaccine offers the advantages of safety and easy inoculation. A variety of virus vectors, such as poxvirus, herpesvirus, adenovirus, and paramyxovirus, have been used in vaccine development.

Recombinant measles virus vector is widely used to develop CHIKV vaccines and performed well in phase I and II clinical trials. Rossi et al. (2019) tested the immunogenicity and efficacy of their new developed measles virus-vectored vaccine on cynomolgus macaques. Serum was examined by plaque reduction neutralization test and enzyme-linked immunosorbent assay (ELISA). The results indicated that a robust immune response was elicited by measles virus-vectored vaccine. There was no obvious difference in hematology and clinical chemical indicators between control and the vaccinated group. The clinical symptoms of the disease, mainly referring to fever here, were not observed either after vaccination or after virus challenge. Macaques were also protected from viremia. The efficacy and safety of this vaccine were confirmed by the outcome of clinical trials. In a randomized, double-blind Phase I clinical trial, the seroconversion rate was 44–92% with a single dose and reached 100% after a second vaccination (Ramsauer et al., 2015). Recently, a double-blind, randomized, placebo-controlled and active-controlled phase II trial was carried out and reported (Reisinger et al., 2019). Participants aged 18–55 respectively received control vaccine (n = 34), MV-CHIK (n = 195), or measles prime and MV-CHIK (n = 34) by intramuscular injections between August 17, 2016, and May 31, 2017. Neutralizing antibodies specifically against CHIKV were detected in MV-CHIK treatment groups, with no serious adverse events reported. Due to its good safety and immunogenicity, MV-CHIK is a promising vaccine candidate for CHIKV.

Most CHIKV vaccine candidates are delivered through injection subcutaneously at the wrist or intramuscularly in the quadriceps muscles. Taking advantage of their platform based on adenovirus 5, the researchers developed an oral CHIKV vaccine (Dora et al., 2019). Preservation in tablets promoted further processing, facilitated non-sterile packaging, shortened the production time, and reduced the economic cost. Oral administration also alleviated the discomfort of vaccination. A replication-deficient 5 type adenovirus (rAd) with a lack of E1 and E3 allowed for the expression of different antigens concurrently, which made it an ideal platform for vaccine development. The researchers have constructed three vaccine candidates with different combinations of CHIKV structural proteins: Ad-CHIKV-SG (expressing C-E3-E2-6K/TF-E1), Ad-CHIKV-E3/E2/E1, and Ad-CHIKV-E3/E2/6K (Dora et al., 2019). All three vaccines induced high IgG titers against CHIKV at week 7, while the former two candidates showed significantly higher titers than Ad-CHIKV-E3/E2/6K. C57BL/6 mice were adopted to test immunogenicity and protection against CHIKV disease. A single dose of 10^8 IU administration intranasally gave rise to neutralizing antibodies and protected mice from viremia and footpad swelling.

Another adenovirus-based study utilized replication-deficient chimpanzee adenovirus. Due to the induction of anti-adenovirus immune response, human adenoviral-vectored vaccines are not suitable for humans. Chimpanzee adenovirus overcomes this problem to maintain vaccine efficacy (Lopez-Camacho et al., 2019). In this study, the full length or capsid-deleted structural proteins of CHIKV were expressed at the adenoviral platform to generated vaccines ChAdOx1 sCHIKV and ChAdOx1 sCHIKV ΔC. A single dose of the two kinds of ChAdOx1 vaccines was injected in BALB/c mice. Two weeks after vaccination, mice that had received either of the two vaccines showed a high T-cell response frequency. ChAdOx1 sCHIKV and ChAdOx1 sCHIKV ΔC also induced a robust humoral response, indicated by a high level of CHIKV-specific IgG. The above results also highlighted that ChAdOx1 sCHIKV did not require an adjuvant to achieve efficacy. Having confirmed the immunogenicity of ChAdOx1 sCHIKV, further studies will be needed to promote preclinical trials.

Vectors are also suitable for bivalent vaccine. ZIKV, an enveloped positive-stranded RNA virus, shares similarities with CHIKV in clinical symptoms and transmission route. Chattopadhyay et al. previously developed a CHIKV vaccine based on VSV vector (VSVΔG-CHIKV), in which the G protein of VSV was replaced by CHIKV E3-E2-6K-E1 envelope polyprotein (Chattopadhyay et al., 2013). They went further to additionally express ZIKV envelope glycoproteins on that platform (VSVΔG-CHIKV-ZIKV) (Chattopadhyay et al., 2018). Vaccination with VSVΔG-CHIKV-ZIKV induced neutralizing antibody in immunocompetent BALB/c mice and type-I IFN receptor-deficient A129 mice. The immune response was sufficient to protect immunized animals from ZIKV and CHIKV infection, with no viremia detectable. Additionally, the deletion of the G protein also eliminated the neurotropism of VSV, making it safer and more efficient.

VLP

Virus-like particle is assembled by expressing viral structural proteins that possess self-assembly capacity. With antigenic epitopes similar to wild-type virus, VLP can induce high neutralizing antibody titer. VLP has high safety due to its deficiency in replicative and infectious ability (DeZure et al., 2016). Although the development of VLP vaccine started later than that of traditional strategies, several prominent VLP vaccine candidates have been developed recently.

Virus-like particle vaccines have shown prospective applications, but the mammalian expression systems in which VLP vaccines have been produced limited productivity and increased cost. *Pichia pastoris*, an ideal platform for protein expression, has been adopted to produce VLP for many viruses. The *Pichia* system not only supplied native circumstance for protein expression but also increased the performance-to-price ratio to a large extent (Vogl et al., 2013). Saraswat et al. (2016) have made a good attempt to utilize a yeast expression system for developing CHIKV VLP vaccine. They successfully introduced the gene expressing CHIKV whole structural proteins into the *Pichia* expression system and confirmed the morphological identity of VLPs with CHIKV by electron microscopy. Next, the potential of this product (CHIK-VLPs) to be a vaccine candidate was extensively evaluated. ELISA and plaque reduction neutralization testing showed that CHIK-VLPs induced high-titered antibodies with super specificity and neutralizing activity. Elevated levels of TNF-α and IL-10 indicated a robust cellular response, which combined with restricted levels of IL-2, IL-4, and IFN-γ to make a balanced response. The humoral and cellular immune response elicited by CHIK-VLPs was consistent with the protection of CHIK-VLP-immunized BALB/c mice against CHIKV pathogenesis.

In another study, researchers evaluated the efficacies of different VLP formulations with or without an adjuvant in protecting adult and aged mice (Arevalo et al., 2019). Although VLP alone was able to protect adult mice against CHIKV disease, the disease was even more serious in aged mice vaccinated by VLP alone or VLP plus QuilA adjuvant. ELISA and microneutralization assays showed that immunization elicited a high level of neutralizing antibody titer specifically against CHIKV in adult mice. However, for aged mice, negligible antibody was detected. This research implied that specific vaccines suitable for the elderly should be developed in the future.

CHIMERIC VACCINE

Chimeric vaccine links the genome or genome fragments of at least two pathogens by genetic engineering to express antigens from multiple pathogens simultaneously. The most attractive advantage of chimera vaccines is a high immune response against multiple pathogens. Besides, since it is constructed by genomic methods, chimeric vaccines are more stable than traditional LAV.

The ideal vaccine would balance safety and immunogenicity; low performance in one or the other is the disadvantage of LAV and inactivated vaccine, respectively. To overcome this issue, Erasmus et al. (2017) creatively used an insect-specific alphavirus, Eilat virus (EILV), to contain CHIKV structural proteins. Its deficiency of replication gave this chimera virus a high level of safety. However, the entry and delivery of RNA during the early stage of virus replication resembled that of wild-type CHIKV. They first identified that EILV/CHIKV virus had an identical structure to wild-type CHIKV. They then chose immunocompetent C57BL/6 mice, immunocompromised A129 IFNα/βR$^{-/-}$ mice, and cynomolgus macaques to conduct *in vivo* experiments. A single dose elicited rapid seroconversion 4 days post-vaccination (DPV). Meanwhile, antigen-specific IFN-γ-producing CD8$^+$ T cells were induced. Challenged by CHIKV at 30 DPV, all C57BL/6 mice vaccinated by EILV/CHIKV were protected from viremia. For IFNα/βR$^{-/-}$ mice, which were utilized for long-term efficacy assessment, EILV/CHIKV vaccination also protected them from weight loss, footpad swelling, viremia, and death. Finally, EILV/CHIKV vaccination was tolerated in cynomolgus macaques. The body temperature remained at baseline level, and viremia was not detectable after CHIKV challenge. In addition, EILV/CHIKV exhibited cross-neutralization against three different strains from the Asian, West African, and Indian Ocean lineages (Erasmus et al., 2017). Another alphavirus, Sindbis virus (SINV), is commonly used as the genetic backbone for chimeric vaccine and successfully protected cynomolgus macaques against lethal eastern equine encephalitis virus (EEEV). However, the Eilat virus is hosted only by insects, further ensuring the safety of the chimeric vaccine.

NUCLEIC ACID VACCINE

DNA vaccine is a novel platform that has been developed in recent years. By introducing exogenous DNA into the host, antigen proteins are synthesized by the host expression system. The obvious advantage of DNA vaccine is its simplicity of production. Additionally, DNA vaccine is stable at low temperature, which makes it convenient to store and transport across long distances (Powers, 2018). However, there are several drawbacks to this strategy. Integrating exogenous DNA may elicit an autoimmune response in the host. The immunogenicity is low in humans, and thus vaccination needs repeated boosters as well as adjuvants (Powers, 2018). Addressing these concerns will enable breakthroughs in DNA vaccine design.

Hidajat et al. have developed a new method called iDNA® infectious clone technology, which generates vaccine from plasmid DNA both *in vitro* and *in vivo* (Hidajat et al., 2016). It is distinct from traditional infectious clone technology, which needed *in vitro* RNA transcription and *in vitro* transfection involving bacteriophage polymerase, in that an iDNA® infectious clone uses a CMV promoter to transcribe genomic RNA from a plasmid in eukaryotic cells (Tretyakova et al., 2013). Taking advantage of this novel technology, they developed a DNA-launching vaccine for CHIKV (pCHIKV-7) that encoded the full-length cDNA of 181/25 vaccine. *In vivo* experiments showed that single-dose vaccination with pCHIKV-7 protected mice from CHIKV disease, with neutralizing antibodies being detectable in all animals (Tretyakova et al., 2014). In 2016, researchers analyzed its genetic stability by next-generation sequencing (NGS) (Hidajat et al., 2016). Illumina HiSeq2000 sequencing revealed that overall pCHIKV-7 was more stable than 181/25. As for E2-12 and E2-82 residues, two previously identified attenuating mutations, the frequencies of reversion in pCHIKV-7 were 0.064 and 0.086%, respectively, much lower than that of 181/25 (0.179 and 0.133%).

Conventional vaccines require a lag phase to allow enough antibody generation, which is not suitable for urgent protective need in response to a virus outbreak. Passive immunotherapy such as monoclonal antibody (mAb) prophylaxis provides effective short-term protection. However, repeated injection

TABLE 1 | Recently developed vaccine candidates against CHIKV.

Type	Vaccine	Antigen/target	Animal model	Dosage	Route	Results	References
LAV	RH-CHIKV EV-CHIKV RHEV-CHIKV	R532H-nsP1 E515V-nsP2	Adult C57BL/6J mice	10^6 PFU, single injection	Injection in the metatarsal region of the footpad	RH-CHIKV and RHEV-CHIKV reduced CHIKV infectivity and alleviated viremia and joint symptoms. Cross-protection against ONNV	Chan et al. (2019)
LAV	Δ5nsP3 DREP-E MVA-CE	nsP3 envelope and capsid	Cynomolgus macaques	10^5 PFU, single injection	Subcutaneous injection in the shoulder and in the upper part of the left wrist	Δ5nsP3 did not induce fever, lymphopenia, or increase in cytokine	Roques et al. (2017)
LAV	ΔC-CHIKV	Capsid deletion	6-week C57BL/6J and IFNAR$^{-/-}$ mice	10^4 PFU, single injection	Subcutaneous injection	Preserves infectivity in BHK-21 cells. Single-dose injection elicited strong protection against CHIKV in both WT and IFNAR$^{-/-}$ mice, without footpad swelling or weight loss	Zhang et al. (2019)
LAV	CHIKV-NoLS	N-terminal region of capsid protein	21-day C57BL/6 mice	10^4 PFU, single injection	Subcutaneous injection	No sign of footpad welling, viremia reduced, and expression of proinflammatory factors decreased. Cross-protection against RRV. Vaccine thermo-stable, and minimal inflammation and tissue damage	Taylor et al. (2017); Abeyratne et al. (2018)
LAV	Stop CHIKV SuperStop CHIKV	Multiple synonymous mutations in genome to reduce mutational robustness	5-week C57BL/6 mice	10^4 PFU, single injection	Footpad injection	No footpad swelling, low viremia, high level of neutralizing antibody	Carrau et al. (2019)
Vector virus	MV-CHIK	Measles-vectored CHIKV structural proteins	18–55-year-old healthy volunteers	5×10^4, 5×10^5 TCID50, twice injection; measle-primed group accepted additional injection at −28 day	Intramuscular injection	Safety and tolerance similar to measle vaccine	Reisinger et al. (2019)
Vector virus	MV-CHIK	Measles-vectored CHIKV structural proteins	Adult cynomolgus macaques	0.35 mL single measle vaccine dose, twice injection at day 0 and day 28	Intramuscular injection in the quadriceps muscles	Viremia low. No signs of disease. Cross-protection against other CHIKV strains	Rossi et al. (2019)
Vector virus	Ad-CHIKV-SG Ad-CHIKV-E3/E2/6K Ad-CHIKV-E3/E2/E1	Structural proteins	6–8-week BALB/c mice 4-week C57BL/6 mice	10^7 infectious units (BALB/c) 10^8 infectious units (C57BL/6)	Intranasal administration	Induced high tighter of CHIKV-specific IgG antibodies	Dora et al. (2019)
Vector virus	ChAdOx1 sCHIKV ChAdOx1 sCHIKV ΔC	Structural polyprotein	6–8-week BALB/c mice	10^8 infectious units with or without adjuvant	Intramuscular injection	High immunogenicity	Lopez-Camacho et al. (2019)

(Continued)

TABLE 1 | Continued

Type	Vaccine	Antigen/target	Animal model	Dosage	Route	Results	References
Vector virus	VSVΔG-CHIKV	CHIKV: E3-E2-6K-E1 envelope polyprotein ZIKV: envelope glycoproteins	6–8-week BALB/c mice 7-week A129 mice	10^7 PFU, single injection	Intramuscular injection	Induced neutralizing antibody responses to both CHIKV and ZIKV. Protected from both CHIKV- and ZIKV-induced diseases	Chattopadhyay et al. (2018)
Chimeric virus	EILV/CHIKV	EILV cDNA clone containing CHIKV structural proteins	4-week C57BL/6 mice; 6-week IFNα/βR$^{-/-}$ mice Cynomolgus macaques	8.8 log10 PFU (C57BL/6) or 8.5 log10 PFU (IFNα/βR$^{-/-}$ mice) of live EILV/CHIKV, single injection	Subcutaneous injection	Protected from viremia and footpad swelling when challenged by virus on day 30 post-vaccination. Exhibited long-term efficacy in IFNα/βR$^{-/-}$ mice. For cynomolgus macaques, held normal, baseline diurnal body temperatures 31 DPC	Erasmus et al. (2017)
VLP	CHIK-VLP	C-E proteins	6–8-week (adult), 18–24-month (aged) C57BL/6 mice	30 μg VLPs with different adjuvants Three-time vaccination with or without adjuvants	Intramuscular injection	CHIK VLP without adjuvant elicited immune responses and protected adult mice but exacerbated disease on aged mice	Arevalo et al. (2019)
VLP	CHIK-VLPs	Structural proteins introduced into yeast expression system	4-week BALB/c mice	10, 20, and 40 μg of yeast-derived CHIK-VLPs (in Freund's adjuvant); boosted at day 14 and day 28	Subcutaneous injection	High level of specific antibody with high neutralization activity. Induced robust humoral and cell-mediated response	Saraswat et al. (2016)
DNA vaccine	dMAb	CHIKV envelope	B6. Cg-Foxn1nu/J mice	100 μg CVM1-Fab plus 25 μg CHIKV Env plasmid injected three times at 2-week intervals	Intramuscular injection	One injection produced antibodies rapidly and neutralized diverse CHIKV clinical isolates	Muthumani et al. (2016)
DNA vaccine	pCHIKV-7	Full-length cDNA of 181/25 vaccine	–	–	–	Genetic stable	Hidajat et al. (2016)
RNA vaccine	CHKV-24	Lipid-encapsulated neutralizing human mAbs	AG129 mice Cynomolgus macaques	10, 2, or 0.4 mg/kg, single injection	Intravenous injection	Protected mice from arthritis, musculoskeletal tissue infection, and lethality and reduced viremia to undetectable levels	Kose et al. (2019)

LAV, live-attenuated virus; VLP, virus-like particles; –, not mentioned.

is necessary due to the short half-life of immunoglobulins. Muthumani et al. (2016) combined the advantages of a passive antibody and vaccination by an *in vivo* delivery method. DNA encoding the biologically active mAb (dMAb) targeting CHIKV envelope was delivered by plasmid rather than virus vector through electroporation. This strategy also circumvented the risk of inducing an immune response against the vector. Immunizing animals by intramuscular injection of dMAb induced antibodies much more rapidly than conventional vaccination methods. Footpad swelling was not observed in immunized animals challenged by the virus. These dMAbs were able to neutralize diverse CHIKV clinical isolates. In conclusion, this study highlighted the advantages of DNA vaccine, which could be combined with other platforms for vaccine development.

A design based on mRNA is one of the newest strategies for CHIKV vaccine. The vaccine can be designed to deliver mAb just like the DNA vaccine introduced above. Kose et al. (2019) isolated neutralizing human mAbs from the B cells of a survivor of CHIKV infection. They introduced the mAb-encoding sequences into lipid-encapsulated mRNA, which was then delivered by infusion. Among all the mAbs being examined, CHKV-24 showed most prominent inhibitory effect in neutralization assay. *In vivo* experiments revealed that infusion of CHKV-24 succeeded in inducing human IgG in both mice and macaques, the latter of which peaked at 24 h after immunization with the dosage varied from 10.1 to 35.9 μg/mL. Compared with proteins, nucleic acids encoding antibodies are easy to produce and cost less. Another strategy for using an mRNA platform is to instruct host cells to express viral antigens for generating antibodies accordingly. A biotech company named Moderna Therapeutics developed an mRNA CHIKV vaccine (mRNA-1388) and made it through to phase I clinical trial, using engineered mRNA that encoded CHIKV structural polyprotein. With a single dose of this mRNA vaccine, a strong immune response was elicited, and 100% protection was achieved in mice (Goyal et al., 2018). This innovation avoided an immune response against engineered mRNA and ensured sufficient protein synthesis.

ANIMAL MODELS

Apart from extensive *ex vivo* studies, *in vivo* experiments are important for developing vaccines. Different animal models have provided platforms for evaluating the efficacy and security of potential CHIKV vaccines. The studies summarized in this paper used cynomolgus macaques and mice of multiple strains involving C57BL/6, BALB/c, and A129.

C57BL/6 mice are immunocompetent animals. Because they are easy to breed and their traits are stable, C57BL/6 mice are widely used to evaluate vaccines. Live-attenuated vaccines evaluated in C57BL/6 mice have included CHIKV-NoLS, RH-CHIKV, EV-CHIKV, RHEV-CHIKV, ΔC-CHIKV, "STOP," and "SuperStop." C57BL/6 mice have also been used to assess CHIK-VLP.

BALB/c mice are easy to breed and display little gender difference in body weight. BALB/c mice have been widely employed to develop DNA vaccines and recombinant vector vaccines (ChOdAx1 sCHIKV, ChOdAx1 sCHIKV ΔC, Ad-CHIKV-SG, Ad-CHIKV-E3/E2/6K, and Ad-CHIKV-E3/E2/E1).

Another murine model used in CHIKV infection is A129. Since they lack type I interferon receptors, A129 mice are deficient in the innate immune response. However, their adaptive immunity is retained so that they are tolerant to virus challenging (Couderc et al., 2008). A129 mice have been involved in immunogenicity studies of the EILV/CHIKV, VSVΔG-CHIKV, and CHKV-24 mRNA vaccines.

The cynomolgus macaque, as a non-human primate, is particularly suitable for studying the pathogenesis of viral infection. Compared with murine models, non-human primates share more similarities with humans in physiology, metabolism, and immunity (Labadie et al., 2010), making them highly effective for predicting the efficacy of human treatment. Despite the high cost and complexity of breeding them, macaques remain an irreplaceable model in vaccine development. Non-human primates have been proved to be susceptible to CHIKV infection (Labadie et al., 2010). Studies on LAV vaccine Δ5nsP3, vector vaccine MV-CHIK, mRNA vaccine CHKV-24, and chimeric vaccine EILV/CHIKV have set cynomolgus macaque as an animal model for immunogenicity assessment.

CONCLUSION

As a rapidly spreading recurrent infectious disease, CHIKF has attracted wide attention. Vaccination is a powerful means to control epidemic diseases including CHIKF, but there is no commercial vaccine against CHIKV at present. The re-outbreak of CHIKF since 2004 boosted CHIKV vaccine development. Researchers have applied a variety of strategies to develop vaccine candidates, some of which have entered the Phase-I or Phase-II stage of clinical trials and show promising application prospects. In this paper, the latest progress in the development and testing of CHIKV vaccine, especially since 2016, was reviewed. The development strategies, immunogenicity evaluation, and protective efficacy against diseases were introduced; the key information is summarized in **Table 1**.

Future studies should pay more attention to the following aspects: (1) Comprehensive consideration of both safety and immunogenicity. This is a common concern for all vaccine production. On the premise of keeping a low rate of revertant mutation of the virus, the vaccine titer should be enhanced to achieve better protection efficacy. (2) Convenience of production and use. Vaccines should be thermostable and easy to produce, transport, and store. In addition, their administration should be convenient, and the discomfort of vaccination should be alleviated. Bivalent and multivalent chimeric vaccines can immunize against more than one virus at one time, which will greatly improve the immune response. (3) Long-term and short-term protection. Vaccines should provide long-term protection. However, acute protection is needed in local areas in times of outbreak. From this point of view, DNA vaccine with both long-term and short-term protective efficacies is a good choice (Muthumani et al., 2016). (4) Different performance in different populations. In one study involving adult and aged mice, vaccines that showed protective efficacies in adult mice exaggerated the symptoms of disease in aged mice (Arevalo et al., 2019). This result suggests that the populations had a significant difference in response to the vaccine. Attention should be paid to the complexity of the social population, especially when determining the dose of vaccine to use. Broadly speaking, most vaccine studies are based on animal models, whether the developed vaccine is suitable for humans has yet to be evaluated. Clinical trials need to be promoted. It is believed that with the progress of new strategies and studies, commercial CHIKV vaccine with high safety, strong immunogenicity, convenient development, and moderate cost can be developed in the near future.

AUTHOR CONTRIBUTIONS

LZ and SS provided the concept. SG drafted the manuscript. SG and LZ revised the manuscript. All authors approved the final version for publication.

FUNDING

This work was supported by grants from the National Key Plan for Research and Development of China (2016YFD0500300), the National Natural Science Foundation of China (81871663 and 81672035), and the Academic Promotion Program of Shandong First Medical University.

REFERENCES

Abeyratne, E., Freitas, J. R., Zaid, A., Mahalingam, S., and Taylor, A. (2018). Attenuation and stability of CHIKV-NoLS, a live-attenuated chikungunya virus vaccine candidate. *Vaccines* 7:E2. doi: 10.3390/vaccines7010002

Arevalo, M. T., Huang, Y., Jones, C. A., and Ross, T. M. (2019). Vaccination with a chikungunya virus-like particle vaccine exacerbates disease in aged mice. *PLoS Negl. Trop. Dis.* 13:e0007316. doi: 10.1371/journal.pntd.0007316

Carrau, L., Rezelj, V. V., Noval, M. G., Levi, L. I., Megrian, D., Blanc, H., et al. (2019). Chikungunya virus vaccine candidates with decreased mutational robustness are attenuated in vivo and have compromised transmissibility. *J. Virol.* 93:e00775-19. doi: 10.1128/JVI.00775-19

Chan, Y. H., Teo, T. H., Utt, A., Tan, J. J., Amrun, S. N., Abu Bakar, F., et al. (2019). Mutating chikungunya virus non-structural protein produces potent live-attenuated vaccine candidate. *EMBO Mol. Med.* 11:e10092. doi: 10.15252/emmm.201810092

Chattopadhyay, A., Aguilar, P. V., Bopp, N. E., Yarovinsky, T. O., Weaver, S. C., and Rose, J. K. (2018). A recombinant virus vaccine that protects against both Chikungunya and Zika virus infections. *Vaccine* 36, 3894–3900. doi: 10.1016/j.vaccine.2018.05.095

Chattopadhyay, A., Wang, E., Seymour, R., Weaver, S. C., and Rose, J. K. (2013). A chimeric vesiculo/alphavirus is an effective alphavirus vaccine. *J. Virol.* 87, 395–402. doi: 10.1128/JVI.01860-12

Couderc, T., Chretien, F., Schilte, C., Disson, O., Brigitte, M., Guivel-Benhassine, F., et al. (2008). A mouse model for Chikungunya: young age and inefficient type-I interferon signaling are risk factors for severe disease. *PLoS Pathog.* 4:e29. doi: 10.1371/journal.ppat.0040029

DeZure, A. D., Berkowitz, N. M., Graham, B. S., and Ledgerwood, J. E. (2016). Whole-Inactivated and virus-like particle vaccine strategies for Chikungunya Virus. *J. Infect. Dis.* 214(Suppl. 5), S497–S499. doi: 10.1093/infdis/jiw352

Dora, E. G., Rossi, S. L., Weaver, S. C., Tucker, S. N., and Mateo, R. (2019). An adjuvanted adenovirus 5-based vaccine elicits neutralizing antibodies and protects mice against chikungunya virus-induced footpad swelling. *Vaccine* 37, 3146–3150. doi: 10.1016/j.vaccine.2019.04.069

Elsinga, J., Gerstenbluth, I., van der Ploeg, S., Halabi, Y., Lourents, N. T., Burgerhof, J. G., et al. (2017). Long-term Chikungunya Sequelae in Curacao: burden, determinants, and a novel classification tool. *J. Infect. Dis.* 216, 573–581. doi: 10.1093/infdis/jix312

Enserink, M. (2007). Infectious diseases. Chikungunya: no longer a third world disease. *Science* 318, 1860–1861. doi: 10.1126/science.318.5858.1860

Erasmus, J. H., Auguste, A. J., Kaelber, J. T., Luo, H., Rossi, S. L., Fenton, K., et al. (2017). A chikungunya fever vaccine utilizing an insect-specific virus platform. *Nat. Med.* 23, 192–199. doi: 10.1038/nm.4253

Goyal, M., Chauhan, A., Goyal, V., Jaiswal, N., Singh, S., and Singh, M. (2018). Recent development in the strategies projected for chikungunya vaccine in humans. *Drug Des. Dev. Ther.* 12, 4195–4206. doi: 10.2147/DDDT.S181574

Harrison, V. R., Eckels, K. H., Bartelloni, P. J., and Hampton, C. (1971). Production and evaluation of a formalin-killed Chikungunya vaccine. *J. Immunol.* 107, 643–647.

Hidajat, R., Nickols, B., Forrester, N., Tretyakova, I., Weaver, S., and Pushko, P. (2016). Next generation sequencing of DNA-launched Chikungunya vaccine virus. *Virology* 490, 83–90. doi: 10.1016/j.virol.2016.01.009

Khan, M., Dhanwani, R., Rao, P. V., and Parida, M. (2012). Subunit vaccine formulations based on recombinant envelope proteins of Chikungunya virus elicit balanced Th1/Th2 response and virus-neutralizing antibodies in mice. *Virus Res.* 167, 236–246. doi: 10.1016/j.virusres.2012.05.004

Kitaoka, M. (1967). Japanese encephalitis vaccine including a preliminary report on dengue fever and chikungunya vaccines. *Jpn. J. Med. Sci. Biol.* 20(Suppl.), 41–56.

Kose, N., Fox, J. M., Sapparapu, G., Bombardi, R., Tennekoon, R. N., de Silva, A. D., et al. (2019). A lipid-encapsulated mRNA encoding a potently neutralizing human monoclonal antibody protects against chikungunya infection. *Sci. Immunol.* 4:eaaw6647. doi: 10.1126/sciimmunol.aaw6647

Kumar, M., Sudeep, A. B., and Arankalle, V. A. (2012). Evaluation of recombinant E2 protein-based and whole-virus inactivated candidate vaccines against chikungunya virus. *Vaccine* 30, 6142–6149. doi: 10.1016/j.vaccine.2012.07.072

Labadie, K., Larcher, T., Joubert, C., Mannioui, A., Delache, B., Brochard, P., et al. (2010). Chikungunya disease in nonhuman primates involves long-term viral persistence in macrophages. *J. Clin. Invest.* 120, 894–906. doi: 10.1172/JCI40104

Langsjoen, R. M., Haller, S. L., Roy, C. J., Vinet-Oliphant, H., Bergren, N. A., Erasmus, J. H., et al. (2018). Chikungunya virus strains show lineage-specific variations in virulence and cross-protective ability in murine and nonhuman primate models. *mBio* 9:e02449-17. doi: 10.1128/mBio.02449-17

Ljungberg, K., and Liljestrom, P. (2015). Self-replicating alphavirus RNA vaccines. *Expert Rev. Vaccines* 14, 177–194. doi: 10.1586/14760584.2015.965690

Lopez-Camacho, C., Kim, Y. C., Blight, J., Lazaro Moreli, M., Montoya-Diaz, E., Huiskonen, J. T., et al. (2019). Assessment of immunogenicity and neutralisation efficacy of viral-vectored vaccines against chikungunya virus. *Viruses* 11:E322. doi: 10.3390/v11040322

Metz, S. W., Geertsema, C., Martina, B. E., Andrade, P., Heldens, J. G., van Oers, M. M., et al. (2011). Functional processing and secretion of Chikungunya virus E1 and E2 glycoproteins in insect cells. *Virol. J.* 8:353. doi: 10.1186/1743-422X-8-353

Metz, S. W., Martina, B. E., van den Doel, P., Geertsema, C., Osterhaus, A. D., Vlak, J. M., et al. (2013). Chikungunya virus-like particles are more immunogenic in a lethal AG129 mouse model compared to glycoprotein E1 or E2 subunits. *Vaccine* 31, 6092–6096. doi: 10.1016/j.vaccine.2013.09.045

Muthumani, K., Block, P., Flingai, S., Muruganantham, N., Chaaithanya, I. K., Tingey, C., et al. (2016). Rapid and long-term immunity elicited by DNA-encoded antibody prophylaxis and DNA vaccination against chikungunya virus. *J. Infect. Dis.* 214, 369–378. doi: 10.1093/infdis/jiw111

Plante, K. S., Rossi, S. L., Bergren, N. A., Seymour, R. L., and Weaver, S. C. (2015). Extended preclinical safety, efficacy and stability testing of a live-attenuated chikungunya vaccine candidate. *PLoS Negl. Trop. Dis.* 9:e0004007. doi: 10.1371/journal.pntd.0004007

Powers, A. M. (2018). Vaccine and therapeutic options to control chikungunya virus. *Clin. Microbiol. Rev.* 31:e00104-16. doi: 10.1128/CMR.00104-16

Ramsauer, K., Schwameis, M., Firbas, C., Mullner, M., Putnak, R. J., Thomas, S. J., et al. (2015). Immunogenicity, safety, and tolerability of a recombinant measles-virus-based chikungunya vaccine: a randomised, double-blind, placebo-controlled, active-comparator, first-in-man trial. *Lancet Infect. Dis.* 15, 519–527. doi: 10.1016/S1473-3099(15)70043-5

Reisinger, E. C., Tschismarov, R., Beubler, E., Wiedermann, U., Firbas, C., Loebermann, M., et al. (2019). Immunogenicity, safety, and tolerability of the measles-vectored chikungunya virus vaccine MV-CHIK: a double-blind, randomised, placebo-controlled and active-controlled phase 2 trial. *Lancet* 392, 2718–2727. doi: 10.1016/S0140-6736(18)32488-7

Roques, P., Ljungberg, K., Kummerer, B. M., Gosse, L., Dereuddre-Bosquet, N., Tchitchek, N., et al. (2017). Attenuated and vectored vaccines protect nonhuman primates against chikungunya virus. *JCI Insight* 2:e83527. doi: 10.1172/jci.insight.83527

Rossi, S. L., Comer, J. E., Wang, E., Azar, S. R., Lawrence, W. S., Plante, J. A., et al. (2019). Immunogenicity and efficacy of a measles virus-vectored chikungunya vaccine in nonhuman primates. *J. Infect. Dis.* 220, 735–742. doi: 10.1093/infdis/jiz202

Rudd, P. A., Raphael, A. P., Yamada, M., Nufer, K. L., Gardner, J., Le, T. T., et al. (2015). Effective cutaneous vaccination using an inactivated chikungunya virus vaccine delivered by Foroderm. *Vaccine* 33, 5172–5180. doi: 10.1016/j.vaccine.2015.07.099

Saraswat, S., Athmaram, T. N., Parida, M., Agarwal, A., Saha, A., and Dash, P. K. (2016). Expression and characterization of yeast derived chikungunya virus like particles (CHIK-VLPs) and its evaluation as a potential vaccine candidate. *PLoS Negl. Trop. Dis.* 10:e0004782. doi: 10.1371/journal.pntd.0004782

Strauss, J. H., and Strauss, E. G. (1994). The alphaviruses: gene expression, replication, and evolution. *Microbiol. Rev.* 58, 491–562.

Taylor, A., Liu, X., Zaid, A., Goh, L. Y., Hobson-Peters, J., Hall, R. A., et al. (2017). Mutation of the N-Terminal region of chikungunya virus capsid protein: implications for vaccine design. *mBio* 8:e01970-16. doi: 10.1128/mBio.01970-16

Tiwari, M., Parida, M., Santhosh, S. R., Khan, M., Dash, P. K., and Rao, P. V. (2009). Assessment of immunogenic potential of Vero adapted formalin inactivated vaccine derived from novel ECSA genotype of chikungunya virus. *Vaccine* 27, 2513–2522. doi: 10.1016/j.vaccine.2009.02.062

Tretyakova, I., Hearn, J., Wang, E., Weaver, S., and Pushko, P. (2014). DNA vaccine initiates replication of live attenuated chikungunya virus in vitro and elicits protective immune response in mice. *J. Infect. Dis.* 209, 1882–1890. doi: 10.1093/infdis/jiu114

Tretyakova, I., Lukashevich, I. S., Glass, P., Wang, E., Weaver, S., and Pushko, P. (2013). Novel vaccine against Venezuelan equine encephalitis combines advantages of DNA immunization and a live attenuated vaccine. *Vaccine* 31, 1019–1025. doi: 10.1016/j.vaccine.2012.12.050

Vogl, T., Hartner, F. S., and Glieder, A. (2013). New opportunities by synthetic biology for biopharmaceutical production in Pichia pastoris. *Curr. Opin. Biotechnol.* 24, 1094–1101. doi: 10.1016/j.copbio.2013.02.024

Zhang, Y. N., Deng, C. L., Li, J. Q., Li, N., Zhang, Q. Y., Ye, H. Q., et al. (2019). Infectious chikungunya virus (CHIKV) with a complete capsid deletion: a new approach for a CHIKV vaccine. *J. Virol.* 93:e00504-19. doi: 10.1128/JVI.00504-19

9

The Current and Future State of Vaccines, Antivirals and Gene Therapies Against Emerging Coronaviruses

Longping V. Tse[1], *Rita M. Meganck*[2], *Rachel L. Graham*[1] *and Ralph S. Baric*[1,3*]

[1] *Department of Epidemiology, The University of North Carolina at Chapel Hill, Chapel Hill, NC, United States,* [2] *Curriculum in Genetics and Molecular Biology, The University of North Carolina at Chapel Hill, Chapel Hill, NC, United States,*
[3] *Department of Microbiology and Immunology, The University of North Carolina at Chapel Hill, Chapel Hill, NC, United States*

Correspondence:
Ralph S. Baric
rbaric@email.unc.edu

Emerging coronaviruses (CoV) are constant global public health threats to society. Multiple ongoing clinical trials for vaccines and antivirals against CoVs showcase the availability of medical interventions to both prevent and treat the future emergence of highly pathogenic CoVs in human. However, given the diverse nature of CoVs and our close interactions with wild, domestic and companion animals, the next epidemic zoonotic CoV could resist the existing vaccines and antivirals developed, which are primarily focused on Severe Acute Respiratory Syndrome Coronavirus (SARS-CoV) and Middle East Respiratory Syndrome Coronavirus (MERS CoV). In late 2019, the novel CoV (SARS-CoV-2) emerged in Wuhan, China, causing global public health concern. In this review, we will summarize the key advancements of current vaccines and antivirals against SARS-CoV and MERS-CoV as well as discuss the challenge and opportunity in the current SARS-CoV-2 crisis. At the end, we advocate the development of a "plug-and-play" platform technologies that could allow quick manufacturing and administration of broad-spectrum countermeasures in an outbreak setting. We will discuss the potential of AAV-based gene therapy technology for *in vivo* therapeutic antibody delivery to combat SARS-CoV-2 outbreak and the future emergence of severe CoVs.

Keywords: coronavirus (CoV), vaccine, antivirals, adeno-associate virus, passive immunization strategy, MERS- and SARS-CoV, 2019 nCoV

INTRODUCTION

The zoonotic transmission and subsequent adaptation to humans of emerging RNA viruses is a global public health concern. In the 21st century alone, coronaviruses (CoV) have been responsible for two separate endemics, the severe acute respiratory syndrome (SARS) and Middle East Respiratory Syndrome (MERS) CoVs (de Wit et al., 2016). In late Dec 2019, a novel SARS-like CoV designated 2019 nCoV emerged in Wuhan China, causing > 60,000 cases and over 1350 deaths in an ongoing epidemic (Hui et al., 2020). Other highly pathogenic threat viruses that have emerged in the 21st century include influenza viruses, Ebola viruses, flaviviruses and paramyxoviruses (Mackenzie and Jeggo, 2013). The high mutation and recombination rate of RNA viruses drives the emergence of new viral strains that can rapidly adapt to new and changing ecologies (Drake and Holland, 1999; Lauring and Andino, 2010). Furthermore, industrialization, globalization and traditional cultural habits potentiate the likelihood of zoonotic transmission and facilitate the spread of viruses in the human population. While new outbreaks from emergent viruses are inevitable, scientists, epidemiologists, and the health care industry are racing to develop new technologies to better predict and minimize the impact of an outbreak by employing global viral surveillance programs and developing vaccines and antivirals (Lipkin and Firth, 2013). A major challenge of vaccine and antiviral development is the elusive nature of the emerging viruses, which oftentimes emerge from highly heterogeneous populations of virus strains that circulate in animal reservoirs (Lauring and Andino, 2010). Therefore, to prepare for future outbreaks, vaccines and antivirals will need to be both potent and broadly effective against multiple potential emerging viruses within and across virus families. Additionally, in order to control and prevent viral spread, treatments must be readily available to affected populations and have a fast response time. In this review, we will focus our discussion on the challenges, as well as current development, of vaccines and antivirals for SARS-CoV and MERS-CoV. At the end, we will also discuss the potential use of AAV-based gene therapy as a quick response to prevent and treat emerging viral infections in the current SARS-CoV-2 and future outbreak situations.

Endemic and Emerging Coronaviruses

Coronaviruses are a diverse group of positive-stranded RNA viruses which infect a wide range of animals from birds to mammals, causing a variety of diseases (Perlman and Netland, 2009; Woo et al., 2009; Peck et al., 2015). Based on sequence identity of the spike protein or the non-structural proteins (nsp), CoVs are classified into four different sub-groups, *alphacoronaviruses*, *betacoronaviruses*, *gammacoronaviruses*, and *deltacoronaviruses* (**Figure 1**). Human coronaviruses (hCoVs), such as 229E, OC43, NL-63 and HKU-1 are highly transmissible respiratory viruses which are responsible for around 10-20% of common cold cases annually (McIntosh et al., 1970; Cabeça et al., 2013). HCoV-related illness is often self-limited in immune competent individuals but may cause more severe upper and lower respiratory tract infections in the young and elderly population (Woo et al., 2005; Lau et al., 2006). In addition, highly pathogenic CoVs may emerge through zoonotic reservoirs. In the past two decades, SARS-CoV and MERS-CoV emerged from bats and spread to humans through intermediate hosts including civet cats and camels, respectively (Raj et al., 2014). SARS-CoV and MERS-CoV belong to the sub-groups 2b and 2c of the *Betacoronavirus* genus (Peck et al., 2015). The latest CoV outbreak is the SARS-CoV-2, a *Betacoronavirus* 2b which emerged from bats and spread to humans (Lu et al., 2020). The mortality rate of these viruses range from 10 to 40% but can exceed 50% in the elderly (Min et al., 2004; Li et al., 2005; Bolles et al., 2011b; Raj et al., 2014; Sharif-Yakan and Kanj, 2014; World Health Organization [WHO], 2018). The unusually high mortality rate is linked to disease progression leading to acute respiratory distress syndrome (ARDS) which causes hypoxemia, pulmonary edema, and infiltration of inflammatory immune cells in the lung (Cabeça et al., 2013; Gralinski and Baric, 2015). If unresolved, the diseases progress to late phase ARDS, leading to end-stage lung disease and death (Ding et al., 2003). Currently, no vaccines or antiviral drugs are approved to prevent or treat severe CoV infection.

The Challenge for Vaccine Development

The CoV *S*-protein is the major envelope glycoprotein and the main determinant of protective immunity. The *S*-protein is composed of two principle subunits, S1 and S2; S1 governs receptor binding and S2 is responsible for membrane fusion (Li, 2016). Similar to other class I fusion proteins, *S*-protein undergoes a major conformational change between pre-fusion and post-fusion which also presents different antigenic epitopes. While able to bind to both conformations, Abs targeting the post-fusion form are not necessary neutralizing; in contrast, Abs targeting the pre-fusion form of the *S*-protein correlate better with neutralization. In particular, vaccines and neutralizing antibodies (nAbs) which target the receptor binding domain (RBD) of the *S*-protein can effectively neutralize the virus (Zhu et al., 2007; Tang et al., 2014). However, due to high selective pressure and tropism determinants, *S*-protein is the most diverse region of CoV. For instance, the *S*-proteins from SARS-CoV and MERS-CoV share only 44% sequence identity (Kandeel, 2018). The majority of differences between *S*-proteins is in the S1 region, which is further separated into the N-terminal Domain (NTD) and RBD. The diverse nature of the RBD between SARS-CoV and MERS-CoV is reflected in the use of different entry receptors, either angiotensin I converting enzyme 2 (ACE2) or dipeptidyl peptidase 4 (DPP4), respectively (Li et al., 2003; Raj et al., 2013). The diversity of *S*-protein also renders vaccines and nAbs unlikely to be cross-protective between existing and emerging CoVs. Surveillance and experimental data have identified multiple animal SARS- and MERS-like CoVs that have significant diversity in *S*-protein and are able to replicate in human cells without adaptation (Menachery et al., 2015, 2016; Luo et al., 2018). Once transmitted to human population, such variation between *S*-protein between the previous and the new emerging CoVs will pose a major challenge on the progress of vaccine development.

CRITERIA FOR GENERATING EFFECTIVE VACCINE FOR CoVs

Vaccine Criteria for SARS and MERS-CoV Viruses

The surface glycoproteins are the main target for vaccine development. In CoV infection, Abs against *S*-protein were shown to be protective in multiple animal studies. Furthermore, in a passive immunization study in camel, the nAb level is directly correlated to lung pathology and survival (Zhao et al., 2015). As such, one of the main goals for CoV vaccines in humans is the ability to elicit a strong humoral immune response against the *S*-protein. Particularly, the pre-fusion form of the *S*-protein is an attractive target for Abs to confer protective immunity.

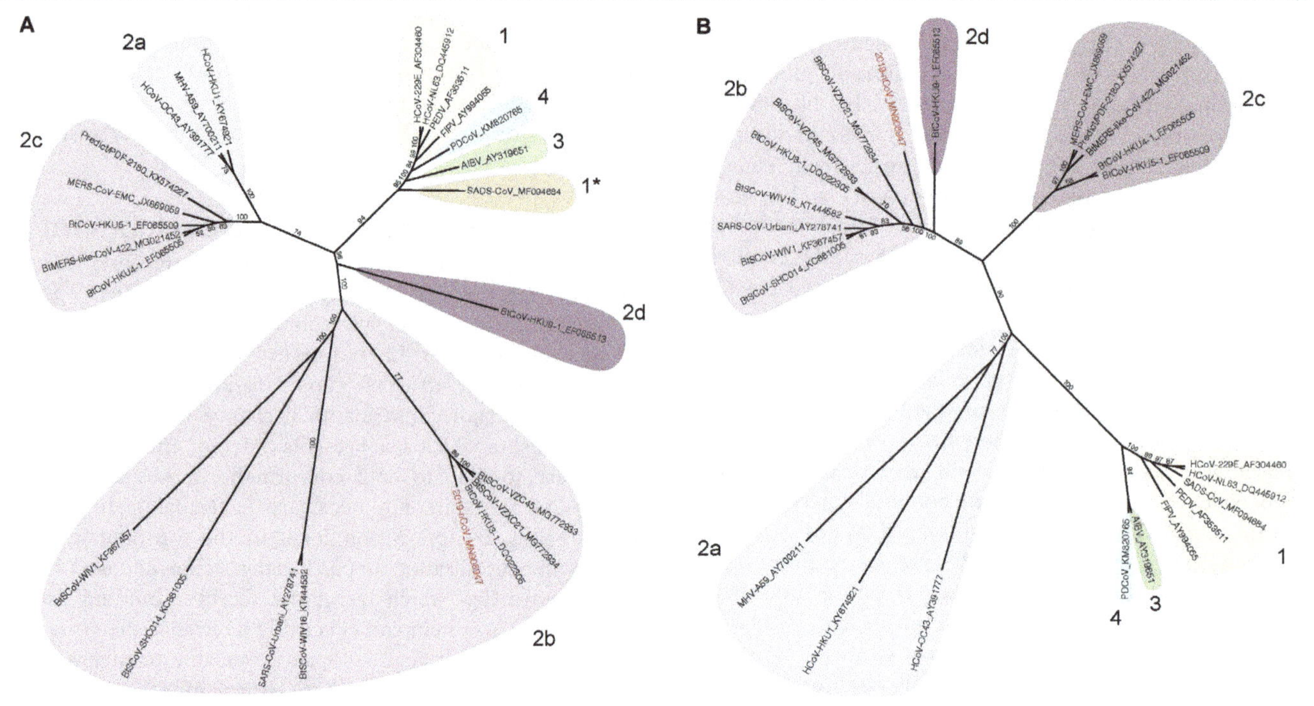

FIGURE 1 | Spike and nsp12 phylogeny of representative coronaviruses. The Spike **(A)** and nsp12 **(B)** protein sequences of selected coronaviruses were aligned and phylogenetically compared. Coronavirus genera are grouped by classic subgroup designations (1, 2a-d, 3, and 4). In the Spike tree in **(A)**, SADS-CoV is designated as 1* because of its distinctive grouping compared with more conserved proteins (e.g., nsp12, see **(B)**). Branches in each tree are labeled with consensus support values (in %). Sequences were aligned using free end gaps with the Blosum62 cost matrix, and the tree was constructed using the neighbor-joining method based on the multiple sequence alignment in Geneious Prime. Numbers following the underscores in each sequence correspond to the GenBank Accession number. The SARS-CoV-2 is highlighted in red. The radial phylogram was exported from Geneious and then rendered for publication using Adobe Illustrator CC 2020.

In order to "lock" the *S*-protein in its antigenic optimal pre-fusion form, two mutations, V1060P and L1061P, were introduced into the MERS-CoV *S*-protein (Pallesen et al., 2017). The resulting MERS S-2P is able to elicit both RBD and non-RBD binding nAbs (Pallesen et al., 2017). The same strategy was also shown to work in the SARS-CoV-2 *S*-protein (Wrapp et al., 2020). Other structural proteins such as E and M and the nsp N also contribute to viral protection and clearance (Channappanavar et al., 2014; Zhao et al., 2016; Deng et al., 2018). Similarly to other respiratory viruses such as influenza, mucosal IgA plays a major role in disease protection and has a synergistic effect with IgG (Belshe et al., 2000; Plotkin, 2010). In order to elicit a strong mucosal IgA immunity, the route of vaccine administration is important. Studies have shown that intranasal inoculation of a recombinant RBD vaccine can elicit greater mucosal IgA production than intramuscular or subcutaneous injection (Ma et al., 2014a). However, the duration of mucosal antibodies is typically shorter lived than systemic IgG responses and the longest longitudinal study of MERS-CoV IgA responses ended after 6 months (Hapfelmeier et al., 2010; Ma et al., 2014a). In comparison, in a natural infection case study, SARS-targeting systemic memory B cells were present up to 6 years for SARS-CoV (Oh et al., 2012; Tang et al., 2019); and up to 34 months post infection for MERS-CoV (Payne et al., 2016). Another important consideration for SARS-CoV and MERS-CoV vaccination is the T cell response against the virus, specifically the N proteins, which is important for viral clearance (Zhao et al., 2010; Channappanavar et al., 2014). A study has shown that adoptive transfer of viral specific T-cells to SCID mice enhances survival and reduces lung titer after SARS-CoV infection (Zhao et al., 2010). Moreover, intranasal vaccination of N protein using the VEEV replicon system elicits CD4+ memory T-cells responses in the airway. Upon challenge, the airway CD4+ memory T cells secrete IFN-γ, which subsequently enhances the innate immune response as well as coordinates the CD8+ T cell priming and migration which protects mice from lethal disease, but not weight loss or virus titers under carefully controlled conditions (Zhao et al., 2016). Interestingly, Rag−/− mice are able to clear SARS-CoV infection, suggesting innate immunity is sufficient for viral clearance (Zhao et al., 2010). However, the mechanism of this viral clearance is still unknown. Another important aspect of emerging CoV vaccine is the breadth of protection. As mentioned previously, the antigenic variation in the *S*-protein between CoVs limits the breadth of cross protection against multiple emerging CoVs, and is especially true for *S*-protein only vaccines (Wang et al., 2018, 2019).

Learning from natural infection, MERS-CoV specific CD4+ and CD8+ T cells are detected in PBMCs in MERS-CoV infected survivors (Zhao et al., 2017). Therefore, a balance of B cell and T cell responses is generally considered the gold standard to prevent and resolve MERS-CoV and SARS-CoV infection. Multiple strategies have been developed to elicit long lasting B and T cell responses for SARS-CoV and MERS-CoV. These include the traditional live attenuated, inactivated, and subunit vaccines, and newer development of nanoparticles, vectorized vaccines, and RNA/DNA vaccines. In this review, we have selected only the vaccine studies that have an *in vivo* challenge model and have summarized the different parameters, including vaccine components, dosage, challenge conditions, animal models and the study outcome in **Table 1**. We will also discuss each type of vaccine strategy and focus on the finished clinical trial targeting SARS-CoV and the 3 ongoing clinical trials targeting MERS-CoV using DNA (Martin et al., 2008; Modjarrad et al., 2019) and vectorized vaccines. Other comprehensive reviews on CoV vaccine development can be found elsewhere (Zhang et al., 2014; Du and Jiang, 2015; Perlman and Vijay, 2016; Schindewolf and Menachery, 2019; Yong et al., 2019).

Current Vaccine Strategies

Inactivated vaccines are the quickest option for vaccine development in an outbreak situation. Multiple chemical and physical methods have been applied singly or in combination to inactivate CoVs, including β-propiolactone, formalin, formaldehyde and UV. While multiple studies have shown the efficacy of inactivated vaccines in hamster, ferret and multiple mouse challenge models (Stadler et al., 2005; See et al., 2006, 2008; Spruth et al., 2006; Roberts et al., 2010), one study suggested a potential vaccine enhanced pathologies (Bolles et al., 2011a). In this study, double inactivation (DIV) of SARS-CoV using formalin and UV+alum elicits a Th2 skewed response and is only partially protective to young mice (6–8 weeks-old) and not protective to experimentally aged mice (12–14 weeks-old) (Bolles et al., 2011a). Furthermore, upon challenge, DIV vaccinated mice show increased infiltration of eosinophils, neutrophils and other inflammatory cell populations in the lung, likely due to the N specific immune response (Bolles et al., 2011a). Further studies have suggested that by replacing alum with TLR agonists such as Poly I:C, Poly U or LPS as adjuvants, the skewed Th2 responses can be alleviated and may reduce the infiltration of eosinophils in the lung (Iwata-Yoshikawa et al., 2014).

Gamma-ray inactivated whole MERS-CoV (WIV) with alum or M59 also suffers from the Th2 skewed immune response and pulmonary eosinophilia upon challenge, suggesting a potential risk of using inactive virus for CoV vaccination (Agrawal et al., 2016). Interestingly, formaldehyde inactivated MERS-CoV co-administered with alum and CpG shows a more balanced Th1/Th2 response and is able to protect mice from a challenge model (Ad5 transduced hDPP4) with reduction in lung viral titer and improved lung pathology. There is no observable vaccine-induced lung pathology or infiltration of eosinophils upon challenge (Deng et al., 2018). The difference in vaccine outcomes indicates an incomplete understanding of the effect of adjuvants on the inactivated SARS and MERS-CoV vaccines. In respiratory syncytial virus (RSV) vaccines, formalin inactivated vaccines presents the post-fusion form predominately and fail to elicit protective immune responses. Whether the same phenomenon exists in inactivated CoV is still unknown, although it could explain the discrepancy between reports. The inconsistent results from different vaccine models also underscores the host genetic elements affecting vaccine outcome. Nevertheless, inactivated vaccine is still one of the most straightforward methods for vaccine development and has the quickest response time in an outbreak situation.

Live attenuated viral vaccines are the closest mimic of natural infection and generally elicit strong B and T cell responses (Zhao et al., 2017). Multiple strategies have been used to genetically attenuate SARS-CoV and MERS-CoV by either deleting or mutating structural, non-structural or accessory proteins. Intranasal immunization of a SARS-CoV lacking E protein (rSARS-CoV-ΔE) has shown complete protection from pulmonary replication in a Golden Syrian hamster model (Lamirande et al., 2008). A similar virus has been generated in the MERS backbone, creating a conditional mutant that requires trans expression of E for productive replication (Almazán et al., 2013). Mutations of the DEDD motif of the 3′ to 5′ exonuclease (ExoN-nsp14) "proof-reading protein" on a mouse-adapted SARS-CoV attenuated the virus both *in vitro* and *in vivo*. A single intranasal immunization is able to elicit strong nAbs (>6-fold protective titers) and completely protect against lethal challenges in an aged mouse model (12 months-old BALB/c) (Graham et al., 2012). Mutations in the nsp 16 (NSP16), a 2′O-methyltransferase, in both SARS-CoV and MERS-CoV have also been shown to attenuate the viruses and to protect BALB/c and CRISPR-Cas humanized DPP4-288-330 mice from lethal challenge (Menachery et al., 2014, 2017, 2018). Moreover, these attenuation strategies can be multiplexed, leading to highly stable live attenuated vaccines with limited capability to undergo recombination and reversion repair (Graham et al., 2018; Menachery et al., 2018). Although the live attenuated vaccine is effective in small animal models, there remain safety concerns about potential revertants and recombination with natural CoVs which hinders their usage in the clinical setting. Furthermore, live attenuated vaccines often require greater time for development and safety testing which lessens utility in an outbreak situation.

Protein-based subunit vaccines are considered the safest format of vaccine. However, the low immunogenicity of subunit vaccines dictates a heavily reliance on adjuvants. Different forms of the S-protein, including the S1 RBD, RBD-Fc (RBD with human IgG Fc fusion), and N-terminal domain (NTD), have demonstrated various degrees of nAb responses and protection in multiple animal models including non-human primates (NHP) (Lan et al., 2015; Zhang et al., 2016; Jiaming et al., 2017; Wang et al., 2017; Deng et al., 2018; Nyon et al., 2018; Adney et al., 2019). For instance, the SARS-CoV S1 subunit vaccine produced from sf9 cells and with the adjuvant saponin or protollin are able to reduce lung viral titer in young or aged mice after challenge, respectively (Bisht et al., 2005; Hu et al., 2007). An RBD subunit of SARS-CoV produced from Chinese hamster ovarian (CHO) cells with Freund's adjuvant is able to protect young BALB/c mice from infection (Du et al., 2010). MERS-CoV-S1 with adjuvants MF59 or Advax HCXL is able to protect alpacas and dromedary camels against MERS-CoV challenge (Adney et al., 2019). Adjuvant selection can affect the vaccine outcome, and combinations of adjuvants can have synergistic effects on the strength of the response. For instance, rRBD with adjuvants alum and CpG ODN together elicits a stronger humoral and cellular T cell response

TABLE 1 | Summary of SARS-CoV and MERS-CoV vaccines studies

SARS-CoV Vaccines	Antigens	Vaccine formulations	Dose, Time of vaccination	Animal models	Challenge dose. Virus strains, Time after last vaccination, Route	Results	References
Whole Inactivated Vaccine	Inactivated	SARS-CoV FRA (*b*-propiolactone) + MF59	5 μg at 0, 2, and 4 weeks, SC	BALB/c	10^4 TCID50 SARS-CoV Urbani, IN	Protection, no virus detected in Lung and Nasal Turbinates	Stadler et al., 2005 EID
	Inactivated	SARS-CoV Tor2 (*b*-propiolactone) + Alum	50 μg at 0 and 4 weeks, SC	6 week old 129S6/SvEv	10^6 pfu SARS-CoV Tor2 at week 3, IN	Protection	See et al., 2006 JGV
	Double Inactive	SARS-CoV (Utah) formaldehyde and UV inactivation + Al(OH)3	0.08 – 0.2 μg at week 0 and 2, SC	6 – 8 weeks CD1 mice	10^5 TCID50 SARS-CoV Utah at week 3 or 11, IN	Protection, no virus detected in lung and trachea	Spruth et al., 2006 Vaccines
	Inactivated	SARS-CoV Tor2 (*b*-propiolactone) + Alum	50 μg at 0 and 4 weeks, SC	8 – 10 month old ferret	10^6 pfu SARS-CoV Tor2 at week 3, IN	Weak protection, slight reduction of viral titer in lung, BAL and nasal wash, slight improvement in lung pathology	See et al., 2008 JGV
	Inactivated	SARS-CoV Urbina (*b*-propiolactone) + AS01B and AS03A	0.15 – 1.5 μg at week 0 and 3, IM	BALB/c	10^5 TCID50 SARS-CoV Urbani at week 3, IN	Protection, no virus detected in lung	Roberts et al., 2010 Viral Immunology
	Inactivated	SARS-CoV Urbina (*b*-propiolactone) + AS01B and AS03A	2.0 μg at week 0 and 3, IM	4 – 8 week old Golden syrian hamsters	10^3 TCID50 SARS-CoV Urbani at week 4 or 18, IN	Partial protection, reduce viral titer in lung	Roberts et al., 2010 Viral Immunology
	Double Inactive	SARS-CoV MA15 formalin and UV inactivated + Alum	0.2 μg at week 0 and 3–4 week, footpad	6 – 8 weeks old BALB/cAnNHsd	10^5 PFU SARS-CoV MA15, SZ61and GD03 at week 5, IN	Partial protection, reduce viral titer in lung and good protection from lethal challenge (MA15)	Bolles et al., 2011a JVI
	Double Inactive	SARS-CoV MA15 formalin and UV inactivated + Alum	0.2 μg at week 0 and 3–4 week, footpad	12 – 14 months old BALB/cAnNHsd	10^5 PFU SARS-CoV MA15, SZ61and GD03 at week 5, IN	Weak protection, small drop in viral titer in lung, weak protection from leathal challenge (MA15)	Bolles et al., 2011a JVI
LAV	SARS-CoV-ΔE (Urbani)	SARS-CoV-ΔE (Urbani)	10^3 TCID50 at 0 week, IN	7 week old Golden syrian hamsters	10^3 TCID50 SARS-CoV Urbani and GD03 at week 4, IN	Protection, no virus detected in lung	Lamirande et al., 2008 JVI
	SARS-COV ExoN (MA15)	SARS-CoV-ExoN (MA15)	$10^{2.5}$ or 10^4 PFU at week	12 months old BALB/c	$10^{2.5}$ TCID50 SARS-CoV MA15 at week 4, IN	Complete survival from lethal challenge, no virus detected in lung	Graham et al., 2012 Nat Med
	SARS-CoV ΔNSP16	SARS-CoV Δ2′-*O*-Methyltransferase	10^2 PFU at week 0, IN	10 weeks old BALB/c and C57BL/6	10^5 PFU SARS-CoV MA15 at week 4, IN	Complete survival from lethal challenge, no viral titer performed	Menachery et al., 2014 JVI
	SARS-CoV ΔNSP16/ExoN	SARS-CoV Δ2′-*O*-Methyltransferase and ExoN mutation	10^2 PFU at week 0, IN	12 months old BALB/c	10^5 PFU SARS-CoV MA15 at week 4, IN	Complete survival from lethal challenge, no virus detected in lung	Menachery et al., 2018 JVI
Subunit	subunit nS Sf9	SARS-CoV S (14-762) Urbani + QS21	10 μg at week 0, 4, and 8, SC	6 weeks old BALB/c	10^5 TCID50 SARS-CoV (Urbani) at week 4, IN	Protection, reduce viral titer in lung and nasal turbinates	Bisht et al., 2005 Virology
	Ectodomain Sf9	SARS-CoV S ectodomain (Urbani) + Protollin	10 or 30 μg at week 0, 2 and 5, IN	~ 1 year old BALB/c	$5x10^4$ TCID50 SARS-CoV Urbani at week 1, IN	Protection, reduce viral titer in lung	Hu et al., 2007 Vaccines

(Continued)

TABLE 1 | Continued

SARS-CoV Vaccines	Antigens	Vaccine formulations	Dose, Time of vaccination	Animal models	Challenge dose. Virus strains, Time after last vaccination, Route	Results	References
	Subunit RBD219 CHO	SARS-CoV RBD (318-536)Tor2 + Freund	20 μg at week 0 and 10 μg at week 3 and 6, SC	4 – 6 weeks old BALB/c	$5x10^5$ TCID50 SARS-CoV GZ50 at 10 day, IN	Protection, no virus detected in lung	Du et al., 2010 viral immunology
Subunit Trimer	Spike trimer	SARS-CoV RBD Spike Trimer Urbani + Alum	50 μg at week 0, 3, and 6, SC	5 weeks old Golden syrian hamsters	10^3 TCID50 SARS-CoV Urbani at week 2, IN	Protection, no virus detected in lung and reduce pneumonitis	Kam et al., 2007 Vaccines
VLP	MHV-S VLP	SARS-CoV S in MHV + Alum	2 μg at 0 and 4 weeks	6 – 8 week old BALB/c	10^6 TCID50 SARS-CoV at week 8, IN	Protect, no virus detected in Lung	Lokugamage et al., 2008 Vaccine
	Flu M1-S	SARS-CoV S Urbani in influenza M1 + Al(OH)3	0.8 or 4 μg at week 0 and 3, IM	6 – 8 weeks old BALB/c	2xLD50 mouse adapted SARS-CoV V2163 at week 3, IN	Complete survival from lethal challenge, no virus detected in lung	Liu et al., 2011 Vaccines
DNA	Plasmid *S*-Ectodomain	Plasmid expressing SARS-CoV S ΔCD or ectodomain (Urbani)	25 μg at week 0, 3, and 6, IM	6 – 8 week old BALB/c	10^4 TCID50 SARS-CoV Urbani, at Day 30, IN	Protection, reduce viral titer in lung and nasal turbinates	Yang et al., 2004 Nature
Vector	BHPIV3 SARS-S	SARS-CoV S or SME Urbani in parainfluenza virus type 3 vector (BHPIV3)	10^6 TCID50 at 0 week, IN	Golden syrian hamsters	10^3 TCID50 SARS-CoV Urbani at week 4, IN	Protection, no virus detected in lung	Buchholz et al., 2004 PNAS
	BHPIV3 SARS-S	SARS-CoV S Urbani in parainfluenza virus type 3 vector (BHPIV3)	10^6 TCID50 each at 0 week, IN and IT	African green monkeys	"A large dose of SARS-CoV" at week 4, IN	Protection, no virus detected in lung	Bukreyev et al., 2004 Lancet
	MVA-SARS-S	SARS-CoV S Urbani in MVA	10^7 at 0 and 4 week, IN	BALB/c	10^4 TCID50 SARS-CoV Urbani, at week 8, IN	Protection, reduce viral titer in lung and nasal turbinates	Bisht et al., 2004 PNAS
	MVA-SARS-S	SARS-CoV S Urbani in MVA	10^7 at 0 and 4 week, IM	BALB/c	10^4 TCID50 SARS-CoV Urbani, at week 8, IN	Protection, reduce viral titer in lung and nasal turbinates	Bisht et al., 2004 PNAS
	MVA-SARS-S	SARS-CoV S and N Tor2 in MVA	10^8 pfu at 0 and 5×10^7 at 2 week, IP and SC	Ferret	10^6 pfu SARS-CoV Tor2 at week 4, IN	No protection according to viral RNA in lung, Ab induction	Czub et al., 2005 Vaccines
	VSV-S	VSV-SARS-S Urbani	1.4×10^4 pfu at week 0, IN	BALB/c	10^4 TCID50 SARS-CoV Urbani at month 1 and 4, IN	Protection, no virus detected in lung and nasal turbinates	Kapadia et al., 2005 Virology
	hAd5 (N+S)	Human Adenovirus 5 with S + Ad5 N gene	3×10^8 pfu each at 0 and 4 weeks, IM	6 week old 129S6/SvEv	10^6 pfu SARS-CoV Tor2 at week 3, IN	No protection despite strong IgG1, IgG2a Ab induction and high IFN-g secretion	See et al., 2006 JGV
	hAd5 (N+S)	Human Adenovirus 5 with S + Ad5 N gene	3×10^8 pfu each at 0 and 4 weeks, IN	6 week old 129S6/SvEv	10^6 pfu SARS-CoV Tor2 at week 3, IN	Partial protection, Induction of IgA	See et al., 2006 JGV

(Continued)

TABLE 1 | Continued

MERS-CoV Vaccines	Antigens	Vaccine formulations	Dose, Time of vaccination	Animal models	Challenge dose. Virus strains, Time after last vaccination, Route	Results	References
	VEEV-S	SARS-CoV GD03 S in VEEV	10^6 IU at 0 week, boost 3 – 5 weeks, footpad	4 – 7 weeks old	10^5 pfu SARS-CoV GD03 and Urbani at week 7 – 8 and week 54, IN	Protection, no virus detected in lung	Deming et al., 2006 PIOS Med
	VEEV-S	SARS-CoV GD03 S in VEEV	10^6 IU at 0 week, boost 3 - 5 week, footpad	> 26 week old	10^5 pfu SARS-CoV GD03 and Urbani at week 7 -8 and week 54, IN	No protection	Deming et al., 2006 PIOS Med
	hAd5-S + AdC7-S	Human Adenovirus 5 with S + Chimpanzee AdC7 with S Tor2	5 × 10^{11} VP/kg at 0 and 1 month, IM	18 – 20 weeks old ferret	10^6 pfu SARS-CoV Tor2 at not specify, IN	Protection, reduce viral titer in lung and nasal turbinates	Kobinger et al., 2007 Vaccines
	hAd5 (N+S)	Human Adenovirus 5 with S + Ad5 N gene	1 × 10^9 pfu each at 0 and 4 weeks, IM	8 - 10 month old ferret	10^6 pfu SARS-CoV Tor2 at week 3, IN	Inconclusive, control hAd5 shows non-specific protection	See et al., 2008 JGV
	hAd5 (N+S)	Human Adenovirus 5 with S + Ad5 N gene	1 × 10^9 pfu each at 0 and 4 weeks, IN	8 – 10 months old ferret	10^6 pfu SARS-CoV Tor2 at week 3, IN	Inconclusive, control hAd5 shows non-specific protection	See et al., 2008 JGV
Whole Inactivaed Vaccine	Inactivated	MERS-CoV (γ-ray) + Alum or MF59	10^6 TCID50 at week 0 and 3, IM	hCD26/DPP4 transgenic mice	10^3 TCID50 (100xLD50) MERS-CoV at week 3, IN	Protection from virus replication, no virus detected in lung, increase lung pathology	Agrawal et al., 2016 Human vaccine and immuno therapy
	Inactivated	MERS-CoV EMC/2012 (formaldehyde) + Alum and CpG	1 µg at week 0, 4 and 8, IM	14 – 16 week old BALB/c transduced with hDPP4 by Ad5	10^5 PFU MERS-CoV (EMC/2012) at week 2, IN	Protection, no virus detected in lung	Deng et al., 2018 Emerging Microbes and infection
LAV	MERSS-CoV ΔNSP16	MERS-CoV Δ2′-*O*-Methyltransferase EMC MA1	10^6 PFU at week 0, IN	10 - 20 week old C57BL/6 288-330+/+	10^6 PFU MERS-CoV EMC MA1 at week 4, IN	Complete survival from lethal challenge, reduce viral titer in lung	Menachery et al., 2017 msphere
Subunit	RBD	MERS-CoV RBD S367-606 (EMC/2012) + alum	200 µg at week 0 and 100 µg at week 8 and 25, IM	Rhesus Macaque	6.5x10^7 TCID50 MERS-CoV (EMC/2012) at week 2, IN	Partial protection, reduce viral titer in lung and trachea	Lan et al., 2015 EBioMedicine
	NTD	MERS-CoV NTD S18-353 (EMC/2012) + alum and CpG	5 or 1 µg at week 0, 4 and 8, IM	16 – 18 weeks old BALB/c transduced with hDPP4 by Ad5	10^5 PFU MERS-CoV (EMC/2012) at week 2, IN	Partial protection, reduce lung and trachea pathologies, no viral titer information	Jiaming et al., 2017 Vaccines
	S ectodomain	MERS-CoV EMC/2012 S ectodomain + Alum and CpG	1 µg at week 0, 4 and 8, IM	14 – 16 week old BALB/c transduced with hDPP4 by Ad5	10^5 PFU MERS-CoV (EMC/2012) at week 2, IN	Protection, reduction in lung viral titer	Deng et al., 2018 Emerging Microbes and infection
	RBD-Fc	MERS-CoV RBD S377-588 Fc (EMC/2012) + MF59	10 µg at week 0, 3, and 6, SC	4 – 6 weeks old BALB/c transduced with hDPP4 by Ad5	10^5 PFU MERS-CoV (EMC/2012) at week 2, IN	Protection, no virus detected in lung	Zhang et al., 2016 Cellular and molecular immunology
	RBD-Fc	MERS-CoV RBD S377-588 Fc (EMC/2012) + Addavax	10 µg at week 0 and 4, IM	hCD26/DPP4 transgenic mice	10^3 TCID50 (100xLD50) MERS-CoV (EMC/2012) at week 4, IN	Complete survival from lethal challenge, no virus detected in lung	Nyon et al., 2018 Vaccines

(Continued)

TABLE 1 | Continued

MERS-CoV Vaccines	Antigens	Vaccine formulations	Dose, Time of vaccination	Animal models	Challenge dose. Virus strains, Time after last vaccination, Route	Results	References
	S1	MERS-CoV ENgland1 S1 + Advax HCXL or Sigma oil-in-water emulsion	400 μg at week 0, 4 and 15, IM	dromedary camel	10^7 TCID50 MERS-CoV (EMC/2012) at ~week 4, IN	Protection, reduce viral titer in lung and nasal turbinate	Adney et al., 2019 Virus
	S1	MERS-CoV ENgland1 S1 + Advax HCXL or Sigma oil-in-water emulsion	400 μg at week 0, 4, and 15, IM	Alpaca	10^7 TCID50 MERS-CoV (EMC/2012) at ~week 4, IN	Protection, no virus detected in lung, nasal turbinate and nasal swabs	Adney et al., 2019 Virus
Subunit Trimer	RBD Trimer	MERS-CoV RBD-Fd (Trimer) + alum	5 μg at week 0 and 4, IM	hCD26/DPP4 transgenic mice	10^4 TCID50 MERS-CoV (EMC/2012) at week 12, IN	Complete survival from lethal challenge, no viral titer performed	Tai et al., 2016 Virology
VLP	S nanoparticles	MERS-CoV Jordan S nanoparticle + Matrix M1	10 μg at week 0 and 3, IM	15 – 17 weeks old BALB/c transduced with hDPP4 by Ad5	2.5 × 10^3 PFU MERS-CoV (Jordan) at week 4, IN	Protection from chalenge, no virus detected in lung	Coleman et al., 2017 Vaccines
	BNSP333-S	MERS-CoV S1 Jordan fused with rabies virus G protein VLP	10 μg at week 0, 1, and 3, IM	15 – 17 weeks old BALB/c transduced with hDPP4 by Ad5	2.5 × 10^3 PFU MERS-CoV (Jordan) at week 4, IN	Protection, no virus detected in lung	Wirblich et al., 2017 JVI
DNA	Plasmid S-protein	Plasmid expressing MERS-CoV S1 (Al-Hasa_1_2013)	0.5 or 2 mg at week 0, 3 and 6, IM	Rhesus macaques	7 × 10^6 TCID50 MERS-CoV (EMC/2012) at week 5, IT, IN, oral and ocular	Protection, reduce viral titer in lung, reduce clinical pathology	Muthumani et al., 2015 STM
	Plasmid S1	Plasmid expressing MERS-CoV S1 (Al-Hasa_15_2013)	100 μg at week 0, 3 and 6, IM	14 - 16 week old BALB/c transduced with hDPP4 by Ad5	10^5 PFU MERS-CoV (EMC/2012) at Day 18, IN	Protection, reduce viral titer in lung	Chi et al., 2017 Vaccines
Vector	MVvca2 S or soluble S	Recombinant measles virus with MERS-CoV (EMC/2012) S or soluble S	10^5 TCID50 at week 0 and 4, IP	6 – 12 week old IFNAR–/– CD46Ge transduced with hDPP4 by Ad5	7 × 10^4 TCID50 MERS-CoV (EMC/2012) at week 6, IN	Protection, reduce viral titer in lung, reduce lung pathology	Malczyk et al., 2015 JVI
	ChAdOx1 MERS	ChAdOx1 with MERS-CoV S-protein (EMC/2012)	10^8 IU at week 0, IN or IM	hCD26/DPP4 transgenic mice	10^4 TCID50 MERS-CoV (EMC/2012) at week 4, IN	Complete survival from lethal challenge, no virus detected in lung, reduce lung pathology	Munster et al., 2017 npj
	MVA-MERS-S	MVA with MERS-CoV S-protein	10^6, 10^7, or 10^8 PFU at week 0, IM or SC	14 – 16 week old BALB/c transduced with hDPP4 by Ad5	7 × 10^4 TCID50 MERS-CoV (EMC/2012) at week 6, IN	Protection, reduce viral RNA genome in lung, reduce lung pathology	Volz et al., 2015 JVI
	rAd5-S1/F/CD40L	hAd5 with MERS-CoV S1 trimer fused with CD40L	10^9 PFU at week 0 and 4, IM	hCD26/DPP4 transgenic mice	10^3 TCID50 (100xLD50) MERS-CoV (EMC/2012) at week 4, IN	Complete survival from lethal challenge, no virus detected in lung, reduce lung pathology	Hashem et al., 2019 JID

Selection criteria: Only animal studies with a challenge model are included. LAV, live attenuated vaccine; VLP, virus like particle; RBD, receptor binding domain; IM, intramuscular; IN, intranasal; SC, subcutaneous; IP, intraperitoneal.

(Lan et al., 2014). Additionally, rNTD with alum is able to reduce lung pathology in a non-lethal MERS-CoV challenge (Jiaming et al., 2017). Instead of adjuvants alone, immune enhancers such as an Fc fragment, which increases the protein half-life when fused with the RBD, can also elicit a stronger IgG nAb and cellular immune response in multiple experimental animals (Du et al., 2013; Ma et al., 2014b; Tang et al., 2015; Nyon et al., 2018). RBD-Fc fusion subunit vaccine is able to protect a lethal challenge of MERS-CoV in adenovirus transduced hCD26/DPP4 mice (Zhang et al., 2016; Wang et al., 2017). While a large amount of work concerning the subunit vaccines has been done in conjunction with different adjuvants, the effect of each adjuvant is not well understood and multi-adjuvant systems (combinatorial admixes) have not been rigorously tested. A more systematic method of studying the effect of different adjuvants on CoV vaccines will be valuable for vaccine development, perhaps using genetic reference populations that more accurately phenocopy human genetic variation (Leist and Baric, 2018).

Trimeric forms of the *S*-protein and RBD have been developed using the T4 trimerization domain to mimic the native conformation of the spike RBD (Kam et al., 2007; Tai et al., 2016). The trimeric RBD antigens are able to elicit a robust nAb response and protect 80% of hDPP4 transgenic mice from lethal MERS-CoV challenge, although most animals still experienced slight weight loss (Tai et al., 2016). Alternatively, the MERS-CoV *S*-protein has been structurally designed to remain in perfusion state by mutating V1060 and L1061 at the tip of the central helix to proline (S-2P) (Kirchdoerfer et al., 2016; Pallesen et al., 2017). The MERS S-2P protein retains the receptor binding properties of the wild-type S and elicits nAbs against at least 3 different S domains, including RBD, NTD, and S2. Intramuscular injection of the MERS S-2P elicits nAb responses in mice comparable to the monomeric S1 and trimeric *S*-protein antigens. (Pallesen et al., 2017).

Similar to subunit vaccines are the viral like particle (VLP) and nanoparticle vaccines. VLP and nanoparticles provide multivalent binding similar to actual viruses without the potential safety concerns. In SARS-CoV, multiple systems were used to generate *S*-protein VLPs, including the mouse hepatitis virus (MHV) and influenza matrix 1 (M1). In the chimeric MHV system, the SARS-CoV protein is co-expressed with the MHV E, M and N proteins to produce MHV-S VLP. Mice vaccinated with the MHV-S VLP and alum have inhibited viral replication in lung after a homologous strain challenge (Lokugamage et al., 2008). Instead of using MHV structural proteins, the influenza system express the SARS-CoV *S*-protein with influenza virus M1 proteins in Sf9 cells to create the M1-S VLP. Immunization of M1-S VLP with aluminum hydroxide can protect mice from a lethal challenge of SARS-CoV (Liu et al., 2011). In MERS-CoV, expression of S, E, and M proteins using the baculovirus system produces VLPs that are morphologically similar to the actual virus (Coleman et al., 2014; Wang et al., 2017b). Other methods such as CPV-based (Wang et al., 2017a), rabies virus (MV)-based (Wirblich et al., 2017), ferritin-based (Seong, 2018), and *S*-protein aggregates (Coleman et al., 2014) are all able to elicit immune responses and reduce viral replication in a mouse model when co-administered with Matrix M1 adjuvant (Coleman et al., 2017). Although all show different degree of immune response in animal, only one study showed a reduction of viral titer *in vivo* via an adenovirus transduced hCD26/DPP4 mouse model (Coleman et al., 2017).

Clinical Trials for SARS- and MERS-CoV Vaccines

A finished phase 1 clinical trial for a SARS-CoV vaccine is a DNA vaccine that encodes the ectodomain of the SARS-CoV *S*-protein (NCT00099463). DNA vaccines rely on a continuous expression of antigen from a DNA plasmid that is injected intramuscularly and electroporated (Muthumani et al., 2015; Wang et al., 2015; Chi et al., 2017). In pre-clinical studies, 3 doses of an intramuscular plasmid injection was able to reduce viral titer in both lung and nasal turbinate in a BALB/c challenge model (Yang et al., 2004). The phase 1 trial showed favorable results; after 3 doses of DNA vaccine, all subjects showed CD4+ T cell responses, while 80% of subjects had nAbs and 20% of subjects showed CD8+ T cell responses. However, there has been no follow-up in the vaccine development, likely due to the end of the SARS-CoV outbreak (Martin et al., 2008). One MERS-CoV vaccine that is currently undergoing clinical trials (NCT03721718) is a DNA-based vaccine (Modjarrad et al., 2019). GLS-5300 is a DNA vaccine based on a consensus full-length *S*-protein from MERS-CoV under the control of a CMV promoter. In preclinical studies, the vaccine was electroporated into mice, camel and rhesus monkeys three times within 1 month. The vaccine elicited B cell responses in all animals at 1 month post vaccination, and extracted IgG was able to neutralize multiple strains of MERS-CoV including England/2/2013, and Al-Hasa/1/2013 and, surprisingly, a group 1b CoV NL63 and a group 2a CoV HKU1 using the pseudotype neutralization assay (Muthumani et al., 2015). T cell responses were assessed in mice and monkeys, with both demonstrating T cell responses as indicated by the presence of IFN-γ, TNFα and IL2-secreting CD4+ and CD8+ T cells after peptide stimulation. Rhesus monkeys were also protected from challenge of the vaccine strain with lower viral titers and lung pathology as assessed by radiography and pathology studies (Muthumani et al., 2015). Currently, GLS-5300 has completed Phase I clinical trials (safety). Three doses (0.67, 2, and 6 mg) of GLS-5300 were electroporated intramuscularly at weeks 0, 4, and 12. Ninety-four percent of subjects were seroconverted and nAbs were detected in 50% of the individuals. Seventy-six percent of subjects developed T-cell responses against peptides derived from MERS-CoV *S*-proteins (Modjarrad et al., 2019). Other than a full *S*-protein DNA vaccine, different designs also show promising results in preclinical mouse models. Notably, a DNA vaccine composed of only the S1 domain showed efficacy when paired with different adjuvants (Chi et al., 2017). Hybrid strategies using a DNA vaccine paired with a protein booster also showed promising results in eliciting more balanced Th1 and Th2 responses (Wang et al., 2015; Al-Amri et al., 2017).

Vector-Based Vaccines

Two out of the three clinical trials for MERS vaccines are vectorized vaccines. Viral vector-based vaccines have multiple advantages over the generic protein or DNA-based subunit vaccines. Firstly, as viral vectors utilize a defined viral entry mechanism, they are more efficient at delivering DNA into cells. Second, the vector itself can serve as an adjuvant which in turn elicits both B- and T-cell responses (Ura et al., 2014). Finally, a wide variety of vector systems including measles viruses (Malczyk et al., 2015; Bodmer et al., 2018), Venezuelan equine encephalitis virus (VEEV) replicon system (Deming et al., 2006; Agnihothram et al., 2014; Zhao et al., 2016), adeno-associated virus (AAV) (Du et al., 2008), parainfluenza type 3 (BHPIV3) (Buchholz et al., 2004; Bukreyev et al., 2004), human and chimpanzee adenovirus (hAd5 and ChAdOx1) (See et al., 2006, 2008; Kobinger et al., 2007; Kim et al., 2014; Guo et al., 2015; Hashem et al., 2019) and modified vaccinia virus Ankara (MVA) (Bisht et al., 2004; Czub et al., 2005; Kapadia et al., 2005; Haagmans et al., 2016) have been previously established for use as vaccine platforms for multiple infectious diseases. Herein, we will focus on the three systems that have been or are currently under clinical trial; all others are summarized in **Table 1**.

Replication-defective adenovirus vectors are one of the most effective choices to deliver vaccine antigens. Human adenovirus 5 (hAd5) and enteric adenovirus type 41 (Ad41) have both been used to deliver MERS-CoV S or S1 proteins. Intramuscular inoculation of the vaccine elicits both B-cell (nAb titer) and T-cell (IFN-γ secreting splenocytes and pulmonary lymphocytes) responses (Guo et al., 2015). However, pre-existing nAbs against hAd5 and 41 in the human population have limited their usage to dromedary camels instead of humans (Chirmule et al., 1999). The pre-existing nAb problem against hAd5 can be circumvented by using a chimpanzee adenovirus. One such platform is ChAdOx1, wherein the adenovirus E1 gene is replaced by a MERS-CoV *S*-protein with an N-terminal secretion peptide from human plasminogen activator (tPA) driven by a CMV promoter. Intramuscular inoculation of the vector successfully elicits nAbs against *S*-protein as quickly as 14 days post infection. Splenic CD8+ T-cells secreting IFN-γ, TNF-α and IL-17 are also present at 28 days post infection (Alharbi et al., 2017). A single intranasal or intramuscular inoculation of ChAdOx1-MERS is able to protect a human DPP4 transgenic mouse from lethal challenge by MERS-CoV, and the vaccine (Munster et al., 2017) is currently under phase 1 clinical trial (NCT03399578). CHAdOx1 has also shown effective protection for Rift Valley Fever Virus in dromedary camels (Warimwe et al., 2016).

The modified vaccinia virus Ankara (MVA) vector is another effective platform for MERS-CoV vaccine development. *S*-protein is inserted into the MAV genome at deletion site III driven by the viral P11 promoter. After a single intramuscular injection, BALB/c mice produce nAbs against both the RBD and S2, as tested *in vitro* (Song et al., 2013). A follow-up study identified IFN-γ secreting splenocytes after peptide S291 stimulation at 56 days post infection, suggesting the vaccine is able to elicit memory CD8+ T cell responses. The vaccine is also able to protect a hDDP4-transduced BALB/c mouse model. RNA genomes in the lungs and lung pathology are drastically reduced compared to mock vaccination (Volz et al., 2015). The MAV based MERS-CoV vaccine has also been tested on dromedary camels and elicits induction of nAbs in sera and nasal swabs. Vaccinated camels also show reduced RNA genomes and gross pathology. The Phase I clinical trial has just been completed and the results are pending (NCT03615911).

ANTIVIRALS

The Challenge for Treatment Windows

The average incubation period for SARS-CoV and MERS-CoV is around 5 days (Zumla et al., 2015; de Wit et al., 2016) and the main site of viral replication is the lower respiratory tract (Corman et al., 2015; Petrovsky, 2016). At 7–10 days after symptomatic onset, viral RNA titer peaks in the upper respiratory tract (Drosten et al., 2004; Corman et al., 2015). For terminal cases, disease lasts for an average of 12 days post symptomatic onset for MERS-CoV and 24 days for SARS-CoV (Zumla et al., 2015). Interestingly, severe symptoms begin as the viral titer is decreasing, suggesting that severe CoV pathogenesis is due to immune complications and the inability to resolve inflammation (Peiris et al., 2003a; Wang et al., 2004). SARS-CoV upregulates pro-inflammatory cytokine production in the lung, including IL1, IL6, IL8, IL10, CXCL10 and TNF-α production (Binnie et al., 2014). Compared to SARS-CoV infected patients with mild diseases, patients with ARDS fail to induce interferon (IFN) expression and the subsequent IFN-stimulated genes (ISGs) that are indicative of adaptive immune responses (Cameron et al., 2007; Binnie et al., 2014). The inability to switch from an innate immune response to the adaptive immune response may lead to uncontrollable inflammation and severe end stage lung disease. Given the rapid progression of symptoms to terminal illness, there is only approximately a 1 week treatment window after the onset of symptoms for antiviral and medical intervention (Widagdo et al., 2017). This treatment window could further compromised by delays in virus diagnosis, causing a challenge for timely medical intervention administration when the virus titers and pathological symptom are relatively mild (Corman et al., 2015; Ahmed, 2019). Unlike humans, experimental animal models have a compressed disease course (<7 days), and it is difficult to differentiate between early and late phase of infection. It would be beneficial for clinical studies to separate the early- (<10 days) and late-phase (>10 days) patients to determine differences in patient response between the groups.

The Challenge for Therapeutic Development

Despite of the presence of a 3′ to 5′ exoribonuclease (exoN) proofreading enzyme, their large genome size (28–30 kb) means that CoVs remain in the category of highly mutating viruses (Eckerle et al., 2007, 2010; Denison et al., 2011). The high mutation rate poses a considerable challenge for antiviral development as drug resistant viruses could arise or already exist within the quasispecies in nature or from an infected individual (Briese et al., 2014). For instance, after a prolonged period of nAb or drug treatments, the CoV can acquire mutations which confer resistance to the therapeutics (Zumla et al., 2016a). The appearance of these "escape viruses" has been confirmed in multiple mouse model studies in well-contained laboratory

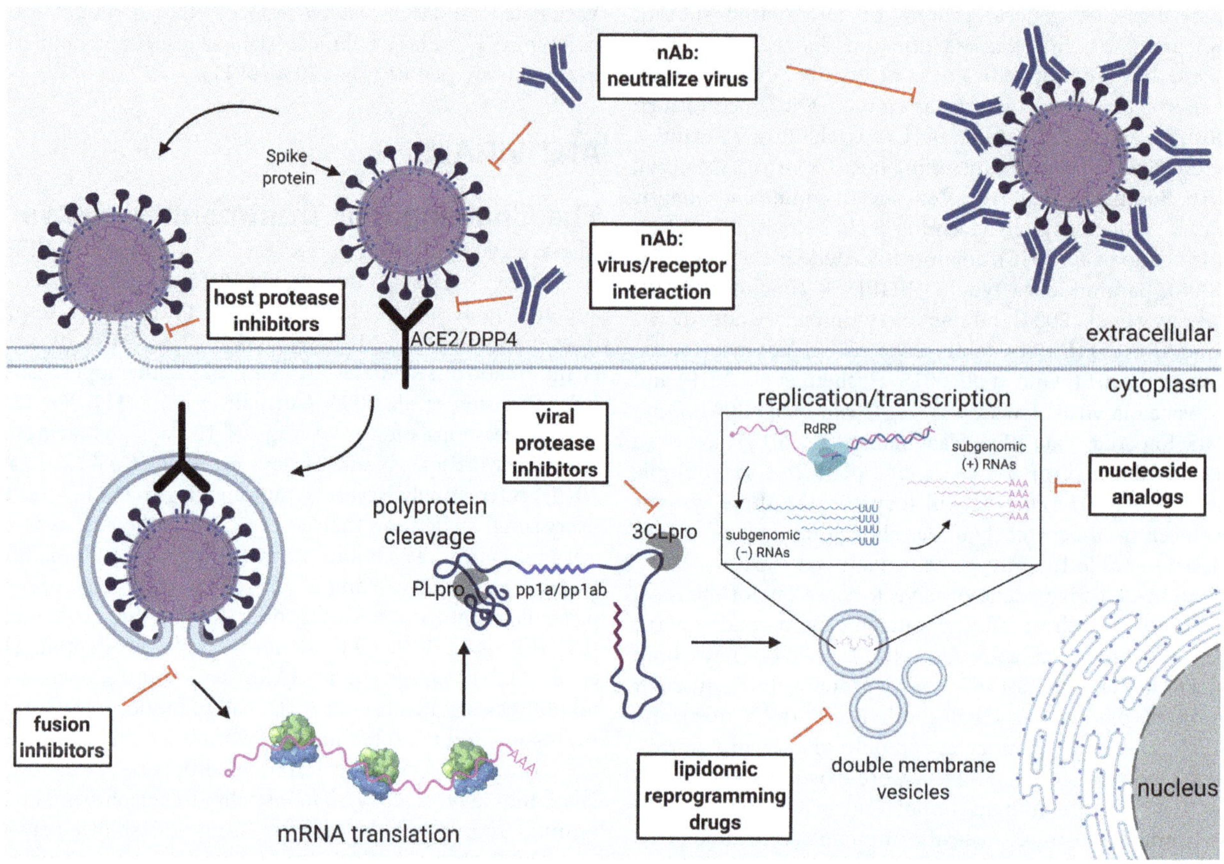

FIGURE 2 | Schematic of the CoV replication cycle and key steps for antiviral targets. White text boxes indicate the subtype of antivirals that work either extracellularly or intracellularly. Different steps of the CoV replication cycle are illustrated in cartoon form, including receptor binding, membrane fusion, viral RNA replication, sub-genomic RNA transcription and translation.

settings as well as in nature (Neuman et al., 2006; Ter Meulen et al., 2006; Huang et al., 2008; Jiang et al., 2014; Tang et al., 2014; Tai et al., 2017; Kleine-Weber et al., 2019). Fortunately, some of the mutations that confer drug resistance also compromise viral fitness and attenuate the virus (Deng et al., 2014; Agostini et al., 2018). Another therapeutic intervention is the use of immune modulators, such as IFN-α2a/2b, IFN-β1b and corticosteroids in treating CoVs (Loutfy et al., 2003; Peiris et al., 2003b; Sung et al., 2004). Although multiple studies have shown efficacy of IFN-α2a/2b and IFN-β1b singly or in combination with off-labeled antivirals such as ribavirin, lopinavir (LPV) and ritonavir (RTV) in treating SARS- and MERS-CoV in mouse, rhesus monkey and marmoset models (Haagmans et al., 2004; Barnard et al., 2006b; Falzarano et al., 2013b; Chan et al., 2015), clinical studies have shown inconclusive results (Momattin et al., 2013; Mo and Fisher, 2016). Currently, a randomized controlled trial is underway to determine the efficacy of a combination of LPV/RTV and IFN-β1b in treating MERS-CoV infection (NCT02845843).

Convalescent Plasma and Monoclonal Antibodies

Although there is no approved drug to treat severe CoV infection, multiple strategies have shown promising results in an experimental setting (**Figure 2**). Convalescent plasma (CP) is derived from patients who have recovered from SARS-CoV and MERS-CoV infection and contains high titer nAbs (Hsueh et al., 2004; Al Kahlout et al., 2019; Shin et al., 2019). Some data suggest that CP use against SARS-CoV infection is safe and, when administered at an early time point, may reduce mortality (Mair-Jenkins et al., 2015). CP neutralizing titers > 1:80 may have a positive impact on infected MERS-CoV patients with respiratory failure (Ko et al., 2018). Unfortunately, CP from convalescent patients is difficult to obtain in large quantities and the Ab titer is too low to have beneficial effects, making it difficult to be used as a main stream therapeutic or for clinical testing (Arabi et al., 2016). As such, no systematic, well-designed clinical trial has formally demonstrated the efficacy of CP in emerging CoV infection. Rather, a clinical trial for testing CP against MERS-CoV infection was withdrawn prior to patient enrollment (NCT02190799).

Although CP from convalescent patients is difficult to obtain, the active component (neutralizing antibodies) can be isolated and subsequently produced in large quantity using recombinant technology (Corti et al., 2016). Passive infusion of neutralizing monoclonal Abs (mAbs) has been used for several diseases with success, including RSV and Ebola virus (Graham and Ambrosino, 2015; Zumla et al., 2016b). Numerous highly potent mAbs against

SARS-CoV and MERS-CoV have been isolated by multiple groups all over the world using different methods such as phage display and direct B cell cloning from immunized animals or convalescent patients (Sui et al., 2004; Traggiai et al., 2004; Greenough et al., 2005; van den Brink et al., 2005; Zhu et al., 2007; Corti et al., 2016). While all of them shows protecting activity *in vitro*, several of them have also shown efficacy in mouse and NHP models (Ter Meulen et al., 2004; Johnson et al., 2016; Chen et al., 2017; van Doremalen et al., 2017; de Wit et al., 2018; Xu et al., 2019). The plethora of potent nAbs have also provided insight into the major antigenic sites on which vaccine development should focus. A list of mAbs that show efficacy *in vivo* against SARS-CoV and MERS-CoV are summarized in **Table 2**. Due to the differences in testing conditions, direct comparison of mAb efficacy should be avoided. Multiple comprehensive review articles on the subject can also be found (Prabakaran et al., 2009; Coughlin and Prabhakar, 2012; Xu et al., 2019).

The binding epitopes of some well-studied mAbs provide valuable information for the neutralization mechanism and clinical implications. The majority of the mAbs target the RBD of the spike protein and prevent viral attachment. For example, mAb 80R is able to protect both *in vitro* and a 16 weeks old mouse model against SARS-CoV Urbani. However, it is unable to protect other strains due to amino acid variations in the RBD (Zhu et al., 2007). On the other hand, S230.15 mimics receptor binding and triggers conformational changes in the SARS *S*-protein, completely protecting young and old mice from SARS-CoV challenge against multiple SARS-CoV, including Urbani, GD03 and SZ16 (Rockx et al., 2008; Walls et al., 2019a). Similar to SARS-CoV, the majority of mAbs targeting MERS-CoV, such as MERS-4, MERS-27 (Jiang et al., 2014), m336 (Ying et al., 2014, 2015) and humanized Ab 4C2 and 2E6 (Li et al., 2015) all target the RBD and prevent the virus from binding to DPP4 with high potency. Interestingly, the mAb LCA60, isolated from a MERS-CoV infected patient, binds to RBD region and confers a broader neutralizing breadth, and is able to neutralize EMC2012 and London1 strains of MERS-CoV (Corti et al., 2015). Non-RBD targeting Abs G2 and G4 recognize the non-RBD region of S1 and S2 of MERS-CoV, respectively, showing cross-reactivity with multiple MERS-CoV variants and can protect hDPP4 transduced mice from challenge (Wang et al., 2015, 2018). Two nanobodies isolated from camelids, NbMS10 and HCAb-83, show potency in hDPP4 transgenic mice by reducing weight loss and increasing survival after challenge. Interestingly, NbMS10 is able to protect mice as a therapeutic treatment 3 days post infection (Raj et al., 2018; Zhao et al., 2018).

While many mAbs show promising properties for clinical use, two mAbs, REGN3048 and REGN3051, have completed phase 1 clinical trials (NCT03301090). These two mAbs were isolated from VelocImmune mice (expressing the variable regions of human Ig heavy and kappa light chain) immunized with MERS *S*-protein. Both mAbs show picomolar binding and inhibition of MERS pseudo particles transduction on Huh7 cells. REGN3048 is able to neutralize seven natural isolates of S variants, and IP injection of the mAb at 1 day before or after challenge reduces MERS-CoV RNA levels and lung pathologies in an hDPP4 transgenic mouse model (Pascal et al., 2015). Given the acute severe phase that is associated with emerging CoV infections, a major hurdle for therapeutic antibodies and drugs is that early administration will likely prove most efficacious in clinical care, as has also been shown with influenza virus, Ebola virus and RSV immunotherapeutics (Olinger et al., 2012; Qiu et al., 2012; Fry et al., 2014; Rezaee et al., 2017).

Fusion and Viral Protease Inhibitors

Another critical step for CoV life cycle is membrane fusion and the subsequent release of the RNA genome for replication (Millet and Whittaker, 2018). Membrane fusion of CoVs is governed by the S2 domain of the *S*-protein (Pallesen et al., 2017; Tortorici and Veesler, 2019). The S2 stem undergoes a major conformational change at the two heptad repeat regions (HR1 and HR2) to bring the host and viral membrane in close proximity for fusion pore formation (Yuan et al., 2017; Walls et al., 2019b). Multiple peptidomimetic fusion inhibitors that mimic the HR1 and HR2 of either SARS-CoV or MERS-CoV block the formation of the helical core and efficiently inhibit membrane fusion in the micromolar range (Gao et al., 2013; Lu et al., 2014; Xia et al., 2019). A single report has shown treatment of HR2 peptide 5h prior to MERS-CoV challenge in an Ad5-hDPP4 transduction mouse model reduces viral lung titer (Channappanavar et al., 2015). The ability of these drugs to protect in lethal, high titer mouse models has yet to be proven.

CoV nsp3 and nsp5 genes encode the papain-like cysteine protease (PLpro) and 3C-like serine protease (3CLpro), respectively (Perlman and Netland, 2009). PLpro cleaves the polyprotein and separates it into nsp1 to 4 while 3CLpro separates nsp4 to 16 (Ziebuhr et al., 2000; Harcourt et al., 2004). Since polyprotein processing is a critical step for CoV replication and transcription, viral proteases are high priority drug targets. Originally developed as HIV protease inhibitors, LPV and RTV have low micromolar activity against 3CLpro of both SARS-CoV and MERS-CoV *in vitro* (Wu et al., 2004; De Wilde et al., 2014). Testing in SARS-CoV infected patients has shown beneficial outcomes, including lowering the viral load, reducing the onset of ARDS, and lowering mortality rates with LPV and RTV (see nucleoside analogs) treatments (Chu et al., 2004). However, most of the drug studies were performed using retrospective control, sometimes with unbalanced gender ratios, and no treatment has proven efficacious in a randomized control trial (Zumla et al., 2016a). In a marmoset model, LPV/RTV treatment suggested a modest improvement in clinical and pathological outcome as well as reduction of viral load (Chan et al., 2015). However, due to different pathological consequences of treated and untreated group, viral titers were measured at different time points post-infection and all the experiments were performed with a relatively small number (n = 3) of single gender (male) animals (Chan et al., 2015). SARS-CoV and MERS-CoV infection has been shown to be heavily biased by age and gender, where elders and males experience more severe complications than females in clinical cases and mouse models (Karlberg et al., 2004; Alghamdi et al., 2014; Channappanavar et al., 2017). A single subject in a case study, an elderly patient, survived a severe MERS-CoV infection using a combination therapy of LPV/RTV,

TABLE 2 | Summary of SAR-CoV and MERS-CoV neutralizating antibodies.

SARS mAbs	Epitopes	Origins	Animal models	Treatment timing, Routes	Dose, route of infection, Strains	Results	References
S3.1	Spike	EBV transformated B cell from SARS patient	8 weeks old BALB/c	24 h pre-infection, prophoylatic, IP	10^4 TCID50, IN, Urbani	Reduce viral titer (lung and nasal turbinates)	Traggiai et al., 2004
80R	RBD	Phage display on naive human antibody library	16 weeks old BALB/c	24 h pre-infection, prophoylatic, IP	10^4 TCID50, IN, Urbani	Reduce viral titer (lung)	Sui et al., 2004
m396	RBD	Naive human antibody library	8 week old BALB/c	24 h pre-infection, prophoylatic, IP	10^5 TCID50, IN, Urbani, GD03, SZ16	Reduce viral titer (lung)	Zhu et al., 2007
S230.15	RBD	EBV transformated B cell from SARS patient	8 weeks old BALB/c	24 h pre-infection, prophoylatic, IP	10^5 TCID50, IN, Urbani, GD03, SZ16	Reduce viral titer (lung)	Zhu et al., 2007
			12 months old BALB/c	24 h pre-infection, prophoylatic, IP	10^6 PFU, IN, Urbani, GZ02, SZ16		Rockx et al., 2008
				Co-administration, IN	10^6 PFU, IN, GZ02	Not conclusive, reduce titer	
				1, 2, and 3 days post-infection, theraputic	10^6 PFU, IN, GZ02	Not protective	
CR3014	RBD	Naive human antibody library	Ferret	24 h pre-infection, prophoylatic, IP	10^4 TCID50, IT, HKU-39849	Reduce viral titer (lung), no lung lesion	van den Brink et al., 2005
				Co-administration	10^3 and 10^4 TCID50, IT, HKU-39849	Reduce viral titer (lung), reduce lung lesion	Ter Meulen et al., 2004
			4 – 6 weeks old BALB/c	24 h pre-infection, prophoylatic, IP	10^5 TCID50, IN, Urbani, GD03, SZ16	Reduce viral titer (lung)	Greenough et al., 2005
m68	Spike (non-RBD)	Transgenic mice with human Ig gene immunized with SARS-CoV Spike	4 – 6 weeks old BALB/c	24 h pre-infection, prophoylatic, IP	10^5 TCID50, IN, Urbani, GD03, SZ16	Reduce viral titer (lung)	Greenough et al., 2005
MERS mAbs	**Epitopes**	**Origins**	**Animal models**	**Treatment timing, Routes**	**Dose, route of infection, Strains**	**Results**	**References**
4C2	RBD	Mice immunized with MERS-CoV RBD	4 – 6 weeks old BALB/c transduced with hDPP4 by Ad5	24 h pre-infection, prophylactic, IV	10^5 PFU, IN, EMC/2012	Reduce viral titer (lung)	Li et al., 2015
				24 h post-infection, theraputic, IV			
Mersmab1	RBD	Mice immunized with MERS-CoV S1	hDPP4 transgenic mice	24 h post-infection, theraputic, IV	$10^{4.6}$ TCID50, IN, EMC/2012	Reduce viral titer (lung)	Du et al., 2014; Qiu et al., 2016
CDC2-C2	RBD	Single B cell cloning from MERS patients	hDPP4 transgenic mice	24 h pre-infection, prophylactic, IP	10^6 TCID50, IN, EMC/2012	Reduce viral titer (lung)	Wang et al., 2015, 2018
G2	Spike (non-RBD)	Mice primed with MERS-CoV DNA and S1 protein	hDPP4 transgenic mice	24 h pre-infection, prophylactic, IP	10^6 TCID50, IN, EMC/2012	Reduce viral titer (lung)	Wang et al., 2015, 2018
G4	S2	Mice primed with MERS-CoV DNA and S1 protein	hDPP4 transgenic mice	24 h pre-infection, prophylactic, IP	10^6 TCID50, IN, EMC/2012	Reduce viral titer (lung)	Wang et al., 2015, 2018
MCA1	RBD	Phage display on naive human antibody library	2 years old common marmosets	24 h pre-infection, prophylactic, IP	5×10^6 PFU, IT, EMC/2012	Reduce viral titer (lung), weight loss and patholicical scores	Chen et al., 2017
				2 or 12 h post-infection, theraputic, IP			

(Continued)

TABLE 2 | Continued

MERS mAbs	Epitopes	Origins	Animal models	Treatment timing, Routes	Dose, route of infection, Strains	Results	References
LCA60	RBD	Single B cell cloning from MERS patients	4 – 6 weeks old BALB/c transduced with hDPP4 by Ad5	24 h pre-infection, prophylactic, IP	10^5 PFU, IN, EMC/2012 and London1/2012	Reduce viral titer (lung), weight loss and pathology	Corti et al., 2015
				24 h post-infection, theraputic, IP			Corti et al., 2015
			2 – 6 years old common marmosets	24 h pre-infection, prophylactic, IP	5.2×10^6 PFU, IN + IT + ocular + orally, EMC/2012	Moderately protective, reduce weight loss and pathology	de Wit et al., 2019
m336	RBD	Phage display on navie human antibody library	hDPP4 transgenic mice	12h pre-infection, prophylactic, IP	10^4 TCID50, IN, EMC/2012	reduce viral titer (lung), weight loss and patholicical scores	Ying et al., 2014, 2015
				12h post-infection, theraputic, IP			Agrawal et al., 2016
			5 – 7 months old Australian white rabbit	24 h pre-infection, prophylactic, IV and IN	10^5 TCID50, IN, EMC/2012	Reduce viral RNA titer and lung inflammation	Houser et al., 2016
			Common marmosets	6 h (IV) and 48 h (SC) post-infection, theraputic	5.2×10^6 PFU, IN + IT + ocular + orally, EMC/2012	Moderately protective, reduce clinical diseases and gross pathology	van Doremalen et al., 2017
NbMS10	RBD	llama immunized with MERS-CoV RBD	hDPP4 transgenic mice	3 days pre-infection, prophylactic, IP	$10^{5.3}$ TCID50, IN, EMC/2012	Reduce weight loss and increase survival	Zhao et al., 2018
				1 or 3 days post-infection, theraputic, IP			Zhao et al., 2018
HCAb-83	RBD	Dromedary camel immunized with MERS-CoV DNA and Spike protein	hDPP4 transgenic mice	6 h pre-infection, prophylactic, IP	10^5 TCID50, IN, EMC/2012	Reduce viral titer (lung), weight loss and increase survival	Raj et al., 2018

IV, intravenous; IN, intranasal; IT, intratracheal; SC, subcutaneous; IP, intraperitoneal.

IFN1α, and ribavirin (Kim et al., 2016). An ongoing clinical trial in Saudi Arabia has begun to use a combination of LPV/RTV and IFNβ-1b for laboratory-confirmed MERS-CoV infection (NCT02845843). Given the importance of 3CLpro I viral life cycle, it is an attractive target for novel drug development (Kumar et al., 2017).

Nucleoside Analogs and RdRp Inhibitors

Ribavirin is a guanosine analog that targets RNA dependent RNA polymerases (RdRp) and has a broad efficacy against RNA viruses (Loustaud-Ratti et al., 2016). The drug inhibits viral RNA synthesis and has shown efficacy against HCV and RSV (De Clercq et al., 2016). Ribavirin inhibits SARS-CoV and MERS-CoV replication at high concentration *in vitro* (Tan et al., 2004; Falzarano et al., 2013a), However, ribavirin enhances viral replication in the mouse lung and prolongs viral persistence in a SARS-CoV mouse model (Barnard et al., 2006a). Although not effective as a monotherapy, ribavirin shows a synergistic effect against SARS-CoV and MERS-CoV when combine with IFN (Momattin et al., 2013). In a rhesus macaque model, MERS-CoV infected monkeys show improvement after treating with ribavirin and IFN-α2b (Falzarano et al., 2013b). Furthermore, ribavirin has been used in clinical settings during SARS-CoV and MERS-CoV outbreaks (Omrani et al., 2014; Khalid et al., 2015; Shalhoub et al., 2015). While some studies report positive outcome after treatment with ribavirin + IFN, others suggest no significant improvement (Dicaro et al., 2004; Khalid et al., 2015). Due to the variation in dosage and time of administration and the lack of control, the efficacy of using ribavirin in patients is inconclusive. Mechanistically, studies show that recombinant CoV with a deleted proof-reading exonucleases N (ExoN) shows higher sensitivity toward ribavirin. These results indirectly suggest that the low activity of ribavirin in CoV could be explained by the presence of a proofreading exonucleases N (ExoN, nsp14) which can excise the drug from the viral mRNA in CoVs (Smith et al., 2013; Ferron et al., 2017).

Two nucleoside analogs, β-D-N4-Hydroxycytidine (NHC) and GS-5734 (remdesivir), have shown high efficacy against CoVs and are less sensitive to ExoN (Sheahan et al., 2017, 2020; Agostini et al., 2018, 2019). NHC is a cytidine analog and has recently been shown to inhibit multiple viruses, including influenza virus, RSV and Ebola virus (Reynard et al., 2015; Urakova et al., 2017;

Yoon et al., 2018). It has micro-molar EC50 against both alpha and beta CoVs including SARS-CoV and MERS-CoV (Barnard et al., 2004; Pyrc et al., 2006; Agostini et al., 2019). Currently under clinical development for Ebola viruses, remdesivir is a nucleoside prodrug that is effective against multiple other RNA viruses including Nipah viruses, RSV, and CoVs (Lo et al., 2017; Sheahan et al., 2017). Remdesivir has sub-micromolar inhibition concentrations in a broad range of CoVs including SARS-CoV, MERS-CoV, and hCoV-NL63, as well as pre-pandemic bat-CoVs WIV1 and SHC014 in an *in vitro* human airway epithelial (HAE) model (Sheahan et al., 2017; Agostini et al., 2018). Prophylactic administration (one day pre-infection) of remdesivir can mitigate disease by reducing the viral titer and lung pathology in lethal mouse models challenged with a mouse adapted SARS-CoV MA15. Remdesivir also shows therapeutic activity when administered early at one day post-infection (corresponding to 7–10 days after the onset of symptoms in human infection). However, treatment initiated two days post infection does not improve disease outcomes, although the murine disease model is more compressed than in humans (Sheahan et al., 2017). Importantly, remdesivir shows excellent prophylactic protection. Rhesus macaques are completely protected from MERS-CoV infection as scored by lung pathology and clinical score as well as inhibited viral growth. Therapeutic treatment 12-h post infection shows moderate improvement of clinical outcomes on NHPs (de Wit et al., 2020). The parental nucleoside of remdesivir, GS-441524, has also shown to be effective for treating FIP, a disease caused by the α-CoV FIPV (Murphy et al., 2018; Pedersen et al., 2019). Currently, NHC and remdesivir are the only broadly effective antiviral drugs against all SARS-like, MERS-like, human contemporary, and animal CoVs (Sheahan et al., 2017; Agostini et al., 2018; Murphy et al., 2018; Pedersen et al., 2019). Some antiviral drugs, such as chloroquine and T-705, also show efficacy *in vitro* and are under consideration for the current COVID-19 outbreak (Wang et al., 2020).

HOST FACTOR INHIBITORS AND IMMUNO-MODULATORS

Host Protease Inhibitors

Like all class I viral fusion proteins, CoV S glycoproteins require proteolytic cleavage by host proteases for membrane fusion and viral entry (Belouzard et al., 2012; White and Whittaker, 2016; Millet and Whittaker, 2018). Two cleavage events have been characterized in SARS-CoV and MERS-CoV. The first cleavage event separates the head (S1) and the fusion stem (S2) by cutting the S1/S2 junction (Millet and Whittaker, 2015). The second cleavage event occurs at the S2' site which is usually located immediately upstream of the fusion peptide (Belouzard et al., 2009). Multiple proteases have been shown to be involved in the cleavage events, including cathepsin-L, trypsin-like serine proteases, transmembrane serine proteases (TTSP) and proprotein convertases such as furin (Millet and Whittaker, 2015). Cathepsin-L inhibitors MDL28170 and SSAA09E1 block SARS-CoV pseudotyped particle infection in pre-treated 293T cells (Simmons et al., 2005; Adedeji et al., 2013). While a peptidomimetic furin substrate, decanoyl-RVKR-chloromethylketone, has been shown to inhibit cleavage of MERS *S*-protein and block infection in multiple cell lines including normal human bronchial epithelial cells (NHBE), the *in vivo* potency of this approach is less certain (Gierer et al., 2014; Millet and Whittaker, 2014; Matsuyama et al., 2018).

Host Receptor Inhibitors

The blocking of receptor interactions is also a target of antiviral development. *N*-(2-aminoethyl)-1 aziridine-ethanamine (NAAE) blocks the interaction of SARS *S*-protein and ACE2 and inhibits S-mediated cell-to-cell fusion at millimolar concentrations (Huentelman et al., 2004). Similarly, an Ab blocking DPP4 can also inhibit MERS-CoV infection on primary bronchial epithelial cells (Raj et al., 2013). Importantly, the *S*-proteins of SARS-CoVs and MERS-CoV interact with their receptors outside of the active sites. Therefore, it would be of interest to develop inhibitors that do not affect the normal function of the host proteins but abolish the interaction of the CoV and receptor. Otherwise, long term inhibition of cellular proteins could have adverse effects on the host. For instance, inhibition of ACE2 may cause hypertension (Danilczyk and Penninger, 2006). Additionally, DPP4 is also responsible for multiple cellular functions including immune homeostasis, stem cell development, metabolism and T-cell regulation, and hence is not an ideal target for MERS-CoV infection (Matteucci and Giampietro, 2016; Ou et al., 2019).

Other Host Factor Inhibitors

Another attractive target to inhibit CoV infection is the host metabolic pathways essential for CoV life cycles. CoVs replicate and transcribe in membrane-bound vesicles derived from the host's rough ER (Snijder et al., 2006; Stertz et al., 2007; Reggiori et al., 2010). MERS-CoV infection upregulates the biosynthetic pathways of multiple major lipogenic enzymes, including fatty acid synthase (FAS), acetyl-CoA carboxylase (ACC) and HMG-CoA synthase (HMGCS) (Yuan et al., 2019). AM580, which targets the major lipid biosynthesis transactivator n-SREBPs by interfering with and downregulating global lipid synthesis (Goldstein et al., 2006; Yuan et al., 2019), inhibits the replication of multiple viruses including influenza virus, Zika virus, Enterovirus-A71 and MERS-CoV (Yuan et al., 2019). Remarkably, MERS-CoV viral titer is reduced by 1,000- to 1,000,000-fold in the presence of AM580 in Huh7 cells or a human intestinal organoid model, respectively, and IP injection of AM580 for 3 days protects a human hDPP4 transgenic mouse model from MERS-CoV lethal challenge (Yuan et al., 2019).

Immune Modulators

Corticosteroids

SARS-CoV and MERS-CoV both cause lung inflammation and can progress into severe respiratory syndrome. Lacking direct antiviral effect, corticosteroids are an immune suppressor which is administrated to severe patients to alleviate lung inflammation. However, immune suppression could also facilitate viral replication. Therefore, corticosteroids are often administrated with antiviral or other immune modulators, such as IFN which can activate the immune system. Retrospective and prospective clinical studies have shown mixed observation in treating SARS-CoV and MERS-CoV patients with corticosteroids, IFN and ribavirin; while some showed a positive effect, others showed no difference.

IFNs

SARS-CoV and MERS-CoV are able to suppress the induction of IFN synthesis by multiple mechanisms including inhibition of the IFN signal transduction pathways and evading detection by pattern recognition receptors (PRRs) and toll-like receptors (TLRs) (Frieman et al., 2008; Lim et al., 2016; Mubarak et al., 2019). Therefore, external administration of IFN regiments could re-initiate the antiviral immune response in the host. During the SARS-CoV and MERS-CoV outbreaks, IFN-α, IFN-β, and IFN-γ were used in combination with various antiviral drugs, including LPV/RTV, ribavirin, corticosteroids and poly I:C (Zumla et al., 2016a). Although most of the clinical reports are positive, there is no consensus on the efficacy of IFN treatment in CoV infection. In animal model studies, IFN treatment is only effective when administrated at early time point for both SARS-CoV and MERS-CoV (Channappanavar et al., 2016, 2019). Furthermore, many of the clinical studies were confounded by multiple factors, including IFN dosages, combination of different antivirals, and the stage of infection (Mo and Fisher, 2016). For instance, some studies targeted patients in the late stage of infection and show a worse survival rate than average (Al-Tawfiq et al., 2014; Khalid et al., 2014). Based on multiple research reports, IFN-β shows the best efficacy in treating MERS-CoV infection (Chan et al., 2013; Hart et al., 2014; Kim et al., 2016). Currently, an open labeled, well controlled clinical study is aiming to test a set dose of LPV/RTV and IFN-β in treating MERS-CoV. The trial will probably provide insight into treating MERS-CoV infection in human population.

THE CURRENT SARS-CoV-2 OUTBREAK: A CHALLENGE, AN OPPORTUNITY

In December 2019, a new CoV outbreak started in Wuhan, China, a megacity with a population of 11 million. With an estimated basic reproduction number (R_0) of 1.4 – 2.5, SARS-CoV-2 quickly spread to every province in China and began to spread globally by the end of January 2020 (Zhou et al., 2020), and was declared a worldwide pandemic in March 2020 by the World Health Organization. SARS-CoV-2 is capable of human-to-human transmission via either symptomatic or asymptomatic patients (Rothe et al., 2020). The high mutation rate of CoVs and the possibility of super-spreader could potentiate the continuous spreading globally. Originally from bat, the SARS-CoV-2 Is 96% identical to a bat CoV designated RaTG13, isolated from a cave in Yunnan Province, China and belongs to the betacoronavirus 2b family, as does SARS-CoV (Zhou et al., 2020). However, the S-proteins between SARS-CoV and 2019 nCoV share only 76–78% sequence similarity, rendering the current experimental vaccines and antivirals unlikely to be fully protective against SARS-CoV-2. As many group 2b SARS-like CoV have pre-epidemic potential, vaccines and countermeasures should be targeted against all of these strains to maximally protect against current and future threats to the global health and economy (Menachery et al., 2015, 2016).

After two CoV outbreaks in the last two decades, the public health officials and clinicians have experience in preventing spread and treating SARS-CoV-2 patients. Prompt communication between governments, quick quarantine procedures, and rapid viral detection assays have helped minimize SARS-CoV-2 cases in other countries thus far. Additionally, the scientific community has developed novel vaccine strategies and experimental antivirals to fight emerging CoV. New vaccines that specifically targeting SARS-CoV-2 are under development. Moderna had started a phase 1 clinical trial on an RNA vaccine (mRNA-1273) that encodes the prefusion stabilized form of SARS-CoV-2 S-protein (NCT04283461). Although there are no published studies of a RNA vaccine platform against CoV, the RNA platform has shown efficacy against multiple other viral infectious diseases including influenza, rabies, Flavivirus, and Ebola viruses in experimental animal models (Zhang et al., 2019). Furthermore, pre-clinical data of the Zika virus mRNA vaccine (mRNA-1893) from Moderna has shown protection against Zika virus and abrogated maternal transmission of Zika virus in pregnant mice (Richner et al., 2017; Jagger et al., 2019). Broad-spectrum antivirals which have shown efficacy against multiple CoVs have the potential to treat SARS-CoV-2 (Sheahan et al., 2017, 2020). Given the high number of infected patients and at risk individuals, the current situation provides an opportunity to initiate clinical trials for (a) vaccine formulation designed to protect uninfected people, (b) broad spectrum antivirals to treat infected individuals and (c) formulation of immune modulators to alleviate clinical pathologies. A well-designed clinical trial could not only ameliorate the current situation, but also lay the foundation for future CoV outbreaks. Supported by a recent study on SARS-CoV-2 (Wang et al., 2020) and multiple research studies on SARS and MERS-CoVs (Sheahan et al., 2017, 2020; de Wit et al., 2020) and a single clinical report (Holshue et al., 2020), remdesivir hold promises as treatment for SARS-CoV-2. The Chinese government has started a clinical trial using remdesivir for treating SARS-CoV-2 patients with mild to severe symptoms (NCT04252664, NCT04257656). On the clinical side, if time and resources permit, a centralized repository that records and digitizes infection cases would aid future medical and epidemiology studies through machine learning programs. Finally, the current situation also provides an opportunity to develop unconventional treatments, such as gene therapy, to target infectious diseases.

UNCONVENTIONAL VACCINES AND THERAPEUTICS – GENE THERAPIES

The field of gene therapy has undergone rapid growth in the last 10 years. Although mainly focused on rare genetic diseases, its potential in treating infectious diseases should not be discounted. One of the leading vectors, adeno-associated virus (AAV), has proven to be safe for human use and multiple AAV-based gene therapy drugs are approved by the FDA and the EMA (Kay et al., 2000; Kaplitt et al., 2007). So far, the only report of use of AAV in CoV is as a DNA vaccine to deliver SARS-CoV spike protein for immunization (Du et al., 2008). Given the recent developments in human antibody cloning technologies, AAV holds a promising potential to be a hybrid of vaccine and therapeutic which acts as a passive immunization vector to provide protection for the outbreak and as a therapeutic in early time scales.

AAV as a Vector for Passive Immunization Against Emerging CoV

The Vectors – Safety

AAV is a non-pathogenic, non-enveloped, 4.7 kb single-stranded DNA virus belonging to the *Dependoparvovirus* genus within the family *Parvoviridae* (Cotmore et al., 2014). AAV infects a wide variety of animals, from bearded dragons to humans. Natural AAV isolates have different tissue tropisms in humans and can be reverse engineered to better fulfill various medical needs. To target SARS-CoV, MERS-CoV and other respiratory virus infections, a human airway tropic AAV is needed. Multiple reports have demonstrated that natural isolates AAV5 (Zabner et al., 2000), AAV6 (Limberis et al., 2009), and AAV9 (Adam et al., 2014) as well as engineered vectors AAV2.5 (Li et al., 2009) and AAV2.5T (Excoffon et al., 2009) are able to transduce human lung epithelial cells, including primary human airway epithelial (HAE) cultures. Although there is a high prevalence of nAbs against AAVs in the human population, new technologies have been developed to engineer AAV to evade humoral immune responses (Tse et al., 2015, 2017). These developments potentially allow for the delivery of CoV vaccines or immunotherapeutic directly to the mucosal compartments of the lung.

The Package – Flexibility

Passive immunization of AAV can be developed as a platform technology in which the nAb can be quickly exchanged to target specific pathogens. Multiple studies have shown passive immunization using AAV is effective against viral infectious diseases such as HIV, (Balazs et al., 2012; Lin and Balazs, 2018) Ebola, (Limberis et al., 2016) influenza, (Balazs et al., 2013; Laursen et al., 2018), and others (Nieto and Salvetti, 2014). The package for delivery is extremely flexible, from authentic immunoglobulins (IgG) to immunoadhesins (IA) to single chain variable fragments (scFv) to bi-specific antibodies (Naso et al., 2017). Furthermore, a combination of Abs, small antiviral peptides and immuno-modulators can be co-delivered at the same time to achieve multidimensional therapy. Although AAV-based passive immunization has not yet been tested as therapeutic, it could serve as a fast-acting prophylactic alternative to traditional vaccines.

The Timing – Quick

The most important aspect to control an outbreak is to reduce the spread by protecting the population from infection. However, there is a lag time between the beginning of an outbreak and the development of an effective vaccine in which the population is completely vulnerable. Prophylactic treatments, such as infusion of Abs and antivirals, could protect individual for a short duration. However, these prophylactic treatments require constant intake to stay effective and are toxic as well as financially impractical for long-term use (Hansel et al., 2010). AAV-based passive immunization could perfectly fill the vacuum by protecting the population before the arrival of a vaccine. Since AAV is a platform technology, anti-viral packages can be swapped and tested quickly, within a month (Strobel et al., 2019). After administration in animals, protection can be achieved in less than a week, faster than any vaccine strategies. In an influenza study, AAV9 delivery of IA via intranasal inoculation protected animals from lethal influenza challenges including H5N1, H1N1 and H1N1 1918 within 3 days of AAV administration (Limberis et al., 2013). Unlike traditional gene therapy in which the transgene lasts for long periods of time, the natural turnover rate of airway epithelia means that the nAb introduction is not permanent, reducing the chance that the host will produce antibodies targeting the therapeutic antibody delivered by AAV (anti-drug antibody responses) (Nieto and Salvetti, 2014). Therefore, AAV-based passive immunization is a quick and excellent option to deploy in an outbreak situation for emerging infectious diseases.

The Challenges

AAV-based gene therapy has great potential for treating viral infectious diseases. However, there are multiple hurdles for AAV-based gene therapy to achieve its full potential. (1) Low transduction efficiency, (2) pre-existing nAb against AAVs, (3) transgene toxicity and loss of expression, and (4) extremely high price tag (Colella et al., 2018; Kaemmerer, 2018). Fortunately, multiple strategies have been developed to address these hurdles (Tse et al., 2015). For instance, through vector engineering, a new generation of AAV vectors can evade pre-existing nAbs while retaining a good transduction profile in the respiratory system (Li et al., 2009; Tse et al., 2017). For rare genetic diseases, life-long gene expression is important for therapeutic purposes but could cause toxicity. On the contrary, for emerging CoVs, the goal is a short-term protection from the virus. Therefore, AAV can target epithelial cells that have a regular turn-over rate, hence providing short-term protection and preventing transgene toxicity. AAV-based therapies are known for their extremely high prices, sometime up to a million US dollar per treatment. However, the prices are inflated due to the small market size of rare genetic diseases and the cost for drug development. Given the huge market size of infectious diseases, the price for AAV-based therapy for infectious diseases should be more reasonable. Unlike rare genetic diseases and other infectious diseases, an emerging CoV outbreak is uniquely suitable for AAV-based passive immunization as a short-term protection therapy before vaccine deployment.

CONCLUSION

The continuous development of vaccines, antivirals, and hopefully gene therapies will provide an arsenal for combating and controlling emerging CoV diseases. For vaccine development, understanding the antigenicity and neutralizing antibody footprints of different CoVs could aid the development of broad-spectrum vaccines and, ultimately, the possibility of a universal CoV vaccine. Vaccine formulation, including dosage and adjuvants, should be tested systemically and, if possible, on animal models that reflects the genetic variation of the human population. A deeper understanding of the basic biology of CoV and host-virus interaction can lead to the discovery of druggable targets. Importantly, we should not overlook the potential of the existing broad-spectrum antivirals and should start clinical trials on these drugs in a timely fashion. Prevention is always the best treatment, and constant viral surveillance of wild animals for potential emerging CoVs is extremely important. Testing the outbreak potential of heterologous SARS- and MERS-like viruses with different spike proteins could better prepare society from the next outbreak. A centralized digital database that collect public health and clinical information of the current outbreak would allow global retrospective studies in the future using machine learning and other big data analysis. On the research side, quick, reliable and easily employed viral testing kits should be developed. Innovative technologies such as gene therapy should be adequately explored for their potential to combat CoVs and act as another line of defense against elusive emerging viral diseases. The current SARS-CoV-2 poses a huge challenge for society; however, given experience with emerging CoVs and global effort, it is hoped that the impact of the outbreak will be minimal.

AUTHOR CONTRIBUTIONS

LT wrote the review. RM, RG, and RB reviewed and revised the final version.

FUNDING

The manuscript presented here were supported by grants from the National Institute of Allergy and Infectious Disease of the United States National Institutes of Health (NIH) by awards AI108197, AI110700, AI132178, and AI149644 (RB). **Figure 2** is generated using biorender (https://biorender.com/).

ACKNOWLEDGMENTS

We thank Dr. Timothy Sheahan and Dr. Yixuan Hou for critical reading of this manuscript and all members in the RB laboratory for helpful discussions.

REFERENCES

Adam, V. S., Crosariol, M., Kumar, S., Ge, M. Q., Czack, S. E., Roy, S., et al. (2014). Adeno-associated virus 9-mediated airway expression of antibody protects old and immunodeficient mice against influenza virus. *Clin. Vaccine Immunol.* 21, 1528–1533. doi: 10.1128/CVI.00572-514

Adedeji, A. O., Severson, W., Jonsson, C., Singh, K., Weiss, S. R., and Sarafianos, S. G. (2013). Novel inhibitors of severe acute respiratory syndrome coronavirus entry that act by three distinct mechanisms. *J. Virol.* 87, 8017–8028. doi: 10.1128/jvi.00998-913

Adney, D. R., Wang, L., Van Doremalen, N., Shi, W., Zhang, Y., Kong, W., et al. (2019). Efficacy of an adjuvanted middle east respiratory syndrome coronavirus spike protein vaccine in dromedary camels and alpacas. *Viruses* 11:212. doi: 10.3390/v11030212

Agnihothram, S., Gopal, R., Yount, B. L. J., Donaldson, E. F., Menachery, V. D., Graham, R. L., et al. (2014). Evaluation of serologic and antigenic relationships between middle eastern respiratory syndrome coronavirus and other coronaviruses to develop vaccine platforms for the rapid response to emerging coronaviruses. *J. Infect. Dis.* 209, 995–1006. doi: 10.1093/infdis/jit609

Agostini, M. L., Andres, E. L., Sims, A. C., Graham, R. L., Sheahan, T. P., Lu, X., et al. (2018). Coronavirus susceptibility to the antiviral remdesivir (GS-5734) is mediated by the viral polymerase and the proofreading exoribonuclease. *mBio* 9, 1–15. doi: 10.1128/mBio.00221-218

Agostini, M. L., Pruijssers, A. J., Chappell, J. D., Gribble, J., Lu, X., Andres, E. L., et al. (2019). Small-molecule antiviral β-d-N4-hydroxycytidine inhibits a proofreading-intact coronavirus with a high genetic barrier to resistance. *J. Virol.* 93:e01348-19. doi: 10.1128/JVI.01348-1319

Agrawal, A. S., Tao, X., Algaissi, A., Garron, T., Narayanan, K., Peng, B. H., et al. (2016). Immunization with inactivated Middle East Respiratory Syndrome coronavirus vaccine leads to lung immunopathology on challenge with live virus. *Hum. Vaccines Immunother.* 12, 2351–2356. doi: 10.1080/21645515.2016.1177688

Ahmed, A. E. (2019). Diagnostic delays in Middle East respiratory syndrome coronavirus patients and health systems. *J. Infect. Public Health* 12, 767–771. doi: 10.1016/j.jiph.2019.04.002

Al Kahlout, R. A., Nasrallah, G. K., Farag, E. A., Wang, L., Lattwein, E., Müller, M. A., et al. (2019). Comparative serological study for the prevalence of Anti-MERS coronavirus antibodies in high- and low-risk groups in qatar. *J. Immunol. Res.* 2019:1386740. doi: 10.1155/2019/1386740

Al-Amri, S. S., Abbas, A. T., Siddiq, L. A., Alghamdi, A., Sanki, M. A., Al-Muhanna, M. K., et al. (2017). Immunogenicity of candidate MERS-CoV DNA vaccines based on the spike protein. *Sci. Rep.* 7:44875. doi: 10.1038/srep44875

Alghamdi, I. G., Hussain, I. I., Almalki, S. S., Alghamdi, M. S., Alghamdi, M. M., and El-Sheemy, M. A. (2014). The pattern of Middle East respiratory syndrome coronavirus in Saudi Arabia: a descriptive epidemiological analysis of data from the Saudi Ministry of Health. *Int. J. Gen. Med.* 7, 417–423. doi: 10.2147/IJGM.S67061

Alharbi, N. K., Padron-Regalado, E., Thompson, C. P., Kupke, A., Wells, D., Sloan, M. A., et al. (2017). ChAdOx1 and MVA based vaccine candidates against MERS-CoV elicit neutralising antibodies and cellular immune responses in mice. *Vaccine* 35, 3780–3788. doi: 10.1016/j.vaccine.2017.05.032

Almazán, F., Dediego, M. L., Sola, I., Zuñiga, S., Nieto-torres, J. L., Marquez-jurado, S., et al. (2013). A Vaccine candidate east respiratory syndrome coronavirus as a vaccine candidate. *mBio* 4, 1–11. doi: 10.1128/mBio.00650-13.Editor

Al-Tawfiq, J. A., Momattin, H., Dib, J., and Memish, Z. A. (2014). Ribavirin and interferon therapy in patients infected with the Middle East respiratory syndrome coronavirus: an observational study. *Int. J. Infect. Dis.* 20, 42–46. doi: 10.1016/j.ijid.2013.12.003

Arabi, Y. M., Hajeer, A. H., Luke, T., Raviprakash, K., Balkhy, H., Johani, S., et al. (2016). Feasibility of using convalescent plasma immunotherapy for MERS-CoV infection, Saudi Arabia. *Emerg. Infect. Dis.* 22, 1554–1561. doi: 10.3201/eid2209.151164

Balazs, A. B., Bloom, J. D., Hong, C. M., Rao, D. S., and Baltimore, D. (2013). Broad protection against influenza infection by vectored immunoprophylaxis in mice. *Nat. Biotechnol.* 31:647. doi: 10.1038/nbt.2618

Balazs, A. B., Chen, J., Hong, C. M., Rao, D. S., Yang, L., and Baltimore, D. (2012). Antibody-based protection against HIV infection by vectored immunoprophylaxis. *Nature* 481, 81–84. doi: 10.1038/nature10660

Barnard, D. L., Day, C. W., Bailey, K., Heiner, M., Montgomery, R., Lauridsen, L., et al. (2006a). Enhancement of the infectivity of SARS-CoV in BALB/c mice by IMP dehydrogenase inhibitors, including ribavirin. *Antiviral Res.* 71, 53–63. doi: 10.1016/j.antiviral.2006.03.001

Barnard, D. L., Day, C. W., Bailey, K., Heiner, M., Montgomery, R., Lauridsen, L., et al. (2006b). Evaluation of immunomodulators, interferons and known in vitro SARS-CoV inhibitors for inhibition of SARS-CoV replication in BALB/c mice. *Antivir. Chem. Chemother.* 17, 275–284. doi: 10.1177/095632020601700505

Barnard, D. L., Hubbard, V. D., Burton, J., Smee, D. F., Morrey, J. D., Otto, M. J., et al. (2004). Inhibition of severe acute respiratory syndrome-associated coronavirus (SARSCoV) by calpain inhibitors and β-D-N4-hydroxycytidine. *Antivir. Chem. Chemother.* 15, 15–22. doi: 10.1177/095632020401500102

Belouzard, S., Chu, V. C., and Whittaker, G. R. (2009). Activation of the SARS coronavirus spike protein via sequential proteolytic cleavage at two distinct sites. *Proc. Natl. Acad. Sci. U.S.A.* 106, 5871–5876. doi: 10.1073/pnas.0809524106

Belouzard, S., Millet, J. K., Licitra, B. N., and Whittaker, G. R. (2012). Mechanisms of coronavirus cell entry mediated by the viral spike protein. *Viruses* 4, 1011–1033. doi: 10.3390/v4061011

Belshe, R. B., Gruber, W. C., Mendelman, P. M., Mehta, H. B., Mahmood, K., Reisinger, K., et al. (2000). Correlates of immune protection induced by live, attenuated, cold-adapted, trivalent, intranasal influenza virus vaccine. *J. Infect. Dis.* 181, 1133–1137. doi: 10.1086/315323

Binnie, A., Tsang, J. L. Y., and Dos Santos, C. C. (2014). Biomarkers in acute respiratory distress syndrome. *Curr. Opin. Crit. Care* 20, 47–55. doi: 10.1097/MCC.0000000000000048

Bisht, H., Roberts, A., Vogel, L., Bukreyev, A., Collins, P. L., Murphy, B. R., et al. (2004). Severe acute respiratory syndrome coronavirus spike protein expressed by attenuated vaccinia virus protectively immunizes mice. *Proc. Natl. Acad. Sci. U.S.A.* 101, 6641–6646. doi: 10.1073/pnas.0401939101

Bisht, H., Roberts, A., Vogel, L., Subbarao, K., and Moss, B. (2005). Neutralizing antibody and protective immunity to SARS coronavirus infection of mice induced by a soluble recombinant polypeptide containing an N-terminal segment of the spike glycoprotein. *Virology* 334, 160–165. doi: 10.1016/j.virol.2005.01.042

Bodmer, B. S., Fiedler, A. H., Hanauer, J. R. H., and Mühlebach, M. D. (2018). Live-attenuated bivalent measles virus-derived vaccines targeting Middle East respiratory syndrome coronavirus induce robust and multifunctional T cell responses against both viruses in an appropriate mouse model. *Virology* 521, 99–107. doi: 10.1016/j.virol.2018.05.028

Bolles, M., Deming, D., Long, K., Agnihothram, S., Whitmore, A., Ferris, M., et al. (2011a). A double-inactivated severe acute respiratory syndrome coronavirus vaccine provides incomplete protection in mice and induces increased eosinophilic proinflammatory pulmonary response upon challenge. *J. Virol.* 85, 12201–12215. doi: 10.1128/jvi.06048-6011

Bolles, M., Donaldson, E., and Baric, R. (2011b). SARS-CoV and emergent coronaviruses: viral determinants of interspecies transmission. *Curr. Opin. Virol.* 1, 624–634. doi: 10.1016/j.coviro.2011.10.012

Briese, T., Mishra, N., Jain, K., East, M., Syndrome, R., Quasispecies, C., et al. (2014). Dromedary camels in Saudi Arabia include homologues of human isolates revealed through whole-genome analysis etc. *mBio* 5, 1–5. doi: 10.1128/mBio.01146-14.Editor

Buchholz, U. J., Bukreyev, A., Yang, L., Lamirande, E. W., Murphy, B. R., Subbarao, K., et al. (2004). Contributions of the structural proteins of severe respiratory syndrome coronavirus to protective immunity. *Proc. Natl. Acad. Sci. U.S.A.* 101, 9804–9809. doi: 10.1073/pnas.0403492101

Bukreyev, A., Lamirande, E. W., Buchholz, U. J., Vogel, L. N., Elkins, W. R., St Claire, M., et al. (2004). Mucosal immunisation of African green monkeys (*Cercopithecus aethiops*) with an attenuated parainfluenza virus expressing the SARS coronavirus spike protein for the prevention of SARS. *Lancet* 363, 2122–2127. doi: 10.1016/S0140-6736(04)16501-X

Cabeça, T. K., Granato, C., and Bellei, N. (2013). Epidemiological and clinical features of human coronavirus infections among different subsets of patients. *Influenza Other Respir. Viruses* 7, 1040–1047. doi: 10.1111/irv.12101

Cameron, M. J., Ran, L., Xu, L., Danesh, A., Bermejo-Martin, J. F., Cameron, C. M., et al. (2007). Interferon-mediated immunopathological events are associated with atypical innate and adaptive immune responses in patients with severe acute respiratory syndrome. *J. Virol.* 81, 8692–8706. doi: 10.1128/jvi.00527-527

Chan, J. F. W., Chan, K. H., Kao, R. Y. T., To, K. K. W., Zheng, B. J., Li, C. P. Y., et al. (2013). Broad-spectrum antivirals for the emerging Middle East respiratory syndrome coronavirus. *J. Infect.* 67, 606–616. doi: 10.1016/j.jinf.2013.09.029

Chan, J. F. W., Yao, Y., Yeung, M. L., Deng, W., Bao, L., Jia, L., et al. (2015). Treatment with lopinavir/ritonavir or interferon-β1b improves outcome of MERSCoV infection in a nonhuman primate model of common marmoset. *J. Infect. Dis.* 212, 1904–1913. doi: 10.1093/infdis/jiv392

Channappanavar, R., Fehr, A. R., Vijay, R., Mack, M., Zhao, J., Meyerholz, D. K., et al. (2016). Dysregulated type I interferon and inflammatory monocyte-macrophage responses cause lethal pneumonia in SARS-CoV-infected mice. *Cell Host Microbe* 19, 181–193. doi: 10.1016/j.chom.2016.01.007

Channappanavar, R., Fehr, A. R., Zheng, J., Wohlford-Lenane, C., Abrahante, J. E., Mack, M., et al. (2019). IFN-I response timing relative to virus replication determines MERS coronavirus infection outcomes. *J. Clin. Invest.* 129, 3625–3639. doi: 10.1172/JCI126363

Channappanavar, R., Fett, C., Mack, M., Ten Eyck, P. P., Meyerholz, D. K., and Perlman, S. (2017). Sex-based differences in susceptibility to severe acute respiratory syndrome coronavirus infection. *J. Immunol.* 198, 4046–4053. doi: 10.4049/jimmunol.1601896

Channappanavar, R., Lu, L., Xia, S., Du, L., Meyerholz, D. K., Perlman, S., et al. (2015). Protective effect of intranasal regimens containing peptidic middle east respiratory syndrome coronavirus fusion Inhibitor against MERS-CoV infection. *J. Infect. Dis.* 212, 1894–1903. doi: 10.1093/infdis/jiv325

Channappanavar, R., Zhao, J., and Perlman, S. (2014). T cell-mediated immune response to respiratory coronaviruses. *Immunol. Res.* 59, 118–128. doi: 10.1007/s12026-014-8534-z

Chen, Z., Bao, L., Chen, C., Zou, T., Xue, Y., Li, F., et al. (2017). Human neutralizing monoclonal antibody inhibition of Middle East respiratory syndrome coronavirus replication in the common marmoset. *J. Infect. Dis.* 215, 1807–1815. doi: 10.1093/infdis/jix209

Chi, H., Zheng, X., Wang, X., Wang, C., Wang, H., Gai, W., et al. (2017). DNA vaccine encoding Middle East respiratory syndrome coronavirus S1 protein induces protective immune responses in mice. *Vaccine* 35, 2069–2075. doi: 10.1016/j.vaccine.2017.02.063

Chirmule, N., Propert, K. J., Magosin, S. A., Qian, Y., Qian, R., and Wilson, J. M. (1999). Immune responses to adenovirus and adeno-associated virus in humans. *Gene Ther.* 6, 1574–1583. doi: 10.1038/sj.gt.3300994

Chu, C. M., Cheng, V. C. C., Hung, I. F. N., Wong, M. M. L., Chan, K. H., Chan, K. S., et al. (2004). Role of lopinavir/ritonavir in the treatment of SARS: initial virological and clinical findings. *Thorax* 59, 252–256. doi: 10.1136/thorax.2003.012658

Colella, P., Ronzitti, G., and Mingozzi, F. (2018). Emerging Issues in AAV-Mediated In Vivo Gene Therapy. *Mol. Ther. Methods Clin. Dev.* 8, 87–104. doi: 10.1016/j.omtm.2017.11.007

Coleman, C. M., Liu, Y. V., Mu, H., Taylor, J. K., Massare, M., Flyer, D. C., et al. (2014). Purified coronavirus spike protein nanoparticles induce coronavirus neutralizing antibodies in mice. *Vaccine* 32, 3169–3174. doi: 10.1016/j.vaccine.2014.04.016

Coleman, C. M., Venkataraman, T., Liu, Y. V., Glenn, G. M., Smith, G. E., Flyer, D. C., et al. (2017). MERS-CoV spike nanoparticles protect mice from MERS-CoV infection. *Vaccine* 35, 1586–1589. doi: 10.1016/j.vaccine.2017.02.012

Corman, V. M., Albarrak, A. M., Omrani, A. S., Albarrak, M. M., Farah, M. E., Almasri, M., et al. (2015). Viral shedding and antibody response in 37 patients with Middle East respiratory syndrome coronavirus infection. *Clin. Infect. Dis.* 62, 477–483. doi: 10.1093/cid/civ951

Corti, D., Passini, N., Lanzavecchia, A., and Zambon, M. (2016). Rapid generation of a human monoclonal antibody to combat Middle East respiratory syndrome. *J. Infect. Public Health* 9, 231–235. doi: 10.1016/j.jiph.2016.04.003

Corti, D., Zhao, J., Pedotti, M., Simonelli, L., Agnihothram, S., Fett, C., et al. (2015). Prophylactic and postexposure efficacy of a potent human monoclonal antibody against MERS coronavirus. *Proc. Natl. Acad. Sci. U.S.A.* 112, 10473–10478. doi: 10.1073/pnas.1510199112

Cotmore, S. F., Agbandje-McKenna, M., Chiorini, J. A., Mukha, D. V., Pintel, D. J., Qiu, J., et al. (2014). The family Parvoviridae. *Arch. Virol.* 159, 1239–1247. doi: 10.1007/s00705-013-1914-1911

Coughlin, M. M., and Prabhakar, B. S. (2012). Neutralizing human monoclonal antibodies to severe acute respiratory syndrome coronavirus: target, mechanism of action, and therapeutic potential. *Rev. Med. Virol.* 22, 2–17. doi: 10.1002/rmv.706

Czub, M., Weingartl, H., Czub, S., He, R., and Cao, J. (2005). Evaluation of modified vaccinia virus Ankara based recombinant SARS vaccine in ferrets. *Vaccine* 23, 2273–2279. doi: 10.1016/j.vaccine.2005.01.033

Danilczyk, U., and Penninger, J. M. (2006). Angiotensin-converting enzyme II in the heart and the kidney. *Circ. Res.* 98, 463–471. doi: 10.1161/01.RES.0000205761.22353.5f

De Clercq, E., Li, G., Clercq, E., and De. (2016). Approved antiviral drugs over the past 50 years. *Clin. Microbiol. Rev.* 29, 695–747. doi: 10.1128/CMR.00102-15. Address

De Wilde, A. H., Jochmans, D., Posthuma, C. C., Zevenhoven-Dobbe, J. C., Van Nieuwkoop, S., Bestebroer, T. M., et al. (2014). Screening of an FDA-approved compound library identifies four small-molecule inhibitors of Middle East respiratory syndrome coronavirus replication in cell culture. *Antimicrob. Agents Chemother.* 58, 4875–4884. doi: 10.1128/AAC.03011-3014

de Wit, E., Feldmann, F., Cronin, J., Jordan, R., Okumura, A., Thomas, T., et al. (2020). Prophylactic and therapeutic remdesivir (GS-5734) treatment in the rhesus macaque model of MERS-CoV infection. *Proc. Natl. Acad. Sci. U.S.A.* 117, 6771–6776. doi: 10.1073/pnas.1922083117

de Wit, E., Feldmann, F., Horne, E., Okumura, A., Cameroni, E., Haddock, E., et al. (2019). Prophylactic efficacy of a human monoclonal antibody against MERS-CoV in the common marmoset. *Antiviral Res.* 163, 70–74. doi: 10.1016/j.antiviral.2019.01.016

de Wit, E., Feldmann, F., Okumura, A., Horne, E., Haddock, E., Saturday, G., et al. (2018). Prophylactic and therapeutic efficacy of mAb treatment against MERS-CoV in common marmosets. *Antiviral Res.* 156, 64–71. doi: 10.1016/j.antiviral.2018.06.006

de Wit, E., Van Doremalen, N., Falzarano, D., and Munster, V. J. (2016). SARS and MERS: Recent insights into emerging coronaviruses. *Nat. Rev. Microbiol.* 14, 523–534. doi: 10.1038/nrmicro.2016.81

Deming, D., Sheahan, T., Heise, M., Yount, B., Davis, N., Sims, A., et al. (2006). Vaccine efficacy in senescent mice challenged with recombinant SARS-CoV bearing epidemic and zoonotic spike variants. *PLoS Med.* 3:e0030525. doi: 10.1371/journal.pmed.0030525

Deng, X., StJohn, S. E., Osswald, H. L., O'Brien, A., Banach, B. S., Sleeman, K., et al. (2014). Coronaviruses resistant to a 3C-like protease inhibitor are attenuated for replication and pathogenesis, revealing a low genetic barrier but high fitness cost of resistance. *J. Virol.* 88, 11886–11898. doi: 10.1128/jvi.01528-1514

Deng, Y., Lan, J., Bao, L., Huang, B., Ye, F., Chen, Y., et al. (2018). Enhanced protection in mice induced by immunization with inactivated whole viruses compare to spike protein of middle east respiratory syndrome coronavirus. *Emerg. Microbes Infect.* 7:60. doi: 10.1038/s41426-018-0056-57

Denison, M. R., Graham, R. L., Donaldson, E. F., Eckerle, L. D., and Baric, R. S. (2011). Coronaviruses: an RNA proofreading machine regulates replication fidelity and diversity. *RNA Biol.* 8, 270–279. doi: 10.4161/rna.8.2.15013

Dicaro, A., Li, Y., Strong, J. E., Aoki, F., Plummer, F., Jones, S. M., et al. (2004). Severe acute respiratory syndrome - related coronavirus is inhibited by interferon- a. *J. Infect. Dis.* 189, 1164–1167. doi: 10.1086/382597

Ding, Y., Wang, H., Shen, H., Li, Z., Geng, J., Han, H., et al. (2003). The clinical pathology of severe acute respiratory syndrome (SARS): a report from China. *J. Pathol.* 200, 282–289. doi: 10.1002/path.1440

Drake, J. W., and Holland, J. J. (1999). Mutation rates among RNA viruses. *Proc. Natl. Acad. Sci. U.S.A.* 96, 13910–13913. doi: 10.1073/pnas.96.24.13910

Drosten, C., Chiu, L. L., Panning, M., Leong, H. N., Preiser, W., Tam, J. S., et al. (2004). Evaluation of advanced reverse transcription-PCR assays and an alternative PCR target region for detection of severe acute respiratory syndrome-associated Coronavirus. *J. Clin. Microbiol.* 42, 2043–2047. doi: 10.1128/JCM.42.5.2043-2047.2004

Du, L., and Jiang, S. (2015). Middle East respiratory syndrome: current status and future prospects for vaccine development. *Expert Opin. Biol. Ther.* 15, 1647–1651. doi: 10.1517/14712598.2015.1092518

Du, L., Kou, Z., Ma, C., Tao, X., Wang, L., Zhao, G., et al. (2013). A truncated receptor-binding domain of MERS-CoV spike protein potently inhibits MERS-CoV infection and induces strong neutralizing antibody responses?: implication for developing therapeutics and vaccines. *PLoS One* 8:e0081587. doi: 10.1371/journal.pone.0081587

Du, L., Zhao, G., Chan, C. C. S., and Li, L. (2010). A 219-mer CHO-Expressing Receptor-Binding Domain. *Viral Immunol.* 23, 211–219. doi: 10.1089/vim.2009.0090

Du, L., Zhao, G., Lin, Y., Sui, H., Chan, C., Ma, S., et al. (2008). Intranasal vaccination of recombinant adeno-associated virus encoding receptor-binding domain of severe acute respiratory syndrome coronavirus (SARS-CoV) spike protein induces strong mucosal immune responses and provides long-term protection against SARS-. *J. Immunol.* 180, 948–956. doi: 10.4049/jimmunol.180.2.948

Du, L., Zhao, G., Yang, Y., Qiu, H., Wang, L., Kou, Z., et al. (2014). A conformation-dependent neutralizing monoclonal antibody specifically targeting receptor-binding domain in Middle East respiratory syndrome coronavirus spike protein. *J. Virol.* 88, 7045–7053. doi: 10.1128/jvi.00433-14

Eckerle, L. D., Becker, M. M., Halpin, R. A., Li, K., Venter, E., Lu, X., et al. (2010). Infidelity of SARS-CoV Nsp14-exonuclease mutant virus replication is revealed by complete genome sequencing. *PLoS Pathog.* 6:e1000896. doi: 10.1371/journal.ppat.1000896

Eckerle, L. D., Lu, X., Sperry, S. M., Choi, L., and Denison, M. R. (2007). High fidelity of murine hepatitis virus replication is decreased in nsp14 exoribonuclease mutants. *J. Virol.* 81, 12135–12144. doi: 10.1128/jvi.01296-1297

Excoffon, K. J. D. A., Koerber, J. T., Dickey, D. D., Murtha, M., Keshavjee, S., Kaspar, B. K., et al. (2009). Directed evolution of adeno-associated virus to an infectious respiratory virus. *Proc. Natl. Acad. Sci. U.S.A.* 106, 3865–3870. doi: 10.1073/pnas.0813365106

Falzarano, D., De Wit, E., Martellaro, C., Callison, J., Munster, V. J., and Feldmann, H. (2013a). Inhibition of novel β coronavirus replication by a combination of interferon-α2b and ribavirin. *Sci. Rep.* 3, 1–6. doi: 10.1038/srep01686

Falzarano, D., de Wit, E., Rasmussen, A. L., Feldmann, F., Okumura, A., Scott, D. P., et al. (2013b). Treatment with interferon-α2b and ribavirin improves outcome in MERS-CoV-infected rhesus macaques. *Nat. Med.* 19, 1313–1317. doi: 10.1038/nm.3362

Ferron, F., Subissi, L., Theresa, A., Morais, S. De, Thi, N., Le, T., et al. (2017). Structural and molecular basis of mismatch correction and ribavirin excision from coronavirus RNA. *Proc. Natl. Acad. Sci. U.S.A.* 115, E162–E171. doi: 10.1073/pnas.1718806115

Frieman, M., Heise, M., and Baric, R. (2008). SARS coronavirus and innate immunity. *Virus Res.* 133, 101–112. doi: 10.1016/j.virusres.2007.03.015

Fry, A. M., Goswami, D., Nahar, K., Sharmin, A. T., Rahman, M., Gubareva, L., et al. (2014). Efficacy of oseltamivir treatment started within 5 days of symptom onset to reduce infl uenza illness duration and virus shedding in an urban setting in Bangladesh?: a randomised placebo-controlled trial. *Lancet Infect. Dis.* 14, 109–118. doi: 10.1016/S1473-3099(13)70267-70266

Gao, J., Lu, G., Qi, J., Li, Y., Wu, Y., Deng, Y., et al. (2013). Structure of the fusion core and inhibition of fusion by a heptad repeat peptide derived from the S protein of middle east respiratory syndrome coronavirus. *J. Virol.* 87, 13134–13140. doi: 10.1128/jvi.02433-2413

Gierer, S., Müller, M. A., Heurich, A., Ritz, D., Springstein, B. L., Karsten, C. B., et al. (2014). Inhibition of proprotein convertases abrogates processing of the middle eastern respiratory syndrome coronavirus spike protein in infected cells but does not reduce viral infectivity. *J. Infect. Dis.* 211, 889–897. doi: 10.1093/infdis/jiu407

Goldstein, J. L., DeBose-Boyd, R. A., and Brown, M. S. (2006). Protein sensors for membrane sterols. *Cell* 124, 35–46. doi: 10.1016/j.cell.2005.12.022

Graham, B. S., and Ambrosino, D. M. (2015). History of passive antibody administration for prevention and treatment of infectious diseases. *Curr. Opin. HIV AIDS* 10, 129–134. doi: 10.1097/COH.0000000000000154

Graham, R. L., Becker, M. M., Eckerle, L. D., Bolles, M., Denison, M. R., and Baric, R. S. (2012). A live, impaired-fidelity coronavirus vaccine protects in an aged, immunocompromised mouse model of lethal disease. *Nat. Med.* 18, 1820–1826. doi: 10.1038/nm.2972

Graham, R. L., Deming, D. J., Deming, M. E., Yount, B. L., and Baric, R. S. (2018). Evaluation of a recombination-resistant coronavirus as a broadly applicable, rapidly implementable vaccine platform. *Commun. Biol.* 1:179. doi: 10.1038/s42003-018-0175-177

Gralinski, L. E., and Baric, R. S. (2015). Molecular pathology of emerging coronavirus infections. *J. Pathol.* 235, 185–195. doi: 10.1002/path.4454

Greenough, T. C., Babcock, G. J., Roberts, A., Hernandez, H. J., and Thomas, W. D. Jr. (2005). Development and characterization of a severe acute respiratory syndrome-associated coronavirus-neutralizing human monoclonal antibody that provides effective immunoprophylaxis in mice. *J. Infect. Dis.* 191, 507–514. doi: 10.1086/427242

Guo, X., Deng, Y., Chen, H., Lan, J., Wang, W., Zou, X., et al. (2015). Systemic and mucosal immunity in mice elicited by a single immunization with human adenovirus type 5 or 41 vector-based vaccines carrying the spike protein of Middle East respiratory syndrome coronavirus. *Immunology* 145, 476–484. doi: 10.1111/imm.12462

Haagmans, B. L., Kuiken, T., Martina, B. E., Fouchier, R. A. M., Rimmelzwaan, G. F., van Amerongen, G., et al. (2004). Pegylated interferon-α protects type 1 pneumocytes against SARS coronavirus infection in macaques. *Nat. Med.* 10, 290–293. doi: 10.1038/nm1001

Haagmans, B. L., van den Brand, J. M. A., Raj, V. S., Volz, A., Wohlsein, P., Smits, S. L., et al. (2016). An orthopoxvirus-based vaccine reduces virus excretion after MERS-CoV infection in dromedary camels. *Science* 351, 77–81. doi: 10.1126/science.aad1283

Hansel, T. T., Kropshofer, H., Singer, T., Mitchell, J. A., and George, A. J. T. (2010). The safety and side effects of monoclonal antibodies. *Nat. Rev. Drug Discov.* 9, 325–338. doi: 10.1038/nrd3003

Hapfelmeier, S., Lawson, M. A. E., Slack, E., Kirundi, J. K., Stoel, M., Heikenwalder, M., et al. (2010). Reversible microbial colonization of germ-free mice reveals the dynamics of IgA immune responses. *Science* 328, 1705–1709. doi: 10.1126/science.1188454

Harcourt, B. H., Jukneliene, D., Kanjanahaluethai, A., Bechill, J., Severson, K. M., Smith, C. M., et al. (2004). Identification of severe acute respiratory syndrome coronavirus replicase products and characterization of papain-like protease activity. *J. Virol.* 78, 13600–13612. doi: 10.1128/JVI.78.24.13600

Hart, B. J., Dyall, J., Postnikova, E., Zhou, H., Kindrachuk, J., Johnson, R. F., et al. (2014). Interferon-β and mycophenolic acid are potent inhibitors of middle east respiratory syndrome coronavirus in cell-based assays. *J. Gen. Virol.* 95, 571–577. doi: 10.1099/vir.0.061911-61910

Hashem, A. M., Algaissi, A., Agrawal, A. S., Al-Amri, S. S., Alhabbab, R. Y., Sohrab, S. S., et al. (2019). A highly immunogenic, protective, and safe adenovirus-based vaccine expressing middle east respiratory syndrome coronavirus S1-CD40L fusion protein in a transgenic human dipeptidyl peptidase 4 mouse model. *J. Infect. Dis.* 220, 1558–1567. doi: 10.1093/infdis/jiz137

Holshue, M. L., DeBolt, C., Lindquist, S., Lofy, K. H., Wiesman, J., Bruce, H., et al. (2020). First case of 2019 novel coronavirus in the United States. *N. Engl. J. Med.* 382, 929–936. doi: 10.1056/nejmoa2001191

Houser, K. V., Gretebeck, L., Ying, T., Wang, Y., Vogel, L., Lamirande, E. W., et al. (2016). Prophylaxis with a Middle East respiratory syndrome coronavirus (MERS-CoV)-specific human monoclonal antibody protects rabbits from MERS-CoV infection. *J. Infect. Dis.* 213, 1557–1561. doi: 10.1093/infdis/jiw080

Hsueh, P. R., Huang, L. M., Chen, P. J., Kao, C. L., and Yang, P. C. (2004). Chronological evolution of IgM, IgA, IgG and neutralisation antibodies after infection with SARS-associated coronavirus. *Clin. Microbiol. Infect.* 10, 1062–1066. doi: 10.1111/j.1469-0691.2004.01009.x

Hu, M. C., Jones, T., Kenney, R. T., Barnard, D. L., Burt, D. S., and Lowell, G. H. (2007). Intranasal Protollin-formulated recombinant SARS S-protein elicits respiratory and serum neutralizing antibodies and protection in mice. *Vaccine* 25, 6334–6340. doi: 10.1016/j.vaccine.2007.06.017

Huang, J. D., Zheng, B. J., and Sun, H. Z. (2008). Helicases as antiviral drug targets. *Hong Kong Med. J.* 14, 36–38.

Huentelman, M. J., Zubcevic, J., Hernández Prada, J. A., Xiao, X., Dimitrov, D. S., Raizada, M. K., et al. (2004). Sructure-based discovery of a novel angiotensin-converting enzyme 2 inhibitor. *Hypertension* 44, 903–906. doi: 10.1161/01.HYP.0000146120.29648.36

Hui, D. S., Azhar, I. E., Madani, T. A., Ntoumi, F., Kock, R., Dar, O., et al. (2020). The continuing 2019-nCoV epidemic threat of novel coronaviruses to global health — The latest 2019 novel coronavirus outbreak in Wuhan. *China Int. J. Infect. Dis.* 91, 264–266. doi: 10.1016/j.ijid.2020.01.009

Iwata-Yoshikawa, N., Uda, A., Suzuki, T., Tsunetsugu-Yokota, Y., Sato, Y., Morikawa, S., et al. (2014). Effects of toll-like receptor stimulation on eosinophilic infiltration in lungs of BALB/c mice immunized with UV-inactivated severe acute respiratory syndrome-related coronavirus vaccine. *J. Virol.* 88, 8597–8614. doi: 10.1128/jvi.00983-914

Jagger, B. W., Dowd, K. A., Chen, R. E., Desai, P., Foreman, B., Burgomaster, K. E., et al. (2019). Protective efficacy of nucleic acid vaccines against transmission of zika virus during pregnancy in mice. *J. Infect. Dis.* 220, 1577–1588. doi: 10.1093/infdis/jiz338

Jiaming, L., Yanfeng, Y., Yao, D., Yawei, H., Linlin, B., Baoying, H., et al. (2017). The recombinant N-terminal domain of spike proteins is a potential vaccine against Middle East respiratory syndrome coronavirus (MERS-CoV) infection. *Vaccine* 35, 10–18. doi: 10.1016/j.vaccine.2016.11.064

Jiang, L., Wang, N., Zuo, T., Shi, X., Poon, K.-M. M. V., Wu, Y., et al. (2014). Potent neutralization of MERS-CoV by human neutralizing monoclonal antibodies to the viral spike glycoprotein. *Sci. Transl. Med.* 6:234ra59. doi: 10.1126/scitranslmed.3008140

Johnson, R. F., Bagci, U., Keith, L., Tang, X., Mollura, D. J., Zeitlin, L., et al. (2016). 3B11-N, a monoclonal antibody against MERS-CoV, reduces lung pathology in rhesus monkeys following intratracheal inoculation of MERS-CoV Jordan-n3/2012. *Virology* 490, 49–58. doi: 10.1016/j.virol.2016.01.004

Kaemmerer, W. F. (2018). How will the field of gene therapy survive its success? *Bioeng. Transl. Med.* 3, 166–177. doi: 10.1002/btm2.10090

Kam, Y. W., Kien, F., Roberts, A., Cheung, Y. C., Lamirande, E. W., Vogel, L., et al. (2007). Antibodies against trimeric S glycoprotein protect hamsters against SARS-CoV challenge despite their capacity to mediate FcgammaRII-dependent entry into B cells *in vitro*. *Vaccine* 25, 729–740. doi: 10.1016/j.vaccine.2006.08.011

Kandeel, M. (2018). Bioinformatics analysis of the recent MERS-CoV with special reference to the virus-encoded Spike protein. *Mol. Enzymol. Drug Targets* 01, 1–10. doi: 10.21767/2572-5475.10001

Kapadia, S. U., Rose, J. K., Lamirande, E., Vogel, L., Subbarao, K., and Roberts, A. (2005). Long-term protection from SARS coronavirus infection conferred by a single immunization with an attenuated VSV-based vaccine. *Virology* 340, 174–182. doi: 10.1016/j.virol.2005.06.016

Kaplitt, M. G., Feigin, A., Tang, C., Fitzsimons, H. L., Mattis, P., Lawlor, P. A., et al. (2007). Safety and tolerability of gene therapy with an adeno-associated virus (AAV) borne GAD gene for Parkinson's disease: an open label, phase I trial. *Lancet* 369, 2097–2105. doi: 10.1016/S0140-6736(07)60982-60989

Karlberg, J., Chong, D. S. Y., and Lai, W. Y. Y. (2004). Do men have a higher case fatality rate of severe acute respiratory syndrome than women do? *Am. J. Epidemiol.* 159, 229–231. doi: 10.1093/aje/kwh056

Kay, M. A., Manno, C. S., Ragni, M. V., Larson, P. J., Couto, L. B., McClelland, A., et al. (2000). Evidence for gene transfer and expression of factor IX in haemophilia B patients treated with an AAV vector. *Nat. Genet.* 24, 257–261. doi: 10.1038/73464

Khalid, M., Al Rabiah, F., Khan, B., Al Mobeireek, A., Butt, T. S., and Al Mutairy, E. (2015). Ribavirin and interferon-alpha2b as primary and preventive treatment for Middle East respiratory syndrome coronavirus: a preliminary report of two cases. *Antivir. Ther.* 20, 87–91. doi: 10.3851/IMP2792

Khalid, M., Khan, B., Al Rabiah, F., Alismaili, R., Saleemi, S., Rehan-Khaliq, A. M., et al. (2014). Middle eastern respiratory syndrome corona virus (MERS CoV): case reports from a tertiary care hospital in Saudi Arabia. *Ann. Saudi Med.* 34, 396–400. doi: 10.5144/0256-4947.2014.396

Kim, E., Okada, K., Kenniston, T., Raj, V. S., AlHajri, M. M., Farag, E. A. B. A. B. A., et al. (2014). Immunogenicity of an adenoviral-based Middle East Respiratory syndrome coronavirus vaccine in BALB/c mice. *Vaccine* 32, 5975–5982. doi: 10.1016/j.vaccine.2014.08.058

Kim, U. J., Won, E.-J., Kee, S.-J., Jung, S.-I., and Jang, H.-C. (2016). Combination therapy with lopinavir/ritonavir, ribavirin and interferon-alpha for Middle East respiratory syndrome. *Antivir. Ther.* 21, 455–459. doi: 10.3851/IMP3002

Kirchdoerfer, R. N., Cottrell, C. A., Wang, N., Pallesen, J., Yassine, H. M., Turner, H. L., et al. (2016). Pre-fusion structure of a human coronavirus spike protein. *Nature* 531, 118–121. doi: 10.1038/nature17200

Kleine-Weber, H., Elzayat, T., Wang, L., Elzayat, M. T., Wang, L., Graham, B. S., et al. (2019). Mutations in the spike protein of Middle East respiratory syndrome coronavirus transmitted in Korea increase. *J. Virol.* 93, 1–14. doi: 10.1128/JVI.01381-1318

Ko, J.-H., Seok, H., Cho, S. Y., Ha, Y. E., Baek, J. Y., Kim, S. H., et al. (2018). Challenges of convalescent plasma infusion therapy in Middle East respiratory coronavirus infection: a single centre experience. *Antivir. Ther.* 23, 617–622. doi: 10.3851/IMP3243

Kobinger, G. P., Figueredo, J. M., Rowe, T., Zhi, Y., Gao, G., Sanmiguel, J. C., et al. (2007). Adenovirus-based vaccine prevents pneumonia in ferrets challenged with the SARS coronavirus and stimulates robust immune responses in macaques. *Vaccine* 25, 5220–5231. doi: 10.1016/j.vaccine.2007.04.065

Kumar, V., Shin, J. S., Shie, J. J., Ku, K. B., Kim, C., Go, Y. Y., et al. (2017). Identification and evaluation of potent Middle East respiratory syndrome coronavirus (MERS-CoV) 3CLPro inhibitors. *Antiviral Res.* 141, 101–106. doi: 10.1016/j.antiviral.2017.02.007

Lamirande, E. W., DeDiego, M. L., Roberts, A., Jackson, J. P., Alvarez, E., Sheahan, T., et al. (2008). A live attenuated severe acute respiratory syndrome coronavirus is immunogenic and efficacious in golden syrian hamsters. *J. Virol.* 82, 7721–7724. doi: 10.1128/jvi.00304-308

Lan, J., Deng, Y., Chen, H., Lu, G., Wang, W., Guo, X., et al. (2014). Tailoring subunit vaccine immunity with adjuvant combinations and delivery routes using the middle east respiratory coronavirus (MERS-CoV) receptor-binding domain as an antigen. *PLoS One* 9:e0112602. doi: 10.1371/journal.pone.0112602

Lan, J., Yao, Y., Deng, Y., Chen, H., Lu, G., Wang, W., et al. (2015). Recombinant receptor binding domain protein induces partial protective immunity in rhesus macaques against Middle East respiratory syndrome coronavirus challenge. *EBioMedicine* 2, 1438–1446. doi: 10.1016/j.ebiom.2015.08.031

Lau, S. K. P., Woo, P. C. Y., Yip, C. C. Y., Tse, H., Tsoi, H. W., Cheng, V. C. C., et al. (2006). Coronavirus HKU1 and other coronavirus infections in Hong Kong. *J. Clin. Microbiol.* 44, 2063–2071. doi: 10.1128/JCM.02614-2615

Lauring, A. S., and Andino, R. (2010). Quasispecies theory and the behavior of RNA viruses. *PLoS Pathog.* 6:e1001005. doi: 10.1371/journal.ppat.1001005

Laursen, N. S., Friesen, R. H. E., Zhu, X., Jongeneelen, M., Blokland, S., Vermond, J., et al. (2018). Universal protection against influenza infection by a multidomain antibody to influenza hemagglutinin. *Science* 362, 598–602. doi: 10.1126/science.aaq0620

Leist, S. R., and Baric, R. S. (2018). Giving the genes a shuffle: using natural variation to understand host genetic contributions to viral infections. *Trends Genet.* 34, 777–789. doi: 10.1016/j.tig.2018.07.005

Li, F. (2016). Structure, function, and evolution of coronavirus spike proteins. *Annu. Rev. Virol.* 3, 237–261. doi: 10.1146/annurev-virology-110615-142301

Li, W., Moore, M. J., Vasilieva, N., Sui, J., Wong, S. K., Berne, M. A., et al. (2003). Angiotensin-converting enzyme 2 is a functional receptor for the SARS coronavirus. *Nature* 426, 450–454. doi: 10.1038/nature02145

Li, W., Shi, Z., Yu, M., Ren, W., Smith, C., Epstein, J. H., et al. (2005). Bats are natural reservoirs of SARS-like coronaviruses. *Science* 310, 676–680. doi: 10.1126/science.1118391

Li, W., Zhang, L., Johnson, J. S., Zhijian, W., Grieger, J. C., Ping-Jie, X., et al. (2009). Generation of novel aav variants by directed evolution for improved cftr delivery to human ciliated airway epithelium. *Mol. Ther.* 17, 2067–2077. doi: 10.1038/mt.2009.155

Li, Y., Wan, Y., Liu, P., Zhao, J., Lu, G., Qi, J., et al. (2015). A humanized neutralizing antibody against MERS-CoV targeting the receptor-binding domain of the spike protein. *Cell Res.* 25, 1237–1249. doi: 10.1038/cr.2015.113

Lim, Y., Ng, Y., Tam, J., and Liu, D. (2016). Human coronaviruses: a review of virus-host interactions. *Diseases* 4, 26. doi: 10.3390/diseases4030026

Limberis, M. P., Adam, V. S., Wong, G., Gren, J., Kobasa, D., Ross, T. M., et al. (2013). Intranasal antibody gene transfer in mice and ferrets elicits broad protection against pandemic influenza. *Sci. Transl. Med.* 5:187ra72. doi: 10.1126/scitranslmed.3006729

Limberis, M. P., Tretiakova, A., Nambiar, K., Wong, G., Racine, T., Crosariol, M., et al. (2016). Adeno-associated virus serotype 9-expressed zmapp in mice confers protection against systemic and airway-acquired ebola virus infection. *J. Infect. Dis.* 214, 1975–1979. doi: 10.1093/infdis/jiw460

Limberis, M. P., Vandenberghe, L. H., Zhang, L., Pickles, R. J., and Wilson, J. M. (2009). Transduction efficiencies of novel AAV vectors in mouse airway epithelium in vivo and human ciliated airway epithelium in vitro. *Mol. Ther.* 17, 294–301. doi: 10.1038/mt.2008.261

Lin, A., and Balazs, A. B. (2018). Adeno-associated virus gene delivery of broadly neutralizing antibodies as prevention and therapy against hiv-1 11 medical and health sciences 1103 clinical sciences 11 medical and health sciences 1108 medical microbiology marit van Gils, m.j.vangils@amc. *Retrovirology* 15, 1–17. doi: 10.1186/s12977-018-0449-447

Lipkin, W. I., and Firth, C. (2013). Viral surveillance and discovery. *Curr. Opin. Virol.* 3, 199–204. doi: 10.1016/j.coviro.2013.03.010

Liu, Y. V., Massare, M. J., Barnard, D. L., Kort, T., Nathan, M., Wang, L., et al. (2011). Chimeric severe acute respiratory syndrome coronavirus (SARS-CoV) S glycoprotein and influenza matrix 1 efficiently form virus-like particles (VLPs) that protect mice against challenge with SARS-CoV. *Vaccine* 29, 6606–6613. doi: 10.1016/j.vaccine.2011.06.111

Lo, M. K., Jordan, R., Arvey, A., Sudhamsu, J., Shrivastava-Ranjan, P., Hotard, A. L., et al. (2017). GS-5734 and its parent nucleoside analog inhibit Filo-, Pneumo-, and Paramyxoviruses. *Sci. Rep.* 7, 1–7. doi: 10.1038/srep43395

Lokugamage, K. G., Yoshikawa-Iwata, N., Ito, N., Watts, D. M., Wyde, P. R., Wang, N., et al. (2008). Chimeric coronavirus-like particles carrying severe acute respiratory syndrome coronavirus (SCoV) S protein protect mice against challenge with SCoV. *Vaccine* 26, 797–808. doi: 10.1016/j.vaccine.2007.11.092

Loustaud-Ratti, V., Debette-Gratien, M., Jacques, J., Alain, S., Marquet, P., Sautereau, D., et al. (2016). Ribavirin: Past, present and future. *World J. Hepatol.* 8, 123–130. doi: 10.4254/wjh.v8.i2.123

Loutfy, M. R., Blatt, L. M., Siminovitch, K. A., Ward, S., Wolff, B., Lho, H., et al. (2003). Interferon alfacon-1 plus corticosteroids in severe acute respiratory syndrome: a preliminary study. *JAMA* 290, 3222–3228. doi: 10.1001/jama.290.24.3222

Lu, L., Liu, Q., Zhu, Y., Chan, K. H., Qin, L., Li, Y., et al. (2014). Structure-based discovery of Middle East respiratory syndrome coronavirus fusion inhibitor. *Nat. Commun.* 5:3067. doi: 10.1038/ncomms4067

Lu, R., Zhao, X., Li, J., Niu, P., Yang, B., Wu, H., et al. (2020). Genomic characterisation and epidemiology of 2019 novel coronavirus: implications for virus origins and receptor binding. *Lancet* 6736, 1–10. doi: 10.1016/S0140-6736(20)30251-30258

Luo, C.-M., Wang, N., Yang, X.-L., Liu, H.-Z., Zhang, W., Li, B., et al. (2018). Discovery of novel bat coronaviruses in south china that use the same receptor as middle east respiratory syndrome coronavirus. *J. Virol.* 92:e00116-18. doi: 10.1128/JVI.00116-118

Ma, C., Li, Y., Wang, L., Zhao, G., Tao, X., Tseng, C.-T. K., et al. (2014a). Intranasal vaccination with recombinant receptor-binding domain of MERS-CoV spike protein induces much stronger local mucosal immune responses than subcutaneous immunization: implication for designing novel mucosal MERS vaccines. *Vaccine* 32, 2100–2108. doi: 10.1016/j.vaccine.2014.02.004

Ma, C., Wang, L., Tao, X., Zhang, N., Yang, Y., Tseng, C.-T. K., et al. (2014b). Searching for an ideal vaccine candidate among different MERS coronavirus receptor-binding fragments—The importance of immunofocusing in subunit vaccine design. *Vaccine* 32, 6170–6176. doi: 10.1016/j.vaccine.2014.08.086

Mackenzie, J. S., and Jeggo, M. (2013). Reservoirs and vectors of emerging viruses. *Curr. Opin. Virol.* 3, 170–179. doi: 10.1016/j.coviro.2013.02.002

Mair-Jenkins, J., Saavedra-Campos, M., Baillie, J. K., Cleary, P., Khaw, F. M., Lim, W. S., et al. (2015). The effectiveness of convalescent plasma and hyperimmune immunoglobulin for the treatment of severe acute respiratory infections of viral etiology: a systematic review and exploratory meta-analysis. *J. Infect. Dis.* 211, 80–90. doi: 10.1093/infdis/jiu396

Malczyk, A. H., Kupke, A., Prüfer, S., Scheuplein, V. A., Hutzler, S., Kreuz, D., et al. (2015). A highly immunogenic and protective Middle East respiratory syndrome coronavirus vaccine based on a recombinant measles virus vaccine platform. *J. Virol.* 89, 11654–11667. doi: 10.1128/jvi.01815-15

Martin, J. E., Louder, M. K., Holman, L. S. A., Gordon, I. J., Enama, M. E., Larkin, B. D., et al. (2008). A SARS DNA vaccine induces neutralizing antibody and cellular immune responses in healthy adults in a Phase I clinical trial. *Vaccine* 26, 6338–6343. doi: 10.1016/j.vaccine.2008.09.026

Matsuyama, S., Shirato, K., Kawase, M., Terada, Y., Kawachi, K., Fukushi, S., et al. (2018). Middle East Respiratory syndrome coronavirus spike protein is not activated directly by cellular furin during viral entry into target cells. *J. Virol.* 92:e00683-18. doi: 10.1128/JVI.00683-618

Matteucci, E., and Giampietro, O. (2016). Dipeptidyl peptidase-4 (CD26): knowing the function before inhibiting the enzyme. *Curr. Med. Chem.* 4, 80–102. doi: 10.2174/978168108249311609 0005

McIntosh, K., Kapikian, A. Z., Turner, H. C., Hartley, J. W., Parrott, R. H., and Chanock, R. M. (1970). Seroepidemiologic studies of coronavirus infection in adults and children. *Am. J. Epidemiol.* 91, 585–592. doi: 10.1093/oxfordjournals.aje.a121171

Menachery, V. D., Gralinski, L. E., Mitchell, H. D., Dinnon, K. H., Leist, S. R., Yount, B. L., et al. (2017). Middle East respiratory syndrome coronavirus nonstructural protein 16 is necessary for interferon resistance and viral pathogenesis. *mSphere* 2, 1–12. doi: 10.1128/msphere.00346-317

Menachery, V. D., Gralinski, L. E., Mitchell, H. D., Dinnon, K. H., Leist, S. R., Yount, B. L., et al. (2018). Combination attenuation offers strategy for live attenuated coronavirus vaccines. *J. Virol.* 92, 1–15. doi: 10.1128/jvi.00710-718

Menachery, V. D., Yount, B. L., Debbink, K., Agnihothram, S., Gralinski, L. E., Plante, J. A., et al. (2015). A SARS-like cluster of circulating bat coronaviruses shows potential for human emergence. *Nat. Med.* 21, 1508–1513. doi: 10.1038/nm.3985

Menachery, V. D., Yount, B. L., Josset, L., Gralinski, L. E., Scobey, T., Agnihothram, S., et al. (2014). Attenuation and restoration of severe acute respiratory syndrome coronavirus mutant lacking 2'-o-methyltransferase activity. *J. Virol.* 88, 4251–4264. doi: 10.1128/jvi.03571-3513

Menachery, V. D., Yount, B. L., Sims, A. C., Debbink, K., Agnihothram, S. S., Gralinski, L. E., et al. (2016). SARS-like WIV1-CoV poised for human emergence. *Proc. Natl. Acad. Sci. U.S.A.* 113, 3048–3053. doi: 10.1073/pnas.1517719113

Millet, J. K., and Whittaker, G. R. (2014). Host cell entry of Middle East respiratory syndrome coronavirus after two-step, furin-mediated activation of the spike protein. *Proc. Natl. Acad. Sci. U.S.A.* 111, 15214–15219. doi: 10.1073/pnas.1407087111

Millet, J. K., and Whittaker, G. R. (2015). Host cell proteases: critical determinants of coronavirus tropism and pathogenesis. *Virus Res.* 202, 120–134. doi: 10.1016/j.virusres.2014.11.021

Millet, J. K., and Whittaker, G. R. (2018). Physiological and molecular triggers for SARS-CoV membrane fusion and entry into host cells. *Virology* 517, 3–8. doi: 10.1016/j.virol.2017.12.015

Min, J., Yu, D., Liang, W., Xu, R., Wang, Z., Fang, L., et al. (2004). Molecular evolution of the SARS coronavirus during the course of the SARS epidemic in China. *Science* 303, 1666–1669. doi: 10.1126/science.1092002

Mo, Y., and Fisher, D. (2016). A review of treatment modalities for Middle East Respiratory Syndrome. *J. Antimicrob. Chemother.* 71, 3340–3350. doi: 10.1093/jac/dkw338

Modjarrad, K., Roberts, C. C., Mills, K. T., Castellano, A. R., Paolino, K., Muthumani, K., et al. (2019). Safety and immunogenicity of an anti-Middle East respiratory syndrome coronavirus DNA vaccine: a phase 1, open-label, single-arm, dose-escalation trial. *Lancet Infect. Dis.* 19, 1013–1022. doi: 10.1016/S1473-3099(19)30266-X

Momattin, H., Mohammed, K., Zumla, A., Memish, Z. A., and Al-Tawfiq, J. A. (2013). Therapeutic Options for Middle East respiratory syndrome coronavirus (MERS-CoV) - possible lessons from a systematic review of SARS-CoV therapy. *Int. J. Infect. Dis.* 17, e792–e798. doi: 10.1016/j.ijid.2013.07.002

Mubarak, A., Alturaiki, W., and Hemida, M. G. (2019). Middle east respiratory syndrome coronavirus (mers-cov): infection, immunological response, and vaccine development. *J. Immunol. Res.* 2019, 1–11. doi: 10.1155/2019/6491738

Munster, V. J., Wells, D., Lambe, T., Wright, D., Fischer, R. J., Bushmaker, T., et al. (2017). Protective efficacy of a novel simian adenovirus vaccine against lethal MERS-CoV challenge in a transgenic human DPP4 mouse model. *NPJ Vaccines* 2, 1–3. doi: 10.1038/s41541-017-0029-21

Murphy, B. G., Perron, M., Murakami, E., Bauer, K., Park, Y., Eckstrand, C., et al. (2018). The nucleoside analog GS-441524 strongly inhibits feline infectious peritonitis (FIP) virus in tissue culture and experimental cat infection studies. *Vet. Microbiol.* 219, 226–233. doi: 10.1016/j.vetmic.2018.04.026

Muthumani, K., Falzarano, D., Reuschel, E. L., Tingey, C., Flingai, S., Villarreal, D. O., et al. (2015). A synthetic consensus anti-spike protein DNA vaccine induces protective immunity against Middle East respiratory syndrome coronavirus in nonhuman primates. *Sci. Transl. Med.* 7:301ra132. doi: 10.1126/scitranslmed.aac7462

Naso, M. F., Tomkowicz, B., Perry, W. L., and Strohl, W. R. (2017). Adeno-associated virus (AAV) as a vector for gene therapy. *BioDrugs* 31, 317–334. doi: 10.1007/s40259-017-0234-235

Neuman, B. W., Stein, D. A., Kroeker, A. D., Bestwick, R. K., Iversen, P. L., Moulton, H. M., et al. (2006). Inhibition and escape of SARS-CoV treated with antisense morpholino oligomers. *Adv. Exp. Med. Biol.* 581, 567–571. doi: 10.1007/978-0-387-33012-9_103

Nieto, K., and Salvetti, A. (2014). AAV vectors vaccines against infectious diseases. *Front. Immunol.* 5:5. doi: 10.3389/fimmu.2014.00005

Nyon, M. P., Du, L., Tseng, C.-T. K. T. K., Seid, C. A., Pollet, J., Naceanceno, K. S., et al. (2018). Engineering a stable CHO cell line for the expression of a MERS-coronavirus vaccine antigen. *Vaccine* 36, 1853–1862. doi: 10.1016/j.vaccine.2018.02.065

Oh, H. J., Gan, S. K., Bertoletti, A., and Tan, Y. (2012). Understanding the T cell immune response in SARS coronavirus infection. *Emerg. Microbes Infect.* 1:e23. doi: 10.1038/emi.2012.26

Olinger, G. G., Pettitt, J., Kim, D., Working, C., Bohorov, O., Bratcher, B., et al. (2012). Delayed treatment of Ebola virus infection with plant-derived monoclonal antibodies provides protection in rhesus macaques. *Proc. Natl. Acad. Sci. U.S.A.* 109, 18030–18035. doi: 10.1073/pnas.1213709109

Omrani, A. S., Saad, M. M., Baig, K., Bahloul, A., Abdul-Matin, M., Alaidaroos, A. Y., et al. (2014). Ribavirin and interferon alfa-2a for severe Middle East respiratory syndrome coronavirus infection: a retrospective cohort study. *Lancet Infect. Dis.* 14, 1090–1095. doi: 10.1016/S1473-3099(14)70920-X

Ou, X., Leary, H. A. O., and Broxmeyer, H. E. (2019). Review Article Implications of DPP4 modi fi cation of proteins that regulate stem / progenitor and more mature cell types. *Blood* 122, 161–170. doi: 10.1182/blood-2013-02-487470.X.O

Pallesen, J., Wang, N., Corbett, K. S., Wrapp, D., Kirchdoerfer, R. N., Turner, H. L., et al. (2017). Immunogenicity and structures of a rationally designed prefusion MERS-CoV spike antigen. *Proc. Natl. Acad. Sci. U.S.A.* 114, E7348–E7357. doi: 10.1073/pnas.1707304114

Pascal, K. E., Coleman, C. M., Mujica, A. O., Kamat, V., Badithe, A., Fairhurst, J., et al. (2015). Pre- and postexposure efficacy of fully human antibodies against Spike protein in a novel humanized mouse model of MERS-CoV infection. *Proc. Natl. Acad. Sci. U.S.A.* 112, 8738–8743. doi: 10.1073/pnas.1510830112

Payne, D. C., Iblan, I., Rha, B., Alqasrawi, S., Haddadin, A., Nsour, M., et al. (2016). Persistence of antibodies against Middle East respiratory syndrome coronavirus. *Emerg. Infect. Dis.* 22, 1824–1826.

Peck, K. M., Burch, C. L., Heise, M. T., and Baric, R. S. (2015). Coronavirus host range expansion and middle east respiratory syndrome coronavirus emergence: biochemical mechanisms and evolutionary perspectives. *Annu. Rev. Virol.* 2, 95–117. doi: 10.1146/annurev-virology-100114-155029

Pedersen, N. C., Perron, M., Bannasch, M., Montgomery, E., Murakami, E., Liepnieks, M., et al. (2019). Efficacy and safety of the nucleoside analog GS-441524 for treatment of cats with naturally occurring feline infectious peritonitis. *J. Feline Med. Surg.* 21, 271–281. doi: 10.1177/1098612X19825701

Peiris, J. S. M., Chu, C. M., Cheng, V. C. C., Chan, K. S. H., Hung, I. F. N., Poon, L. L. M., et al. (2003a). Clinical progression and viral load in a community outbreak of coronavirus-associated SARS pneumonia: a prospective study. *Lancet* 361, 1767–1772. doi: 10.1016/S0140-6736(03)13412-13415

Peiris, J. S. M., Lai, S. T., Poon, L. L. M., Guan, Y., Yam, L. Y. C., Lim, W., et al. (2003b). Coronavirus as a possible cause of severe acute respiratory syndrome. *Lancet* 361, 1319–1325. doi: 10.1016/S0140-6736(03)13077-13072

Perlman, S., and Netland, J. (2009). Coronaviruses post-SARS: update on replication and pathogenesis. *Nat. Rev. Microbiol.* 7, 439–450. doi: 10.1038/nrmicro2147

Perlman, S., and Vijay, R. (2016). Middle East respiratory syndrome vaccines. *Int. J. Infect. Dis.* 47, 23–28. doi: 10.1016/j.ijid.2016.04.008

Petrovsky, N. (2016). SARS coronavirus infections of the lower respiratory tract and their prevention. *Microbiol. Respir. Syst. Infect.* 2016, 45–53. doi: 10.1016/B978-0-12-804543-5.00003-8

Plotkin, S. A. (2010). Correlates of protection induced by vaccination. *Clin. Vaccine Immunol.* 17, 1055–1065. doi: 10.1128/CVI.00131-110

Prabakaran, P., Zhu, Z., Xiao, X., Biragyn, A., Dimitrov, A. S., Broder, C. C., et al. (2009). Potent human monoclonal antibodies against SARS CoV, Nipah and Hendra viruses. *Expert Opin. Biol. Ther.* 9, 355–368. doi: 10.1517/14712590902763755

Pyrc, K., Bosch, B. J., Berkhout, B., Jebbink, M. F., Dijkman, R., Rottier, P., et al. (2006). Inhibition of human coronavirus NL63 infection at early stages of the replication cycle. *Antimicrob. Agents Chemother.* 50, 2000–2008. doi: 10.1128/AAC.01598-1595

Qiu, H., Sun, S., Xiao, H., Feng, J., Guo, Y., Tai, W., et al. (2016). Single-dose treatment with a humanized neutralizing antibody affords full protection of a human transgenic mouse model from lethal Middle East respiratory syndrome (MERS)-coronavirus infection. *Antiviral Res.* 132, 141–148. doi: 10.1016/j.antiviral.2016.06.003

Qiu, X., Audet, J., Wong, G., Pillet, S., Bello, A., Cabral, T., et al. (2012). Successful treatment of ebola virus - infected cynomolgus macaques with monoclonal antibodies. *Sci. Transl. Med.* 4, 1–12.

Raj, V. S., Mou, H., Smits, S. L., Dekkers, D. H. W., Müller, M. A., Dijkman, R., et al. (2013). Dipeptidyl peptidase 4 is a functional receptor for the emerging human coronavirus-EMC. *Nature* 495, 251–254. doi: 10.1038/nature 12005

Raj, V. S., Okba, N. M. A., Gutierrez-Alvarez, J., Drabek, D., van Dieren, B., Widagdo, W., et al. (2018). Chimeric camel/human heavy-chain antibodies protect against MERS-CoV infection. *Sci. Adv.* 4, 1–10. doi: 10.1126/sciadv. aas9667

Raj, V. S., Osterhaus, A. D. M. E., Fouchier, R. A. M., and Haagmans, B. L. (2014). MERS: emergence of a novel human coronavirus. *Curr. Opin. Virol.* 5, 58–62. doi: 10.1016/j.coviro.2014.01.010

Reggiori, F., Monastyrska, I., Verheije, M. H., Calì, T., Ulasli, M., Bianchi, S., et al. (2010). Coronaviruses hijack the LC3-I-positive EDEMosomes, ER-derived vesicles exporting short-lived ERAD regulators, for replication. *Cell Host Microbe* 7, 500–508. doi: 10.1016/j.chom.2010.05.013

Reynard, O., Nguyen, X. N., Alazard-Dany, N., Barateau, V., Cimarelli, A., and Volchkov, V. E. (2015). Identification of a new ribonucleoside inhibitor of ebola virus replication. *Viruses* 7, 6233–6240. doi: 10.3390/v7122934

Rezaee, F., Linfield, D. T., Harford, T. J., and Piedimonte, G. (2017). Ongoing developments in RSV prophylaxis?: a clinician's analysis. *Curr. Opin. Virol.* 112781, 70–78. doi: 10.1016/j.coviro.2017.03.015

Richner, J. M., Himansu, S., Dowd, K. A., Butler, S. L., Salazar, V., Fox, J. M., et al. (2017). Modified mRNA vaccines protect against zika virus infection. *Cell* 168, 1114.e10–1125.e10. doi: 10.1016/j.cell.2017.02.017

Roberts, A., Lamirande, E. W., Vogel, L., Baras, B., Goossens, G., Knott, I., et al. (2010). Immunogenicity and protective efficacy in mice and hamsters of a β-propiolactone inactivated whole virus SARS-CoV vaccine. *Viral Immunol.* 23, 509–519. doi: 10.1089/vim.2010.0028

Rockx, B., Corti, D., Donaldson, E., Sheahan, T., Stadler, K., Lanzavecchia, A., et al. (2008). Structural basis for potent cross-neutralizing human monoclonal antibody protection against lethal human and zoonotic severe acute respiratory syndrome coronavirus challenge. *J. Virol.* 82, 3220–3235. doi: 10.1128/jvi. 02377-2377

Rothe, C., Schunk, M., Sothmann, P., Bretzel, G., Froeschl, G., Wallrauch, C., et al. (2020). Transmission of 2019-nCoV infection from an asymptomatic contact in Germany. *N. Engl. J. Med.* 382, 970–971. doi: 10.1056/nejmc2001468

Schindewolf, C., and Menachery, V. D. (2019). Middle east respiratory syndrome vaccine candidates: cautious optimism. *Viruses* 11:74. doi: 10.3390/v11010074

See, R. H., Petric, M., Lawrence, D. J., Mok, C. P. Y., Rowe, T., Zitzow, L. A., et al. (2008). Severe acute respiratory syndrome vaccine efficacy in ferrets: whole killed virus and adenovirus-vectored vaccines. *J. Gen. Virol.* 89, 2136–2146. doi: 10.1099/vir.0.2008/001891-1890

See, R. H., Zakhartchouk, A. N., Petric, M., Lawrence, D. J., Mok, C. P. Y., Hogan, R. J., et al. (2006). Comparative evaluation of two severe acute respiratory syndrome (SARS) vaccine candidates in mice challenged with SARS coronavirus. *J. Gen. Virol.* 87, 641–650. doi: 10.1099/vir.0.81579-81570

Seong, B. L. (2018). Chaperna-mediated assembly of ferritin-based middle east respiratory syndrome-coronavirus nanoparticles. *Front. Immunol.* 9:1093. doi: 10.3389/fimmu.2018.01093

Shalhoub, S., Farahat, F., Al-Jiffri, A., Simhairi, R., Shamma, O., Siddiqi, N., et al. (2015). IFN-α2a or IFN-β1a in combination with ribavirin to treat Middle East respiratory syndrome coronavirus pneumonia: a retrospective study. *J. Antimicrob. Chemother.* 70, 2129–2132. doi: 10.1093/jac/ dkv085

Sharif-Yakan, A., and Kanj, S. S. (2014). Emergence of MERS-CoV in the middle east: origins, transmission, treatment, and perspectives. *PLoS Pathog.* 10:e1004457. doi: 10.1371/journal.ppat.1004457

Sheahan, T. P., Sims, A. C., Graham, R. L., Menachery, V. D., Gralinski, L. E., Case, J. B., et al. (2017). Broad-spectrum antiviral GS-5734 inhibits both epidemic and zoonotic coronaviruses. *Sci. Transl. Med.* 9, 1–11. doi: 10.1126/scitranslmed. aal3653

Sheahan, T. P., Sims, A. C., Leist, S. R., Schäfer, A., Won, J., Brown, A. J., et al. (2020). Comparative therapeutic efficacy of remdesivir and combination lopinavir, ritonavir, and interferon beta against MERS-CoV. *Nat. Commun.* 11:222. doi: 10.1038/s41467-019-13940-13946

Shin, H. S., Kim, Y., Kim, G., Lee, J. Y., Jeong, I., Joh, J. S., et al. (2019). Immune responses to middle east respiratory syndrome coronavirus during the acute and convalescent phases of human infection. *Clin. Infect. Dis.* 68, 984–992. doi: 10.1093/cid/ciy595

Simmons, G., Gosalia, D. N., Rennekamp, A. J., Reeves, J. D., Diamond, S. L., and Bates, P. (2005). Inhibitors of cathepsin L prevent severe acute respiratory syndrome coronavirus entry. *Proc. Natl. Acad. Sci. U.S.A.* 102, 11876–11881. doi: 10.1073/pnas.0505577102

Smith, E. C., Blanc, H., Surdel, M. C., Vignuzzi, M., and Denison, M. R. (2013). Coronaviruses lacking exoribonuclease activity are susceptible to lethal mutagenesis: evidence for proofreading and potential therapeutics. *PLoS Pathog.* 9:e1003565. doi: 10.1371/journal.ppat.1003565

Snijder, E. J., van der Meer, Y., Zevenhoven-Dobbe, J., Onderwater, J. J. M., van der Meulen, J., Koerten, H. K., et al. (2006). Ultrastructure and origin of membrane vesicles associated with the severe acute respiratory syndrome coronavirus replication complex. *J. Virol.* 80, 5927–5940. doi: 10.1128/jvi.02501-2505

Song, F., Fux, R., Provacia, L. B., Volz, A., Eickmann, M., Becker, S., et al. (2013). Middle east respiratory syndrome coronavirus spike protein delivered by modified vaccinia virus ankara efficiently induces virus-neutralizing antibodies. *J. Virol.* 87, 11950–11954. doi: 10.1128/jvi.01672-1613

Spruth, M., Kistner, O., Savidis-Dacho, H., Hitter, E., Crowe, B., Gerencer, M., et al. (2006). A double-inactivated whole virus candidate SARS coronavirus vaccine stimulates neutralising and protective antibody responses. *Vaccine* 24, 652–661. doi: 10.1016/j.vaccine.2005.08.055

Stadler, K., Roberts, A., Becker, S., Vogel, L., Eickmann, M., Kolesnikova, L., et al. (2005). SARS vaccine protective in mice [2]. *Emerg. Infect. Dis.* 11, 1312–1314. doi: 10.3201/eid1108.041003

Stertz, S., Reichelt, M., Spiegel, M., Kuri, T., Martínez-Sobrido, L., García-Sastre, A., et al. (2007). The intracellular sites of early replication and budding of SARS-coronavirus. *Virology* 361, 304–315. doi: 10.1016/j.virol.2006.11.027

Strobel, B., Zuckschwerdt, K., Zimmermann, G., Mayer, C., Eytner, R., Rechtsteiner, P., et al. (2019). Standardized, Scalable, and Timely Flexible Adeno-Associated Virus Vector Production Using Frozen High-Density HEK-293 Cell Stocks and CELLdiscs. *Hum. Gene Ther. Methods* 30, 23–33. doi: 10.1089/hgtb.20 18.228

Sui, J., Li, W., Murakami, A., Tamin, A., Matthews, L. J., Wong, S. K., et al. (2004). Potent neutralization of severe acute respiratory syndrome (SARS) coronavirus by a human mAb to S1 protein that blocks receptor association. *Proc. Natl. Acad. Sci. U.S.A.* 101, 2536–2541. doi: 10.1073/pnas.0307140101

Sung, J. J. Y., Wu, A., Joynt, G. M., Yuen, K. Y., Lee, N., Chan, P. K. S., et al. (2004). Severe acute respiratory syndrome: report of treatment and outcome after a major outbreak. *Thorax* 59, 414–420. doi: 10.1136/thx.2003.014076

Tai, W., Wang, Y., Fett, C. A., Zhao, G., Li, F., Perlman, S., et al. (2017). Recombinant receptor-binding domains of multiple middle east respiratory syndrome coronaviruses (MERS-CoVs) induce cross-neutralizing antibodies against divergent human and camel MERS-CoVs and antibody escape mutants. *J. Virol.* 91:e01651-16. doi: 10.1128/JVI.01651-1616

Tai, W., Zhao, G., Sun, S., Guo, Y., Wang, Y., Tao, X., et al. (2016). A recombinant receptor-binding domain of MERS-CoV in trimeric form protects human dipeptidyl peptidase 4 (hDPP4) transgenic mice from MERS-CoV infection. *Virology* 499, 375–382. doi: 10.1016/j.virol.2016.10.005

Tan, E. L. C., Ooi, E. E., Lin, C. Y., Tan, H. C., Ling, A. E., Lim, B., et al. (2004). Inhibition of SARS coronavirus infection in vitro with clinically approved antiviral drugs. *Emerg. Infect. Dis.* 10, 581–586. doi: 10.3201/eid1004.030458

Tang, F., Quan, Y., Xin, Z., Wrammert, J., Ma, M., Lv, H., et al. (2019). Lack of peripheral memory B cell responses in recovered patients with severe acute respiratory syndrome: a six-year follow-up study. *J. Immunol.* 186, 7264–7268. doi: 10.4049/jimmunol.0903490

Tang, J., Zhang, N., Tao, X., Zhao, G., Guo, Y., Tseng, C. K., et al. (2015). Optimization of antigen dose for a receptor- binding domain-based subunit vaccine against MERS coronavirus. *Hum. Vaccines Immunother.* 11, 1244–1250. doi: 10.1080/21645515.2015.1021527

Tang, X. C., Agnihothram, S. S., Jiao, Y., Stanhope, J., Graham, R. L., Peterson, E. C., et al. (2014). Identification of human neutralizing antibodies against MERS-CoV and their role in virus adaptive evolution. *Proc. Natl. Acad. Sci. U.S.A.* 111, E2018–E2026. doi: 10.1073/pnas.1402074111

Ter Meulen, J., Bakker, A. B. H., Van Den Brink, E. N., Weverling, G. J., Martina, B. E. E., Haagmans, B. L., et al. (2004). Human monoclonal antibody as prophylaxis for SARS coronavirus infection in ferrets. *Lancet* 363, 2139–2141. doi: 10.1016/S0140-6736(04)16506-16509

Ter Meulen, J., Van Den Brink, E. N., Poon, L. L. M., Marissen, W. E., Leung, C. S. W., Cox, F., et al. (2006). Human monoclonal antibody combination against SARS coronavirus: synergy and coverage of escape mutants. *PLoS Med.* 3:e237. doi: 10.1371/journal.pmed.0030237

Tortorici, M. A., and Veesler, D. (2019). *Structural Insights into Coronavirus Entry*, 1st Edn. Amsterdam: Elsevier.

Traggiai, E., Becker, S., Subbarao, K., Kolesnikova, L., Uematsu, Y., Gismondo, M. R., et al. (2004). An efficient method to make human monoclonal antibodies from memory B cells: potent neutralization of SARS coronavirus. *Nat. Med.* 10, 871–875. doi: 10.1038/nm1080

Tse, L. V., Klinc, K. A., Madigan, V. J., Castellanos Rivera, R. M., Wells, L. F., Havlik, L. P., et al. (2017). Structure-guided evolution of antigenically distinct adeno-associated virus variants for immune evasion. *Proc. Natl. Acad. Sci. U.S.A.* 114, E4812–E4821. doi: 10.1073/pnas.1704766114

Tse, L. V., Moller-Tank, S., and Asokan, A. (2015). Strategies to circumvent humoral immunity to adeno-associated viral vectors. *Expert Opin. Biol. Ther.* 15, 845–855. doi: 10.1517/14712598.2015.1035645

Ura, T., Okuda, K., and Shimada, M. (2014). Developments in viral vector-based vaccines. *Vaccines* 2, 624–641. doi: 10.3390/vaccines2030624

Urakova, N., Kuznetsova, V., Crossman, D. K., Sokratian, A., Guthrie, D. B., Kolykhalov, A. A., et al. (2017). β-D- N 4 -hydroxycytidine is a potent anti-alphavirus compound that induces a high level of mutations in the viral genome. *J. Virol.* 92, 1–22. doi: 10.1128/jvi.01965-1917

van den Brink, E. N., ter Meulen, J., Cox, F., Jongeneelen, M. A. C., Thijsse, A., Throsby, M., et al. (2005). Molecular and biological characterization of human monoclonal antibodies binding to the spike and nucleocapsid proteins of severe acute respiratory syndrome coronavirus. *J. Virol.* 79, 1635–1644. doi: 10.1128/jvi.79.3.1635-1644.2005

van Doremalen, N., Falzarano, D., Ying, T., de Wit, E., Bushmaker, T., Feldmann, F., et al. (2017). Efficacy of antibody-based therapies against Middle East respiratory syndrome coronavirus (MERS-CoV) in common marmosets. *Antiviral Res.* 143, 30–37. doi: 10.1016/j.antiviral.2017.03.025

Volz, A., Kupke, A., Song, F., Jany, S., Fux, R., Shams-Eldin, H., et al. (2015). Protective efficacy of recombinant modified vaccinia virus ankara delivering middle east respiratory syndrome coronavirus spike glycoprotein. *J. Virol.* 89, 8651–8656. doi: 10.1128/jvi.00614-615

Walls, A. C., Xiong, X., Park, Y. J., Tortorici, M. A., Snijder, J., Quispe, J., et al. (2019a). Unexpected receptor functional mimicry elucidates activation of coronavirus fusion. *Cell* 176, 1026.e15–1039.e15. doi: 10.1016/j.cell.2018.12.028

Walls, A. C., Xiong, X., Rey, A., Park, Y., Corti, D., Veesler, D., et al. (2019b). Activation of coronavirus fusion unexpected receptor functional mimicry elucidates activation of coronavirus fusion. *Cell* 176, 1026–1039.

Wang, C., Zheng, X., Gai, W., Wong, G., Wang, H., Jin, H., et al. (2017a). Novel chimeric virus-like particles vaccine displaying MERS-CoV receptor-binding domain induce specific humoral and cellular immune response in mice. *Antiviral Res.* 140, 55–61. doi: 10.1016/j.antiviral.2016.12.019

Wang, C., Zheng, X., Gai, W., Zhao, Y., Gao, Y., Yang, S., et al. (2017b). MERS-CoV virus-like particles produced in insect cells induce specific humoural and cellular imminity in rhesus macaques. *Oncotarget* 8, 12686–12694.

Wang, Y., Tai, W., Yang, J., Zhao, G., Sun, S., Tseng, C.-T. K., et al. (2017). Receptor-binding domain of MERS-CoV with optimal immunogen dosage and immunization interval protects human transgenic mice from MERS-CoV infection. *Hum. Vaccin. Immunother.* 13, 1615–1624. doi: 10.1080/21645515.2017.1296994

Wang, L., Shi, W., Chappell, J. D., Joyce, M. G., Zhang, Y., Kanekiyo, M., et al. (2018). Importance of neutralizing monoclonal antibodies targeting multiple antigenic sites on the middle east respiratory syndrome coronavirus spike glycoprotein to avoid neutralization escape. *J. Virol.* 92, 1–21. doi: 10.1128/jvi.02002-2017

Wang, L., Shi, W., Joyce, M. G., Modjarrad, K., Zhang, Y., Leung, K., et al. (2015). Evaluation of candidate vaccine approaches for MERS-CoV. *Nat. Commun.* 6, 1–11. doi: 10.1038/ncomms8712

Wang, M., Cao, R., Zhang, L., Yang, X., Liu, J., Xu, M., et al. (2020). Remdesivir and chloroquine effectively inhibit the recently emerged novel coronavirus (2019-nCoV) *in vitro*. *Cell Res.* 30, 269–271. doi: 10.1038/s41422-020-0282-280

Wang, N., Rosen, O., Wang, L., Turner, H. L., Stevens, L. J., Corbett, K. S., et al. (2019). Structural Definition of a Neutralization-Sensitive Epitope on the MERS-CoV S1-NTD. *Cell Rep.* 28, 3395.e6–3405.e6. doi: 10.1016/j.celrep.2019.08.052

Wang, W., Chen, S., Liu, I., Kao, C., Chen, H., Chiang, B., et al. (2004). Temporal relationship of viral load, ribavirin, interleukin (IL)-6, IL-8, and clinical progression in patients with severe acute respiratory syndrome. *Clin. Infect. Dis.* 39, 1071–1075. doi: 10.1086/423808

Warimwe, G. M., Gesharisha, J., Carr, B. V., Otieno, S., Otingah, K., Wright, D., et al. (2016). Chimpanzee adenovirus vaccine provides multispecies protection against rift valley fever. *Sci. Rep.* 6, 1–7. doi: 10.1038/srep20617

White, J. M., and Whittaker, G. R. (2016). Fusion of enveloped viruses in endosomes. *Traffic* 17, 593–614. doi: 10.1111/tra.12389

Widagdo, W., Okba, N. M. A., Stalin Raj, V., and Haagmans, B. L. (2017). MERS-coronavirus: from discovery to intervention. *One Heal.* 3, 11–16. doi: 10.1016/j.onehlt.2016.12.001

Wirblich, C., Coleman, C. M., Kurup, D., Abraham, T. S., Bernbaum, J. G., Jahrling, P. B., et al. (2017). One-health: a safe, efficient, dual-use vaccine for humans and animals against middle east respiratory syndrome coronavirus and rabies virus. *J. Virol.* 91, 1–15.

Woo, P. C. Y., Lau, S. K. P., Huang, Y., and Yuen, K. Y. (2009). Coronavirus diversity, phylogeny and interspecies jumping. *Exp. Biol. Med.* 234, 1117–1127. doi: 10.3181/0903-MR-94

Woo, P. C. Y., Lau, S. K. P., Tsoi, H., Huang, Y., Poon, R. W. S., Chu, C., et al. (2005). Clinical and molecular epidemiological features of coronavirus HKU1-associated community-acquired pneumonia. *J. Infect. Dis.* 192, 1898–1907. doi: 10.1086/497151

World Health Organization [WHO] (2018). *WHO MERS Global Summary and Assessment of Risk*. Geneva: WHO.

Wrapp, D., Wang, N., Corbett, K. S., Goldsmith, J. A., Hsieh, C.-L., Abiona, O., et al. (2020). Cryo-EM structure of the 2019-nCoV spike in the prefusion conformation. *Science* 1263, 1260–1263. doi: 10.1126/science.abb2507

Wu, C. Y., Jan, J. T., Ma, S. H., Kuo, C. J., Juan, H. F., Cheng, Y. S. E., et al. (2004). Small molecules targeting severe acute respiratory syndrome human coronavirus. *Proc. Natl. Acad. Sci. U.S.A.* 101, 10012–10017. doi: 10.1073/pnas.0403596101

Xia, S., Yan, L., Xu, W., Agrawal, A. S., Algaissi, A., Tseng, C. T. K., et al. (2019). A pan-coronavirus fusion inhibitor targeting the HR1 domain of human coronavirus spike. *Sci. Adv.* 5:eaav4580. doi: 10.1126/sciadv.aav4580

Xu, J., Jia, W., Wang, P., Zhang, S., Shi, X., Wang, X., et al. (2019). Antibodies and vaccines against Middle East respiratory syndrome coronavirus. *Emerg. Microbes Infect.* 8, 841–856. doi: 10.1080/22221751.2019.1624482

Yang, Z. Y., Kong, W. P., Huang, Y., Roberts, A., Murphy, B. R., Subbarao, K., et al. (2004). A DNA vaccine induces SARS coronavirus neutralization and protective immunity in mice. *Nature* 428, 561–564. doi: 10.1038/nature02463

Ying, T., Du, L., Ju, T. W., Prabakaran, P., Lau, C. C. Y., Lu, L., et al. (2014). Exceptionally potent neutralization of middle east respiratory syndrome coronavirus by human monoclonal antibodies. *J. Virol.* 88, 7796–7805. doi: 10.1128/jvi.00912-914

Ying, T., Prabakaran, P., Du, L., Shi, W., Feng, Y., Wang, Y., et al. (2015). Junctional and allele-specific residues are critical for MERS-CoV neutralization by an exceptionally potent germline-like antibody. *Nat. Commun.* 6:8223. doi: 10.1038/ncomms9223

Yong, C. Y., Ong, H. K., Yeap, S. K., Ho, K. L., and Tan, W. S. (2019). Recent advances in the vaccine development against middle east respiratory syndrome-coronavirus. *Front. Microbiol.* 10:1781. doi: 10.3389/fmicb.2019.01781

Yoon, J. J., Toots, M., Lee, S., Lee, M. E., Ludeke, B., Luczo, J. M., et al. (2018). Orally efficacious broad-spectrum ribonucleoside analog inhibitor of influenza and respiratory syncytial viruses. *Antimicrob. Agents Chemother.* 62, 1–18. doi: 10.1128/AAC.00766-718

Yuan, S., Chu, H., Chan, J. F. W., Ye, Z. W., Wen, L., Yan, B., et al. (2019). SREBP-dependent lipidomic reprogramming as a broad-spectrum antiviral target. *Nat. Commun.* 10:120. doi: 10.1038/s41467-018-08015-x

Yuan, Y., Cao, D., Zhang, Y., Ma, J., Qi, J., Wang, Q., et al. (2017). Cryo-EM structures of MERS-CoV and SARS-CoV spike glycoproteins reveal the dynamic receptor binding domains. *Nat. Commun.* 8:15092. doi: 10.1038/ncomms15092

Zabner, J., Seiler, M., Walters, R., Kotin, R. M., Fulgeras, W., Davidson, B. L., et al. (2000). Adeno-associated virus type 5 (AAV5) but not AAV2 binds to the apical surfaces of airway epithelia and facilitates gene transfer. *J. Virol.* 74, 3852–3858. doi: 10.1128/JVI.74.8.3852-3858.2000

Zhang, C., Maruggi, G., Shan, H., and Li, J. (2019). Advances in mRNA vaccines for infectious diseases. *Front. Immunol.* 10:594. doi: 10.3389/fimmu.2019.00594

Zhang, N., Channappanavar, R., Ma, C., Wang, L., Tang, J., Garron, T., et al. (2016). Identification of an ideal adjuvant for receptor-binding domain-based subunit vaccines against Middle East respiratory syndrome coronavirus. *Cell. Mol. Immunol.* 13, 180–190. doi: 10.1038/cmi.2015.03

Zhang, N., Jiang, S., and Du, L. (2014). Current advancements and potential strategies in the development of MERS-CoV vaccines. *Expert Rev. Vaccines* 13, 761–774. doi: 10.1586/14760584.2014.912134

Zhao, G., He, L., Sun, S., Qiu, H., Tai, W., Chen, J., et al. (2018). A novel nanobody targeting middle east respiratory syndrome coronavirus (MERS-CoV) receptor-binding domain has potent cross-neutralizing activity and protective efficacy against MERS-CoV. *J. Virol.* 92:e00837-18. doi: 10.1128/JVI.00837-818

Zhao, J., Alshukairi, A. N., Baharoon, S. A., Ahmed, W. A., Bokhari, A. A., Nehdi, A. M., et al. (2017). Recovery from the Middle East respiratory syndrome is associated with antibody and T cell responses. *Sci. Immunol.* 5393, 1–11.

Zhao, J., Perera, R. A. P. M., Kayali, G., Meyerholz, D., Perlman, S., and Peiris, M. (2015). Passive immunotherapy with dromedary immune serum in an experimental animal model for middle east respiratory syndrome. *J. Virol.* 89, 6117–6120. doi: 10.1128/JVI.00446-415

Zhao, J., Zhao, J., and Perlman, S. (2010). T cell responses are required for protection from clinical disease and for virus clearance in severe acute respiratory syndrome coronavirus-infected mice ?. *J. Virol.* 84, 9318–9325. doi: 10.1128/JVI.01049-1010

Zhao, J. J. J., Zhao, J. J. J., Mangalam, A. K., Channappanavar, R., Fett, C., Meyerholz, D. K., et al. (2016). Airway memory CD4+ T cells mediate protective immunity against emerging respiratory coronaviruses. *Immunity* 44, 1379–1391. doi: 10.1016/j.immuni.2016.05.006

Zhou, P., Yang, X.-L., Wang, X.-G., Hu, B., Zhang, L., Zhang, W., et al. (2020). A pneumonia outbreak associated with a new coronavirus of probable bat origin. *Nature* 579, 270–273. doi: 10.1038/s41586-020-2012-2017

Zhu, Z., Chakraborti, S., He, Y., Roberts, A., Sheahan, T., Xiao, X., et al. (2007). Potent cross-reactive neutralization of SARS coronavirus isolates by human monoclonal antibodies. *Proc. Natl. Acad. Sci. U.S.A.* 104, 12123–12128. doi: 10.1073/pnas.0701000104

Ziebuhr, J., Snijder, E. J., and Gorbalenya, A. E. (2000). Virus-encoded proteinases and proteolytic processing in the nidovirales. *J. Gen. Virol.* 81(Pt 4), 853–879.

Zumla, A., Chan, J. F. W. W., Azhar, E. I., Hui, D. S. C. C., and Yuen, K. Y. (2016a). Coronaviruses-drug discovery and therapeutic options. *Nat. Rev. Drug Discov.* 15, 327–347. doi: 10.1038/nrd.20 15.37

Zumla, A., Hui, D. S., Perlman, S., To, C., and Stanley, P. (2015). Middle east respiratory syndrome HHS public access. *Lancet* 386, 995–1007. doi: 10.1016/S0140-6736(15)60454-60458

Zumla, A., Rao, M., Wallis, R. S., Kaufmann, S. H. E., Rustomjee, R., Mwaba, P., et al. (2016b). Host-directed therapies for infectious diseases: current status, recent progress, and future prospects. *Lancet Infect. Dis.* 16, e47–e63. doi: 10. 1016/S1473-3099(16)00078-75

10

Designing a B Cell-Based Vaccine Against a Highly Variable Hepatitis C Virus

Thomas R. Fuerst[1,2], Brian G. Pierce[1,2], Zhen-Yong Keck[3] and Steven K. H. Foung[3*]*

[1] *Institute for Bioscience and Biotechnology Research, University of Maryland, Rockville, MD, United States,* [2] *Department of Cell Biology and Molecular Genetics, University of Maryland, College Park, MD, United States,* [3] *Department of Pathology, Stanford University School of Medicine, Stanford, CA, United States*

***Correspondence:**
Thomas R. Fuerst
tfuerst@umd.edu
Steven K. H. Foung
sfoung@stanford.edu

The ability to use structure-based design and engineering to control the molecular shape and reactivity of an immunogen to induce protective responses shows great promise, along with corresponding advancements in vaccine testing and evaluation systems. We describe in this review new paradigms for the development of a B cell-based HCV vaccine. Advances in test systems to measure *in vitro* and *in vivo* antibody-mediated virus neutralization include retroviral pseudotype particles expressing HCV E1E2 glycoproteins (HCVpp), infectious cell culture-derived HCV virions (HCVcc), and surrogate animal models mimicking acute HCV infection. Their applications have established the role of broadly neutralizing antibodies to control HCV infection. However, the virus has immunogenic regions in the viral envelope glycoproteins that are associated with viral escape or non-neutralizing antibodies. These regions serve as immunologic decoys that divert the antibody response from less prominent conserved regions mediating virus neutralization. This review outlines the immunogenic regions on E2, which are roughly segregated into the hypervariable region 1 (HVR1), and five clusters of overlapping epitopes designated as antigenic domains A-E. Understanding the molecular architecture of conserved neutralizing epitopes within these antigenic domains, and how other antigenic regions or decoys deflect the immune response from these conserved regions will provide a roadmap for the rational design of an HCV vaccine.

Keywords: hepatitis C virus, vaccine design, epitopes, virus neutralization, antigenic domains, human monoclonal antibodies

INTRODUCTION

Chronic hepatitis C virus (HCV) infection often leads to chronic hepatitis, liver failure and hepatocellular carcinoma (Mohd Hanafiah et al., 2013). The virus has infected 3% of the global population with an annual rate of 3–4 million new infections. The number of deaths associated with HCV infection in the United States has been increasing, and it is the primary indication for liver transplantation in the Western world (Rosen, 2011; Ly et al., 2016). While advances in HCV treatment with direct-acting antivirals (DAA) have led to cure rates over 90% with HCV treatment, high costs limit access to these drugs in developing and in developed countries (Cox and Thomas, 2013; Callaway, 2014; Chung and Baumert, 2014). Diagnosis of HCV infection often occurs at a late stage and successful DAA treatment will not alter the risk for cancer. DAA treatment is also less successful with genotype 3 infection, decompensated liver disease and transplant recipients. In addition, reinfection remains a problem even after successful treatment in subjects with continued at risk behavior such as injection drug use. For these reasons, an effective prophylactic vaccine is needed.

The genetic diversity of HCV of at least seven HCV genotypes that differ up to 30% in nucleotide sequence, which can be further subdivided into 67 subtypes (Tarr et al., 2015), poses a major challenge to develop a pan-genotypic vaccine (Walker, 2017). Another hurdle is that immune correlates of protection have yet to be defined for HCV. Nonetheless, B cell immunity contributes to the host defense against HCV infection, although it is more complex than sterilizing immunity as observed for hepatitis A, B and E vaccines (Walker, 2017). During acute infection, a robust neutralizing antibody response correlates with spontaneous resolution of infection (Saito et al., 1990; Lavillette et al., 2005; Pestka et al., 2007; Dowd et al., 2009; Lawitz et al., 2013; Osburn et al., 2014; Walker and Grakoui, 2015). Passive immunization with anti-HCV antibodies before HCV challenge prevented infection in animal models (Farci et al., 1996; Law et al., 2008; Dorner et al., 2011; Morin et al., 2012; Bukh et al., 2015). However, passive immunization of chimpanzees with antibodies that neutralized infectivity of several HCV genotypes in cell culture only delayed infection with homologous virus challenge and failed to protect against heterologous virus strains (Bukh et al., 2015). Other complicating factors for vaccine development include viral envelope proteins of low immunogenicity as suggested by a slow antibody response during acute infection (Logvinoff et al., 2004; Dowd et al., 2009; Liang, 2013) and antibody responses directed at regions of the viral envelope that have a high mutational rate of change (Weiner et al., 1992; Shimizu et al., 1994). In addition, antibody responses in an infected individual tend to lag behind the contemporaneous strains of virus in circulation (von Hahn et al., 2007).

Making it more challenging, accessibility to specific antigenic regions and the induction of neutralizing antibodies to these regions can be hindered by glycan shielding (Helle et al., 2007, 2010). Moreover, direct cell-to-cell transmission of the virus, circulating virions in complex with lipoproteins and downregulation of major histocompatibility complex (MHC) expression are other mechanisms for the virus to escape protective immunity (For review see, André et al., 2002; Cashman et al., 2014; Dunlop et al., 2015; Pierce et al., 2016a). Development of an effective vaccine for HCV must consider these factors.

CHALLENGES OF ANTIGENICALLY VARIABLE VIRUSES

The genetic diversity of HCV is high and commensurate with other antigenically variable viruses. Based on alignments of amino acid reference sequences (represented as phylogenetic trees in **Figure 1**), HCV shows 23% median sequence divergence within genotypes and 33% divergence across genotypes. In contrast, HIV gp120/gp41 (env) has moderately lower sequence variability with 21% median divergence within subtypes and 28% across subtypes, while influenza A virus hemagglutinin has lower variability within hemagglutinin subtype (5%), and much higher sequence variability across subtypes (58%). While specific percent divergence values can vary somewhat based on composition of reference sets, there are clear distinctions in overall glycoprotein sequence diversity among these viruses. Within an infected host, HCV actively avoids immune surveillance (von Hahn et al., 2007) and evolves into a large number of quasispecies through error-prone replication (Tarr et al., 2015) that have up to 10% sequence variations (Simmonds et al., 2005). The lack of proofreading capacity by the viral polymerase leads to a mutational rate of 10^{-5}-10^{-4} nucleotides per replication cycle that is a magnitude higher than that for HIV and HBV (Duffy et al., 2008).

Critical to the development of an effective vaccine is the identification and characterization of conserved epitopes associated with viral neutralization, particularly in the E1 and E2 glycoproteins that are the primary neutralizing antibody (nAb) targets (Ball et al., 2014). The E1 and E2 glycoproteins form a heterodimer (E1E2) (Vieyres et al., 2014), and recent evidence suggests that E1 forms trimers on the virion, mediated by the E1 transmembane region, resulting in higher order assemblies containing three E1E2 heterodimers (Falson et al., 2015). These glycoproteins are associated with viral entry via interactions with several cellular receptors, including scavenger receptor class B type 1 (SR-B1) (Scarselli et al., 2002; Fauvelle et al., 2016) and the tetraspanin CD81 (Pileri et al., 1998), as well as fusion with the endosomal membrane once the virus has been internalized by clathrin-mediated endocytosis (Lindenbach and Rice, 2013). The underlying genetic variability occurs despite the requirement for essential interactions between the envelope glycoproteins and cellular receptors necessary for viral entry, and such interactions have been mapped to highly conserved residues in the E2 protein (Drummer et al., 2006; Owsianka et al., 2006; Grove et al., 2008; Rothwangl et al., 2008).

The sequence variability of E1 and E2 is not uniform within the protein coding regions (Pierce et al., 2016a). As shown in **Figure 2**, E1 and E2 include pronounced regions of high amino acid conservation, as well as other regions with considerable sequence variability; the latter category includes hypervariable region 1 (HVR1, aa 384-410), hypervariable region 2 (HVR2, aa 460-485), and intergenotypic variable region (igVR, aa 570-580) on E2. HVR1 (highlighted in **Figure 2**) is located at the N-terminus of E2 and is under constant immunological pressure. HVR1 serves as a major "immunologic decoy" of the virus (Weiner et al., 1992; Dowd et al., 2009). Other regions of E2 exhibit moderate to complete sequence conservation such as residues 412-423 (antigenic domain E, highlighted in **Figure 2**) which contains linear epitopes targeted by well-characterized broadly nAbs (Owsianka et al., 2005; Broering et al., 2009; Keck et al., 2013), and residues 441-443 and 523-535 which have been reported to be important for recognition of host entry receptors and broadly neutralizing antibodies (Keck et al., 2008, 2012).

MAPPING ANTIGENIC DETERMINANTS OF BROAD VIRUS NEUTRALIZATION

Cross-competition analyses and epitope mapping of broadly neutralizing human monoclonal antibodies (HMAbs) derived

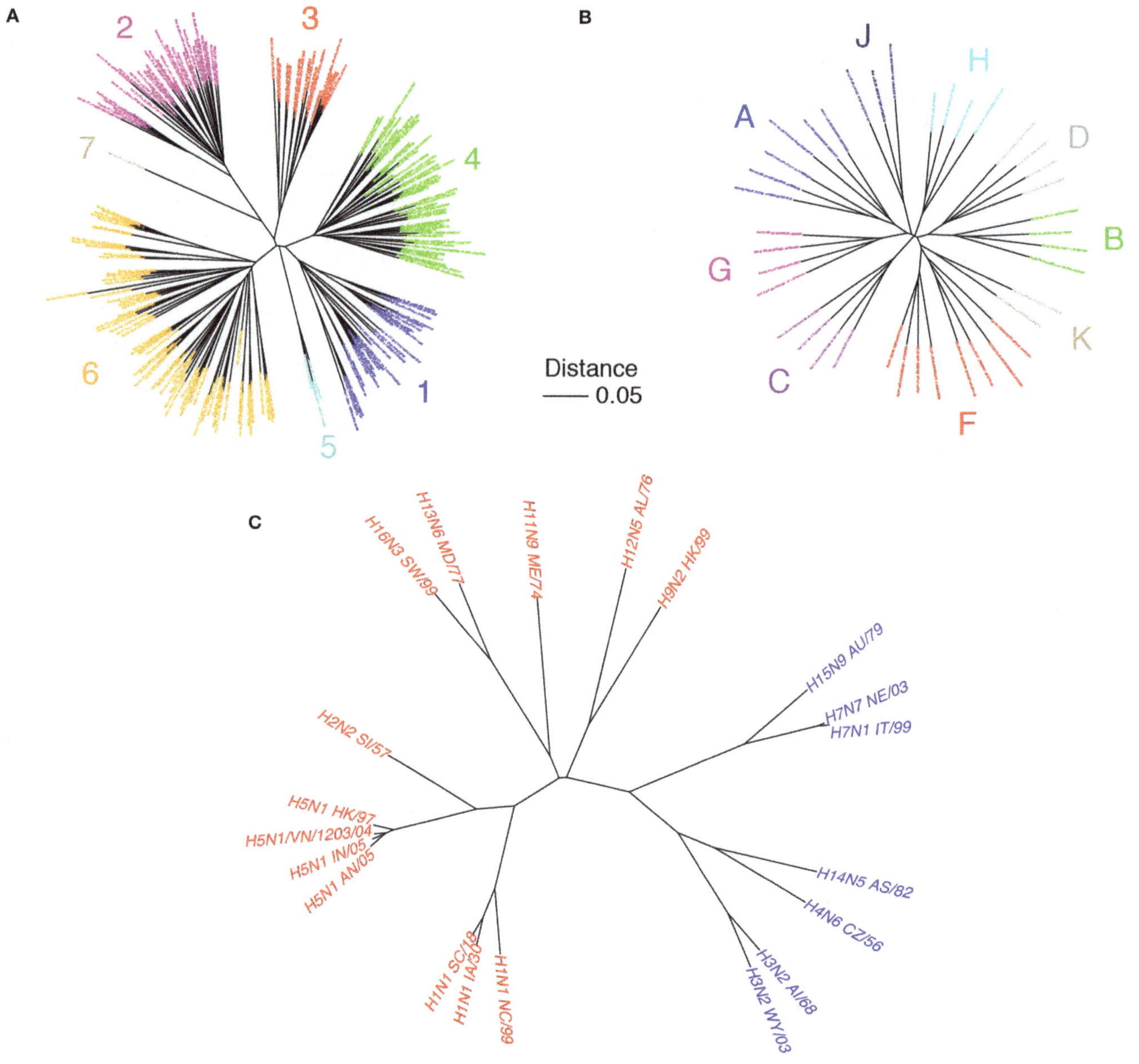

FIGURE 1 | Sequence variability of HCV in comparison with other viruses. Phylogenetic trees of HCV E1E2 **(A)**, HIV env (gp41/gp120; **B**), and influenza hemagglutinin (HA; **C**) are shown. E1E2 amino acid reference sequences (*N* = 204) were downloaded from the LANL HCV database (Kuiken et al., 2005), HIV env reference sequences (*N* = 39) were downloaded from the LANL HIV database (http://www.hiv.lanl.gov), and influenza A HA clones were from Corti et al. (2011), with amino acid sequences downloaded from the Influenza Research Database (Zhang et al., 2017). Multiple sequence alignments were performed using MAFFT software (Katoh and Standley, 2013). Phylogenetic trees were built using the neighbor joining method, and visualized using the APE package (Paradis et al., 2004) in R. Sequence names are labeled, and are colored according to HCV genotype **(A)**, HIV subtype **(B)**, and influenza group (**C**; red = group 1, blue = group 2). Scale bar represents 5% sequence divergence.

from B cells of subjects with chronic HCV infections have identified at least seven clusters of overlapping epitopes on HCV E1E2. Four clusters, designated as antigenic domains A-D, are composed of conformational epitopes on E2 (**Table 1**) (Keck et al., 2012). Two additional clusters, designated as antigenic regions (AR) 4 and 5, are composed of conformational epitopes on E1E2 (Kong et al., 2012); representative antibodies AR4A and AR5A had binding determinants mapped to residues in both E1 and E2 using alanine scanning, and did not engage soluble E2 or denatured E1E2 (Kong et al., 2012). It should be noted that the major antigenic region on E2, designated as AR3, overlaps substantially with antigenic domain B by cross-competition and epitope mapping studies (Law et al., 2008). Interestingly, AR5 overlaps with an antigenic domain C HMAb,

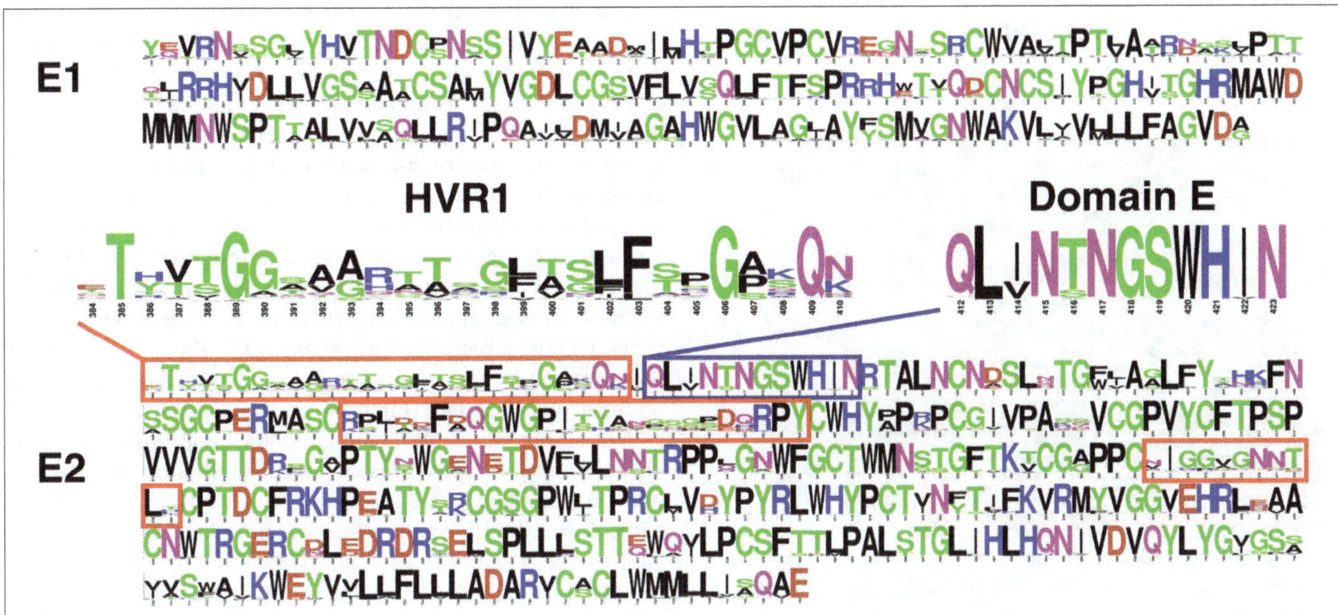

FIGURE 2 | Amino acid sequence variability of HCV envelope glycoproteins E1 and E2 Sequence logos (Crooks et al., 2004) were generated using a multiple sequence alignment of approximately 400 complete E1E2 amino acid sequences downloaded from the Los Alamos HCV database (Kuiken et al., 2005). This gives amino acid propensities at each E1 and E2 position (residues 192-383 and 384-746, respectively, based on the H77 isolate numbering), with total height at each position representing sequence conservation (more variable positions have lower height). Hypervariable regions of E2 are shown in red boxes, and hypervariable region 1 (HVR1; aa 384-410) is highlighted. Antigenic domain E (aa 412-423) is shown in blue box and highlighted. Figure adapted from Pierce et al. (2016a).

TABLE 1 | E2 antigenic domains, representative monoclonal antibodies, and representative structures of antibody-epitope complexes in the Protein Data Bank (PDB) (Rose et al., 2011).

Antigenic domain	Residues	Antibodies	PDB structures
HVR1	384-410	H77.16	–
A	581-584, 627-633	CBH-4D, CBH-4G, CBH-20	–
B	431-439, 529-535	HC-1, HC-11, CBH-5, AR3C	4MWF (Kong et al., 2013)
C	544-549	CBH-7, CBH-23	–
D	420-428, 441-443	HC84.1, HC84.26	4JZN (Krey et al., 2013), 4JZO (Krey et al., 2013)
E	412-423	HCV1, AP33, HC33.1	4DGY (Kong et al., 2012), 4GAJ (Potter et al., 2012), 4XVJ (Li et al., 2015)

CBH-7, by competition analysis and epitope mapping, although CBH-7 binds to E2 and does not require E1 (Giang et al., 2012). A seventh cluster of broadly neutralizing antibodies contains overlapping linear epitopes that are located adjacent to HVR1 on E2. This cluster is designated as antigenic domain E and encompasses amino acids 412-423 (Keck et al., 2014). In addition, there are several sites on E1 alone that have been identified as epitopes of neutralizing monoclonal antibodies, including the E1 N-terminus (aa 192-202) which is targeted by antibody H-111 (Keck et al., 2004), and a separate site (aa 313-328) targeted by HMAbs IGH505 and IGH526 (Meunier et al., 2008), the latter of which was characterized structurally in complex with its E1 epitope (Kong et al., 2015b).

Global alanine scanning of E2 has recently been reported using E2-binding HMAbs and site-directed mutagenesis of the E1E2 coding sequence, and ELISA readout assays to compare mutant binding levels to wild-type (**Figure 3**; Pierce et al., 2016b). This analysis provided many new insights into the E2 3D structure and determinants of antibody recognition. Although some key binding residues were located on the E2 surface, a large portion of them were buried in E2 core structures (Kong et al., 2013; Khan et al., 2014), including cysteines in disulfide bonds and large hydrophobic residues. These residues are not likely to contact the antibodies directly but rather influence recognition through effects on E2 local or global stability. Computational alanine scanning using the E2 core crystal structure (Kong et al., 2013) to predict E2 stability determinants largely agreed with key E2 sites from global alanine scanning (Pierce et al., 2016b), and also highlighted several positions in a dynamic region targeted by neutralizing antibodies and CD81. Correlations between residues from global alanine scanning were used to predict possible contacts between E2 residues in the native structure; these predictions may be useful in computational modeling of the full E2 and E1E2 glycoprotein structures (recent studies in this regard are noted below). Epitope mapping by alanine substitution studies identified two highly conserved E2 residues Gly530 and Asp535 that are required for binding by all antigenic domain B HMAbs (Keck et al., 2008). Additional residues were identified, Gly523 and Trp529, that are also required for binding by some, but not all, of these antibodies. Importantly, Trp529, Gly530, and Asp535 were previously reported to participate

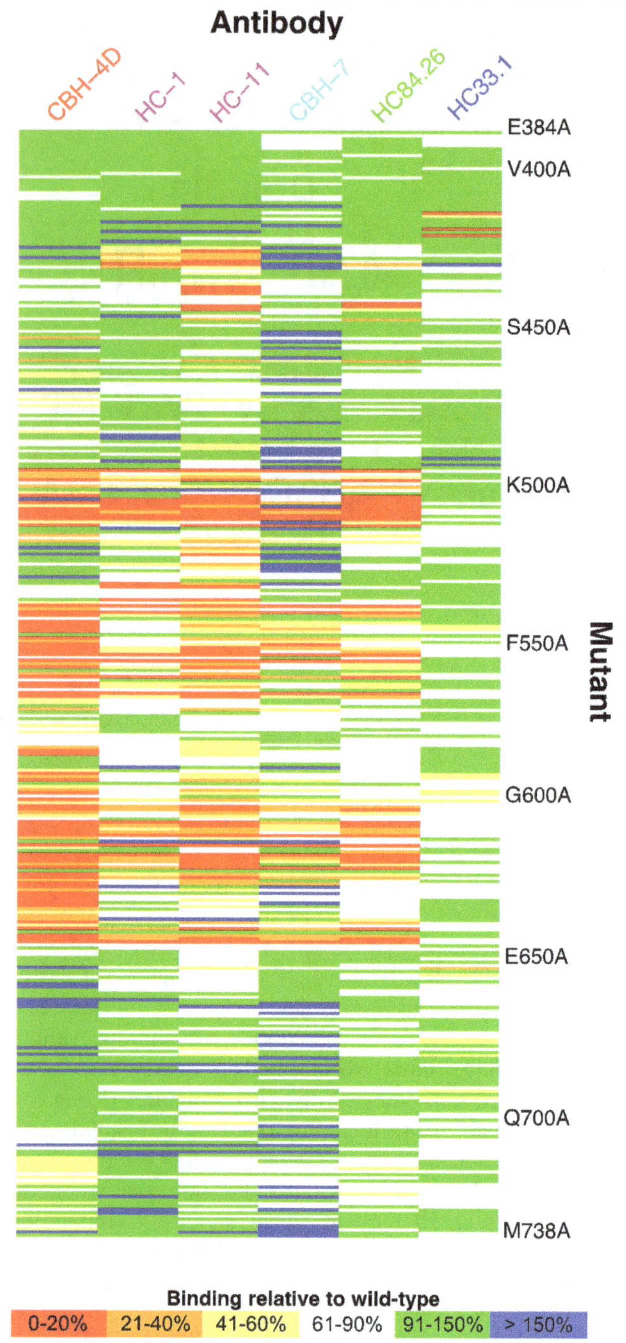

FIGURE 3 | Global E2 alanine scanning, shown as heat map. E2 alanine mutants are on the vertical axis, while HMAbs are on the horizontal axis, colored by antigenic domain (domain A, red; domain B, magenta; domain C, cyan; domain D, green; domain E, blue). Heat map colors represent measured affinity compared with wild-type (H77) E2 as detailed in the legend. Figure adapted from Pierce et al. (2016b).

in the interaction of E2 with CD81 (Owsianka et al., 2006). Thus, the broad neutralizing activity of antigenic domain B HMAbs is mediated by competing with CD81 for binding to conserved residues on E2 that are necessary for virus entry. Similarly, three highly conserved residues form a core region for antigenic domain D epitopes at Leu441, Phe442, and Tyr443 (Keck et al., 2012). Leu441 and Tyr443 are absolutely conserved among all known HCV isolates. Phe442, however, is only 60% conserved. Similar to domain B, the domain D region is also involved in interaction with CD81. For AR4- and AR5-specific epitopes that require association of the E1E2 heterodimer, antibodies binding to this region do not mediate neutralization by inhibiting E2 interaction with CD81, but rather potentially block E1E2 engagement with another co-receptor and/or prevent the necessary conformational change in the E1E2 structure required for virus entry (Giang et al., 2012). With the elucidation of the E2 core structure (Kong et al., 2013), the vast majority of these antibodies, antigenic domain B and D, and AR3, are located on the neutralizing face (**Figure 4**).

Not all broadly neutralizing antibodies share the same antiviral characteristics. In virus co-culture studies, some antigenic domain B antibodies are associated with viral escape, with and without compromising viral fitness, and others are resistant to viral escape. For instance, at a critical antibody concentration, HC-1, a domain B HMAb, can eliminate infectious virions in cell culture with no viral escape mutants detected. Other antibodies, such as CBH-2 and HC-11 that target the same antigenic domain, permitted viral escape through specific mutations in a region of domain B after repeated passages in the presence of increasing concentrations of the antibodies (Keck et al., 2011). Antibodies to antigenic domain E (aa 412-423) are also associated with different patterns of viral escape. Escape from virus neutralization with AP33 and HCV1 nAbs occurs when there is an N-glycan shift from Asn417 to Asn415 (Chung et al., 2013). This glycan shift, however, does not affect neutralization by other antigenic domain E HMAbs, such as HC33.1 (Keck et al., 2014). Interestingly, escape from antigenic domain D HMAbs has not been observed in co-culture studies even though a critical residue, Phe442, is only 60% conserved (Pierce et al., 2016b). Structural studies provided an explanation of the lack of viral escape in that three residues, located at 441-443, form a hydrophobic protrusion that serves as the binding site for domain D HMAbs (Pierce et al., 2016b). When there is a mutation from F442I or F442L, the interaction with the paratope formed by the heavy chain CDRs leads to a decrease in binding energy of the complex that can be compensated by increasing the antibody concentrations. Taken together, functional and biochemical characterization of broadly reactive nAbs creates a high-resolution database and functional map of neutralizing epitopes that can be strategically used in rational vaccine design.

HCV ENVELOPE STRUCTURE AND ANTIBODY RECOGNITION

As noted previously, the E1 and E2 glycoproteins form a heterodimer (Op De Beeck et al., 2000), though E2 is the primary, albeit not the exclusive, target of the antibody response. This suggests that E2 is more exposed than E1 in the context of the virion. E2 is heavily glycosylated, typically containing 11 N-glycans at specific sites, while E1 has up to 5 N-glycans (Vieyres et al., 2014). These N-glycans have been characterized

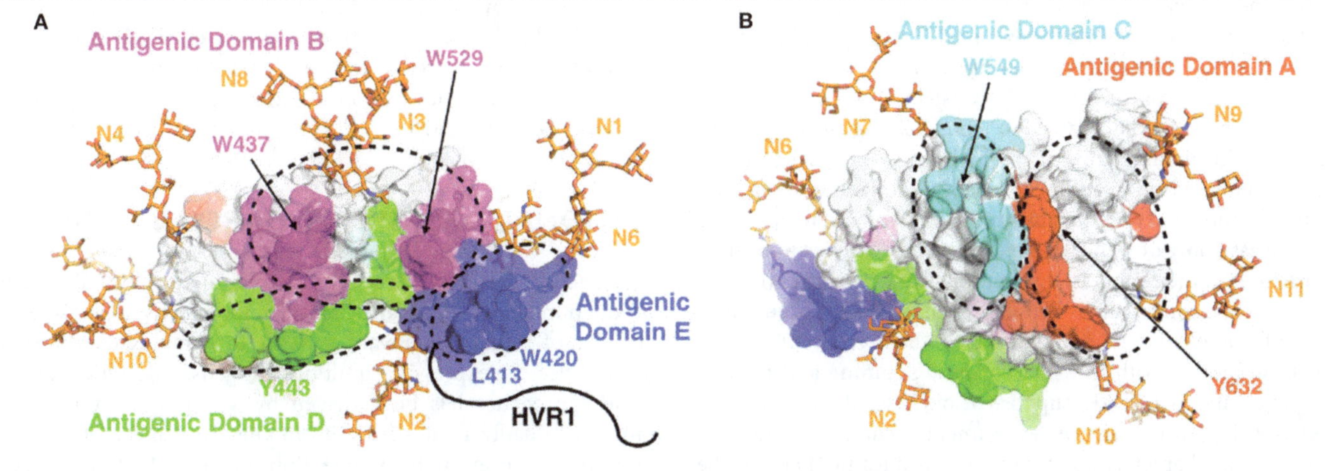

FIGURE 4 | Antigenic domains mapped to the surface of E2. Antigenic domains are colored and labeled on the neutralizing (front layer; **A**) and non-neutralizing (back layer; **B**) face of the E2 core structure (PDB code 4MWF), with key epitope residues shown in space-fill and a subset of those residues labeled. Basic N-glycans were modeled at all 10 sites present in the E2 core structure (N1-N4, N6-N11) using the GlyProt web server (Bohne-Lang and von der Lieth, 2005), and are shown as orange sticks. As the E2 core structure does not include coordinates for the majority of domain E (residues 412-423; of which 412-420 are not present), the domain E coordinates from the domain E-HCV1 complex structure (PDB code 4DGY) were modeled at that site. Hypervariable region 1 (HVR1), which is located at the N-terminus of E2 and also is not represented in the E2 core structure, is shown as a black line for reference. Figure adapted from Fauvelle et al. (2016).

using mass spectroscopy (Iacob et al., 2008), and a number of studies have shown that glycans modulate antibody recognition of E2 *in vitro* (Falkowska et al., 2007; Helle et al., 2007) and *in vivo* (Li et al., 2016; Ren et al., 2016). Notably, one E2 N-glycan (N3; position Asn 430) interacts directly with a broadly neutralizing antibody (AR3C), albeit in the interface periphery, in the crystallographic structure of the AR3C-E2 complex (Kong et al., 2013). Additionally, there are four predicted O-glycans on E2, two of which are located in HVR1 (Bräutigam et al., 2013).

Over the past 5 years, a number of studies have helped to elucidate structural features of E1 and E2, as noted in recent reviews (Khan et al., 2015; Kong et al., 2015a; Pierce et al., 2016a). These have collectively shown that key epitopes targeted by broadly neutralizing antibodies on the "front layer" of E2, which corresponds to the CD81 binding face, exhibit structural heterogeneity, in particular E2 antigenic domain E (Kong et al., 2012; Li et al., 2015; Meola et al., 2015), as well as antigenic domains B and D (Kong et al., 2013; Deng et al., 2014; Keck et al., 2016b; Vasiliauskaite et al., 2017). This has been underscored by a recent study, which combined experimental structural and biophysical characterization with simulations to characterize mobility of the CD81 binding region of E2 (Kong et al., 2016).

Two independently determined structures of the E2 glycoprotein "core" region, corresponding to truncations of glycoprotein ectodomains (Kong et al., 2013; Khan et al., 2014), provide major insights into the tertiary structure of E2. Despite the use of distinct monoclonal antibodies, engineered truncations, expression systems, and represented genotypes (1a and 2a), these structures are highly similar overall (approximately 0.8 Å root mean square distance between Cα residues), revealing a globular fold stabilized by numerous disulfide bonds. However, as noted by others in separate reviews (Castelli et al., 2014; Khan et al., 2015), a number of questions remain largely due to (1) discrepancy between disulfide bonds between the current E2 core crystal structures, (2) large critical regions of E2 absent from these structures due to disordered residues or truncation, including HVR1 (aa 384-410), domain E (aa 412-423), HVR2 and flanking residues (aa 453-485), and the ectodomain C-terminal region (aa 646-717), and (3) absence of the E1 portion of the heterodimer. The two studies describing the E2 core crystal structures did include electron microscopy (Kong et al., 2013) and small angle x-ray scattering (Khan et al., 2014) characterization of the larger E2 ectodomains, but their limited resolution does not permit a view of residue interactions, surface residues, or secondary structures, which collectively would be of potential interest for rational vaccine design.

Characterization of the E1 structure has been limited to nuclear magnetic resonance (NMR) structures of short helical regions (Op De Beeck et al., 2000; Spadaccini et al., 2010), an antibody-epitope complex (Kong et al., 2015b), and the N-terminal region of E1, which displayed an unexpected dimeric assembly (El Omari et al., 2014); follow up studies on the latter would help to confirm its representation of the structure of native E1 on the viral envelope. While the above studies have provided key details on the structure and dynamics of key sites, high-resolution structural determination of uncharacterized regions of E1, E2, and, in particular, the E1E2 heterodimer, will be greatly informative for rational vaccine design efforts and understanding of viral assembly.

COMPUTATIONAL MODELING OF E1E2 ASSEMBLY

Due to the absence of experimentally determined structures of the E1E2 heterodimer, two recent studies have used computational modeling methods to predict the structure of this assembly (Castelli et al., 2017; Freedman et al., 2017).

These models were generated with distinct methods, specifically residue co-evolution analysis based on E1E2 sequence alignments (referred to as evolutionary coupling) to infer residue contacts and guide modeling in one study (Castelli et al., 2017), and a combination of template-based modeling, folding and docking in the other (Freedman et al., 2017). The latter work also employed constraints based on experimental data to guide modeling, and included a model of the transmembrane regions and the putative trimeric assembly of E1E2. As neither of these studies published coordinates of their models, it is not possible to compare directly the extent of convergence between their predicted structures. Both of these studies cross-reference their respective E1E2 structural models with measured alanine scanning and epitope mapping data to provide support, though validation of these models using, for example, experimental characterization of previously uncharacterized mutants of residues predicted to be determinants of E1E2 stability, would provide more conclusive model confirmation. In fact, one of these studies did present pairs of key predicted E1 and E2 interacting residues (Freedman et al., 2017), though no new mutants were tested experimentally in either study. Cross-validation against experimental findings from additional studies, for example recent identification of E1 residues W239, I262, and D263 as putative interface residues with E2 (Haddad et al., 2017), would also help to validate and refine such models.

HCV HOST IMMUNE EVASION STRATEGIES

Mechanisms of HCV evasion from the immune system have been described in several recent reviews (Cashman et al., 2014; Dunlop et al., 2015; Pierce et al., 2016a). Extreme levels of viral sequence variability, leading to millions of quasispecies within infected individuals, permit the virus to escape antibody and T cell responses through disruption of immune molecular recognition. A salient example of this mechanism was observed during clinical trials of the HCV1 monoclonal antibody in humans, where initial viral suppression was followed by rebound where isolates exhibited specific amino acid variants at residues N415 and N417 (the latter resulting a shift in glycosylation from residue 417 to residue 415). These variants severely disrupted the ability of HCV1 to bind E2 and neutralize virus, and were rare or undetectable prior to treatment and in patients receiving placebo (Chung et al., 2013; Babcock et al., 2014). Other viral escape mechanisms include epitope shielding by viral glycans, and the presence of hypervariable "decoy" epitopes that elicit antibodies that compete with broadly neutralizing antibodies (Keck et al., 2016a) are summarized in reviews as noted previously.

Recent studies have highlighted the role of E2 co-receptor recognition in the evasion of the antibody response. Using an analysis of monoclonal antibody resistance among a large set of genotype 1 isolates, El-Diwany et al. identified key sites on E2 that permitted escape through modulation of E2 binding to SR-B1 (El-Diwany et al., 2017). Another study found that a set of growth-adapted mutants, isolated from a large library of genotype 2 clones based on the JFH-1 isolate, exhibited increased neutralization by monoclonal antibodies and lower dependence on SR-B1 binding for infectivity (Zuiani et al., 2016). These findings possibly correlate to the observation of a correlation of viral infectivity with overall neutralizing antibody resistance (Urbanowicz et al., 2015).

RATIONAL DESIGN OF AN HCV VACCINE

Approaches for HCV vaccine development have included production of HCV E2 and E1E2 recombinant envelope proteins and use of immuno-adjuvant systems to complex engineering of viral vectors expressing multiple antigens. The rationale for these approaches has been driven by a requirement to elicit multiple broadly neutralizing antibodies to achieve sterilizing immunity to prevent HCV infection and how best to achieve such immunity. Extensive human and animal studies have been performed with a recombinant genotype 1a E1E2 vaccine (Frey et al., 2010; Ray et al., 2010; Wong et al., 2014; Logan et al., 2017). Houghton and his colleagues showed that recombinant E1E2 proteins adjuvanted with an oil-in-water emulsion (MF59C) is safe in humans (Frey et al., 2010) and elicits broadly neutralizing antibodies in both humans and animals (Ray et al., 2010; Wong et al., 2014), as defined by competition analyses of immunized sera from goats and mice against well-established broadly neutralizing MAbs (Wong et al., 2014; Logan et al., 2017). The problem is that a substantial portion of the human antibody responses to this vaccine is directed at the hypervariable region-1 on E2 (Ray et al., 2010) and these antibodies, while neutralizing, are isolate-specific. Taken together, a design approach to direct the antibody responses against conserved epitopes mediating virus neutralization will be advantageous.

The correlation of host antibody response to HCV with viral clearance and recent successes in structure-based vaccine design for other viruses, such as HIV (Jardine et al., 2013; Correia et al., 2014), RSV (McLellan et al., 2013), and influenza (Yassine et al., 2015), suggest that a rationally designed vaccine that elicits neutralizing antibody responses to conserved epitopes is a viable route to an effective B cell based HCV vaccine. Recently, several engineered E1, E2, and E1E2 antigens have been described, including structure-based epitope designs (He et al., 2015; Sandomenico et al., 2016; Pierce et al., 2017). Although the conditions differed for assessing relative immunogenicity in mice, further studies can define the correlates of the magnitude of responses and breadth of protection by neutralization assays for epitope-based and full-length protein-based antigens with designs to minimize viral escape while exploiting the potential Achilles heel of conserved envelope residues. The recent development of an immune competent mouse model with an HCV-related hepacivirus presents a possible means to evaluate and compare such vaccine design strategies (Billerbeck et al., 2017).

Given recent evidence of mobility of key E2 epitopes associated targeted by neutralizing antibodies (Deng et al., 2014; Li et al., 2015; Meola et al., 2015; Kong et al., 2016; Vasiliauskaite et al., 2017), as noted above, stabilization of these epitopes is an intriguing option for future vaccine design efforts, particularly in light of promising recent studies in this regard for other viruses. Recent studies on engineering HIV SOSIP gp140 trimers include designing a stabilized closed protein conformation while decreasing exposure of non-neutralizing epitopes (de Taeye et al., 2015), as well as generation of new "hyperstable" SOSIP designs with engineered disulfide bonds that elicit improved neutralizing antibodies (Torrents de la Peña et al., 2017). Stabilized RSV F immunogens were recently redesigned to further optimize their stability through iterative structure-based design and experimental biophysical and immunological characterization, yielding next-generation RSV immunogens with markedly improved capacity to induce neutralizing antibodies vs. the original designs (Joyce et al., 2016). In that work, the authors noted that their structure-based vaccine design paradigm to optimize antigenic structure and stability "may have utility in the optimization of other vaccine antigens"; HCV E2 would be one promising target in this regard.

CONCLUSIONS

The medical burden of hepatitis C has decreased by the introduction of effective antiviral therapies. However, control of this insidious disease will require the successful development of an effective preventative vaccine. To achieve this goal, the complex interplay between virus and host during acute infection that leads to spontaneous clearance needs to be better understood to provide clues of protective immunity. The criteria for what constitutes a successful immune response leading to viral clearance in designing at vaccine that is broadly cross protective across the genotypes and long lasting will be the holy grail of such vaccine development efforts. Recent insights from deep sequencing, antibody-antigen interactions, structural biology, and immunogenicity studies provide the basis for novel vaccine designs for this challenging target. While accounting for the primary mechanisms of viral escape, namely sequence variability within the viral envelope glycoproteins including prominent decoy epitopes such as HVR1, immunogens can be designed to enhance their capacity to induce potent neutralizing antibodies to conserved epitopes on the viral envelope. These approaches, combined with novel adjuvant formulations capable of eliciting robust and long-lasting humoral and cellular responses, will significantly advance vaccine development efforts to successfully address this daunting medical challenge.

AUTHOR CONTRIBUTIONS

All authors listed have made a substantial, direct and intellectual contribution to the work, and approved it for publication.

ACKNOWLEDGMENTS

This work was supported in part by National Institute of Allergy and Infectious Diseases/NIH grants R21-AI126582 (SKHF and BGP), U19-AI123862 (SKHF) and R01-AI132213 (TRF, BGP, and SKHF), as well as startup funding from the University of Maryland to BGP.

REFERENCES

André, P., Komurian-Pradel, F., Deforges, S., Perret, M., Berland, J. L., Sodoyer, M., et al. (2002). Characterization of low- and very-low-density hepatitis C virus RNA-containing particles. *J. Virol.* 76, 6919–6928. doi: 10.1128/JVI.76.14.6919-6928.2002

Babcock, G. J., Iyer, S., Smith, H. L., Wang, Y., Rowley, K., Ambrosino, D. M., et al. (2014). High-throughput sequencing analysis of post-liver transplantation HCV E2 glycoprotein evolution in the presence and absence of neutralizing monoclonal antibody. *PLoS ONE* 9:e100325. doi: 10.1371/journal.pone.0100325

Ball, J. K., Tarr, A. W., and McKeating, J. A. (2014). The past, present and future of neutralizing antibodies for hepatitis C virus. *Antiviral Res.* 105, 100–111. doi: 10.1016/j.antiviral.2014.02.013

Billerbeck, E., Wolfisberg, R., Fahnøe, U., Xiao, J. W., Quirk, C., Luna, J. M., et al. (2017). Mouse models of acute and chronic hepacivirus infection. *Science* 357, 204–208. doi: 10.1126/science.aal1962

Bohne-Lang, A., and von der Lieth, C. W. (2005). GlyProt: in silico glycosylation of proteins. *Nucleic Acids Res.* 33, W214–W219. doi: 10.1093/nar/gki385

Bräutigam, J., Scheidig, A. J., and Egge-Jacobsen, W. (2013). Mass spectrometric analysis of hepatitis C viral envelope protein E2 reveals extended microheterogeneity of mucin-type O-linked glycosylation. *Glycobiology* 23, 453–474. doi: 10.1093/glycob/cws171

Broering, T. J., Garrity, K. A., Boatright, N. K., Sloan, S. E., Sandor, F., Thomas, W. D. Jr., et al. (2009). Identification and characterization of broadly neutralizing human monoclonal antibodies directed against the E2 envelope glycoprotein of hepatitis C virus. *J. Virol.* 83, 12473–12482. doi: 10.1128/JVI.01138-09

Bukh, J., Engle, R. E., Faulk, K., Wang, R. Y., Farci, P., Alter, H. J., et al. (2015). Immunoglobulin with high-titer *in vitro* cross-neutralizing hepatitis C virus antibodies passively protects chimpanzees from homologous, but not heterologous, challenge. *J. Virol.* 89, 9128–9132. doi: 10.1128/JVI.01194-15

Callaway, E. (2014). Hepatitis C drugs not reaching poor. *Nature* 508, 295–296. doi: 10.1038/508295a

Cashman, S. B., Marsden, B. D., and Dustin, L. B. (2014). The humoral immune response to HCV: understanding is key to vaccine development. *Front. Immunol.* 5:550. doi: 10.3389/fimmu.2014.00550

Castelli, M., Clementi, N., Pfaff, J., Sautto, G. A., Diotti, R. A., Burioni, R., et al. (2017). A biologically-validated HCV E1E2 heterodimer structural model. *Sci. Rep.* 7:214. doi: 10.1038/s41598-017-00320-7

Castelli, M., Clementi, N., Sautto, G. A., Pfaff, J., Kahle, K. M., Barnes, T., et al. (2014). HCV E2 core structures and mAbs: something is still missing. *Drug Discov. Today* 19, 1964–1970. doi: 10.1016/j.drudis.2014.08.011

Chung, R. T., and Baumert, T. F. (2014). Curing chronic hepatitis C–the arc of a medical triumph. *N. Engl. J. Med.* 370, 1576–1578. doi: 10.1056/NEJMp1400986

Chung, R. T., Gordon, F. D., Curry, M. P., Schiano, T. D., Emre, S., Corey, K., et al. (2013). Human monoclonal antibody MBL-HCV1 delays HCV viral rebound following liver transplantation: a randomized controlled study. *Am. J. Transplant.* 13, 1047–1054. doi: 10.1111/ajt.12083

Correia, B. E., Bates, J. T., Loomis, R. J., Baneyx, G., Carrico, C., Jardine, J. G., et al. (2014). Proof of principle for epitope-focused vaccine design. *Nature* 507, 201–206. doi: 10.1038/nature12966

Corti, D., Voss, J., Gamblin, S. J., Codoni, G., Macagno, A., Jarrossay, D., et al. (2011). A neutralizing antibody selected from plasma cells that binds to group 1 and group 2 influenza A hemagglutinins. *Science* 333, 850–856. doi: 10.1126/science.1205669

Cox, A. L., and Thomas, D. L. (2013). Hepatitis C virus vaccines among people who inject drugs. *Clin. Infect. Dis.* 57(Suppl. 2), S46–S50. doi: 10.1093/cid/cit329

Crooks, G. E., Hon, G., Chandonia, J. M., and Brenner, S. E. (2004). WebLogo: a sequence logo generator. *Genome Res.* 14, 1188–1190. doi: 10.1101/gr.849004 de Taeye, S. W., Ozorowski, G., Torrents de la Peña A., Guttman, M., Julien, J. P., van den Kerkhof, T. L., et al. (2015). Immunogenicity of stabilized HIV-1 envelope trimers with reduced exposure of non-neutralizing epitopes. *Cell* 163, 1702–1715. doi: 10.1016/j.cell.2015.11.056.

Deng, L., Ma, L., Virata-Theimer, M. L., Zhong, L., Yan, H., Zhao, Z., et al. (2014). Discrete conformations of epitope II on the hepatitis C virus E2 protein for antibody-mediated neutralization and nonneutralization. *Proc. Natl. Acad. Sci. U.S.A.* 111, 10690–10695. doi: 10.1073/pnas.1411317111

Dorner, M., Horwitz, J. A., Robbins, J. B., Barry, W. T., Feng, Q., Mu, K., et al. (2011). A genetically humanized mouse model for hepatitis C virus infection. *Nature* 474, 208–211. doi: 10.1038/nature10168

Dowd, K. A., Netski, D. M., Wang, X. H., Cox, A. L., and Ray, S. C. (2009). Selection pressure from neutralizing antibodies drives sequence evolution during acute infection with hepatitis C virus. *Gastroenterology* 136, 2377–2386. doi: 10.1053/j.gastro.2009.02.080

Drummer, H. E., Boo, I., Maerz, A. L., and Poumbourios, P. (2006). A conserved Gly436-Trp-Leu-Ala-Gly-Leu-Phe-Tyr motif in hepatitis C virus glycoprotein E2 is a determinant of CD81 binding and viral entry. *J. Virol.* 80, 7844–7853. doi: 10.1128/JVI.00029-06

Duffy, S., Shackelton, L. A., and Holmes, E. C. (2008). Rates of evolutionary change in viruses: patterns and determinants. *Nat. Rev. Genet.* 9, 267–276. doi: 10.1038/nrg2323

Dunlop, J., Owsianka, A., Cowton, V., and Patel, A. (2015). Current and future prophylactic vaccines for hepatitis C virus. *Vaccine: Dev. Ther.* 2015, 31–44. doi: 10.2147/VDT.S48437

El-Diwany, R., Cohen, V. J., Mankowski, M. C., Wasilewski, L. N., Brady, J. K., Snider, A. E., et al. (2017). Extra-epitopic hepatitis C virus polymorphisms confer resistance to broadly neutralizing antibodies by modulating binding to scavenger receptor B1. *PLoS Pathog* 13:e1006235. doi: 10.1371/journal.ppat.1006235

El Omari, K., Iourin, O., Kadlec, J., Sutton, G., Harlos, K., Grimes, J. M., et al. (2014). Unexpected structure for the N-terminal domain of hepatitis C virus envelope glycoprotein E1. *Nat. Commun.* 5:4874. doi: 10.1038/ncomms5874

Falkowska, E., Kajumo, F., Garcia, E., Reinus, J., and Dragic, T. (2007). Hepatitis C virus envelope glycoprotein E2 glycans modulate entry, CD81 binding, and neutralization. *J. Virol.* 81, 8072–8079. doi: 10.1128/JVI.00459-07

Falson, P., Bartosch, B., Alsaleh, K., Tews, B. A., Loquet, A., Ciczora, Y., et al. (2015). Hepatitis C virus envelope glycoprotein E1 forms trimers at the surface of the virion. *J. Virol.* 89, 10333–10346. doi: 10.1128/JVI.00991-15

Farci, P., Shimoda, A., Wong, D., Cabezon, T., De Gioannis, D., Strazzera, A., et al. (1996). Prevention of hepatitis C virus infection in chimpanzees by hyperimmune serum against the hypervariable region 1 of the envelope 2 protein. *Proc. Natl. Acad. Sci. U.S.A.* 93, 15394–15399. doi: 10.1073/pnas.93.26.15394

Fauvelle, C., Colpitts, C. C., Keck, Z. Y., Pierce, B. G., Foung, S. K., and Baumert, T. F. (2016). Hepatitis C virus vaccine candidates inducing protective neutralizing antibodies. *Expert Rev Vacc.* 15, 1535–1544. doi: 10.1080/14760584.2016.1194759

Freedman, H., Logan, M. R., Hockman, D., Koehler Leman, J., Law, J. L., and Houghton, M. (2017). Computational prediction of the heterodimeric and higher-order structure of gpE1/gpE2 envelope glycoproteins encoded by hepatitis C virus. *J. Virol.* 91, e02309–e02316. doi: 10.1128/JVI.02 309-16

Frey, S. E., Houghton, M., Coates, S., Abrignani, S., Chien, D., Rosa, D., et al. (2010). Safety and immunogenicity of HCV E1E2 vaccine adjuvanted with MF59 administered to healthy adults. *Vaccine* 28, 6367–6373. doi: 10.1016/j.vaccine.2010.06.084

Giang, E., Dorner, M., Prentoe, J. C., Dreux, M., Evans, M. J., Bukh, J., et al. (2012). Human broadly neutralizing antibodies to the envelope glycoprotein complex of hepatitis C virus. *Proc. Natl. Acad. Sci. U.S.A.* 109, 6205–6210. doi: 10.1073/pnas.1114927109

Grove, J., Nielsen, S., Zhong, J., Bassendine, M. F., Drummer, H. E., Balfe, P., et al. (2008). Identification of a residue in hepatitis C virus E2 glycoprotein that determines scavenger receptor BI and CD81 receptor dependency and sensitivity to neutralizing antibodies. *J. Virol.* 82, 12020–12029. doi: 10.1128/JVI.01569-08

Haddad, J. G., Rouillé, Y., Hanoulle, X., Descamps, V., Hamze, M., Dabboussi, F., et al. (2017). Identification of novel functions for hepatitis C virus envelope glycoprotein E1 in virus entry and assembly. *J. Virol.* 91, e00048–e00017. doi: 10.1128/JVI.00048-17

He, L., Cheng, Y., Kong, L., Azadnia, P., Giang, E., Kim, J., et al. (2015). Approaching rational epitope vaccine design for hepatitis C virus with meta-server and multivalent scaffolding. *Sci. Rep.* 5:12501. doi: 10.1038/srep12501

Helle, F., Goffard, A., Morel, V., Duverlie, G., McKeating, J., Keck, Z. Y., et al. (2007). The neutralizing activity of anti-hepatitis C virus antibodies is modulated by specific glycans on the E2 envelope protein. *J. Virol.* 81, 8101–8111. doi: 10.1128/JVI.00127-07

Helle, F., Vieyres, G., Elkrief, L., Popescu, C. I., Wychowski, C., Descamps, V., et al. (2010). Role of N-linked glycans in the functions of hepatitis C virus envelope proteins incorporated into infectious virions. *J. Virol.* 84, 11905–11915. doi: 10.1128/JVI.01548-10

Iacob, R. E., Perdivara, I., Przybylski, M., and Tomer, K. B. (2008). Mass spectrometric characterization of glycosylation of hepatitis C virus E2 envelope glycoprotein reveals extended microheterogeneity of N-glycans. *J. Am. Soc. Mass Spectrom* 19, 428–444. doi: 10.1016/j.jasms.2007.11.022

Jardine, J., Julien, J. P., Menis, S., Ota, T., Kalyuzhniy, O., McGuire, A., et al. (2013). Rational HIV immunogen design to target specific germline B cell receptors. *Science* 340, 711–716. doi: 10.1126/science.1234150

Joyce, M. G., Zhang, B., Ou, L., Chen, M., Chuang, G. Y., Druz, A., et al. (2016). Iterative structure-based improvement of a fusion-glycoprotein vaccine against RSV. *Nat. Struct. Mol. Biol.* 23, 811–820. doi: 10.1038/nsmb.3267

Katoh, K., and Standley, D. M. (2013). MAFFT multiple sequence alignment software version 7: improvements in performance and usability. *Mol. Biol. Evol.* 30, 772–780. doi: 10.1093/molbev/mst010

Keck, Z., Wang, W., Wang, Y., Lau, P., Carlsen, T. H., Prentoe, J., et al. (2013). Cooperativity in virus neutralization by human monoclonal antibodies to two adjacent regions located at the amino terminus of hepatitis C virus E2 glycoprotein. *J. Virol.* 87, 37–51. doi: 10.1128/JVI.01941-12

Keck, Z. Y., Angus, A. G., Wang, W., Lau, P., Wang, Y., Gatherer, D., et al. (2014). Non-random escape pathways from a broadly neutralizing human monoclonal antibody map to a highly conserved region on the hepatitis C virus E2 glycoprotein encompassing amino acids 412-423. *PLoS Pathog* 10:e1004297. doi: 10.1371/journal.ppat.1004297

Keck, Z. Y., Girard-Blanc, C., Wang, W., Lau, P., Zuiani, A., Rey, F. A., et al. (2016a). Antibody response to hypervariable region 1 interferes with broadly neutralizing antibodies to hepatitis C virus. *J. Virol.* 90, 3112–3122. doi: 10.1128/JVI.02458-15

Keck, Z. Y., Li, T. K., Xia, J., Gal-Tanamy, M., Olson, O., Li, S. H., et al. (2008). Definition of a conserved immunodominant domain on hepatitis C virus E2 glycoprotein by neutralizing human monoclonal antibodies. *J. Virol.* 82, 6061–6066. doi: 10.1128/JVI.02475-07

Keck, Z. Y., Saha, A., Xia, J., Wang, Y., Lau, P., Krey, T., et al. (2011). Mapping a region of hepatitis C virus E2 that is responsible for escape from neutralizing antibodies and a core CD81-binding region that does not tolerate neutralization escape mutations. *J. Virol.* 85, 10451–10463. doi: 10.1128/JVI.05259-11

Keck, Z. Y., Sung, V. M., Perkins, S., Rowe, J., Paul, S., Liang, T. J., et al. (2004). Human monoclonal antibody to hepatitis C virus E1 glycoprotein that blocks virus attachment and viral infectivity. *J. Virol.* 78, 7257–7263. doi: 10.1128/JVI.78.13.7257-7263.2004

Keck, Z. Y., Wang, Y., Lau, P., Lund, G., Rangarajan, S., Fauvelle, C., et al. (2016b). Affinity maturation of a broadly neutralizing human monoclonal antibody that prevents acute hepatitis C virus infection in mice. *Hepatology* 64, 1922–1933. doi: 10.1002/hep.28850

Keck, Z. Y., Xia, J., Wang, Y., Wang, W., Krey, T., Prentoe, J., et al. (2012). Human monoclonal antibodies to a novel cluster of conformational epitopes on HCV E2 with resistance to neutralization escape in a genotype 2a isolate. *PLoS Pathog* 8:e1002653. doi: 10.1371/journal.ppat.1002653

Khan, A. G., Miller, M. T., and Marcotrigiano, J. (2015). HCV glycoprotein structures: what to expect from the unexpected. *Curr. Opin. Virol.* 12, 53–58. doi: 10.1016/j.coviro.2015.02.004

Khan, A. G., Whidby, J., Miller, M. T., Scarborough, H., Zatorski, A. V., Cygan, A., et al. (2014). Structure of the core ectodomain of the hepatitis C virus envelope glycoprotein 2. *Nature* 509, 381–384. doi: 10.1038/nature13117

Kong, L., Giang, E., Nieusma, T., Kadam, R. U., Cogburn, K. E., Hua, Y., et al. (2013). Hepatitis C virus E2 envelope glycoprotein core structure. *Science* 342, 1090–1094. doi: 10.1126/science.1243876

Kong, L., Giang, E., Robbins, J. B., Stanfield, R. L., Burton, D. R., Wilson, I. A., et al. (2012). Structural basis of hepatitis C virus neutralization by broadly neutralizing antibody HCV1. *Proc Natl Acad Sci U.S.A.* 109, 9499–9504. doi: 10.1073/pnas.1202924109

Kong, L., Jackson, K. N., Wilson, I. A., and Law, M. (2015a). Capitalizing on knowledge of hepatitis C virus neutralizing epitopes for rational vaccine design. *Curr. Opin. Virol.* 11, 148–157. doi: 10.1016/j.coviro.2015.04.001

Kong, L., Kadam, R. U., Giang, E., Ruwona, T. B., Nieusma, T., Culhane, J. C., et al. (2015b). Structure of hepatitis C virus envelope glycoprotein E1 antigenic site 314-324 in complex with antibody IGH526. *J. Mol. Biol.* 427, 2617–2628. doi: 10.1016/j.jmb.2015.06.012

Kong, L., Lee, D. E., Kadam, R. U., Liu, T., Giang, E., Nieusma, T., et al. (2016). Structural flexibility at a major conserved antibody target on hepatitis C virus E2 antigen. *Proc. Natl. Acad. Sci. U.S.A.* 113, 12768–12773. doi: 10.1073/pnas.1609780113

Krey, T., Meola, A., Keck, Z. Y., Damier-Piolle, L., Foung, S. K., and Rey, F. A. (2013). Structural basis of HCV neutralization by human monoclonal antibodies resistant to viral neutralization escape. *PLoS Pathog* 9:e1003364. doi: 10.1371/journal.ppat.1003364

Kuiken, C., Yusim, K., Boykin, L., and Richardson, R. (2005). The Los Alamos hepatitis C sequence database. *Bioinformatics* 21, 379–384. doi: 10.1093/bioinformatics/bth485

Lavillette, D., Morice, Y., Germanidis, G., Donot, P., Soulier, A., Pagkalos, E., et al. (2005). Human serum facilitates hepatitis C virus infection, and neutralizing responses inversely correlate with viral replication kinetics at the acute phase of hepatitis C virus infection. *J. Virol.* 79, 6023–6034. doi: 10.1128/JVI.79.10.6023-6034.2005

Law, M., Maruyama, T., Lewis, J., Giang, E., Tarr, A. W., Stamataki, Z., et al. (2008). Broadly neutralizing antibodies protect against hepatitis C virus quasispecies challenge. *Nat. Med.* 14, 25–27. doi: 10.1038/nm1698

Lawitz, E., Mangia, A., Wyles, D., Rodriguez-Torres, M., Hassanein, T., Gordon, S. C., et al. (2013). Sofosbuvir for previously untreated chronic hepatitis C infection. *N. Engl. J. Med.* 368, 1878–1887. doi: 10.1056/NEJMoa1214853

Li, D., von Schaewen, M., Wang, X., Tao, W., Zhang, Y., Li, L., et al. (2016). Altered glycosylation patterns increase immunogenicity of a subunit hepatitis C virus vaccine, inducing neutralizing antibodies which confer protection in mice. *J. Virol.* 90, 10486–10498. doi: 10.1128/JVI.01462-16

Li, Y., Pierce, B. G., Wang, Q., Keck, Z. Y., Fuerst, T. R., Foung, S. K., et al. (2015). Structural basis for penetration of the glycan shield of hepatitis C virus E2 glycoprotein by a broadly neutralizing human antibody. *J. Biol. Chem.* 290, 10117–10125. doi: 10.1074/jbc.M115.643528

Liang, T. J. (2013). Current progress in development of hepatitis C virus vaccines. *Nat. Med.* 19, 869–878. doi: 10.1038/nm.3183

Lindenbach, B. D., and Rice, C. M. (2013). The ins and outs of hepatitis C virus entry and assembly. *Nat. Rev. Micro.* 11, 688–700. doi: 10.1038/nrmicro3098

Logan, M., Law, J., Wong, J. A., Hockman, D., Landi, A., Chen, C., et al. (2017). Native folding of a recombinant gpE1/gpE2 heterodimer vaccine antigen from a precursor protein fused with Fc IgG. *J. Virol.* 91:e01552-16. doi: 10.1128/JVI.01552-16

Logvinoff, C., Major, M. E., Oldach, D., Heyward, S., Talal, A., Balfe, P., et al. (2004). Neutralizing antibody response during acute and chronic hepatitis C virus infection. *Proc. Natl. Acad. Sci. U.S.A.* 101, 10149–10154. doi: 10.1073/pnas.0403519101

Ly, K. N., Hughes, E. M., Jiles, R. B., and Holmberg, S. D. (2016). Rising mortality associated with hepatitis C virus in the United States, 2003-2013. *Clin. Infect. Dis.* 62, 1287–1288. doi: 10.1093/cid/ciw111

McLellan, J. S., Chen, M., Joyce, M. G., Sastry, M., Stewart-Jones, G. B., Yang, Y., et al. (2013). Structure-based design of a fusion glycoprotein vaccine for respiratory syncytial virus. *Science* 342, 592–598. doi: 10.1126/science.1243283

Meola, A., Tarr, A. W., England, P., Meredith, L. W., McClure, C. P., Foung, S. K., et al. (2015). Structural flexibility of a conserved antigenic region in hepatitis C virus glycoprotein E2 recognized by broadly neutralizing antibodies. *J. Virol.* 89, 2170–2181. doi: 10.1128/JVI.02190-14

Meunier, J. C., Russell, R. S., Goossens, V., Priem, S., Walter, H., Depla, E., et al. (2008). Isolation and characterization of broadly neutralizing human monoclonal antibodies to the e1 glycoprotein of hepatitis C virus. *J. Virol.* 82, 966–973. doi: 10.1128/JVI.01872-07

Mohd Hanafiah, K., Groeger, J., Flaxman, A. D., and Wiersma, S. T. (2013). Global epidemiology of hepatitis C virus infection: new estimates of age-specific antibody to HCV seroprevalence. *Hepatology* 57, 1333–1342. doi: 10.1002/hep.26141

Morin, T. J., Broering, T. J., Leav, B. A., Blair, B. M., Rowley, K. J., Boucher, E. N., et al. (2012). Human monoclonal antibody HCV1 effectively prevents and treats HCV infection in chimpanzees. *PLoS Pathog* 8:e1002895. doi: 10.1371/journal.ppat.1002895

Op De Beeck, A., Montserret, R., Duvet, S., Cocquerel, L., Cacan, R., Barberot, B., et al. (2000). The transmembrane domains of hepatitis C virus envelope glycoproteins E1 and E2 play a major role in heterodimerization. *J. Biol. Chem.* 275, 31428–31437. doi: 10.1074/jbc.M003003200

Osburn, W. O., Snider, A. E., Wells, B. L., Latanich, R., Bailey, J. R., Thomas, D. L., et al. (2014). Clearance of hepatitis C infection is associated with the early appearance of broad neutralizing antibody responses. *Hepatology* 59, 2140–2151. doi: 10.1002/hep.27013

Owsianka, A., Tarr, A. W., Juttla, V. S., Lavillette, D., Bartosch, B., Cosset, F. L., et al. (2005). Monoclonal antibody AP33 defines a broadly neutralizing epitope on the hepatitis C virus E2 envelope glycoprotein. *J. Virol.* 79, 11095–11104. doi: 10.1128/JVI.79.17.11095-11104.2005

Owsianka, A. M., Timms, J. M., Tarr, A. W., Brown, R. J., Hickling, T. P., Szwejk, A., et al. (2006). Identification of conserved residues in the E2 envelope glycoprotein of the hepatitis C virus that are critical for CD81 binding. *J. Virol.* 80, 8695–8704. doi: 10.1128/JVI.00271-06

Paradis, E., Claude, J., and Strimmer, K. (2004). APE: analyses of phylogenetics and evolution in R language. *Bioinformatics* 20, 289–290. doi: 10.1093/bioinformatics/btg412

Pestka, J. M., Zeisel, M. B., Bläser, E., Schürmann, P., Bartosch, B., Cosset, F. L., et al. (2007). Rapid induction of virus-neutralizing antibodies and viral clearance in a single-source outbreak of hepatitis C. *Proc. Natl. Acad. Sci. U.S.A.* 104, 6025–6030. doi: 10.1073/pnas.0607026104

Pierce, B. G., Boucher, E. N., Piepenbrink, K. H., Ejemel, M., Rapp, C. A., Thomas, W. D. Jr., et al. (2017). Structure-based design of hepatitis C virus vaccines that elicit neutralizing antibody responses to a conserved epitope. *J. Virol.* 91, 01032–01017. doi: 10.1128/JVI.01032-17

Pierce, B. G., Keck, Z.-Y., and Foung, S. K. (2016a). Viral evasion and challenges of hepatitis C virus vaccine development. *Curr. Opin. Virol.* 20, 55–63. doi: 10.1016/j.coviro.2016.09.004

Pierce, B. G., Keck, Z.-Y., Lau, P., Fauvelle, C., Gowthaman, R., Baumert, T. F., et al. (2016b). Global mapping of antibody recognition of the hepatitis C virus E2 glycoprotein: implications for vaccine design. *Proc. Natl. Acad. Sci. U.S.A.* 113, E6946–E6954. doi: 10.1073/pnas.1614942113

Pileri, P., Uematsu, Y., Campagnoli, S., Galli, G., Falugi, F., Petracca, R., et al. (1998). Binding of hepatitis C virus to CD81. *Science* 282, 938–941. doi: 10.1126/science.282.5390.938

Potter, J. A., Owsianka, A. M., Jeffery, N., Matthews, D. J., Keck, Z. Y., Lau, P., et al. (2012). Toward a hepatitis C virus vaccine: the structural basis of hepatitis C virus neutralization by AP33, a broadly neutralizing antibody. *J. Virol.* 86, 12923–12932. doi: 10.1128/JVI.02052-12

Ray, R., Meyer, K., Banerjee, A., Basu, A., Coates, S., Abrignani, S., et al. (2010). Characterization of antibodies induced by vaccination with hepatitis C virus envelope glycoproteins. *J. Infect. Dis.* 202, 862–866. doi: 10.1086/655902

Ren, Y., Min, Y. Q., Liu, M., Chi, L., Zhao, P., and Zhang, X. L. (2016). N-glycosylation-mutated HCV envelope glycoprotein complex enhances antigen-presenting activity and cellular and neutralizing antibody responses. *Biochimica et biophysica acta* 1860, 1764–1775. doi: 10.1016/j.bbagen.2015.08.007

Rose, P. W., Beran, B., Bi, C., Bluhm, W. F., Dimitropoulos, D., Goodsell, D. S., et al. (2011). The RCSB protein data bank: redesigned web site and web services. *Nucleic Acids Res.* 39, D392–D401. doi: 10.1093/nar/gkq1021

Rosen, H. R. (2011). Chronic hepatitis C infection. *N. Engl. J. Med.* 364, 2429–2438. doi: 10.1056/NEJMcp1006613

Rothwangl, K. B., Manicassamy, B., Uprichard, S. L., and Rong, L. (2008). Dissecting the role of putative CD81 binding regions of E2 in mediating HCV entry: putative CD81 binding region 1 is not involved in CD81 binding. *Virol. J.* 5:46. doi: 10.1186/1743-422X-5-46

Saito, I., Miyamura, T., Ohbayashi, A., Harada, H., Katayama, T., Kikuchi, S., et al. (1990). Hepatitis C virus infection is associated with the development of hepatocellular carcinoma. *Proc. Natl. Acad. Sci. U.S.A.* 87, 6547–6549. doi: 10.1073/pnas.87.17.6547

Sandomenico, A., Leonardi, A., Berisio, R., Sanguigno, L., Focà, G., Focà, A., et al. (2016). Generation and characterization of monoclonal antibodies against a cyclic variant of hepatitis C virus E2 Epitope 412-422. *J. Virol.* 90, 3745–3759. doi: 10.1128/JVI.02397-15

Scarselli, E., Ansuini, H., Cerino, R., Roccasecca, R. M., Acali, S., Filocamo, G., et al. (2002). The human scavenger receptor class B type I is a novel candidate receptor for the hepatitis C virus. *EMBO J.* 21, 5017–5025. doi: 10.1093/emboj/cdf529

Shimizu, Y. K., Hijikata, M., Iwamoto, A., Alter, H. J., Purcell, R. H., and Yoshikura, H. (1994). Neutralizing antibodies against hepatitis C virus and the emergence of neutralization escape mutant viruses. *J. Virol.* 68, 1494–1500.

Simmonds, P., Bukh, J., Combet, C., Deléage, G., Enomoto, N., Feinstone, S., et al. (2005). Consensus proposals for a unified system of nomenclature of hepatitis C virus genotypes. *Hepatology* 42, 962–973. doi: 10.1002/hep.20819

Spadaccini, R., D'Errico, G., D'Alessio, V., Notomista, E., Bianchi, A., Merola, M., et al. (2010). Structural characterization of the transmembrane proximal region of the hepatitis C virus E1 glycoprotein. *Biochim. Biophys Acta* 1798, 344–353. doi: 10.1016/j.bbamem.2009.10.018

Tarr, A. W., Khera, T., Hueging, K., Sheldon, J., Steinmann, E., Pietschmann, T., et al. (2015). Genetic diversity underlying the envelope glycoproteins of hepatitis C virus: structural and functional consequences and the implications for vaccine design. *Viruses* 7, 3995–4046. doi: 10.3390/v7072809

Torrents de la Peña, A., Julien, J. P., de Taeye, S. W., Garces, F., Guttman, M., Ozorowski, G., et al. (2017). Improving the immunogenicity of native-like HIV-1 envelope trimers by hyperstabilization. *Cell Rep.* 20, 1805–1817. doi: 10.1016/j.celrep.2017.07.077

Urbanowicz, R. A., McClure, C. P., Brown, R. J. P., Tsoleridis, T., Persson, M. A. A., Krey, T., et al. (2015). A diverse panel of hepatitis C virus glycoproteins for use in vaccine research reveals extremes of monoclonal antibody neutralization resistance. *J. Virol.* 90, 3288–3301. doi: 10.1128/JVI.02700-15

Vasiliauskaite, I., Owsianka, A., England, P., Khan, A. G., Cole, S., Bankwitz, D., et al. (2017). Conformational flexibility in the immunoglobulin-like domain of the hepatitis C virus glycoprotein E2. *MBio* 8:e00382-17. doi: 10.1128/mBio.00382-17

Vieyres, G., Dubuisson, J., and Pietschmann, T. (2014). Incorporation of hepatitis C virus E1 and E2 glycoproteins: the keystones on a peculiar virion. *Viruses* 6, 1149–1187. doi: 10.3390/v6031149

von Hahn, T., Yoon, J. C., Alter, H., Rice, C. M., Rehermann, B., Balfe, P., et al. (2007). Hepatitis C virus continuously escapes from neutralizing antibody and T-cell responses during chronic infection *in vivo*. *Gastroenterology* 132, 667–678. doi: 10.1053/j.gastro.2006.12.008

Walker, C. M. (2017). Designing an HCV vaccine: a unique convergence of prevention and therapy? *Curr. Opin. Virol.* 23, 113–119. doi: 10.1016/j.coviro.2017.03.014

Walker, C. M., and Grakoui, A. (2015). Hepatitis C virus: why do we need a vaccine to prevent a curable persistent infection? *Curr. Opin. Immunol.* 35, 137–143. doi: 10.1016/j.coi.2015.06.010

Weiner, A. J., Geysen, H. M., Christopherson, C., Hall, J. E., Mason, T. J., Saracco, G., et al. (1992). Evidence for immune selection of hepatitis C virus (HCV) putative envelope glycoprotein variants: potential role in chronic HCV infections. *Proc. Natl. Acad. Sci. U.S.A.* 89, 3468–3472. doi: 10.1073/pnas.89.8.3468

Wong, J. A., Bhat, R., Hockman, D., Logan, M., Chen, C., Levin, A., et al. (2014). Recombinant hepatitis C virus envelope glycoprotein vaccine elicits antibodies targeting multiple epitopes on the envelope glycoproteins associated with broad cross-neutralization. *J. Virol.* 88, 14278–14288. doi: 10.1128/JVI.01911-14

Yassine, H. M., Boyington, J. C., McTamney, P. M., Wei, C. J., Kanekiyo, M., Kong, W. P., et al. (2015). Hemagglutinin-stem nanoparticles generate heterosubtypic influenza protection. *Nat. Med.* 21, 1065–1070. doi: 10.1038/nm.3927

Zhang, Y., Aevermann, B. D., Anderson, T. K., Burke, D. F., Dauphin, G., Gu, Z., et al. (2017). Influenza research database: an integrated bioinformatics resource for influenza virus research. *Nucleic Acids Res.* 45, D466–D474. doi: 10.1093/nar/gkw857

Zuiani, A., Chen, K., Schwarz, M. C., White, J. P., Luca, V. C., Fremont, D. H., et al. (2016). A library of infectious hepatitis C viruses with engineered mutations in the E2 gene reveals growth-adaptive mutations that modulate interactions with scavenger receptor class B Type I. *J. Virol.* 90, 10499–10512. doi: 10.1128/JVI.01011-16

11

Inhibition by Marine Algae of Chikungunya Virus Isolated from Patients in a Recent Disease Outbreak in Rio de Janeiro

Claudio Cesar Cirne-Santos[1,2], Caroline de Souza Barros[1], Caio Cesar Richter Nogueira[1,3], Renata Campos Azevedo[4], Kristie Aimi Yamamoto[4], Guilherme Louzada Silva Meira[4], Zilton Farias Meira de Vasconcelos[5], Norman Arthur Ratcliffe[6], Valéria Laneuville Teixeira[3,7], Jonas Schmidt-Chanasit[8], Davis Fernandes Ferreira[4,9]† and Izabel Christina Nunes de Palmer Paixão[1]*†*

[1] Laboratório de Virologia Molecular e Biotecnologia Marinha, Programa de Pós-graduação em Ciências e Biotecnologia, Departamento de Biologia Celular e Molecular, Instituto de Biologia, Universidade Federal Fluminense, Niterói, Brazil, [2] Departamento de Ensino, Curso de Farmácia na Universidade Salgado de Oliveira, Niterói, Brazil, [3] Laboratório de Produtos Naturais de Algas Marinhas (ALGAMAR), Departamento de Biologia Marinha, Instituto de Biologia, Universidade Federal Fluminense, Niterói, Brazil, [4] Instituto de Microbiologia Paulo de Góes (IMPPG), Departamento de Virologia, Universidade Federal do Rio de Janeiro, Rio de Janeiro, Brazil, [5] Instituto Fernandes Figueira (IFF), Fundação Oswaldo Cruz (Fiocruz), Rio de Janeiro, Brazil, [6] Department of Biosciences, College of Science, Swansea University, Swansea, United Kingdom, [7] Laboratório de Biologia e Taxonomia de Algas (LABIOTAL), Programa de Pós-graduação em Biodiversidade Neotropical, Instituto de Biociencias, Universidade Federal do Estado do Rio de Janeiro, Rio de Janeiro, Brazil, [8] Bernhard Nocht Institute for Tropical Medicine, WHO Collaborating Centre for Arbovirus and Haemorrhagic Fever Reference and Research, Hamburg, Germany, [9] Department of Molecular and Structural Biochemistry, North Carolina State University, Raleigh, NC, United States

***Correspondence:**
Davis Fernandes Ferreira
davisf@micro.ufrj.br
Izabel Christina Nunes de Palmer Paixão
izabeluff@gmail.com

Chikungunya virus (CHIKV) infection is one of the most challenging re-emergent diseases caused by a virus, and with no specific antiviral treatment it has now become a major public health concern. In this investigation, 25 blood samples were collected from patients with characteristic CHIKV symptoms and submitted to a virus isolation protocol, which detected 3 CHIKV isolates. These samples were evaluated by sequencing for the characterization of the strains and any homology to viruses circulating in Brazil during a recent outbreak. These viruses were used for the development of antiviral assays. Subsequently, the inhibitory effects of seaweed extracts on CHIKV replication were studied. The marine species of algae tested were *Bryothamnion triquetrum, Caulerpa racemosa, Laurencia dendroidea, Osmundaria obtusiloba*, *Ulva fasciata*, and *Kappaphycus alvarezii,* all of which are found in different countries including Brazil. The results revealed high levels of CHIKV inhibition, including extracts of *O. obtusiloba* with inhibition values of 1.25 μg/mL and a selectivity index of 420. Viral inhibition was dependent on the time of addition of extract of *O. obtusiloba* to the infected cells, with the optimal inhibition occurring up to 16 h after infection. Neuron evaluations with *O. obtusiloba* were performed and demonstrated low toxicity, and in infected neurons we observed high inhibitory activity in a dose-dependent manner. These results indicate that the algal extracts may be promising novel candidates for the development of therapeutic agents against CHIKV infections.

Keywords: chikungunya, arbovirus, seaweed, antiviral, crude extracts

INTRODUCTION

First described in Tanzania in the African continent in 1952 and later definitively identified in Thailand in 1958, Chikungunya virus (CHIKV) has become a serious public health problem. CHIKV is a reemerging arbovirus infection, with significant human morbidity, and until now one million suspected cases have occurred worldwide (Burt et al., 2012; Presti et al., 2014; Brasil, 2018). CHIKV is mainly transmitted by *Aedes albopictus* and *Aedes aegypti*. Infection causes a self-limited febrile illness known as chikungunya fever with symptoms that include myalgia, fever, rash and debilitating joint symptoms such as persistent polyarthritis, which has been reported to last for many months or even years (Schilte et al., 2013). During a mild course of infection, symptoms usually appear after 4–7 days incubation and disappear after about 1 week from onset of symptoms (Grischott et al., 2016; Purpura et al., 2016).

Although CHIKV had not yet been considered a neurotropic virus, there is evidence now of its involvement as a cause of neurological diseases at different ages, although the maternal-child stage has been described as the main target in the manifestations of encephalopathy by this virus. Further studies are needed for the neurotropic correlation of CHIKV, although there is evidence of some probable neurological complications including encephalitis, myelopathy, peripheral neuropathy, melopoeia, and myopathy (Arpino et al., 2009; Chandak et al., 2009).

Arboviruses have symptoms that may be very difficult to differentiate because of their high overlapping characteristics, and thus clinical diagnosis has become a major challenge, mainly due to the current lack of effective methodologies for more accurate diagnosis. Some tests may be more decisive for CHIKV characterization, such as the reduction of platelet numbers and the presence of eruptions. However, the clinical signs and symptoms of CHIKV are indistinguishable from those of dengue fever, and both diseases are transmitted by *Aedes* mosquitoes (Rudolph et al., 2014). Therefore, steps should be taken to minimize misleading diagnosis during patient examination.

Arbovirus outbreaks, mainly of Zika virus (ZIKV), CHIKV, and dengue (DENV), have been frequently reported. In Thailand, CHIKV outbreaks were first documented in the early 1960s, and the latest outbreak was reported in 2008–2009 (Dash et al., 2007; Montagnier, 2010). Studies have shown that CHIKV was transmitted to Europe, in south-eastern France, between 2010 and 2014. However, in 2013, the first cases of autochthonous transmission in the French Caribbean were reported. Throughout 2018, the distribution of CHIKV in the Americas was also observed, reaching more than one million people (Leparc-Goffart et al., 2014; Powers, 2015).

The first autochthonous cases of CHIKV infection in Brazil were confirmed in 2014, in Oiapoque, Amapá (Rudolph et al., 2014). In 2017, there were 161,346 probable cases of CHIKV fever. In 2018, as of June 23, there were 53,089 probable cases of chikungunya fever in this country. Until this latter date, 11 deaths were confirmed from CHIKV while in the same period of 2017, 160 deaths were recorded (Brasil, 2018). To date, four CHIKV genotypes have been described, namely, East-Central-South African (ECSA), Asian, Indian Ocean, and West African (Weaver and Forrester, 2015). The Asian genotype was first detected in the Caribbean region in late 2013 and then spread throughout Central America. Nine months later, the first autochthonous cases in Brazil were detected in Oiapoque City, Amapá State and also in Feira de Santana, Bahia State, which are more than 2,000 Km from each other. Curiously, the ECSA genotype may be circulating in Feira de Santana and this has been shown to be from an individual who had recently returned from Angola and had a symptomatic contact in Feira de Santana (Nunes et al., 2015).

Chikungunya virus is an alphavirus of the Togaviridae family and has an 11.8 kb genome positive-sense single-stranded RNA. Alphavirus particles are enveloped, have a diameter of 70 nm, tend to be spherical (though slightly pleomorphic) and have an isometric nucleocapsid of 40 nm. The central region of the nucleocapsid has about 240 copies of the capsid protein that surrounds the viral genome. In addition, studies have shown that a number of host factors can be added to the nucleocapsid (Sokoloski et al., 2013). The lipid bilayer is strictly from the host and the source of the viral budding site (Strauss and Strauss, 1994; Lu and Kielian, 2000). Alphaviruses encode four non-structural proteins (nspl, nsp2, nsp3, and nsp4), which are fundamental for viral genome replication, and also the structural proteins that include the capsid, and are related to the viral assembly process (Strauss and Strauss, 1994).

There are no vaccines or specific treatments available for the high morbidity rate caused by CHIKV. The most effective treatments are only symptomatic and use analgesics or anti-inflammatories. Therefore, new compounds are urgently required that can act on the CHIKV infection, reducing the high morbidity and mortality rates resulting from this virus. In this present study, natural products derived from marine algae have been tested against CHIKV as a new strategy since, previously, these extracts have been shown to have high activity against different microorganisms and also to be non-toxic for mammalian cells (Bourjot et al., 2012; Abdelnabi et al., 2015; Ching et al., 2015).

MATERIALS AND METHODS

Seaweed Material and Extraction

The project obtained a permit for scientific purposes on 01/07/2012 at SISBIO/IBAMA number 3534 (VLT) and access to genetic heritage (register SISGEN - IBAMA) from the Universiade Federal Fluminense number A05E653 (VLT) in 01/11/2018.

The seaweeds were collected by snorkeling at a depth 1–3 m in various sites from the Brazilian coast. *Bryothamnion triquetrum* (S. G. Gmelin) M. Howe was collected at Atol das Rocas reef, Rio Grande do Norte State (lat. 03° 51′03″, long. 33° 40′29″), *Caulerpa racemosa* (Forsskål) J. Agardh was collected at Baía da Ribeira, Angra dos Reis, Rio de Janeiro State (lat. 22° 98′33″, long. 44° 38′33″), *Kappaphycus alvarezii* (Doty) Doty ex P. C. Silva was harvested from mariculture at Praia Grande, Paraty, Rio de Janeiro State (lat. 23° 16′15″, long. 44° 34′48″), *Laurencia dendroidea* J. Agardh was collected at Orla Bardot, Armação de Búzios, Rio de Janeiro State (lat. 22° 05′03″, long. 41° 53′ 01″), *Osmundaria obtusiloba* (C. Agardh) R. E. Norris was collected at Rasa Beach, Armação de Búzios, Rio de Janeiro State (lat. 22° 45′40″, long. 41° 54′ 32″) and *Ulva fasciata* Delile was collected at Itaipú Beach, Niterói, Rio de Janeiro State (lat. 22o 58′26″, long. 43° 02′ 46″).

The seaweeds were separated from sediments, epiphytes and other associated organisms, washed with sea water and air-dried (approximate temperature 28–30°C for 7–10 days) until the total evaporation of any water.

Air-dried seaweeds (approximately 100 g) were powdered and exhaustively extracted three times using different organic solvents (PA.) each time for 72 h. *Bryothamnion triquetrum* was extracted with dichloromethane, *Caulerpa racemosa* was extracted with acetone, *Kappaphycus alvarezii* was extracted with ethanol, *Laurencia dendroidea* was extracted with hexane, and *Osmundaria obtusiloba* and *Ulva fasciata* were extracted with ethanol.

The extracts were evaporated under reduced pressure, yielding crude extracts of each species (15–20 mg), of which 2–5 mg were used in tests against the CHIKV. The extracts were chosen according to their chemical composition, and by the presence of different classes of active substances (terpenes, sterols, fatty acids, polysaccharides, alkaloids, aromatic compounds) from these algae as indicated by previous studies (Santos et al., 2010; de Souza Barros et al., 2016; Lira et al., 2016). Analytical TLC was performed on Merck Kieselgel GF_{254} plates, spot detection was obtained by spraying with a 2% solution of Ce(SO4) in 2N H_2SO_4 followed by heating for 5 min at 150°C. The extracted compounds were examined by ^{1}H NMR for detection of the majority of substances in each extract. ^{1}H NMR was determined on a Varian-VNMRS apparatus at 300 and 500 MHz. Spectra were recorded in $CDCl_3$ solutions using TMS as internal standard.

The thin layer chromatographic (TLC) used silica gel GF_{254} and various solvents systems as eluents and Nuclear Magnetic Resonance Proton (^{1}H NMR) analyses demonstrated the majority presence of fatty acids and sterols in *B. triquetrum*, the caulerpin; a pigment bis-indole alkaloid from *C. racemosa;* the sterols, mainly cholesterol, from *K. alvarezii;* elatol, a halogenated sesquiterpene from *Laurencia dendroidea*; bromo-phenols from *Osmundaria obtusiloba*; and palmitic acid and other fatty acids from *U. fasciata*. All the products mentioned were obtained in previous studies (Rocha et al., 2007).

For the *in vitro* experiments the crude extracts were diluted in 100% DMSO and then added with culture medium to the final concentration of 0.01% DMSO.

Cell Lines

VERO cells (African green monkey kidney) VERO-ATCCCCL81 were plated in Eagle's minimum essential medium (MEM) (GIBCO) supplemented with 5% Fetal Bovine Serum (FBS). C6/36 mosquito cell line from *Aedes albopictus*, adapted to grow at 33 °C, was cultured in L-15 Medium (Leibovitz) supplemented with 0.3% tryptose phosphate broth, 0.02% glutamine, 1% MEM non-essential amino acids solution and 5% FBS. Purified cultures of retinal neurons were prepared according to earlier descriptions (Mejía-García and Paes-de-Carvalho, 2007). Retinas of 8-day-old chicken embryos were excised, incubated with 0.1% trypsin and then the cells were dissociated in medium with the help of a conical Pasteur pipette. Subsequently, the cells were seeded on 24 well plastic plates coated with poly-L-ornithine at a density of 830 cells/mm in BME containing 2.5% fetal calf serum, 100 U/ml penicillin, 100 mg/ml streptomycin and 2 mM glutamine and incubated at 37°C for 3 days in a 5% CO2 atmosphere. These purified cultures of retinal neurons were firstly described by Adler et al. (1984). In this work, they showed that almost 100% of the cells possess a neuronal identity using techniques such as phase-contrast microscopy, lectin staining and electron microscopy. After that, some groups have been working with this kind of culture to study different effects on neuronal cells, such as (Ferreira and Paes-de-Carvalho, 2001; Paes-de-Carvalho et al., 2003; Mejía-García et al., 2013) among others. More recently, Anccasi et al. (2013) demonstrated by immunocytochemistry assays that these cells are positive to Tuj1 (beta-tubulin III), which is a protein only found in neurons and considered as a neuronal marker, but negative to a glial marker 2M6.

Virus Isolation

Between the months of March and April 2016, 25 samples of 5 mL venous whole blood were collected in a tube containing EDTA anticoagulant. Samples were taken from selected patients who had clear clinical symptoms of arbovirus infections, mainly joint symptoms and fever, and were treated at a hospital in Niteroi, RJ. The patients were interviewed and agreed to blood collection by signing the free and informed consent form, approved by the ethics committee with approved registration – CAAE: 61845416.0.0000.5289. After collection, all samples were submitted to RT-PCR analysis to determine if the patients had other viral infections, either Flavivirus or Alfavirus, and not only CHIKV. Samples were centrifuged for 5 min, and the leukocyte pellet was removed and added to 24-well plates at 90% confluence in VERO cells. After 24 h, the blood cells were removed from the VERO cell monolayer, fresh media was added, containing 5% FBS, and incubated in an atmosphere of 5% CO_2 at 37°C for 3 to 5 days. The cell culture plates were evaluated daily in order to determine any cytopathic effect as a result of viral infection.

RNA Detection by RT-qPCR and Virus Sequence

RNA from samples presenting cytopathic effects was extracted using the commercial kit QIAamp viral RNA mini (QIAGEN, Valencia, CA, United States) according to the manufacturer's instructions. Isolation was confirmed by reverse transcription real-time PCR (RT-PCR) using primers targeting the structural polyprotein (forward TATCCTGACCATCCGACCCT/reverse GGCTCTTGTCCTTGCACTCT) and Superscript III One-Step RT PCR Kit (Invitrogen Carlsbad, CA, United States), according to the manufacturer's instructions. Amplification was performed in the PeqStar (PeqLab, Erlangen, Germany). PCR conditions were as follows: 60°C for 1 min, 50°C for 45 min, 94°C for 2 min followed by 45 cycles of 95°C for 15 s, 55°C for 30 s and 68°C for 60 s.

The resulting amplicons were sequenced in the ABI 3730 genetic analyzer (Applied Biosystems) following the manufacturer's protocol. Raw sequence data were aligned, edited and assembled using the Assembler tool Bioedit Sequence Aligner Editor. The identity was confirmed by using the Basic Local Alignment Search Tool (Blast) and compared to other CHIKV sequences. Phylogenetic tree was constructed using MEGA 7 program. The sequences were deposited in GenBank under accession numbers MK910738 (BRA/RJ/1F), MK910739 (BRA/RJ/18), and MK910740 (BRA/RJ/23). For the antiviral activity assays the strain with deposit number MK910739 was used.

Plaque Reduction Assay

VERO cells were cultured in growth medium DMEM. The cells were then incubated with CHIKV for 2 h, washed with PBS and a mixture of 2% (w/v) carboxymethylcellulose (Sigma-Aldrich) and DMEM supplemented with 5% FCS, 5 mM L-glutamine and 0.20% sodium bicarbonate was added. Serial dilutions of compounds without overlap medium were done. Cells were fixed with 10% formaldehyde subsequently stained with 1% violet crystal. The infectious virus titer (PFU/ml) was determined using the following formula: plaque count × dilution factor × (1/inoculation volume).

Antiviral Assay

Antiviral activity was evaluated using a virus plaque reduction assay. Vero cells and Neurons were grown in 24-well plates, as described above, and subsequently infected with MOI of 0.1 CHIKV in the absence or presence of different concentrations of the compounds. After 1 h of adsorption at 37°C, the residual inoculum was replaced by MEM containing 1% methyl-cellulose and the corresponding dose of each compound. Plaques were counted after 5–10 days of incubation at 37°C, at 5% CO_2. Uninfected and treated neurons were incubated for 48 to 72 h, and the cells were evaluated daily for cytopathic effects and the culture supernatant was collected to determine the reduction of viral RNA production by RT-PCR. For VERO cells, the inhibitory concentration 50% (EC_{50}) was calculated as the compound concentration reducing virus plaques by 50%. The Selective Index (SI) is derived from the relationship between the CC_{50} and the EC_{50} and reflects the potency and possible future selectivity for future drug development. All determinations were performed twice and each in triplicate.

Time of Addition

VERO cells were infected with CHIKV at a MOI of 0.1 and incubated for 2 h. Afterward, the viruses were removed and the medium was replaced. In addition, 2.5 mg/mL of *C. racemosa* and *O. obtusiloba* crude extracts were added at different points of virus replication at 3, 2 or 1 h before infection, time 0 (immediately after virus added) or 1, 2, 4, 8, 12, 16, 20 or 24 h after infection. These cells were incubated in 5% CO_2 atmosphere at 37°C for 72 h, and then viral replication was measured by plaque assay. Titration at all times was performed at the end of the experiment.

Virucidal Effect

A CHIKV suspension containing 10^6 PFU/mL was incubated with different concentrations of *C. racemosa*, *O. obtusiloba*, and *K. alvarezii* (2.5, 5 or 10 μg/mL) for 2 h at 37°C. The CHIKV suspension was also incubated with the same volume of solvent in the extracts (0.01% DMSO). Then, the samples were diluted in MEM and the remaining infectivity was titrated by plaque formation after 48 h. The important point about the extracts is that the sample dilution effectively reduced the drug concentration incubated with the cells by at least 200-fold to confirm that the titer reduction was only due to cell-free virion inactivation. The 50% relative virucidal effect defined inactivation compared to the controls.

Statistical Analysis

The data were analyzed by the Tukey test or Dunnett test comparing all with the controls (ribavirin and DMSO) using the GraphPad Instat version 3 program. A p-value of <0.05 was considered statistically significant. The values of $p < 0.05$ and $p < 0.01$ are shown in the figures.

RESULTS

RT-PCR of the Isolated Samples and Sequencing

C6/36 mosquito cell line from *Aedes albopictus* was exposed to blood samples from patients suspected of infection by ZIKV or CHIKV and observed daily. At each passage in the C6/36 cells, 50 μL of the supernatant was removed and added into VERO cell cultures in which, at the fourth passage after the supernatant was added, the cytopathic effect was observed after 48 h. Of the 25 samples evaluated from patients who exhibited symptoms characteristic of CHIKV, such as fever, rash, muscular pains, joint pains, and headache, 3 presented cytopathic effects so that the culture supernatants were removed and analyzed by RT-PCR. All 3 samples were positive for CHIKV by PCR, but in order to confirm identity, nucleotide sequencing was performed to characterize the chikungunya strains. Phylogenetic Analysis confirmed the presence of the ECSA genotype in Rio de Janeiro. All viral infection experiments were performed with only one isolate as we determined in an initial experiment that there was no difference in the results obtained for each isolate. The isolates were closely related to strains previously detected in Bahia, Pernambuco and Rio de Janeiro (**Figure 1**).

Cytotoxicity in VERO and Neuron Cells

The cytotoxicity (CC_{50}) of algae extracts in Vero and neuron cells was assessed by MTT [3-(4,5-dimethylthiazole-2-yl)-2,5-diphenyltetrazolium bromide] (Sigma-Aldrich), as previously described (Mosmann, 1983) using 10^5 cells in 96-well plates. Vero cells were exposed to increasing concentrations of the compounds (50, 100, 200, 400, 800, and 1000 μg/mL) and incubated for 72 h to determine cell viability. The results in **Table 1** show that in Vero cells the CC_{50} values for the extracts ranged from 178 to 732 μg/mL. In the

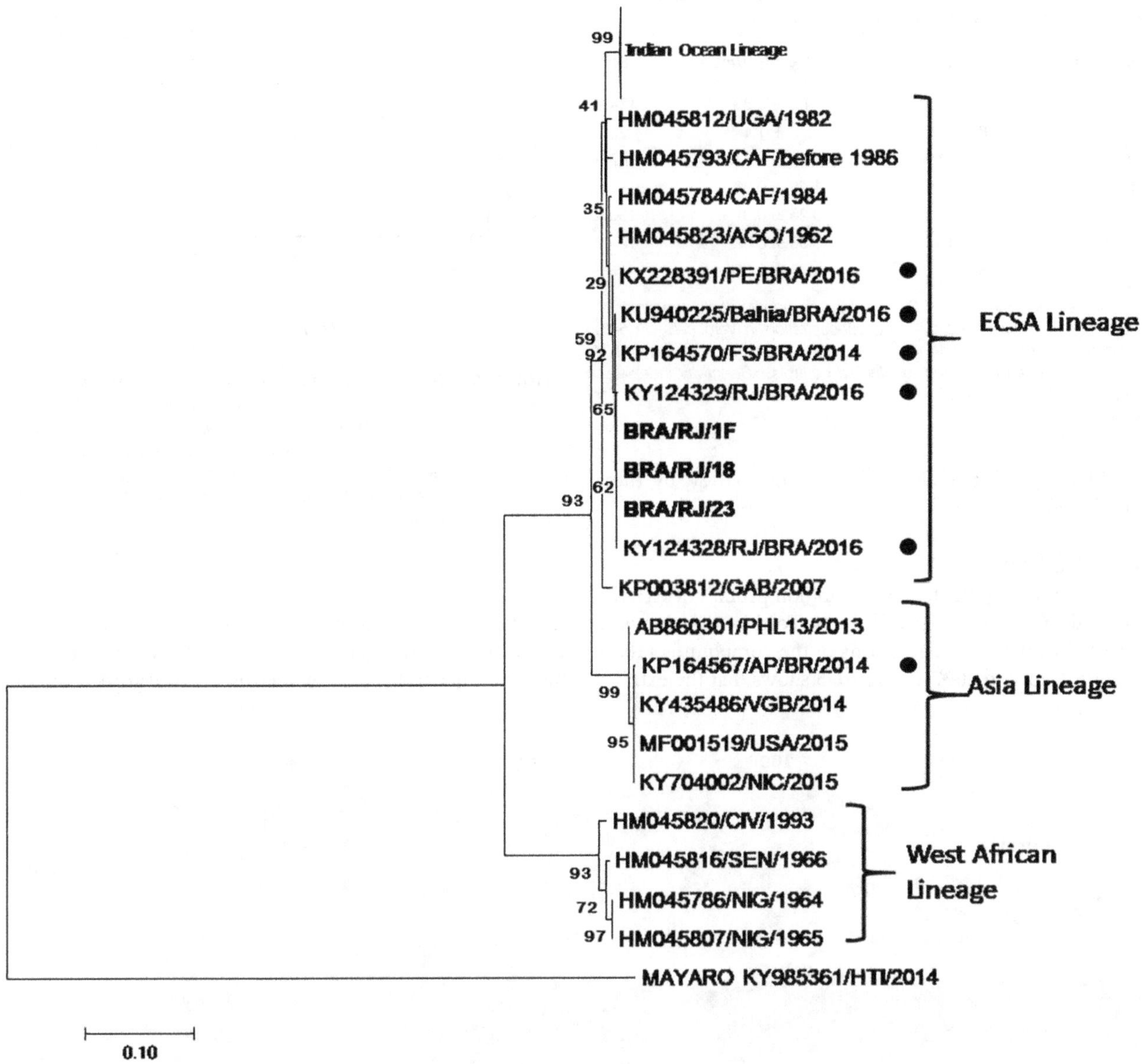

FIGURE 1 | Phylogenetic tree was construct for partial non-structural protein (710 pb). Performed by using the Maximum Likelihood method based on the Kimura 2-parameter model. The analysis involved 69 nucleotide sequences. One fragment of sequences described in this studied is in bold, BRA/RJ/1F, BRA/RJ/18, and BRA/RJ/23 (GenBank access numbers MK910738; MK910739; MK910740). Dots mark the Brazilian isolates.

neurons exposed to the *O. obtusiloba* extracts, there was low cytotoxicity with high viability maintained in concentrations up to 200 μg/mL. In contrast, ribavirin presented cytotoxicity from 100 μg/mL (**Figure 2**).

Inhibition of Chikungunya Virus by Marine Algae

To evaluate the potential of the extracts to inhibit CHIKV replication, Vero cells and neurons were infected in 96-well plates with 0.1 CHIKV MOI, incubated for 1 h for viral adsorption and, subsequently, treated with increasing concentrations of algae extracts. **Figure 3** shows that all the extracts inhibited the replication of CHIKV in a dose-dependent manner. *C. racemosa*, *O. obtusiloba* and *K. alvarezii* inhibited 30 to 98% of CHIKV replication at concentrations from 1.25 to 50 μg/ml. However, the *O. obtusiloba* extract had the highest EC_{50} value (viral inhibition) at 1.25 μg/mL and had a CC_{50} of 525 μg/mL ± 3.11, generating a selectivity index (SI) of 420. In contrast, *C. racemosa* and *K. alvarezii* had lower SIs at 174.2 and 130.1, respectively. Ribavirin, which was used as a control, had an EC_{50} value of 1.73 ± 0.55 μg/mL and was less potent than *O. obtusiloba* extract in inhibiting CHIKV replication (**Table 1**). In infected neurons treated with *O. obtusiloba* extract, there was a significant reduction in the production of copies of viral RNA, demonstrating a

TABLE 1 | Cytotoxicity (CC_{50}) in Vero Cells, anti-CHIKV profile (EC_{50}) and selectivity index (SI) of crude extracts from six seaweeds and ribavirin.

Crude extracts	CC_{50}[a] (μg/mL)	EC_{50}[b] (μg/mL)	SI[c]
C. racemosa	732 ± 18.1	4.2 ± 0.83	174.2
L. dendroidea	178 ± 8.2	7.78 ± 1.1	22.9
U. fasciata	245 ± 11.6	18.9 ± 3.8	12.9
O. obtusiloba	525 ± 15.4	1.25 ± 0.36	420
K. alvarezii	423 ± 19.4	3.25 ± 0.9	130.1
B. triquetrum	400 ± 13.5	3.30 ± 0.82	121.2
Ribavirin	118 ± 5.88	1.73 ± 0.55	68

Data represented as mean ± SD from three independent experiments. [a]Concentration that reduced the cytotoxic concentration in Vero cells by 50% when compared to untreated controls. [b]Concentration that reduced the CHIKV replication by 50% when compared to infected controls. [c]Selectivity index was defined as the ratio between CC_{50} and EC_{50} and represents the safety for in vitro assays.

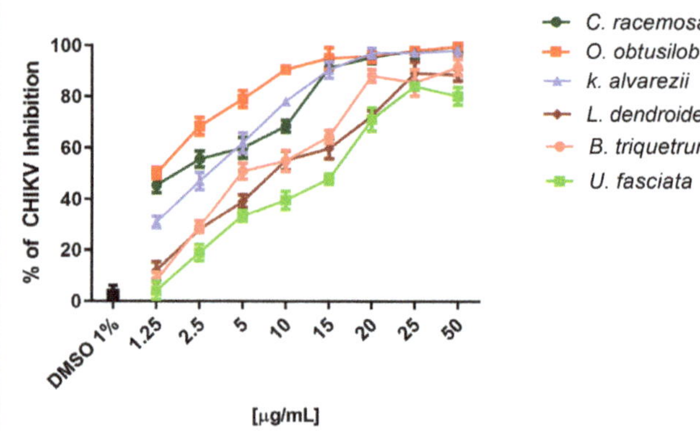

FIGURE 3 | Effect of six seaweeds crude extracts on CHIKV replication. Vero cells were infected with CHIKV (10^6 PFU/mL) at MOI of 0.1 and treated with different concentrations of the extracts, namely, 1.25, 2.5, 5, 10, 15, 20, 25, and 50 μM. The results were evaluated by plaque assay. Error bars indicate the standard deviation and experiments were performed in triplicate. DMSO used as solvent remained at the final concentration of 0.01% showing no activity on CHIKV replication.

strong inhibitory effect of the replication of CHIKV by these compounds (**Figure 4**).

Virucidal Effect

The extracts exhibiting the highest inhibition profiles of CHIKV were selected to test for virucidal effects. To this end, the virus was subjected to three concentrations of the compounds (10, 5, and 2.5 μg/ml) for 2 h at 37°C. **Figure 5** shows that the extracts tested had limited virucidal potentials. However, *O. obtusiloba* was able to inhibit about 40% of CHIKV replication in the highest concentration of extract used (10 μg/mL). In contrast,

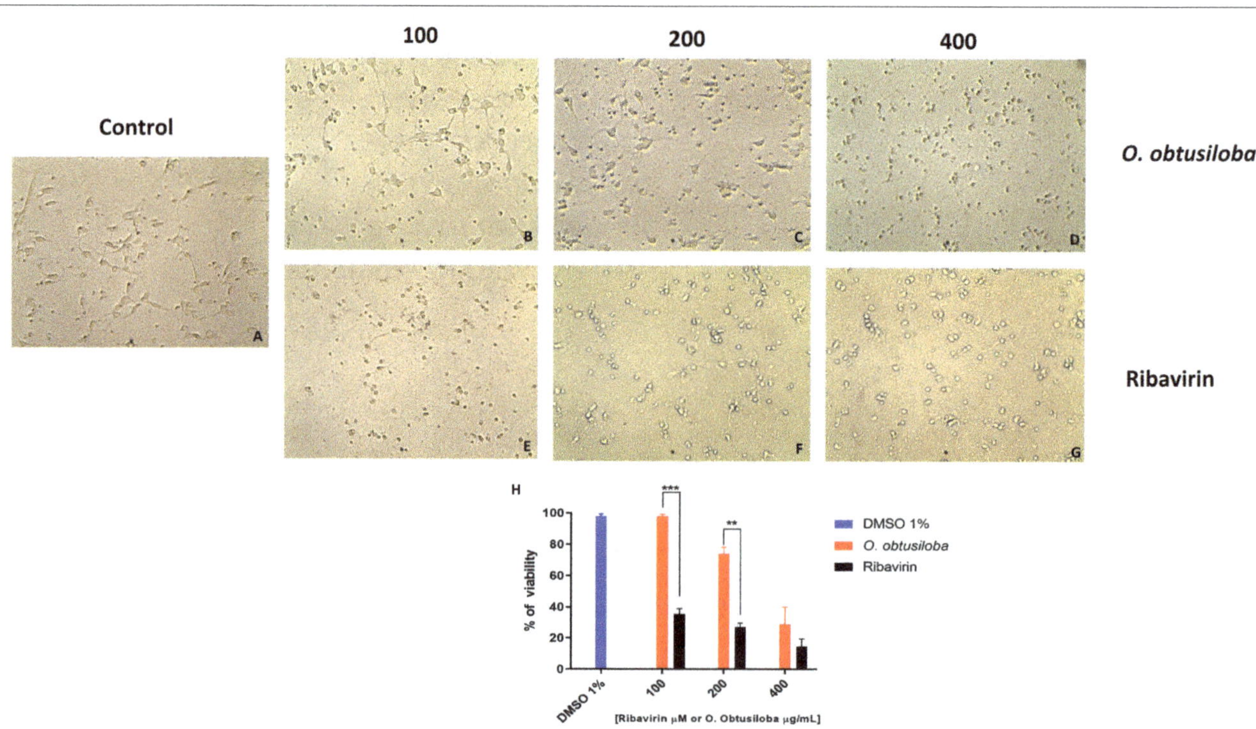

FIGURE 2 | Cytotoxicity of *O. obtusiloba* extract and ribavirin in chick retina neurons in 4-day-old purified cultures. **(A)** Control culture. **(B,C,D)** Cultures incubated with *O. obtusiloba* at concentrations of **(B)** 100 μg/mL, **(C)** 200 μg/mL and **(D)** 400 μg/mL. **(E,F,G)** Cultures incubated with *ribavirin* at concentrations of **(E)** 100 μM, **(F)** 200 μM and **(G)** 400 μM. **(H)** Graphical representation showing the percentage of viability of treated cells with *O. obtusiloba* (blue bar) and percentage of viability of treated cells with ribavirin (dark bar). The results were evaluated by MTT assay and showed that the exposure to the *O. obtusiloba* extract presented low cytotoxicity maintaining high viability in concentrations up to 200 μg/mL. Error bars indicate the standard deviation and experiments were performed in triplicate. $^{**}p < 0.01$; $^{***}p < 0.001$ in Tukey test.

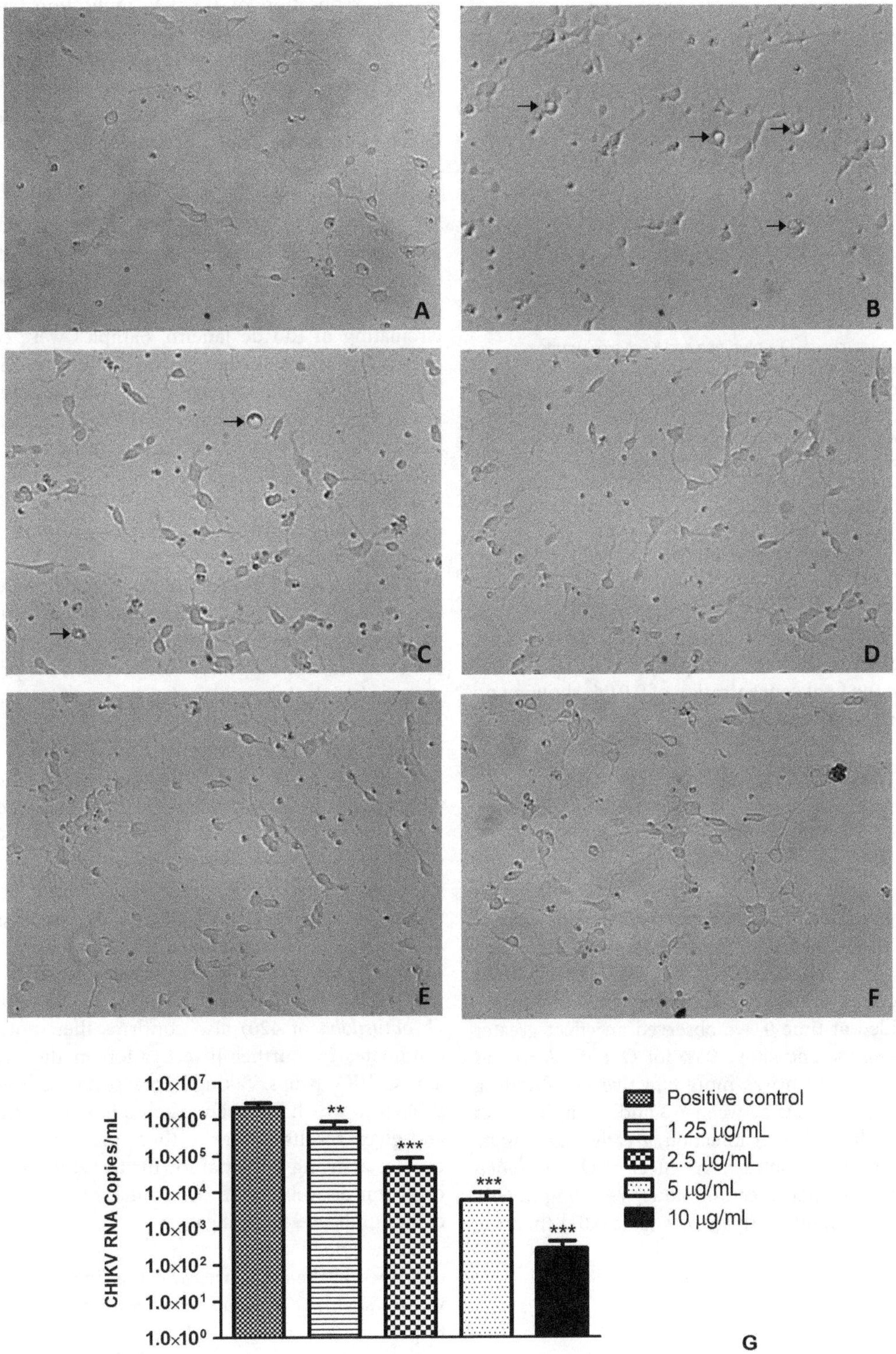

FIGURE 4 | Effect of *O. obtusiloba* extract on CHIKV replication in chick retina neurons in 4-day-old purified cultures. **(A)** Uninfected culture with normal morphology. **(B)** CHIKV-infected culture presenting cytopathic effect (arrow). **(C)** CHIKV-infected culture incubated with 1.25 μg/mL of *O. obtusiloba* presenting cytopathic effect (arrow). **(D)** CHIKV-infected culture incubated with 2.5 μg/mL of *O. obtusiloba* with normal morphology. **(E)** CHIKV-infected culture incubated with 5 μg/mL of *O. obtusiloba* with normal morphology. **(F)** CHIKV-infected culture incubated with 10 μg/mL of *O. obtusiloba* with normal morphology. Chick retina neurons were infected with CHIKV (10^6 PFU/mL) at MOI of 0.1. **(G)** Graphical representation showing the effect of *O. obtusiloba* extract at concentrations of 1.25, 2.5, 5, and 10 μg/mL on CHIKV genomic RNA by quantitative PCR. The results showed that all treatments with the extract showed a significant reduction of RNA copies. Error bars indicate the standard deviation and experiments were performed in triplicate. $**p < 0.01$; $***p < 0.001$ in Tukey test.

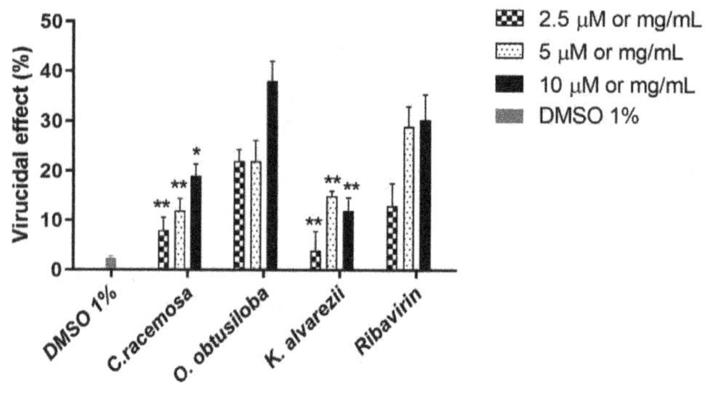

FIGURE 5 | Effect of C. racemosa, O. obtusiloba and K. alvarezii crude extracts on infectivity of CHIKV. To assess potential virucidal activity, we incubated stock CHIKV [CHIKV (106 PFU/mL) at MOI of 0.1] directly with each compound separately at different concentrations for 1 h or with vehicle/DMEM, after which we determined virus titers by standard plaque assays in Vero cells. Experiments were performed independently in triplicate with duplicate plate assays. Error bars indicate the standard deviation and experiments were performed in triplicate. $*p < 0.05$; $**p < 0.01$ in Dunnett test vs. control (Ribavirin). DMSO used as solvent remained at the final concentration of 0.01%, showing no virucidal activity on CHIKV.

Ribavirin used as a control at the same concentration, only inhibited 29% of the production of viral plaques. DMSO used as solvent remained at the final concentration of 0.01%, showing no virucidal activity on CHIKV.

Time of Drug Addition

In order to investigate the mechanism of action of the tested compounds, a time of addition assay was performed using extracts of *C. racemosa* or *O. obtusiloba*, which showed more promising results. For this, VERO cells were treated with *C. racemosa* or *O. obtusiloba* using the antiviral drug Ribavirin, as a control. **Figure 6** shows that when *C. racemosa* or *O. obtusiloba* extracts were added prior to infection of the cells, they produced a pretreatment effect inhibiting about 40% of viral replication. However, when added at time 0, we observed an effect greater than 60% for *C. racemosa* and above 90% for *O. obtusiloba* and Ribavirin. Although Ribavirin was more effective in inhibiting the virus than seaweed extracts between −3 and −1 h, its effect decreased steadily within 2 h after infection, greatly reducing its effects on post infection. In contrast, the effect of *O. obtusiloba* persisted for at least 16 h after infection, slowly reducing to 60% at 20 and 24 h and was significantly greater ($p < 0.01$) than the Ribavirin controls.

DISCUSSION

There are no effective antivirals or vaccines against CHIKV, and as a result this infection has had a significant public health impact, particularly in Brazil and the Americas between 2014 and 2015 (Tan et al., 2018), affecting large numbers of people (Ching et al., 2015; Ahmadi et al., 2016). Numerous studies have been undertaken to discover effective drugs to control this infection, and as a result certain drugs with inhibitory potential for the replication of CHIKV replication, such as Ribavirin, Favipiravir and chloroquine, were developed (Delang et al., 2014; Lani et al., 2015; Ahmadi et al., 2016; Varghese et al., 2016). In the present study, *O. obtusiloba* showed promising results in inhibiting the replication of CHIKV compared to Ribavirin, which has been described as a potential choice for the treatment of CHIKV infection and was used as a control for our studies (Rothan et al., 2015).

The experiments evaluated blood samples of patients suspected of CHIKV infection in the second half of 2016 and who did not travel during this period. This allowed the identification of patients who had been infected by the CHIKV that was circulating in Rio de Janeiro. Samples were collected from 25 patients from Rio de Janeiro who had characteristic chikungunya symptoms and, after extensive attempts, successfully isolated the CHIKV from three patients. RT-PCR and sequencing confirmed that these CHIKV were the same as those in circulation in Brazil and that were initially identified in Bahia to later migrate to Rio de Janeiro (Nunes et al., 2015). This CHIKV were used for *in vitro* studies to test the inhibition of viral replication using seaweed extracts.

Marine organisms, including algae, have undergone many demographic studies as well as analyses of their antimicrobial, antifungal, antiviral, anti-inflammatory activities, and are sources of new therapeutic agents. More recently, the promising antiviral potential of algal derivatives has been targeted in pharmaceutical research, especially for HIV infections (Cirne-Santos et al., 2008; Ahmadi et al., 2015; Pérez et al., 2016).

In the present study, the algal extracts studied had low cytotoxicity in VERO cells with CC_{50} at concentrations higher than 170 μg/mL. The extracts of the algae, *C. racemosa* and *O. obtusiloba,* clearly showed particularly promising results with CC_{50} of 732 and 525 μg/mL, respectively. In relation to the inhibitory effect on CHIKV replication, the EC_{50} of *O. obtusiloba* extract was 1.25 μg/mL, considerably lower than the result obtained with the *C. racemosa* extract, which was 4.2 μg/mL. Comparing the SI levels of both (*C. racemosa* of 174.2 and *O. obtusiloba* of 420) also confirms their potential as possible candidates for further investigation in the discovery of novel anti-CHIKV drugs. Taking into account the inhibitory effects of Ribavirin, which has been inserted in several studies as a control and given results similar to those presented by the extracts, we can see a strong potential for further studies of the mechanism of action as well as the determination of the respective active compounds present in algae.

Some evidence of compounds derived from algae has been well described in the literature, showing significant effects on various viruses such as *Caulerpa racemosa* extract, where alkaloids and terpenoids are found, and in the acetonic extract the main component is caulerpine, which has antiviral activity against HSV-1 (Macedo et al., 2012; Pinto et al., 2012). Antiviral activity against HSV-1 and HSV-2 has also been described for glycolipids extracted from *O. obtusiloba* with EC_{50} values of 42 μg/mL and 12 μg/mL, respectively (de Souza et al., 2012). *O. obtusiloba* ethanolic extract also showed potent antiviral activity against ZIKV (EC_{50} = 1.82) (Cirne-Santos Claudio et al., 2018). De Alencar et al. (2016) showed that the 70%

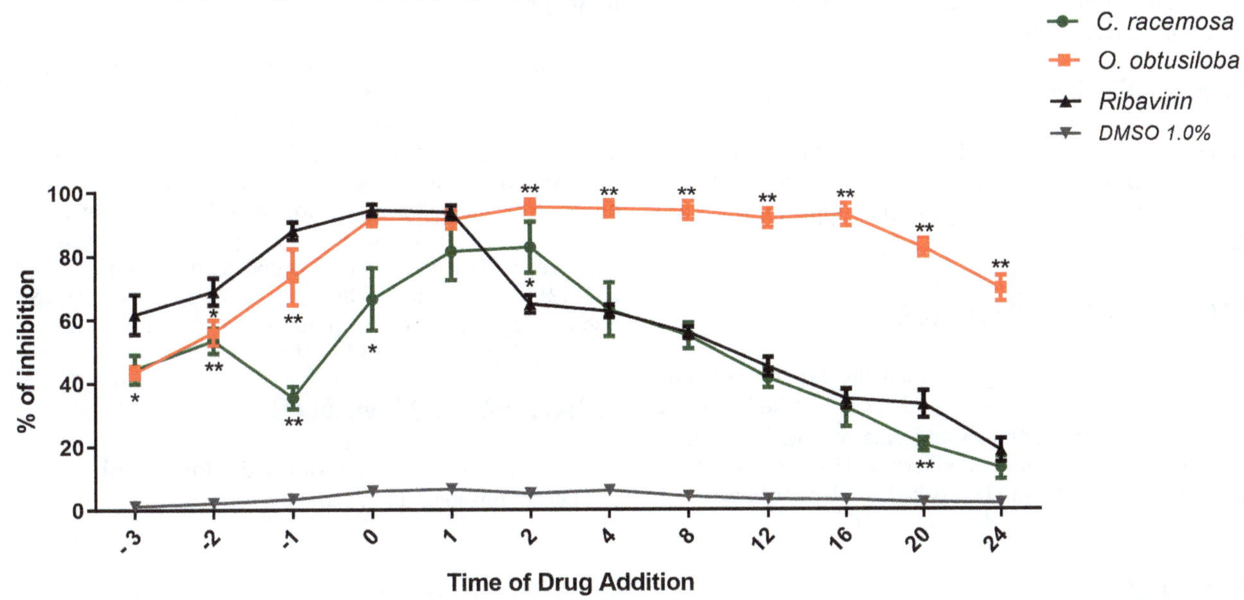

FIGURE 6 | Time of drug addiction studies with *C. racemosa*, *O. obtusiloba*, and *K. alvarezii* crude extracts on CHIKV replication. Vero cells were infected with CHIKV (10^6 PFU/mL) on MOI of 0.1 following each treatment (before the infection, −3, −2, and −1 h; during the infection, 0h; and after the infection, +1, +2, +4, +8, +12, +16, +20, and +24 h), the results were evaluated by plaque assay. Experiments were performed in triplicate. Ribavirin (5 μM) was used as a positive control. *$p < 0.05$; **$p < 0.01$ in Dunnett test vs. control (Ribavirin). DMSO used as solvent remained at the final concentration of 0.01% showing no activity on CHIKV replication.

EtOH was the most effective solvent for extracting phenolic compounds from red seaweeds when compared to hexane, and *O. obtusiloba* EtOH extract presented high antioxidant activity. Seven substances were identified in Brazilian *O. obtusiloba*: three sulfated bromophenols, two bromophenols, one sterol and one glyceride (Carvalho et al., 2006). Given that *O. obtusiloba* ethanolic extract is rich in bromophenols, it is possible that these compounds may be responsible for the inhibitory effects of CHIKV replication.

The extract-tested compounds also had low virucidal potentials (**Figure 5**), with only *O. obtusiloba* resulting in about 40% virucidal activity at 10 μg/mL, although it was superior to the effect of the same concentration of Ribavirin that was used as a control. The study of compounds with this activity is highly relevant because virucidal compounds are chemicals that attack and inactivate viral particles outside the cell (virions), although it is possible that damage to the viral structure occurs (Galabov, 2007).

Several studies have also demonstrated the ability of CHIKV to infect neurons and glial cells with associated neurological complications, suggesting the neurotropic nature of the virus (Chandak et al., 2009; Das et al., 2010; Dhanwani et al., 2012). The results demonstrated that the CHIKV cytopathic effects on infected neurons can be reduced by treatment with *O. obtusiloba* (**Figure 4**). Increasing concentrations of *O. obtusiloba* have higher antiviral activity so that treatment with this compound should be more widely studied, as this may contribute to the reduction of morbidity and mortality of the clinical conditions such as encephalopathies and bone and joint disorders related to CHIKV. Thus, the observation of the reduction in viral RNA production demonstrated by O. obtusiloba tells us the important role of this compound in inhibiting CHIKV replication not only in summer cells but also in primary neurons (**Figure 4**).

Finally, the virus replication inhibition assays by varying the time of extract addition (**Figure 6**) showed that the addition of *O. obtusiloba* at time zero, at the same time as the virus, inhibited viral replication at a rate greater than 80%. This effect was maintained even if the extracts were added up to 16 h after CHIKV infection. There was a small decline in the inhibitory effect after this time, but the extract still inhibited CHIKV replication above 60% if the compound was added within 24 h post-infection. This demonstrates a protective effect even after prolonged contact of the VERO cells with the virus. Pretreatment with these same algal compounds exhibits inhibition of viral replication (approximately 40%), emphasizing the possibility of a virucidal and somewhat protective effect. Importantly, as observed in the time of drug addiction assays, the *O. obtusiloba* extract inhibited viral replication for a longer time than the Ribavirin used as control and also maintains its inhibitory effect for long periods post-infection. This may be vital in many clinical settings where the diagnosis takes some time.

Considering the promising results of the *O. obtusiloba* extract and the previous work of our group demonstrating the low toxicity of this extract administered orally in BALB/c mice (Barros et al., 2018), the extract of this alga becomes a good candidate for further studies. In addition, the possibility of oral treatment with the extract, or the active ingredient isolated from the extract, can also be tested, as was done with dolabelladienetriol (20 mg/Kg/dose; twice a day) against HSV-1 in BALB/c (Garrido et al., 2017).

ETHICS STATEMENT

This project was submitted to the research ethics committee of ASSOCIACAO SALGADO DE OLIVEIRA DE EDUCACAO E CULTURA and obtained the registration approval - CAAE: 61845416.0.0000.5289.

AUTHOR CONTRIBUTIONS

CC-S, CB, KY, GM, and CN performed the experiments and wrote the manuscript. RA, ZV, and JS-C worked on the implementation of methodologies and data review. VT worked on the supply of natural product. NR worked on the revision of English and in writing. DF and IP worked as job coordinators.

FUNDING

The authors are grateful to CNPq (Conselho Nacional de Desenvolvimento Científico e Tecnológico) for financial support and for Productivity Fellowships to IP and VT (443930/2014-7 and 304070/2014-9). IP and VT (E-26/201.442/2014) also thank the FAPERJ (Fundação de Amparo à Pesquisa do Estado do Rio de Janeiro) for the Cientista do Nosso Estado Fellowship. CC-S thanks CAPES (Coordenação de Aperfeiçoamento de Pessoal de Nível Superior) for the Postdoc fellowship and CB thanks FAPERJ for the Postdoc fellowship (E-26/201.344/2016). Support also came from the postgraduate program in sciences and biotechnology of UFF (PPBI-UFF).

ACKNOWLEDGMENTS

The authors would like to acknowledge for the technical support of Thereza Elizabeth P. P. Garcia.

REFERENCES

Abdelnabi, R., Neyts, J., and Delang, L. (2015). Towards antivirals against chikungunya virus. *Antiviral Res.* 121, 59–68. doi: 10.1016/j.antiviral.2015.06.017

Adler, R., Lindsey, J. D., and Elsner, C. L. (1984). Expression of cone-like properties by chick embryo neural retina cells in glial-free monolayer cultures. *J. Cell Biol.* 99, 1173–1178. doi: 10.1083/jcb.99.3.1173

Ahmadi, A., Hassandarvish, P., Lani, R., Yadollahi, P., Jokar, A., Bakar, S. A., et al. (2016). Inhibition of chikungunya virus replication by hesperetin and naringenin. *RSC Adv.* 6, 69421–69430. doi: 10.1039/c6ra16640g

Ahmadi, A., Zorofchian Moghadamtousi, S., Abubakar, S., and Zandi, K. (2015). Antiviral potential of algae polysaccharides isolated from marine sources: a review. *BioMed Res. Int.* 2015:825203. doi: 10.1155/2015/825203

Anccasi, R. M., Ornelas, I. M., Cossenza, M., Persechini, P. M., and Ventura, A. L. M. (2013). ATP induces the death of developing avian retinal neurons in culture via activation of P2X7 and glutamate receptors. *Purinergic Signal.* 9, 15–29. doi: 10.1007/s11302-012-9324-5

Arpino, C., Curatolo, P., and Rezza, G. (2009). Chikungunya and the nervous system: what we do and do not know. *Rev. Med. Virol.* 19, 121–129. doi: 10.1002/rmv.606

Barros, C. D. S., Gomes, M. W. L., Gomes, R. D. S. P., Melchiades, V., Nogueira, C. C. R., Cirne-Santos, C. C., et al. (2018). Acute toxicity evaluation of ethanol extract of red algae, Osmundaria obtusiloba, in BALB/c mice. *J. Med. Plants Res.* 12, 217–221. doi: 10.5897/jmpr2018.6582

Bourjot, M., Delang, L., Nguyen, V. H., Neyts, J., GuéRitte, F. O., Leyssen, P., et al. (2012). Prostratin and 12-O-tetradecanoylphorbol 13-acetate are potent and selective inhibitors of chikungunya virus replication. *J. Nat. Prod.* 75, 2183–2187. doi: 10.1021/np300637t

Brasil. (2018). *Boletim epidemiológico*. Brazil: Ministério da Saúde.

Burt, F. J., Rolph, M. S., Rulli, N. E., Mahalingam, S., and Heise, M. T. (2012). Chikungunya: a re-emerging virus. *Lancet* 379, 662–671. doi: 10.1016/s0140-6736(11)60281-x

Carvalho, L. R. D., Guimarães, S. M., and Roque, N. F. (2006). Sulfated bromophenols from Osmundaria obtusiloba (C. Agardh) RE Norris (*Rhodophyta, Ceramiales*). *Braz. J. Bot.* 29, 453–459.

Chandak, N. H., Kashyap, R. S., Kabra, D., Karandikar, P., Saha, S. S., Morey, S. H., et al. (2009). Neurological complications of Chikungunya virus infection. *Neurol. India* 57, 177–180. doi: 10.4103/0028-3886.51289

Ching, K.-C., Kam, Y.-W., Merits, A., Ng, L. F., and Chai, C. L. (2015). Trisubstituted thieno [3, 2-b] pyrrole 5-carboxamides as potent inhibitors of alphaviruses. *J. Med. Chem.* 58, 9196–9213. doi: 10.1021/acs.jmedchem.5b01047

Cirne-Santos, C. C., Souza, T. M. L., Teixeira, V. L., Fontes, C. F. L., Rebello, M. A., Castello-Branco, L. R. R., et al. (2008). The dolabellane diterpene dolabelladienetriol is a typical noncompetitive inhibitor of HIV-1 reverse transcriptase enzyme. *Antiviral Res.* 77, 64–71. doi: 10.1016/j.antiviral.2007.08.006

Cirne-Santos Claudio, C., Souza Barros Caroline, D., Richter Nogueira Caio, C., Santos Correa Amorim Leonardo, D., Mendonca Campos Renata, D., Ratcliffe Norman, A., et al. (2018). Antiviral effect of the seaweed osmundaria obtusiloba against the Zika virus. *J. Med. Plants Res* 12, 387–395. doi: 10.5897/JMPR2018.6624

Das, T., Jaffar-Bandjee, M. C., Hoarau, J. J., Trotot, P. K., Denizot, M., Lee-Pat-Yuen, G., et al. (2010). Chikungunya fever: CNS infection and pathologies of a re-emerging arbovirus. *Prog. Neurobiol.* 91, 121–129. doi: 10.1016/j.pneurobio.2009.12.006

Dash, P., Parida, M., Santhosh, S., Verma, S., Tripathi, N., Ambuj, S., et al. (2007). East Central South African genotype as the causative agent in reemergence of Chikungunya outbreak in India. *Vector Borne Zoonotic Dis.* 7, 519–528. doi: 10.1089/vbz.2007.7272

De Alencar, D. B., De Carvalho, F. C. T., Rebouças, R. H., Dos Santos, D. R., Dos Santos Pires-Cavalcante, K. M., De Lima, R. L., et al. (2016). Bioactive extracts of red seaweeds pterocladiella capillacea and osmundaria obtusiloba (*Floridophyceae*: *Rhodophyta*) with antioxidant and bacterial agglutination potential. *Asian Pac. J. Trop. Med.* 9, 372–379. doi: 10.1016/j.apjtm.2016.03.015

de Souza, L. M., Sassaki, G. L., Romanos, M. T. V., and Barreto-Bergter, E. (2012). Structural characterization and anti-HSV-1 and HSV-2 activity of glycolipids from the marine algae osmundaria obtusiloba isolated from Southeastern Brazilian coast. *Mar. Drugs* 10, 918–931. doi: 10.3390/md10040918

de Souza Barros, C., Garrido, V., Melchiades, V., Gomes, R., Gomes, M. W. L., Teixeira, V. L., et al. (2016). Therapeutic efficacy in BALB/C mice of extract from marine alga Canistrocarpus cervicornis (*Phaeophyceae*) against herpes simplex virus type 1. *J. Appl. Phycol.* 29, 769–773. doi: 10.1007/s10811-016-0865-9

Delang, L., Segura Guerrero, N., Tas, A., Quérat, G., Pastorino, B., Froeyen, M., et al. (2014). Mutations in the chikungunya virus non-structural proteins cause resistance to favipiravir (T-705), a broad-spectrum antiviral. *J. Antimicrob. Chemother.* 69, 2770–2784. doi: 10.1093/jac/dku209

Dhanwani, R., Khan, M., Bhaskar, A., Singh, R., Patro, I., Rao, P., et al. (2012). Characterization of Chikungunya virus infection in human neuroblastoma SH-SY5Y cells: role of apoptosis in neuronal cell death. *Virus Res.* 163, 563–572. doi: 10.1016/j.virusres.2011.12.009

Ferreira, J. M., and Paes-de-Carvalho, R. (2001). Long-term activation of adenosine A2a receptors blocks glutamate excitotoxicity in cultures of avian retinal neurons. *Brain Res.* 900, 169–176. doi: 10.1016/s0006-8993(01) 02279-x

Galabov, A. S. (2007). Virucidal agents in the eve of manorapid synergy®. *GMS Krankenhaushyg. Interdiszip.* 2, 1–8.

Garrido, V., Barros, C., Melchiades, V. A., Fonseca, R. R., Pinheiro, S., Ocampo, P., et al. (2017). Subchronic toxicity and anti-HSV-1 activity in experimental animal of dolabelladienetriol from the seaweed, dictyota pfaffii. *Regul. Toxicol. Pharmacol.* 86, 193–198. doi: 10.1016/j.yrtph.2017.03.007

Grischott, F., Puhan, M., Hatz, C., and Schlagenhauf, P. (2016). Non-vector-borne transmission of Zika virus: a systematic review. *Travel Med. Infect. Dis.* 14, 313–330. doi: 10.1016/j.tmaid.2016.07.002

Lani, R., Hassandarvish, P., Chiam, C. W., Moghaddam, E., Chu, J. J. H., Rausalu, K., et al. (2015). Antiviral activity of silymarin against chikungunya virus. *Sci. Rep.* 5, 11421. doi: 10.1038/srep11421

Leparc-Goffart, I., Nougairede, A., Cassadou, S., Prat, C., and De Lamballerie, X. (2014). Chikungunya in the Americas. *Lancet* 383:514.

Lira, M.-L. F., Lopes, R., Gomes, A. P., Barcellos, G., Verícimo, M., Osako, K., et al. (2016). Anti-leishmanial activity of Brazilian green, brown, and red algae. *J. Appl. Phycol.* 28, 591–598. doi: 10.1007/s10811-015-0538-0

Lu, Y. E., and Kielian, M. (2000). Semliki forest virus budding: assay, mechanisms, and cholesterol requirement. *J. Virol.* 74, 7708–7719. doi: 10.1128/jvi.74.17.7708-7719.2000

Macedo, N. R. P. V., Ribeiro, M. S., Villaça, R. C., Ferreira, W., Pinto, A. M., Teixeira, V. L., et al. (2012). Caulerpin as a potential antiviral drug against herpes simplex virus type 1. *Rev. Bras. Farmacogn.* 22, 861–867. doi: 10.1590/s0102-695x2012005000072

Mejía-García, T., and Paes-de-Carvalho, R. (2007). Nitric oxide regulates cell survival in purified cultures of avian retinal neurons: involvement of multiple transduction pathways. *J. Neurochem.* 100, 382–394. doi: 10.1111/j.1471-4159.2006.04244.x

Mejía-García, T. A., Portugal, C. C., Encarnação, T. G., Prado, M. A. M., and Paes-De-Carvalho, R. (2013). Nitric oxide regulates AKT phosphorylation and nuclear translocation in cultured retinal cells. *Cell. Signal* 25, 2424–2439. doi: 10.1016/j.cellsig.2013.08.001

Montagnier, L. (2010). 25 years after HIV discovery: prospects for cure and vaccine. *Virology* 397, 248–226.

Mosmann, T. (1983). Rapid colorimetric assay for cellular growth and survival: application to proliferation and cytotoxicity assays. *J. Immunol. Methods* 65, 55–63. doi: 10.1016/0022-1759(83)90303-4

Nunes, M. R. T., Faria, N. R., De Vasconcelos, J. M., Golding, N., Kraemer, M. U., De Oliveira, L. F., et al. (2015). Emergence and potential for spread of Chikungunya virus in Brazil. *BMC Med.* 13:102. doi: 10.1186/s12916-015-0348-x

Paes-de-Carvalho, R., Maia, G., and Ferreira, J. (2003). Adenosine regulates the survival of avian retinal neurons and photoreceptors in culture. *Neurochem. Res.* 28, 1583–1590.

Pérez, M. J., Falqué, E., and Domínguez, H. (2016). Antimicrobial action of compounds from marine seaweed. *Mar. Drugs* 14:E52.

Pinto, A. M. V., Leite, J. P. G., Ferreira, W. J., Cavalcanti, D. N., Villaça, R. C., Giongo, V., et al. (2012). Marine natural seaweed products as potential antiviral drugs against bovine viral diarrhea virus. *Rev. Bras. Farmacogn.* 22, 813–817. doi: 10.1590/s0102-695x2012005000060

Powers, A. M. (2015). Risks to the Americas associated with the continued expansion of chikungunya virus. *J. Gen. Virol.* 96, 1–5. doi: 10.1099/vir.0.070136-0

Presti, A. L., Lai, A., Cella, E., Zehender, G., and Ciccozzi, M. (2014). Chikungunya virus, epidemiology, clinics and phylogenesis: a review. *Asian Pac. J. Trop. Med.* 7, 925–932. doi: 10.1016/S1995-7645(14)60164-4

Purpura, L. J., Choi, M. J., and Rollin, P. E. (2016). Zika virus in semen: lessons from Ebola. *Lancet Infect. Dis.* 16, 1107–1108. doi: 10.1016/s1473-3099(16)30330-9

Rocha, F. D., Soares, A. R., Houghton, P. J., Pereira, R. C., Kaplan, M. A. C., and Teixeira, V. L. (2007). Potential cytotoxic activity of some Brazilian seaweeds on human melanoma cells. *Phytother. Res.* 21, 170–175. doi: 10.1002/ptr.2038

Rothan, H. A., Bahrani, H., Mohamed, Z., Teoh, T. C., Shankar, E. M., Rahman, N. A., et al. (2015). A combination of doxycycline and ribavirin alleviated chikungunya infection. *PLoS One* 10:e0126360. doi: 10.1371/journal.pone.0126360

Rudolph, K. E., Lessler, J., Moloney, R. M., Kmush, B., and Cummings, D. A. (2014). Incubation periods of mosquito-borne viral infections: a systematic review. *Am. J. Trop. Med. Hyg.* 90, 882–891. doi: 10.4269/ajtmh.13-0403

Santos, A. O. D., Veiga-Santos, P., Ueda-Nakamura, T., Sudatti, D. B., Bianco, ÉM., Pereira, R. C., et al. (2010). Effect of elatol, isolated from red seaweed Laurencia dendroidea, on Leishmania amazonensis. *Mar. Drugs* 8, 2733–2743. doi: 10.3390/md8112733

Schilte, C., Staikovsky, F., Couderc, T., Madec, Y., Carpentier, F., Kassab, S., et al. (2013). Chikungunya virus-associated long-term arthralgia: a 36-month prospective longitudinal study. *PLoS Neg.l Trop. Dis.* 7:e2137. doi: 10.1371/journal.pntd.0002137

Sokoloski, K. J., Snyder, A. J., Liu, N. H., Hayes, C. A., Mukhopadhyay, S., and Hardy, R. W. (2013). Encapsidation of host-derived factors correlates with enhanced infectivity of Sindbis virus. *J. Virol.* 87, 12216–12226. doi: 10.1128/JVI.02437-13

Strauss, J. H., and Strauss, E. G. (1994). The alphaviruses: gene expression, replication, and evolution. *Microbiol. Rev.* 58, 491–562.

Tan, Y., Pickett, B. E., Shrivastava, S., Gresh, L., Balmaseda, A., Amedeo, P., et al. (2018). Differing epidemiological dynamics of Chikungunya virus in the Americas during the 2014-2015 epidemic. *PLoS Negl. Trop. Dis.* 12:e0006670. doi: 10.1371/journal.pntd.0006670

Varghese, F. S., Kaukinen, P., Gläsker, S., Bespalov, M., Hanski, L., Wennerberg, K., et al. (2016). Discovery of berberine, abamectin and ivermectin as antivirals against chikungunya and other alphaviruses. *Antiviral Res.* 126, 117–124. doi: 10.1016/j.antiviral.2015.12.012

Weaver, S. C., and Forrester, N. L. (2015). Chikungunya: evolutionary history and recent epidemic spread. *Antiviral Res.* 120, 32–39. doi: 10.1016/j.antiviral.2015.04.016

12

Antiviral Drugs Against Severe Fever with Thrombocytopenia Syndrome Virus Infection

*Mutsuyo Takayama-Ito and Masayuki Saijo**

Department of Virology I, National Institute of Infectious Diseases, Tokyo, Japan

***Correspondence:**
Masayuki Saijo
msaijo@nih.go.jp

Severe fever with thrombocytopenia syndrome (SFTS) is an emerging tick-borne infectious disease caused by SFTS virus (SFTSV), which is a novel bunyavirus. SFTSV was first isolated from patients who presented with fever, thrombocytopenia, leukocytopenia, and multiorgan dysfunction in China. Subsequently, it was found to be widely distributed in Southeast Asia (Korea, Japan, and Vietnam). SFTSV can be transmitted not only from ticks but also from domestic animals, companion animals, and humans. Because the case fatality rate of SFTS is high (6–30%), development of specific and effective treatment for SFTS is required. Studies of potential antiviral drugs for SFTS-specific therapy have been conducted on existing or newly discovered agents *in vitro* and *in vivo*, with ribavirin and favipiravir being the most promising candidates. While animal experiments and retrospective studies have demonstrated the limited efficacy of ribavirin, it was also speculated that ribavirin would be effective in patients with a viral load $<1 \times 10^6$ copies/mL. Favipiravir showed higher efficacy than ribavirin against SFTSV in *in vitro* assays and greater efficacy in animal models, even administrated 3 days after the virus inoculation. Although clinical trials evaluating the efficacy of favipiravir in SFTS patients in Japan are underway, this has yet to be confirmed. Other drugs, including hexachlorophene, calcium channel blockers, 2′-fluoro-2′-deoxycytidine, caffeic acid, amodiaquine, and interferons, have also been evaluated for their inhibitory efficacy against SFTSV. Among them, calcium channel blockers are promising because in addition to their efficacy *in vitro* and *in vivo*, retrospective clinical data have indicated that nifedipine, one of the calcium channel blockers, reduced the case fatality rate by >5-fold. Although further research is necessary to develop SFTS-specific therapy, considerable progress has been achieved in this area. Here we summarize and discuss recent advances in antiviral drugs against SFTSV.

Keywords: severe fever with thrombocytopenia syndrome, severe fever with thrombocytopenia syndrome virus, antiviral, ribavirin, favipiravir

INTRODUCTION

Severe fever with thrombocytopenia syndrome (SFTS) is an emerging tick-borne infectious disease caused by SFTS virus (SFTSV), a novel bunyavirus classified into the genus *Phlebovirus* and family *Bunyaviridae* according to the previous nomenclature by the International Committee of Taxonomy of Viruses (ICTV). However, according to the nomenclature by the ICTV, SFTSV has been classified into the Genus *Banyangvirus*, Family *Phenuiviridae* and re-named as *Huaiyangshan banyangvirus*. In this review article, we have referred to it as "SFTSV." SFTSV is a negative-stranded RNA virus and its genome comprises of three segments, designated as large (L), medium (M), and small (S). The L and M segments encode the RNA dependent RNA polymerase (RdRp) and glycoprotein precursors (Gn and Gc), respectively, and S segment encodes nucleoprotein and nonstructural proteins. The RdRp of SFTSV is responsible for viral replication and is a major target of nucleoside analogs, which are used as therapeutic antiviral drugs. The Gn and Gc are presented on the surface of the virion and are the main targets of neutralizing antibodies. SFTSV was first isolated from patients who presented with fever, thrombocytopenia, leukocytopenia, and multiorgan dysfunction in Hubei and Henan provinces in Central China (Yu et al., 2011). Subsequently, the virus was isolated from sick patients in Japan and South Korea, indicating that SFTSV was endemic not only to China, but also to South Korea and Japan (Kim et al., 2013; Takahashi et al., 2014). In addition, recent studies have reported SFTS as endemic to Vietnam (Tran et al., 2019) and Xinjiang, China (Zhu et al., 2019), indicating that the distribution of SFTSV in Southeast Asia might be much more extensive than expected. Humans become infected mainly via tick-bites, but through close contact with animals such as cats, and dogs and human-to-human transmission has also been reported (Gai et al., 2012; Niu et al., 2013; Kida et al., 2019). The case fatality rate of SFTS is found to vary between 6 and 30% in Japan and South Korea, with a fatality rate of approximately 30% (Choi et al., 2016; Kato et al., 2016). Although World Health Organization listed SFTS as a disease requiring urgent research and development (World Health Organization, 2017), there is no available effective SFTS treatment.

The development of vaccines against SFTSV infection has been attempted (Dong et al., 2019; Kwak et al., 2019). The development of specific treatment for SFTS is crucial because SFTSV infection is relatively rare and the affected patients are mainly elderly. Some proposed treatments for SFTS include steroid pulse therapy (Nakamura et al., 2018), plasma exchange (Oh et al., 2014; Yoo et al., 2019), and antiviral drugs (Saijo, 2018); however, their effectiveness remains unclear.

SFTSV infects a variety of cultured cells, including L929, Vero E6, Vero, and DH82 cells (Yu et al., 2011). Several studies have been conducted to identify effective antiviral agents against SFTSV by screening compound libraries or testing agents that are effective against other viruses (**Table 1**). Because it has been suggested that antiviral drugs may potentially be effective in treatment of multiple viral infections, testing approved drugs is considered as a reasonable strategy (De Clercq and Li, 2016).

Sufficient animal models are required to evaluate the efficacy of antiviral drugs in the treatment of SFTSV infections. However, adult mice and hamsters are not susceptible to SFTSV infection (Jin et al., 2012) and non-human primate models show only mild symptoms similar to those of SFTS in humans (Jin et al., 2015). Only several immunodeficient or immature animal models are available (Gowen and Hickerson, 2017). Mice deficient in α/β interferon receptor ($IFNAR^{-/-}$) (Liu et al., 2014; Tani et al., 2016) and mice and Syrian hamsters deficient for the gene encoding signal transducer and the activator of transcription 2 ($STAT2^{-/-}$) (Gowen et al., 2017; Yoshikawa et al., 2019) were found to be susceptible to SFTSV infection following subcutaneous inoculation, and newborn mice and rats were susceptible to SFTSV infection when inoculated intracerebrally (Chen et al., 2012; Zivcec et al., 2013; Ning et al., 2019). **Table 2** presents animal models that have been used to determine the efficacy of antiviral drugs against SFTSV infections.

In this review article, we summarize and discuss recent advancements made in SFTSV treatment using antiviral drugs.

POTENTIAL THERAPEUTIC DRUGS AGAINST SFTS

Ribavirin

Ribavirin, a nucleotide analog, exerts a broad spectrum of antiviral activity against various viruses, such as respiratory syncytial virus, influenza, measles, herpesvirus, human immunodeficiency virus, Lassa virus, and [in combination with interferon (IFN)-α] hepatitis C virus. Ribavirin can be administered orally, intravenously, or via a nebulizer (Snell, 2001). The proposed mechanisms of action of ribavirin against viruses are indirect (inosine monophosphate dehydrogenase inhibition and immunomodulatory effects) as well as direct (interference with RNA capping, polymerase inhibition, and lethal mutagenesis) (Graci and Cameron, 2006).

Shimojima et al. (2014) first reported the efficacy of ribavirin *in vitro* using three cell lines: monkey kidney-derived Vero, human hepatoma-derived Huh7, and human osteosarcoma-derived U2OS cells. When treated with ribavirin before and during infection with SFTSV, the 99% inhibitory concentration (IC_{99}) of ribavirin was 263, 83, and 78 μM in Vero, Huh7, and U2OS cells, respectively (**Table 1**). However, when Vero cells were treated with ribavirin 3 days after the inoculation, the inhibitory effect was dramatically decreased, suggesting that ribavirin could be used as post-exposure prophylaxis for the prevention of SFTS and also mentioned that ribavirin could be effective as part of a combination therapy to treat SFTS patients (Shimojima et al., 2014). The efficacy of ribavirin against SFTSV replication was also observed in another study, where Vero cells infected with a Korean SFTSV strain were treated at 24 and 48 h post inoculation, and the 50% inhibitory concentration (IC_{50}) range was 3.69–8.72 μg/mL (Lee et al., 2017) (**Table 1**). Despite several differences in viral strains and treatment procedure, ribavirin suppressed SFTS replication, suggesting that it was effective against various SFTSVs for at least 48 h after SFTSV inoculation.

Shimojima et al. (2015) investigated the improvement in efficacy when ribavirin was used in combination with IFNs. All IFNs showed dose-dependent inhibitory effects when used alone. The IC_{90} of IFNα, IFNβ, and IFNγ was 29 U/ml, 24 U/ml, and 12 ng/ml, respectively, and that of ribavirin was 43 μg/mL (**Table 1**). When IFNs were combined with ribavirin at IC_{90}, significant inhibitory effects were observed, with reductions of $>3\ log_{10}$ in viral titers. This study suggested that the combination

TABLE 1 | Efficacy of anti-SFTSV drugs *in vitro*.

Agent	Cells	Study design	Strain of SFTSV	$IC_{50/90/99}$	CC_{50}	References
Ribavirin	Vero	Yield reduction	Chinese strain (HB29)	$IC_{99} = 263\,\mu M$	>1,929 μM	Shimojima et al., 2014
	Huh7			$IC_{99} = 83\,\mu M$		
	U2OS			$IC_{99} = 78\,\mu M$		
	Vero	Yield reduction	Japanese strain (SPL030)	$IC_{99} = 424\,\mu M$	>1,929 μM	
	Huh7			$IC_{99} = 63\,\mu M$		
	U2OS			$IC_{99} = 73\,\mu M$		
	Vero	Yield reduction	Japanese strain (SPL030)	$IC_{90} = 176\,\mu M$*	>2,000 μM	Shimojima et al., 2015
		Yield reduction	Korean isolate strain	$IC_{50} = 15.1–35.7\,\mu M$	>128 μM	Lee et al., 2017
		Yield reduction**	Japanese isolate strain	$IC_{50} = 40.1\,\mu M$	>100 μM	Baba et al., 2017
		Yield reduction	Chinese strain (HB29)	$IC_{50} = 49.7\,\mu M$	>320 μM	Smee et al., 2018
Favipiravir	Vero	Yield reduction	Japanese strain (SPL010)	$IC_{50} = 6\,\mu M$, $IC_{90} = 22\,\mu M$	>1,000 μM	Tani et al., 2016
		Yield reduction**	Japanese isolate strain	$IC_{50} = 25\,\mu M$	>100 μM	Baba et al., 2017
Hexachlorophene	Vero, Huh7	Yield reduction**	Chinese strain (HB29)	$IC_{50} = 1.3\,\mu M$	24.3 μM	Yuan et al., 2019
				$IC^{99} = 7.5\,\mu M$		
Benidipine	Vero	Yield reduction**	Chinese strain	$IC_{50} = 1.412\,\mu M$	96.92 μM	Li et al., 2019
Nifedipine	Vero	Yield reduction**	Chinese strain	$IC_{50} = 98\,\mu M$	>250 μM	
2′-Fluoro-2′-deoxycytidine	Vero	Yield reduction	Chinese strain (HB29)	$IC_{90} = 3.7\,\mu M$	>320 μM	Smee et al., 2018
Caffeic acid	Huh7.5.1-8	Yield reduction**	Chinese strain (HB29)	$IC_{50} = 48\,\mu M$	7.6 mM	Ogawa et al., 2018
Amodiaquine	Vero	Yield reduction**	Japanese isolates strain	$IC_{50} = 19.1\,\mu M$	>100 μM	Baba et al., 2017
IFNα	Vero	Yield reduction	Japanese strain (SPL030)	$IC_{90} = 29$ U/ml	>5,000 U/mL	Shimojima et al., 2015
IFNβ				$IC_{90} = 24$ U/ml	>5,000 U/mL	
IFNγ				$IC_{90} = 12$ ng/ml	>2,000 ng/mL	

Combination with ribavirin and IFNs, virus titers were reduced from 3.2–3.6 log.
***Titers were determined by RT-PCR of the virus genome.*

of ribavirin with IFNs or other agents that function via different mechanisms might be useful in treating patients with SFTS. Ribavirin has shown a limited protective effect in lethal SFTSV challenges in animal experiments (Tani et al., 2016; Gowen et al., 2017) (**Table 2**). The Chinese Ministry of Health initially approved the use of ribavirin to treat SFTS based on the results of *in vitro* studies (Ministry of Health People's Republic of China, 2011). However, a clinical study in China showed that the case fatality rate was similar between patients who received ribavirin and those who did not (Liu et al., 2013). This study included 311 patients, of whom 54 died; in those who received ribavirin therapy, the platelet counts did not increase and the viral loads did not decrease in comparison with those who did not receive the therapy. Furthermore, although the differences were not statistically significant, it was unexpectedly observed that the patients who received ribavirin therapy had lower platelet counts than those who did not.

Another study reported that two patients, in whom plasma exchange and ribavirin treatment were initiated early, recovered from rapidly progressing SFTS (Oh et al., 2014). In these patients, the platelet counts began to gradually recover after initiating ribavirin treatment. Furthermore, according to a large-scale epidemiological study in China including 2096 patients with laboratory-confirmed SFTS between 2011 and 2017, ribavirin therapy was effective in reducing the case fatality rate from 6.25% (15/240 patients) to 1.16% (2/173 patients) in patients with viral loads of $<1 \times 10^6$ copies/mL (Li et al., 2018). However, no effect was observed among those with a viral load of $>1 \times 10^6$ copies/mL.

Favipiravir

Favipiravir (T-705), which was discovered and synthesized by Toyama Chemical Co., Ltd., exerts a broad spectrum of activity against various RNA viruses, including the influenza virus, arenaviruses, bunyaviruses, West Nile virus, yellow fever virus, and foot-and-mouth disease virus (Furuta et al., 2009). Favipiravir is converted to its active form, ribofuranosyl-5-triphosphate, by host enzymes and inhibits viral RNA polymerase in the host cells. Only a few reports have indicated resistance to favipiravir *in vitro* (Delang et al., 2014; Goldhill et al., 2018). As shown in **Tables 1**, **2** favipiravir significantly inhibits SFTSV replication *in vitro* (Tani et al., 2016; Baba et al., 2017) and *in vivo* (Tani et al., 2016, 2018; Gowen et al., 2017; Smee et al., 2018). Furthermore, the IC_{90} of favipiravir (22 μM) in Vero cells (Tani et al., 2016) was lower than that of ribavirin (263 μM) (Shimojima et al., 2014).

The efficacy of favipiravir *in vivo* has been examined using animal models (**Table 2**). The intraperitoneal (i.p.) administration of favipiravir at a dose of 60 or 300 mg/kg/day for 5 days completely protected mice from death upon SFTSV infection, causing only a slight reduction in weight (Tani et al., 2016). On the other hand, ~40% of the mice treated with

TABLE 2 | Efficacy of anti-SFTSV drugs *in vivo* animal model.

Agent	Animals	Dose of agent (times/day)	Route	Treatment	Strain	Dose of virus	Route	Survival (%)	References
Ribavirin	STAT2$^{-/-}$hamster	75 mg/kg/day (twice)	p.o.	Day 1–11	Chinese strain (HB29)	50 PFU	s.c.	0	Gowen et al., 2017
	IFNAR$^{-/-}$C57BL/6	25 mg/kg/day (once)	i.p.	Day 0–5	Japanese strain (SPL010)	10^6 TCID$_{50}$	s.c.	70	Tani et al., 2016
		100 mg/kg/day (once)		Day 0–5				66	
Favipiravir	IFNAR$^{-/-}$C57BL/6	60 mg/kg/day (once)	i.p.	Day 0–5	Japanese strain (SPL010)	10^6 TCID$_{50}$	s.c.	100	Tani et al., 2016
		300 mg/kg/day (once)						100	
		60 mg/kg/day (once)	p.o.					100	
		300 mg/kg/day (once)						100	
		300 mg/kg/day (once)	p.o.	Day 1–6				100	
				Day 2–7				100	
				Day 3–8				100	
				Day 4–9				83	
				Day 5–10				50	
		120 mg/kg/day (twice)	p.o.	Day 0–4	Japanese strain (SPL010)	10^6 TCID$_{50}$	s.c.	100	Tani et al., 2018
				Day 1–5				100	
				Day 2–6				100	
				Day 3–7				100	
				Day 4–8				67	
				Day 5–9				0	
		200 mg/kg/day (twice)	p.o.	Day 0–4				100	
				Day 1–5				100	
				Day 2–6				100	
				Day 3–7				100	
				Day 4–8				100	
				Day 5–9				20	
		100 mg/kg/day (twice)	i.p.	Day 0–8	Chinese strain (HB29)	3 PFU	s.c.	90	Smee et al., 2018
	STAT2$^{-/-}$hamster	300 mg/kg/day (twice)	p.o.	Day 1–11	Chinese strain (HB29)	50 PFU	s.c.	100	Gowen et al., 2017
		150 mg/kg/day (twice)						100	
Benidipine	C57BL/6	15 mg/kg/day (once)	i.g.	Day 0–7	Chinese strain	10^5 TCID$_{50}$	i.p.	100*	Li et al., 2019
	Humanized mouse			Day 0–10				83.3**	
Nifedipine	C57BL/6	100 mg/kg/day (once)	i.g.	Day 0–7	Chinese strain	10^5 TCID$_{50}$	i.p.	100*	
	Humanized mice			Day 0–10				100**	
2′-FdC***	IFNAR$^{-/-}$C57BL/6	50 mg/kg/day (twice)	i.p.	Day 0–8	Chinese strain (HB29)	3 PFU	s.c.	80	Smee et al., 2018
		100 mg/kg/day (twice)		Day 0–8				100	
		200 mg/kg/day (twice)		Day 0–8				80	
IFN-γ	3 days old ICR	0.5 μg/animal (once)	i.p.	Day −1	unknown	1.5 × 10^3 TCID$_{50}$	i.c.	25	Ning et al., 2019
		0.05 μg/animal (once)						25	
		0.5 μg/animal (once)		Day +1	unknown	1.5 × 10^3 TCID$_{50}$		0	
		0.05 μg/animal (once)							0

**Non-lethal model. The viral loads in spleen and serum were significantly reduced.*

***The fatality rate of the vehicle control group was 57.1%.*

****2′-Fluoro-2′-deoxycytidine.*

i.g., inguinal; i.p., intraperitoneal; PFU, plaque-forming unit; p.o., oral; s.c., subcutaneous; TCID, tissue culture infective dose.

ribavirin (i.p.) at a dose of 25 or 100 mg/kg/day lost body weight and died from SFTSV infection with reduction of the case fatality rate. All favipiravir-treated mice survived when the treatment was initiated on or earlier than 3 days post infection, whereas the mice treated at 4 and 5 days post infection exhibited 83% and 50% survival, respectively (Tani et al., 2016). These results demonstrated that favipiravir would be potentially effective for prophylactic use and also for treating of SFTSV infections.

Generally, favipiravir is orally administrated to humans. The oral administration (p.o.) of favipiravir showed similar efficacy to that of i.p. administration in a mouse model (Tani et al., 2016). Furthermore, treatment with favipiravir (300 or 150 mg/kg/day) provided complete protection against a lethal SFTSV challenge in a STAT2 knockout golden Syrian hamster model (Gowen et al., 2017). Additionally, the efficacy of favipiravir at practical dosages of 120 and 200 mg/kg/day p.o. was investigated in a mouse infection model, and all the mice survived when the treatment was initiated at no later than 4 days post infection (Tani et al., 2018).

Hexachlorophene

Yuan et al. (2019) screened an FDA-approved drug library that contained 1,528 drug compounds and identified five that inhibited SFTSV replication at concentrations of $<10\,\mu M$, including two antibacterial and antifungal disinfectants (hexachlorophene and triclosan), a multi-kinase inhibitor for the treatment of advanced solid organ tumors (regorafenib), a small molecule agonist of the C-mannosylation of thrombopoietin receptor (c-Mpl) for the treatment of immune thrombocytopenic purpura and aplastic anemia (eltrombopag), and an antiprotozoal agent (broxyquinoline). Of them, hexachlorophene was the most potent, with an IC_{50} of $1.3 \pm 0.3\,\mu M$ (RNA load) and $2.6 \pm 0.14\,\mu M$ (plaque reduction) and the highest selectivity index (50% cytotoxic concentration $[CC_{50}]/IC_{50}$, 18.7), which was lower than that of the other four antiviral drugs identified (**Table 1**). Furthermore, the results indicated that hexachlorophene treatment interfered with SFTSV entry without affecting virus-host cell attachment to the cells and virus infectivity (Yuan et al., 2019). It was predicted that hexachlorophene would bind to the deep hydrophobic pocket between domains I and III of the SFTSV Gc glycoprotein and would interfere with cell membrane fusion.

Hexachlorophene is an antibacterial compound, a common constituent of soaps and scrubs and is experimentally used as a cholinesterase inhibitor (Hsu et al., 2004). It was reported that hexachlorophene inhibited the viral replication of severe acute respiratory syndrome-related coronavirus *in vitro* by inhibiting 3C-like protease, which is essential for its lifecycle (Hsu et al., 2004).

Calcium Channel Blockers

Calcium channel blockers (CCBs) reduce the intracellular Ca^{2+} level and are widely used for treating various cardiovascular diseases, including hypertension, angina, and supraventricular arrhythmias. Recently, the antiviral activity of CCBs against ebolavirus (Sakurai et al., 2015), marburgvirus (Dewald et al., 2018), Junín virus (Lavanya et al., 2013), West Nile virus (Scherbik and Brinton, 2010), and Japanese encephalitis virus (Wang et al., 2017) has been reported.

Screening a library of 700 FDA-approved drugs identified the CCBs benidipine hydrochloride and nifedipine as inhibitors of SFTSV replication *in vitro* by impairing virus internalization and reducing genome replication during the post-entry phase (Li et al., 2019). This mechanism did not affect viral binding, fusion, and budding. The results of *in vitro* study suggested that treatment with benidipine hydrochloride or nifedipine inhibited SFTSV replication by reducing virus induced Ca^{2+} influx. The anti-SFTSV effect of these two CCBs was further analyzed in C57BL/6 mice and humanized mouse models (**Table 2**), revealing treatment effects of a reduced viral load, increased platelet count, and decreased fatality rate in the humanized mouse model.

Notably, nifedipine is one of the most widely used drugs for treating hypertension and atherosclerosis in China. Thus, Li et al. (2019) performed a retrospective clinical investigation on a large cohort of 2087 patients with SFTS comprising 83 nifedipine-treated, who received nifedipine before admission and during hospitalization, 48 non-nifedipine-treated ones who received nifedipine before admission but not during hospitalization, and 249 general SFTS patients who did not receive nifedipine at all. The case fatality rate was decreased by >5-fold in the nifedipine-treated group (3.6%) compared with the general SFTS group (19.7%) or non-nifedipine treated group (20.8%) (Li et al., 2019). In contrast with ribavirin, a significant decrease in the case fatality rate was also observed in the nifedipine-treated patients (2.4%) with a high viral load ($>10^6$ copies/mL) when compared with the general SFTS patients (29.0%) and non-nifedipine-treated patients (34.5%). Hematemesis, one of the hemorrhagic manifestations that are closely related to death, was found to occur less frequently in the nifedipine-treated group. In this article, the authors clearly showed the inhibitory effect of benidipine hydrochloride or nifedipine in cultured cells and an animal model. Most importantly, it was found that the nifedipine administration enhanced virus clearance and improved clinical recovery.

2′-Fluoro-2′-deoxycytidine

2′-Fluoro-2′-deoxycytidine (2′-FdC) is a nucleoside inhibitor used in anticancer drugs. It inhibits various RNA and DNA viruses *in vitro*, such as Borna virus (Bajramovic et al., 2004), Lassa virus (Welch et al., 2016), Crimean-Congo hemorrhagic fever virus (Welch et al., 2017), influenza virus (Kumaki et al., 2011), and herpesviruses (Wohlrab et al., 1985).

Smee et al. (2018) has shown the antiviral activity of 2′-FdC against various bunyaviruses, such as La Crosse virus, Maporal virus, Punta Toro virus, Rift Valley fever virus, San Angelo virus, Heartland virus, and SFTSV. The IC_{90} of 2′-FdC against SFTSV was $3.7\,\mu M$ in an *in vitro* assay (**Table 1**). This value was much lower than that of ribavirin ($49.7\,\mu M$) in the same study and favipiravir ($22\,\mu M$) in the study conducted by Tani et al. (2016). In an *in vivo* study using $IFNAR^{-/-}$ mice, a 100 mg/kg/day treatment with 2′-FdC was 100% protective against death caused by SFTSV (**Table 2**). However, all the mice treated with 2′-FdC experienced substantial weight loss after SFTSV inoculation, whereas the favipiravir-treated mice displayed very little weight loss, suggesting that favipiravir was more effective than 2′-FdC in controlling morbidity during the infection (Smee et al., 2018). It was also found that treatments with 100 mg/kg/day of either 2′-FdC or favipiravir significantly reduced the viral titers in the serum. Furthermore, there was a slight discrepancy both in the survival rates and virus titers between mice treated with 100 mg/kg/day of 2′-FdC and those with 200 mg/kg/day of 2′-FdC. The survival rate was 80 vs. 100% for 200- and 100-mg/kg/day treatments, respectively; and the virus titer in the serum of 200 mg/kg/day-treated mice was higher than that of mice receiving the 100-mg/kg/day treatment. It was speculated that this was caused by the limited sample size ($n = 4$ or 5).

Caffeic Acid

Caffeic Acid (CA) is a coffee-related polyphenol organic compound that can be found in various plants, including coffee beans. Single cup of coffee contains 70–350 mg chlorogenic acid, the ester of caffeic acid (Clifford, 1999). It exerts a variety of biological effects, including the suppression of cancer cells (Tang et al., 2017; Bułdak et al., 2018) and antiviral properties (Wang et al., 2009; Utsunomiya et al., 2014; Ding et al., 2017; Langland et al., 2018).

Ogawa et al. (2018) showed that CA dose-dependently inhibited SFTSV replication in an *in vitro* assay using Huh7.5.1-8 cells, a highly permissive derivative of human hepatoma Huh7 cells. The IC_{50} of CA against SFTSV was 48 μM, and its CC_{50} was 7.6 mM (**Table 1**). Interestingly, pretreatment of SFTSV with CA prior to inoculation effectively reduced the virus copy number in the supernatant of infected cells at 72 h post infection, and the inhibitory effect was significantly reduced when the cells were treated with CA after SFTSV inoculation. Thus, the authors speculated that CA mainly acted on the viral particles or influenced the early stages of SFTSV infection, although it could act on the host cells to inhibit viral genome replication.

Amodiaquine

Amodiaquine is a novel compound that is routinely prescribed as an antimalarial drug is reported to show antiviral effects against ebolavirus (Gignoux et al., 2016; Sakurai et al., 2018), dengue virus (Boonyasuppayakorn et al., 2014), and zika virus (Balasubramanian et al., 2017). The mechanism of inhibitory activity of amodiaquine against malaria and those viruses remains unclear.

Baba et al. (2017) investigated the effect of amodiaquine and other halogen molecules (fluorine, bromine, and iodine) against the replication of SFTSV *in vitro*. All the derivatives also displayed anti-SFTSV activity, and the IC_{50} was 36.6, 31.1, and 15.6 μM for fluorine bromine, and iodine, respectively (**Table 1**). Among the compounds tested, amodiaquine was identified as a selective inhibitor against SFTSV replication. The CC_{50} and the IC_{50} of amodiaquine was >100 and 19.1 μM, respectively. The IC_{50} of amodiaquine was lower than those of ribavirin (40.1 μM) and favipiravir (25.0 μM).

IFN-γ

IFN-γ is the only member of type II IFNs. It stimulates macrophage and dendritic cells to induce direct antimicrobial activities by regulating antigen processing and presentation pathways. It was initially thought that activated T cells and activated natural killer cells were the only relevant source of IFN-γ; however, macrophages and dendritic cells can also be stimulated to produce IFN-γ *in vitro* under certain conditions (Thäle and Kiderlen, 2005). Because IFN-γ can directly stimulate the expression of some potential antiviral IFN-stimulating proteins by the STAT1 signaling, it plays an important role in viral infection.

Ning et al. (2019) used enzyme-linked immunosorbent assays to demonstrate that SFTSV infection caused a substantial production of serum IFN-γ in patients with SFTS. In turn, IFN-γ exhibited a robust anti-SFTSV activity in cultured cells. Thereafter, they evaluated the efficacy of IFN-γ as an anti-SFTSV drug *in vivo* in a suckling mouse model, which showed that IFN-γ treatment prior to SFTSV infection significantly reduced mortality, protecting ~25% of animals from death, whereas all the untreated mice died within 13 days of the SFTSV challenge. When IFN-γ was administrated post SFTSV infection, 100% of the mice died from the virus.

DISCUSSION

Since then, a considerable number of studies regarding its epidemiological and virological characteristics have been conducted. Ribavirin, one of a broad-spectrum antiviral drug (Beaucourt and Vignuzzi, 2014), is recommended for patients with SFTS in China, and it has been used to treat a considerable number of patients (Ministry of Health People's Republic of China, 2011). The *in vitro* and *in vivo* studies on ribavirin (Shimojima et al., 2014, 2015; Tani et al., 2016; Gowen et al., 2017; Lee et al., 2017) showed the considerable effect. The results of the clinical study conducted by Liu et al. (2013), which showed that ribavirin did not reduce the fatality rate of patients with SFTS, discouraged us from considering ribavirin treatment for treating patients with SFTS. However, Li et al. (2018) reported that ribavirin is effective for early-stage patients with a low viral titer or for the pretreatment of exposed individuals. Nevertheless, in cases of ribavirin administration, patients should be intensely monitored because of the possible adverse events induced by ribavirin such as anemia and hyperamylasemia (Lu et al., 2015).

Favipiravir exhibited higher effectiveness than ribavirin in *in vitro* and *in vivo* studies (Tani et al., 2016, 2018). Meanwhile, favipiravir remained effective when it was used following SFTSV infection in animal models (Tani et al., 2016, 2018; Gowen et al., 2017) indicating its potential as an effective drug for treating SFTS patient. Currently, clinical trials are underway to evaluate the efficacy of favipiravir for treating patients with SFTS in Japan (Cyranoski, 2018; Spengler et al., 2018). Besides, it would be desirable to use intravenous administration because SFTS patients with severe symptoms could have difficulty in taking drugs orally.

Hexachlorophene, an antibacterial compound, was found to be effective for SFTSV in *in vitro* screening using an FDA-approved drug library (Yuan et al., 2019). Because hexachlorophene can cause acute and subacute neurotoxicity in laboratory animals and humans (Kimbrough, 1973; Ramu et al., 2016), further *in vitro* and *in vivo* studies must be conducted.

CCBs, which are used to control cardiovascular diseases, have demonstrated significant effects against SFTSV replication both *in vitro* and *in vivo* (Li et al., 2019). Notably, retrospectively conducted clinical study suggested that nifedipine remarkably reduced the case fatality rate in SFTS patients (Li et al., 2019). Although nifedipine is administrated consistently for patients with cardiac disease, these findings are valuable for developing potential CCB-based therapeutics for SFTS. It is considered that the efficacy of nifedipine in treating patients with SFTS should be evaluated in a prospective manner. For clinical use, careful consideration of the risk-to-benefit value to the patient would be required because an overdose of CCBs has a high-risk of side effects, such as edema, liver damage, and death. The dose used for *in vivo* mouse study (100 mg/kg/day) was extremely higher than the dose generally used for humans (~0.2–1.5 mg/kg/day). Still, these findings indicated the potential therapeutic effect of CCB treatment in patients with SFTS.

2′-FdC is considered a viable candidate therapeutic agent against SFTS. Although, 2′-FdC was more effective than favipiravir *in vitro*, *in vivo* efficacy was less than that of favipiravir (Smee et al., 2018). The administration protocol of 2′-FdC should be considered in future studies.

CA shows inhibitory effects against SFTSV *in vitro*. Little is known about the mechanism of the action, but it was considered that CA interacts with the viral particles, showing inhibitory effects (Ogawa et al., 2018). Because there are limited reports regarding antiviral effects of CA or chlorogenic acid *in vivo* (Wang et al., 2009; Ding et al., 2017), further studies are needed.

Baba et al. (2017) showed that amodiaquine and other halogen molecules effectively inhibited the propagation of SFTSV *in vitro*. Amodiaquine is widely used as an antimalarial drug and can be administered at a low cost. The efficacy of amodiaquine *in vivo* should be evaluated.

The anti-SFTSV efficacy of IFN-γ both *in vitro* and *in vivo* (Ning et al., 2019) was reported. Because IFN-γ is an FDA-approved drug, it has been suggested as a candidate antiviral drug for SFTSV alone or in combination with other drugs (Shimojima et al., 2015).

The efficacy of antibody-based treatment has been studied against SFTS disease. Generally, antibodies play a critical role in the treating a wide variety of viral diseases; such as acquired immunodeficiency syndrome (Ferrari et al., 2016), diseases caused by ebola virus (Mendoza et al., 2017) and influenza (Nachbagauer and Krammer, 2017). Antibody drugs neutralize viruses or bind to the virion to enhance antigen uptake by cytotoxic T cells, making them highly specific for the target virus. It was reported that antiserum of a patient recovered from SFTS completely protected mice from the lethal infection of SFTSV (Shimada et al., 2015). It was also shown that antibodies against SFTSV Gn protein significantly reduced the fatality rate in mice infected with SFTSV, even when treatment was initiated from 3 days post inoculation (Kim et al., 2019). These reports suggested that antibodies alone or in combination with antiviral drugs could be used to treat patients with SFTS.

There are two studies for developing vaccines against SFTSV infection (Dong et al., 2019; Kwak et al., 2019). A recombinant vesicular stomatitis virus expressing SFTSV antigen completely protected mice from SFTSV infection (Dong et al., 2019). A DNA vaccine expressing antigens of SFTSV, elicited both neutralizing antibody response and SFTSV-specific T cell response and protected aged-ferrets from the lethal SFTSV infection (Kwak et al., 2019). Safe and effective vaccines against SFTS should be developed.

Because all these mentioned drugs have inhibitory effect on SFTSV replication, combination therapies with some drugs, which have different mechanisms of action should be considered. Although, it should be considered that an antiviral drug against SFTS would be administrated to a pre-symptomatic exposed individual, the main targets of these drugs are certainly patients with suggestive symptoms of SFTS. SFTSV circulates between mammals and ticks in Southeast Asia, indicating that we cannot escape the risk of being infected with SFTSV. SFTS is classified in a disease category of viral hemorrhagic fever with high case fatality rate. Recently, cases of SFTS have been reported, wherein the patients were infected with SFTSV from cats, which might be infected with SFTSV from tick (Kida et al., 2019). Therefore, we are hopeful that specific treatments with antiviral agents will be developed and approved for patients with SFTS as early as possible.

AUTHOR CONTRIBUTIONS

MS and MT-I conceptualized and designed the study. MT-I collected and assembled the data and drafted the manuscript. MS critically revised the manuscript.

FUNDING

Some part of this review article was obtained through the studies financially supported from the Ministry of Health, Labour, and Welfare (grant number H25-Shinko-Shitei-009), Japan Agency for Medical Research and Development (AMED, 16fk0108002j, 17fk0108202j, 18fk0108002j, 19fk0108081j, 19fk0108072). The funders had no role in study design, data collection and analysis, decision to publish, or preparation of the manuscript.

ACKNOWLEDGMENTS

We thank all the staff members working for the research project for SFTS in Japan, especially, Dr. Hideki Tani, Dr. Masayuki Shimojima, Dr. Takeshi Kurosu, Dr. Tomoki Yoshikawa, Dr. Hirofumi Kato, Dr. Masaaki Satoh, Department of Virology 1, National Institute of Infectious Diseases, Tokyo, Japan. The present affiliate of Dr. Hideki Tani is the Department of Virology, Graduate School of Medicine and Pharmaceutical Sciences, University of Toyama, Toyama, Japan.

REFERENCES

Baba, M., Toyama, M., Sakakibara, N., Okamoto, M., Arima, N., and Saijo, M. (2017). Establishment of an antiviral assay system and identification of severe fever with thrombocytopenia syndrome virus inhibitors. *Antivir. Chem. Chemother.* 25, 83–89. doi: 10.1177/2040206617740303

Bajramovic, J. J., Volmer, R., Syan, S., Pochet, S., and Gonzalez-Dunia, D. (2004). 2'-fluoro-2'-deoxycytidine inhibits Borna disease virus replication and spread. *Antimicrob. Agents Chemother.* 48, 1422–1425. doi: 10.1128/AAC.48.4.1422-1425.2004

Balasubramanian, A., Teramoto, T., Kulkarni, A. A., Bhattacharjee, A. K., and Padmanabhan, R. (2017). Antiviral activities of selected antimalarials against dengue virus type 2 and Zika virus. *Antiviral Res.* 137, 141–150 doi: 10.1016/j.antiviral.2016.11.015

Beaucourt, S., and Vignuzzi, M. (2014). Ribavirin: a drug active against many viruses with multiple effects on virus replication and propagation. Molecular basis of ribavirin resistance. *Curr. Opin. Virol.* 8, 10–15. doi: 10.1016/j.coviro.2014.04.011

Boonyasuppayakorn, S., Reichert, E. D., Manzano, M., Nagarajan, K., and Padmanabhan, R. (2014). Amodiaquine, an antimalarial drug, inhibits dengue virus type 2 replication and infectivity. *Antiviral Res.* 106, 125–134. doi: 10.1016/j.antiviral.2014.03.014

Bułdak, R. J., Hejmo, T., Osowski, M., Bułdak, Ł., Kukla, M., Polaniak, R., et al. (2018). The impact of coffee and its selected bioactive compounds on the development and progression of colorectal cancer *in vivo* and *in vitro*. *Molecules* 23:E3309. doi: 10.3390/molecules23123309

Chen, X. P., Cong, M. L., Li, M. H., Kang, Y. J., Feng, Y. M., Plyusnin, A., et al. (2012). Infection and pathogenesis of Huaiyangshan virus (a novel tick-borne bunyavirus) in laboratory rodents. *J. Gen. Virol.* 93, 1288–1293. doi: 10.1099/vir.0.041053-0

Choi, S. J., Park, S. W., Bae, I. G., Kim, S. H., Ryu, S. Y., Kim, H. A., et al. (2016). Severe fever with thrombocytopenia syndrome in South Korea, 2013-2015. *PLoS Negl. Trop. Dis.* 10:e0005264. doi: 10.1371/journal.pntd.0005264

Clifford, M. N. (1999). Chlorogenic acids and other cinnamates– nature, occurrence and dietary burden. *J. Sci. Food. Agric.* 79:362–372. doi: 10.1002/(SICI)1097-0010(19990301)79:3<362::AID-JSFA256>3.0.CO;2-D

Cyranoski, D. (2018). East Asia braces for surge in deadly tick-borne virus news. *Nature* 556, 282–283. doi: 10.1038/d41586-018-04486-6

De Clercq, E., and Li, G. (2016). Approved antiviral drugs over the past 50 years. *Clin. Microbiol. Rev.* 29, 695–747. doi: 10.1128/CMR.00102-15

Delang, L., Guerrero, N. S., Tas, A., Quérat, G., Pastorino, B., Froeyen, M., et al. (2014). Mutations in the chikungunya virus non-structural proteins cause resistance to favipiravir (T-705), a broad-spectrum antiviral. *J. Antimicrob. Chemother.* 69, 2770–2784. doi: 10.1093/jac/dku209

Dewald, L. E., Dyall, J., Sword, J. M., Torzewski, L., Zhou, H., Postnikova, E., et al. (2018). The calcium channel blocker bepridil demonstrates efficacy in the murine model of marburg virus disease. *J. Infect. Dis.* 22, S588–S591. doi: 10.1093/infdis/jiy332

Ding, Y., Cao, Z., Cao, L., Ding, G., Wang, Z., and Xiao, W. (2017). Antiviral activity of chlorogenic acid against influenza A (H1N1/H3N2) virus and its inhibition of neuraminidase. *Sci. Rep.* 7, 1–11. doi: 10.1038/srep45723

Dong, F., Li, D., Wen, D., Li, S., Zhao, C., Qi, Y., et al. (2019). Single dose of a rVSV-based vaccine elicits complete protection against severe fever with thrombocytopenia syndrome virus. *NPJ Vaccines* 4:5. doi: 10.1038/s41541-018-0096-y

Ferrari, G., Haynes, B. F., Koenig, S., Nordstrom, J. L., Margolis, D. M., and Tomaras, G. D. (2016). Envelope-specific antibodies and antibody-derived molecules for treating and curing HIV infection. *Nat. Rev. Drug Discov.* 15, 823–834. doi: 10.1038/nrd.2016.173

Furuta, Y., Takahashi, K., Shiraki, K., Sakamoto, K., Smee, D. F., Barnard, D. L., et al. (2009). T-705 (favipiravir) and related compounds: novel broad-spectrum inhibitors of RNA viral infections. *Antiviral Res.* 82, 95–102. doi: 10.1016/j.antiviral.2009.02.198

Gai, Z., Liang, M., Zhang, Y., Zhang, S., Jin, C., Wang, S. W., et al. (2012). Person-to-person transmission of severe fever with thrombocytopenia syndrome bunyavirus through blood contact. *Clin. Infect. Dis.* 54, 249–252. doi: 10.1093/cid/cir776

Gignoux, E., Azman, A. S., De Smet, M., Azuma, P., Massaquoi, M., Job, D., et al. (2016). Effect of artesunate.amodiaquine on mortality related to Ebola virus disease. *N. Engl. J. Med.* 374, 23–32. doi: 10.1056/NEJMoa1504605

Goldhill, D. H., Te Velthuis, A. J. W., Fletcher, R. A., Langat, P., Zambon, M., Lackenby, A., et al. (2018). The mechanism of resistance to favipiravir in influenza. *Proc. Natl. Acad. Sci. U.S.A.* 115, 11613–11618. doi: 10.1073/pnas.1811345115

Gowen, B. B., and Hickerson, B. T. (2017). Hemorrhagic fever of bunyavirus etiology: disease models and progress towards new therapies. *J. Microbiol.* 55, 183–195. doi: 10.1007/s12275-017-7029-8

Gowen, B. B., Westover, J. B., Miao, J., Van Wettere, A. J., Rigas, J. D., Hickerson, B. T., et al. (2017). Modeling severe fever with thrombocytopenia syndrome virus infection in golden syrian hamsters: importance of STAT2 in preventing disease and effective treatment with favipiravir. *J. Virol.* 91, e01942–e01916. doi: 10.1128/JVI.01942-16

Graci, J. D., and Cameron, C. E. (2006). Mechanisms of action of ribavirin against distinct viruses. *Rev. Med. Virol.* 16, 37–48. doi: 10.1002/rmv.483

Hsu, J. T. A., Kuo, C. J., Hsieh, H. P., Wang, Y. C., Huang, K. K., Lin, C. P. C., et al. (2004). Evaluation of metal-conjugated compounds as inhibitors of 3CL protease of SARS-CoV. *FEBS Lett.* 574, 116–120. doi: 10.1016/j.febslet.2004.08.015

Jin, C., Jiang, H., Liang, M., Han, Y., Gu, W., Zhang, F., et al. (2015). SFTS virus infection in nonhuman primates. *J. Infect. Dis.* 211, 915–925. doi: 10.1093/infdis/jiu564

Jin, C., Liang, M., Ning, J., Gu, W., Jiang, H., Wu, W., et al. (2012). Pathogenesis of emerging severe fever with thrombocytopenia syndrome virus in C57/BL6 mouse model. *Proc. Natl. Acad. Sci. U.S.A.* 109, 10053–10058. doi: 10.1073/pnas.1120246109

Kato, H., Yamagishi, T., Shimada, T., Matsui, T., Shimojima, M., Saijo, M., et al. (2016). Epidemiological and clinical features of severe fever with thrombocytopenia syndrome in Japan, 2013-2014. *PLoS ONE* 11:e0165207. doi: 10.1371/journal.pone.0165207

Kida, K., Matsuoka, Y., Shimoda, T., Matsuoka, H., Yamada, H., Saito, T., et al. (2019). A case of cat-to-human transmission of severe fever with thrombocytopenia syndrome virus. *Jpn. J. Infect. Dis.* 72, 356–358. doi: 10.7883/yoken.JJID.2018.526

Kim, K. H., Kim, J., Ko, M., Chun, J. Y., Kim, H., Kim, S., et al. (2019). An anti-Gn glycoprotein antibody from a convalescent patient potently inhibits the infection of severe fever with thrombocytopenia syndrome virus. *PLoS Pathog.* 15:e1007375. doi: 10.1371/journal.ppat.1007375

Kim, K. H., Yi, J., Kim, G., Choi, S. J., Jun, K. I., Kim, N. H., et al. (2013). Severe fever with thrombocytopenia syndrome, South Korea, 2012. *Emerg. Infect. Dis.* 19, 1892–1894 doi: 10.3201/eid1911.130792

Kimbrough, R. D. (1973). Review of the toxicity of hexachlorophene, including its neurotoxicity. *J. Clini. Pharmacol.* 13, 439–444. doi: 10.1002/j.1552-4604.1973.tb00196.x

Kumaki, Y., Day, C. W., Smee, D. F., Morrey, J. D., and Barnard, D. L. (2011). *In vitro* and *in vivo* efficacy of fluorodeoxycytidine analogs against highly pathogenic avian influenza H5N1, seasonal, and pandemic H1N1 virus infections. *Antiviral Res.* 92, 329–340. doi: 10.1016/j.antiviral.2011.09.001

Kwak, J. E., Kim, Y. I., Park, S. J., Yu, M. A., Kwon, H. I., Eo, S., et al. (2019). Development of a SFTSV DNA vaccine that confers complete protection against lethal infection in ferrets. *Nat. Commun.* 10, 1–11. doi: 10.1038/s41467-019-11815-4

Langland, J., Jacobs, B., Wagner, C. E., Ruiz, G., and Cahill, T. M. (2018). Antiviral activity of metal chelates of caffeic acid and similar compounds towards herpes simplex, VSV-Ebola pseudotyped and vaccinia viruses. *Antiviral Res.* 160, 143–150. doi: 10.1016/j.antiviral.2018.10.021

Lavanya, M., Cuevas, C. D., Thomas, M., Cherry, S., and Ross, S. R. (2013). siRNA screen for genes that affect Junín virus entry uncovers voltage-gated calcium channels as a therapeutic target. *Sci. Transl. Med.* 5:204ra131. doi: 10.1126/scitranslmed.3006827

Lee, M. J., Kim, K. H., Yi, J., Choi, S. J., Choe, P. G., Park, W. B., et al. (2017). *In vitro* antiviral activity of ribavirin against severe fever with thrombocytopenia syndrome virus. *Korean J. Intern. Med.* 32, 731–737. doi: 10.3904/kjim.2016.109

Li, H., Lu, Q., Bin, X. B., Zhang, S. F., Liu, K., Du, J., et al. (2018). Epidemiological and clinical features of laboratory-diagnosed severe fever with thrombocytopenia syndrome in China, 2011–17: a prospective observational study. *Lancet Infect. Dis.* 18, 1127–1137. doi: 10.1016/S1473-3099(18)30293-7

Li, H., Zhang, L. K., Li, S. F., Zhang, S. F., Wan, W. W., Zhang, Y. L., et al. (2019). Calcium channel blockers reduce severe fever with thrombocytopenia syndrome virus (SFTSV) related fatality. *Cell Res.* 29, 739–753. doi: 10.1038/s41422-019-0214-z

Liu, W., Lu, Q. B., Cui, N., Li, H., Wang, L. Y., Liu, K., et al. (2013). Case-fatality ratio and effectiveness of ribavirin therapy among hospitalized patients in china who had severe fever with thrombocytopenia syndrome. *Clin. Infect. Dis.* 57, 1292–1299. doi: 10.1093/cid/cit530

Liu, Y., Wu, B., Paessler, S., Walker, D. H., Tesh, R. B., and Yu, X. J. (2014). The pathogenesis of severe fever with thrombocytopenia syndrome virus infection in alpha/beta interferon knockout mice: insights into the pathologic mechanisms of a new viral hemorrhagic fever. *J. Virol.* 88, 1781–1786. doi: 10.1128/JVI.02277-13

Lu, Q. B., Zhang, S. Y., Cui, N., Hu, J. G., Fan, Y. D., Guo, C. T., et al. (2015). Common adverse events associated with ribavirin therapy for Severe fever with thrombocytopenia syndrome. *Antiviral Res.* 119, 19–22. doi: 10.1016/j.antiviral.2015.04.006

Mendoza, E. J., Racine, T., and Kobinger, G. P. (2017). The ongoing evolution of antibody-based treatments for Ebola virus infection. *Immunotherapy.* 9, 435–450. doi: 10.2217/imt-2017-0010

Ministry of Health and People's Republic of China (2011). Guideline for prevention and treatment of severe fever with thrombocytopenia syndrome (2010 version). *Chinese J. Clin. Infect. Dis.* 4, 193—194.

Nachbagauer, R., and Krammer, F. (2017). Universal influenza virus vaccines and therapeutic antibodies. *Clin. Microbiol. Infect.* 23, 222–228. doi: 10.1016/j.cmi.2017.02.009

Nakamura, S., Azuma, M., Maruhashi, T., Sogabe, K., Sumitani, R., Uemura, M., et al. (2018). Steroid pulse therapy in patients with encephalopathy associated with severe fever with thrombocytopenia syndrome. *J. Infect. Chemother.* 24, 389–392. doi: 10.1016/j.jiac.2017.11.004

Ning, Y., Mo, Q., Feng, K., Min, Y. Q., Li, M., Hou, D., et al. (2019). Interferon-γ-directed inhibition of a novel high-pathogenic phlebovirus and viral antagonism of the antiviral signaling by targeting STAT1. *Front. Immunol.* 10:1182. doi: 10.3389/fimmu.2019.01182

Niu, G., Li, J., Liang, M., Jiang, X., Jiang, M., Yin, H., et al. (2013). Severe fever with thrombocytopenia syndrome virus among domesticated animals, China. *Emerg. Infect. Dis.* 19, 756–763. doi: 10.3201/eid1905.120245

Ogawa, M., Shirasago, Y., Ando, S., Shimojima, M., Saijo, M., and Fukasawa, M. (2018). Caffeic acid, a coffee-related organic acid, inhibits infection by severe fever with thrombocytopenia syndrome virus *in vitro*. *J. Infect. Chemother.* 24, 597–601. doi: 10.1016/j.jiac.2018.03.005

Oh, W. S., Heo, S. T., Kim, S. H., Choi, W. J., Han, M. G., and Kim, J. Y. (2014). Plasma exchange and ribavirin for rapidly progressive severe fever with thrombocytopenia syndrome. *Int. J. Infect. Dis.* 18, 84–86. doi: 10.1016/j.ijid.2013.08.011

Ramu, J., Konak, T., Paule, M. G., Hanig, J. P., and Liachenko, S. (2016). Longitudinal diffusion tensor imaging of the rat brain after hexachlorophene exposure. *Neurotoxicology* 56, 225–232. doi: 10.1016/j.neuro.2016.08.011

Saijo, M. (2018). Pathophysiology of severe fever with thrombocytopenia syndrome and development of specific antiviral therapy. *J. Infect. Chemother.* 24, 773–781. doi: 10.1016/j.jiac.2018.07.009

Sakurai, Y., Kolokoltsov, A. A., Chen, C. C., Tidwell, M. W., Bauta, W. E., Klugbauer, N., et al. (2015). Two-pore channels control Ebola virus host cell entry and are drug targets for disease treatment. *Science.* 347, 995–998. doi: 10.1126/science.1258758

Sakurai, Y., Sakakibara, N., Toyama, M., Baba, M., and Davey, R. A. (2018). Novel amodiaquine derivatives potently inhibit Ebola virus infection. *Antiviral Res.* 160, 175–182. doi: 10.1016/j.antiviral.2018.10.025

Scherbik, S. V., and Brinton, M. A. (2010). Virus-induced Ca^{2+} influx extends survival of west nile virus-infected cells. *J. Virol.* 84, 8721–8731. doi: 10.1128/JVI.00144-10

Shimada, S., Posadas, H. G., Aoki, K., Morita, K., and Hayasaka, D. (2015). Therapeutic effect of post-exposure treatment with antiserum on severe fever with thrombocytopenia syndrome (SFTS) in a mouse model of SFTS virus infection. *Virology* 482, 19–27. doi: 10.1016/j.virol.2015.03.010

Shimojima, M., Fukushi, S., Tani, H., Taniguchi, S., Fukuma, A., and Saijo, M. (2015). Combination effects of ribavirin and interferons on severe fever with thrombocytopenia syndrome virus infection. *Virol. J.* 12:181. doi: 10.1186/s12985-015-0412-3

Shimojima, M., Fukushi, S., Tani, H., Yoshikawa, T., Fukuma, A., Taniguchi, S., et al. (2014). Effects of ribavirin on severe fever with thrombocytopenia syndrome virus *in vitro*. *Jpn. J. Infect. Dis.* 67, 423–427. doi: 10.7883/yoken.67.423

Smee, D. F., Jung, K. H., Westover, J., and Gowen, B. B. (2018). 2′-Fluoro-2′-deoxycytidine is a broad-spectrum inhibitor of bunyaviruses *in vitro* and in phleboviral disease mouse models. *Antiviral Res.* 160, 48–54. doi: 10.1016/j.antiviral.2018.10.013

Snell, N. J. (2001). Ribavirin - current status of a broad spectrum antiviral agent. *Expert Opin. Pharmacother.* 2, 1317–1324. doi: 10.1517/14656566.2.8.1317

Spengler, J. R., Bente, D. A., Bray, M., Burt, F., Hewson, R., Korukluoglu, G., et al. (2018). Second international conference on Crimean-Congo hemorrhagic fever. *Antiviral Res.* 150, 137–147. doi: 10.1016/j.antiviral.2017.11.019

Takahashi, T., Maeda, K., Suzuki, T., Ishido, A., Shigeoka, T., Tominaga, T., et al. (2014). The first identification and retrospective study of severe fever with thrombocytopenia syndrome in Japan. *J. Infect. Dis.* 209, 816–827. doi: 10.1093/infdis/jit603

Tang, H., Yao, X., Yao, C., Zhao, X., Zuo, H., and Li, Z. (2017). Anti-colon cancer effect of caffeic acid p-nitro-phenethyl ester *in vitro* and *in vivo* and detection of its metabolites. *Sci. Rep.* 7:7599. doi: 10.1038/s41598-017-07953-8

Tani, H., Fukuma, A., Fukushi, S., Taniguchi, S., Yoshikawa, T., Iwata-yoshikawa, N., et al. (2016). Efficacy of T-705 (Favipiravir) in the treatment of infections with lethal severe fever with thrombocytopenia syndrome virus. *mSphere* 1, e00061–e00015. doi: 10.1128/mSphere.00061-15

Tani, H., Komeno, T., Fukuma, A., Fukushi, S., Taniguchi, S., Shimojima, M., et al. (2018). Therapeutic effects of favipiravir against severe fever with thrombocytopenia syndrome virus infection in a lethal mouse model: dose-efficacy studies upon oral administration. *PLoS ONE* 13:e0206416. doi: 10.1371/journal.pone.0206416

Thäle, C., and Kiderlen, A. F. (2005). Sources of interferon-gamma (IFN-γ) in early immune response to Listeria monocytogenes. *Immunobiology* 210, 673–683. doi: 10.1016/j.imbio.2005.07.003

Tran, X. C., Yun, Y., An,L., Van, Kim, S. H., Thao, N. T. P., Man, P. K. C., et al. (2019). Endemic severe fever with thrombocytopenia syndrome, Vietnam. *Emerg. Infect. Dis.* 25, 1029–1031. doi: 10.3201/eid2505.181463

Utsunomiya, H., Ichinose, M., Ikeda, K., Uozaki, M., Morishita, J., Kuwahara, T., et al. (2014). Inhibition by caffeic acid of the influenza a virus multiplication *in vitro*. *Int. J. Mol. Med.* 34, 1020–1024. doi: 10.3892/ijmm.2014.1859

Wang, G. F., Shi, L. P., Ren, Y. D., Liu, Q. F., Liu, H. F., Zhang, R. J., et al. (2009). Anti-hepatitis B virus activity of chlorogenic acid, quinic acid and caffeic acid *in vivo* and *in vitro*. *Antiviral Res.* 83, 186–190. doi: 10.1016/j.antiviral.2009.05.002

Wang, S., Liu, Y., Guo, J., Wang, P., Zhang, L., Xiao, G., et al. (2017). Screening of FDA-approved drugs for inhibitors of Japanese encephalitis virus infection. *J. Virol.* 91, e01055–e01017. doi: 10.1128/JVI.01055-17

Welch, S. R., Guerrero, L. W., Chakrabarti, A. K., McMullan, L. K., Flint, M., Bluemling, G. R., et al. (2016). Lassa and Ebola virus inhibitors identified using minigenome and recombinant virus reporter systems. *Antiviral Res.* 136, 9–18. doi: 10.1016/j.antiviral.2016.10.007

Welch, S. R., Scholte, F. E. M., Flint, M., Chatterjee, P., Nichol, S. T., Bergeron, É., et al. (2017). Identification of 2′-deoxy-2′-fluorocytidine as a potent inhibitor of Crimean-Congo hemorrhagic fever virus replication using a recombinant fluorescent reporter virus. *Antiviral Res.* 147, 91–99. doi: 10.1016/j.antiviral.2017.10.008

Wohlrab, F., Jamieson, A. T., Hay, J., Mengel, R., and Guschlbauer, W. (1985). The effect of 2′-fluoro-2′-deoxycytidine on herpes virus growth. *Biochim. Biophys. Acta* 824, 233–242. doi: 10.1016/0167-4781(85)90053-3

World Health Organization (2017). *Annual Review of Diseases Prioritized Under the Research and Development Blueprint, 2017.* Available online at: http://www.who.int/blueprint/what/research-development/2017-Prioritization-Long-Report.pdf?ua=1 (accessed February 7, 2020).

Yoo, J. R., Kim, S. H., Kim, Y. R., Lee, K. H., Oh, W. S., and Heo, S. T. (2019). Application of therapeutic plasma exchange in patients having severe fever with thrombocytopenia syndrome. *Korean J. Intern. Med.* 34, 902–909. doi: 10.3904/kjim.2016.194

Yoshikawa, R., Sakabe, S., Urata, S., and Yasuda, J. (2019). Species-specific pathogenicity of severe fever with thrombocytopenia syndrome virus is determined by anti-STAT2 activity of NSs. *J. Virol.* 93, e02226–e02218. doi: 10.1128/JVI.02226-18

Yu, X. J., Liang, M. F., Zhang, S. Y., Liu, Y., Li, J. D., Sun, Y. L., et al. (2011). Fever with thrombocytopenia associated with a novel bunyavirus in China. *N. Engl. J. Med.* 364, 1523–1532. doi: 10.1056/NEJMoa1010095

Yuan, S., Chan, J. F. W., Ye, Z. W., Wen, L., Tsang, T. G. W., Cao, J., et al. (2019). Screening of an FDA-approved drug library with a two-tier system identifies an entry inhibitor of severe fever with thrombocytopenia syndrome virus. *Viruses* 11:E385. doi: 10.3390/v11040385

Zhu, L., Yin, F., Moming, A., Zhang, J., Wang, B., Gao, L., et al. (2019). First case of laboratory-confirmed severe fever with thrombocytopenia syndrome disease revealed the risk of SFTSV infection in Xinjiang, China. *Emerg. Microbes Infect.* 8, 1122–1125. doi: 10.1080/22221751.2019.1645573

Zivcec, M., Safronetz, D., and Feldmann, H. (2013). Animal models of tick-borne hemorrhagic fever viruses. *Pathogens* 2, 402–421. doi: 10.3390/pathogens2020402

13

Virus-Like Particles Derived from a Virulent Strain of Pest des Petits Ruminants Virus Elicit a more Vigorous Immune Response in Mice and Small Ruminants than those from a Vaccine Strain

Feihu Yan[1†], Entao Li[1,2†], Ling Li[3†], Zachary Schiffman[4,5], Pei Huang[1,6], Shengnan Zhang[1,7], Guohua Li[1,8], Hongli Jin[1,9], Hualei Wang[9], Xinghai Zhang[1,9], Yuwei Gao[1], Na Feng[1], Yongkun Zhao[1*], Chengyu Wang[1*] and Xianzhu Xia[1,2,6]*

[1] Key Laboratory of Jilin Province for Zoonosis Prevention and Control, Changchun Veterinary Research Institute, Chinese Academy of Agricultural Sciences, Changchun, China, [2] College of Veterinary Medicine, South China Agricultural University, Guangzhou, China, [3] National Research Center for Exotic Animal Diseases, China Animal Health and Epidemiology Center, Qingdao, China, [4] Department of Medical Microbiology and Infectious Diseases, University of Manitoba, Winnipeg, MB, Canada, [5] National Microbiology Laboratory, Special Pathogens Program, Public Health Agency of Canada, Winnipeg, MB, Canada, [6] College of Veterinary Medicine, Jilin Agricultural University, Changchun, China, [7] College of Wildlife Resources, Northeast Forestry University, Harbin, China, [8] College of Animal Science and Technology, Shihezi University, Shihezi, China, [9] College of Veterinary Medicine, Jilin University, Changchun, China

***Correspondence:**
Na Feng
fengna0308@126.com
Yongkun Zhao
zhaoyongkun1976@126.com
Chengyu Wang
wangchengyu2019103@163.com

Peste des petits ruminants (PPRs) is highly contagious, acute or subacute disease of small ruminants caused by peste des petits ruminants virus (PPRV). To date, several studies have designed and evaluated PPRV-like particles (VLPs) as a vaccine candidate for the prevention and control of PPR, with the majority of these VLPs constructed using sequences derived from a PPRV vaccine strain due to its high immunogenicity. However, because of the lack of available genetic material and certain structural proteins and/or the alteration of posttranslational glycosylation modifications, the immunogenicity of VLPs derived from a vaccine strain is not always optimal. In this study, two PPRV VLP candidates, derived from either the lineage IV Tibet/30 virulent strain or the lineage II Nigeria 75/1 vaccine strain, were generated using a baculovirus system through the coexpression of the PPRV matrix (M), hemagglutinin (H), and fusion (F) proteins in the high expression level cell line High Five. These VLPs were then used to immunize mice, goats, and sheep followed by two boosts after primary immunization. Both VLPs were found to induce a potent humoral immune response as demonstrated by the high ratio of immunoglobulin G1 (IgG1) to IgG2a. In all animals, both VLPs induced high titers of virus-neutralizing antibodies (VNAs), as well as H- and F-specific antibodies, with the Tibet/30 VLPs yielding higher antibody titers by comparison to the Nigeria 75/1 VLPs. Studies in mice also demonstrated that the Tibet/30 VLPs induced a more robust interleukin 4 and interferon γ response than the Nigeria 75/1 VLPs. Goats and sheep immunized with both VLPs exhibited a robust humoral and cell-mediated immune response. Furthermore, our results demonstrated that the VLPs derived from the virulent lineage IV Tibet/30 strain were more immunogenic, inducing a more potent and robust humoral and cell-mediated immune response in vaccinated animals by comparison to the lineage II Nigeria 75/1 vaccine strain VLPs. In addition, VNA titers were significantly higher among animals vaccinated with the Tibet/30 VLPs by comparison to the Nigeria 75/1 VLPs. Taken together, these findings suggest that VLPs derived from the virulent lineage IV Tibet/30 strain are more immunogenic by comparison to those derived from the lineage II Nigeria 75/1 vaccine strain and thus represent a promising vaccine candidate for the control and eradication of PPR.

Keywords: peste des petits ruminants virus, virus-like particles, small ruminants, virulent strain, vaccine strain, immune response

INTRODUCTION

Peste des petits ruminants virus (PPRV), renamed to small ruminant morbillivirus in 2017 (referred to as PPRV throughout this study) (Amarasinghe et al., 2017), is the etiological agent of peste des petits ruminants (PPRs), a highly contagious and devastating transboundary disease, which affects nearly 30 million animals, mainly goats and sheep, annually across more than 70 countries worldwide. Peste des petits ruminants virus (genus *Morbillivirus*, family Paramyxoviridae) is a non-segmented, negative-sense RNA virus with a genome of ~16 kb that encodes a total of six structural proteins [nucleocapsid (N), phosphoprotein (P), matrix (M), fusion (F), hemagglutinin (H), and polymerase (L)] and two non-structural proteins (V and C) (Gibbs et al., 1979; Bailey et al., 2005). Coexpression of the PPRV M, F, and H proteins results in the efficient assembly and release of virus-like particles (VLPs) (Wang et al., 2017). The M protein is the most abundant structural protein within the mature virion and plays a critical role in viral morphogenesis, acting as a driving force of virus budding (Haffar et al., 1999; Pohl et al., 2007). Proteins F and H are two surface expressed glycoproteins, which play an important role in attachment to the host cell, as well as mediating fusion of the viral envelope with the host cell membrane (Baron et al., 2016). While both the F and H proteins are potent inducers of a protective host immune response, the H protein is more immunogenic compared to F, ultimately stimulating a more robust humoral immune response, with the majority of virus-neutralizing antibodies (VNAs) being directed against the H protein (Sinnathamby et al., 2001; Renukaradhya et al., 2002; Rahman et al., 2003; Diallo et al., 2007).

Peste des petits ruminant is classified by the World Organization for Animal Health (OIE) as a notifiable terrestrial animal disease and is estimated to result in economic losses of US $1.4 million to $2.1 billion annually, mostly in Africa and Asia, mainly due to morbidity, mortality, production losses, and treatment costs. Furthermore, PPR also has severe negative impacts on food and job security, as well as livelihood, especially among women and children, exacerbating poverty and malnutrition, particularly among highly vulnerable rural communities (Kumar et al., 2014).

Following the successful global eradication of rinderpest in 2011, a global consensus was reached on the need to eradicate PPR (Taylor, 2016). In April 2015, a PPR global control and eradication strategy were endorsed during a conference in Côte d'Ivoire with the aim of eradicating PPR globally by 2030 (OIE and FAO, 2015). To implement this strategy, the Food and Agriculture Organization of the United Nations (FAO) and OIE, 2016 launched, in October 2016, an initial PPR global eradication program for 2017–2021. In accordance with this strategy, the Chinese government issued in December 2015 the National Eradication Program for PPR (2016–2020), with the goal of eradicating PPR countrywide by 2020 (Liu et al., 2018). Lessons learned from the global eradication of rinderpest in 2011 demonstrated that the use of a highly efficacious vaccine was critical to the campaign's success, and as such, vaccination has been identified as the most suitable option for the control and eradication of PPR.

Sequence-based phylogenetic analysis has classified PPRV into four distinct lineages (I, II, III, and IV) (Forsyth and Barrett, 1995; Couacy-Hymann et al., 2002), but only one serotype exists. Lineages I, II, and III are most prominent among African and Middle Eastern countries, whereas lineage IV is most prominent among Asian countries (Wu et al., 2016) and more recently several African countries previously reporting only a single lineage (Kwiatek et al., 2011; Munir, 2015). Although there is only one serotype of PPRV, there are quantitative and qualitative differences in immune responses among different lineages (Hodgson et al., 2018). While PPRV VLPs derived from lineage II vaccine strains have proven promising as a differentiating infected from vaccinated animals (DIVA) vaccine candidate, the immunogenicity of VLPs derived from virulent strains still remains largely unknown (Li et al., 2014; Liu et al., 2015; Wang et al., 2017; Yan et al., 2019).

To this effect, we constructed two VLP vaccine candidates derived from the lineage IV Tibet/30 virulent strain and lineage II–attenuated Nigeria 75/1 vaccine strain respectively using a baculovirus system for the simultaneous coexpression of the codon-optimized M, F, and H proteins in insect cells. These VLPs were subsequently used to immunize mice, goats, and sheep, and the results revealed that the Tibet/30 VLPs were highly immunogenic, eliciting a more potent humoral and cell-mediated immune response among vaccinated animals by comparison to the Nigeria 75/1 VLPs and thus represents a prospective candidate vaccine for the control and eradication of PPR.

MATERIALS AND METHODS

Cells and Viruses

Adherent *Spodoptera frugiperda* (Sf9) insect cells used for baculovirus rescue and propagation were maintained in Grace's Insect Medium (Life Technologies, San Diego, CA, United States) and cultured at 27°C. High Five insect cells (BTI-TN-5B1-4) used for VLP production were grown in suspension in Express Five serum-free media (Thermo Fisher Scientific, Saint Louis, MO, United States) and cultured at 27°C on a temperate orbital shaker at 200 rpm. Propagation and titration of PPRV were done on African green monkey kidney cells (Vero), which were cultured in Dulbecco modified Eagle medium supplemented with 10% heat inactivated fetal bovine serum at 37°C with 5% CO_2. Peste des petits ruminants virus vaccine strain Nigeria 75/1 was stored in our laboratory.

Construction of Bacmid Transfer Plasmid

Codon optimized open reading frames for the PPRV M, F, and H genes from the PPRV virulent strain China/Tibet/Geg/07-30 (GenBank FJ905304.1) and vaccine strain Nigeria 75/1 (GenBank HQ197753.1) with restriction enzyme sequences (**Table 1**) were synthesized by Sangon Biotech (Shanghai, China) Co., Ltd. The synthetic codon optimized genes were cloned into Puc57-Simple plasmid, respectively. The M gene was inserted into a modified pFastBacDual vector under a p10 promoter flanked by *Rsr*II and *Stu*I restriction sites yielding the recombinant plasmid pFBD-M. Then the H gene was cloned into pFBD-M under a polyhedrin (pH) promoter digested with *Sal*I and *Hing*III to yield the recombinant plasmid pFBD-M-H. Subsequently, the F gene was cloned into the recombinant plasmid pFBD-M-H vector under the second pH promoter digested with *Nhe*I and *Sph*I yielding the recombinant transfer plasmid pFBD-M-F-H (**Figure 1A**). Bacmid transfer plasmids were transformed into *Escherichia coli* DH10TMBac competent cells (Life Technologies, United States) containing the AcMNPV baculovirus genome to obtain recombinant bacmids containing M, F, and H genes of the PPRV Tibet/30 and Nigeria 75/1 strains, respectively. Recombinant bacmids were identified by polymerase chain reaction using three pairs of gene specific primers for the two PPRV strains. The sequences of all primers used in this study are summarized in **Table 1**.

TABLE 1 | Sequences of primers used in the present study.

Primer	Sequence (5′–3′)	Restriction enzyme site
$M_{Tibet}F$	ACAC<u>CGGTCCG</u>ATGACCGAAATCTACGACTT	*Rsr*II
$M_{Tibet}R$	ACAC<u>AGGCCT</u>TTAGAGAATTTTAAAGAGGCC	*Stu*I
$F_{Tibet}F$	ACAC<u>GTCGAC</u>ATGACCAGGGTTGCTATC	*Sal*I
$F_{Tibet}R$	ACAC<u>AAGCTT</u>TTACAGAGAGCGAACGTAAG	*Hing*III
$H_{Tibet}F$	ACAC<u>GCTAGC</u>ATGTCCGCTCAAAGGGAGAG	*Nhe*I
$H_{Tibet}R$	ACAC<u>GCATGC</u>TTACACGGGATTGCAAGTGAC	*Sph*I
$M_{Nigeria}F$	ACAC<u>GGTCCG</u>ATGACCGAGATCTACGAT	*Rsr*II
$M_{Nigeria}R$	ATAC<u>AGGCCT</u>TTACAGGATCTTGAACAG	*Stu*I
$F_{Nigeria}F$	ACA<u>GTCGAC</u>ATGACACGGGTCGCAACC	*Sal*I
$F_{Nigeria}R$	ATAC<u>AAGCTT</u>CTACAGTGATCTCACGTA	*Hing*III
$H_{Nigeria}F$	ACA<u>GCTAGC</u>ATGTCCGCACAAAGGGAA	*Nhe*I
$H_{Nigeria}R$	ATAC<u>GCATGC</u>TCAGACTGGATTACATGT	*Sph*I

[a] *Restriction enzyme sites are underlined.*

Generation and Identification of Recombinant Baculoviruses

Recombinant baculoviruses (rBVs) expressing PPRV M, F, and H proteins from either the virulent Tibet/30 strain or vaccine Nigeria 75/1 strain were rescued using the Cellfectin II Reagent (Life Technologies, United States) as previously described (Yan et al., 2019). Briefly, Sf9 cells were seeded 24 h prior to transfection in a 6-well plate at a density of 8×10^5 cells/well to achieve a confluency of 80–90%. For transfection, 3 μg of recombinant bacmid DNA diluted in 100 μL unsupplemented Grace's Insect Medium was combined with 100 μL diluted Cellfectin II Reagent (8 μL Cellfectin II Reagent diluted in unsupplemented Grace's Medium) vortexed briefly and subsequently incubated at room temperature for 15–30 min. The DNA–lipid mixture was then added onto the Sf9 cells and incubated at 27°C. After 72 h, first-generation rBVs (P1) were harvested and subsequently passaged for several generations in order to obtain high-titer baculovirus.

To confirm expression of the M, F, and H proteins, both rBVs were subjected to immunofluorescence assay (IFA) and Western blot (WB) as previously described (Yan et al., 2019). Briefly, Sf9 cells were infected with the two rBVs, as well as wild-type baculovirus at a multiplicity of infection (MOI) of 1. Fourth-eight hours after infection, the cells were either fixed with 80% acetone and subjected to IFA analysis or lysed in sodium dodecyl sulfate–polyacrylamide gel electrophoresis sample buffer followed by WB analysis.

Generation and Purification of PPRV VLPs

To generate PPRV VLPs, suspension High Five cells were infected with the rBVs at an MOI of 5 and the supernatants harvested at 120 h after infection and subjected to centrifugation at 7,000 rpm for 30 min to pellet cells and debris. The resulting clarified supernatant was then subjected to ultracentrifugation at a speed of 30,000 rpm for 1.5 h at 4°C to pellet the VLPs. The VLPs were then purified by ultracentrifugation at 35,000 rpm for 1.5 h at 4°C using a sucrose density gradient of 20–40–60% (wt/vol) prepared in phosphate-buffered saline (PBS). Protein bands between 20 and 40% corresponding to the purified VLPs were harvested and subsequently subjected to ultracentrifugation at 35,000 rpm for 1.5 h at 4°C to remove the sucrose. Lastly, the concentration of the VLPs was quantified using the BCA protein assay kit as per the manufacturer's protocol (Beyotime, Nanjing, China).

Electron and Immunoelectron Microscopy

The presence and morphology of PPRV VLPs were evaluated by negative staining electron microscopy as previously described

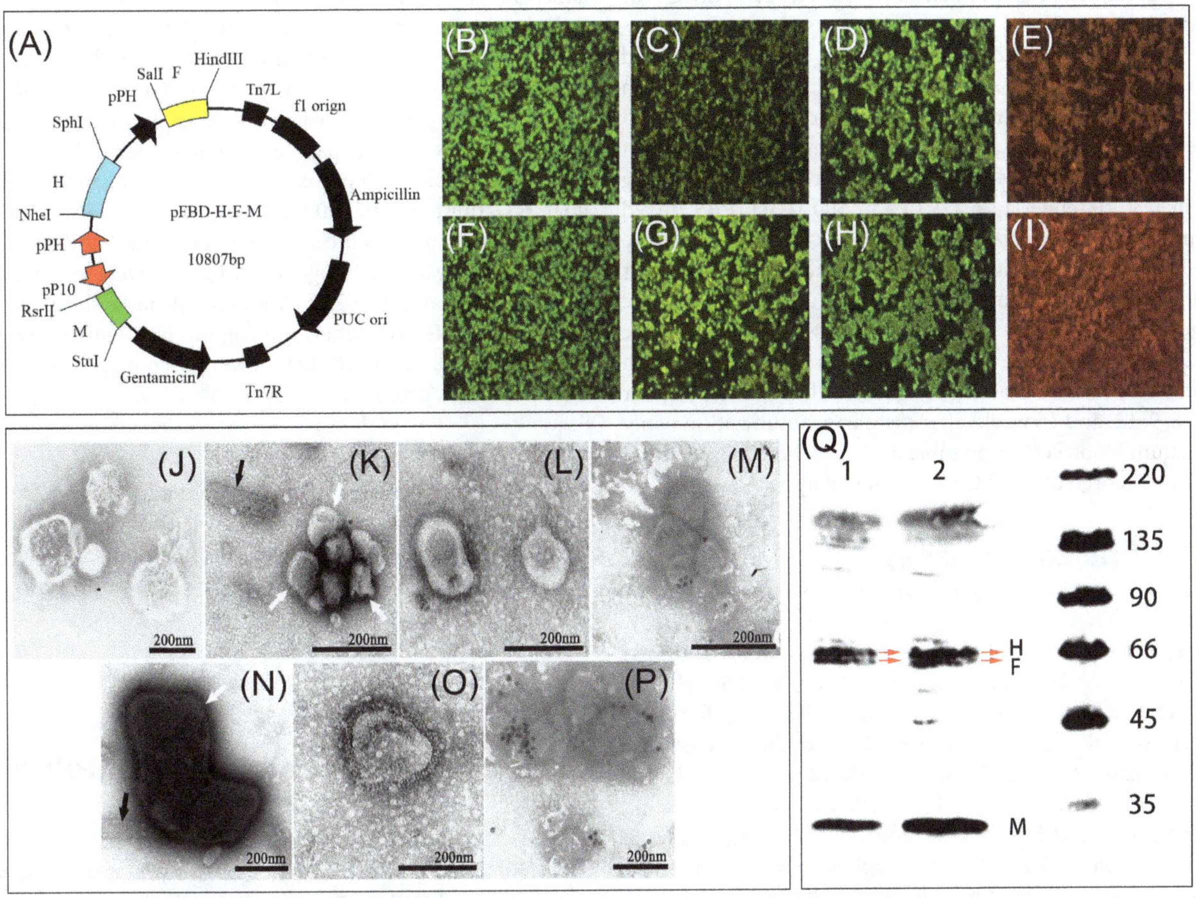

FIGURE 1 | Generation and characterization of PPRV VLPs. **(A)** Schematic diagram for the recombinant plasmids pFBD-M-F-H. **(B–I)** Detection of the expression of M, F, and H. Sf9 cells were mock-infected or infected with rBVs rpFBD-M-F-H or wild-type baculovirus. Expression was evaluated by IFA using mouse anti-PPRV M, F, and H polyclonal antibody, respectively. Nigeria 75/1 M protein **(B)**, Nigeria 75/1 F protein **(C)**, Nigeria 75/1 H protein **(D)**, Tibet/30 M protein **(E)**, Tibet/30 F protein **(F)**, Tibet/30 H protein **(G)**, wild-type baculovirus-infected control **(H)**, and mock-infected control **(I)**. **(J–P)** Transmission electron microscopy images of virus and VLP preparations. Native PPRV particles **(J)**, residual baculoviruses (indicated by black triangles) in preparations of Nigeria 75/1 VLPs (indicated by white arrow) **(K)**, purified Nigeria 75/1 PPRV VLPs **(L)**, and immunogold-labeled Nigeria 75/1 VLPs stained with mouse anti-PPRV H polyclonal antibody followed by gold-labeled goat anti-mouse IgG antibody **(M)**. Residual baculoviruses (indicated by black triangles) in preparations of Tibet/30 VLPs (indicated by white arrow) **(N)**, purified Tibet/30 PPRV VLPs **(O)**, and immunogold-labeled Tibet/30 VLPs stained with mouse anti-PPRV H polyclonal antibody followed by gold-labeled goat anti-mouse IgG antibody **(P)**. **(Q)** Western blot depicting (1) Nigeria 75/1 and (2) Tibet/30 VLP protein expression using sheep polyclonal antibody. However, M, F, and H proteins incorporation in both VLPs were confirmed by Western blot analysis, which demonstrated both M (38 kDa), F (59 kDa), and H (68 kDa) consistent with their respective molecular sizes.

(Qi et al., 2015). For immunoelectron microscopy, PPRV VLPs were applied to a copper–rhodium (Cu-Rh) grid and incubated at room temperature for 60 min followed by incubation with sheep anti-PPRV antibodies (1:200 dilution) at 37°C for 60 min. The copper mesh was then incubated with a 1:50 diluted 10 nm gold-labeled mouse anti-sheep immunoglobulin G (IgG) antibody at 37°C for 30 min (Abcam, Cambridge, MA, United States), and the copper mesh subsequently observed under a transmission electron microscope.

Immunization of Mice, Goats, and Sheep and Sera Collection

All live animal work was performed in accordance with guidelines from the Animal Welfare and Ethics Committee of the Changchun Veterinary Research Institute (permit no. SCXK-2012-017). The environment and housing facilities satisfied the National Standards of Laboratory Animal Requirements (GB 14925-2001) of China.

Eight-week-old female BALB/c mice were purchased from the Changchun Institute of Biological Products Co., Ltd., China, and randomly separated into three groups of 10. Mice were vaccinated intramuscularly in the gastrocnemius muscle with 50 μg PPRV Tibet/30 or Nigeria 75/1 VLPs in 50 μL PBS mixed with 50 μL AddaVax adjuvant. Mice in the control group were given 50 μL PBS mixed with 50 μL AddaVax adjuvant. All groups received a second and third booster immunization at 2 and 4 weeks following the primary immunization. For mice, whole blood was collected 2, 4, 6, and 8 weeks following primary immunization, and the sera subsequently separated and stored at −80°C for further analysis.

Nine outbred goats (12–24 months old) and nine outbred sheep (8–16 months old) were fed by the Zhaoyuan Gaojiatan Goat Farm (Shandong, China) and independently randomized into three groups of three animals each. Goats were multipoint vaccinated subcutaneously (s.c.) in the neck skin with 300 μg PPRV Tibet/30 or Nigeria 75/1 VLPs in 500 μ μL PBS mixed with 1 mL AddaVax adjuvant. Goats in the control group were given 500 μL PBS mixed with 1 mL AddaVax adjuvant. All groups received a second and third booster immunization at three and 6 weeks following the primary immunization. Sheep were immunized using the same exact approach as for goats. For both goats and sheep, whole blood was collected through the jugular vein at 3, 6, 9, 12, and 15 weeks after primary immunization using 10 mL vacuum blood collection tubes and the serum subsequently separated and stored at −80°C for further analysis.

Virus Neutralization Assay

Serum samples from mice, goats, and sheep were analyzed for PPRV-specific VNA titers using a microneutralization assay. Briefly, 50 μL 2-fold serial diluted inactivated sera were combined with 50 μL PPRV Nigeria 75/1 ($100TCID_{50}$) in 96-well cell culture plate and incubated at 37°C and 5% CO_2 for 1 h. Virus-only control wells and uninfected-cell control wells were included. Following incubation, 100 μL (2×10^5 cells) of Vero cell suspension was added to each well, and cytopathic effect (CPE) observed 8 days after infection. Virus neutralizing antibody titers were defined as the highest serum dilution at which the CPE was inhibited by at least 50% (Yan et al., 2019).

Enzyme-Linked Immuneospot Assays for Cytokine Production in Mice

Mouse splenocytes were harvested 2 weeks following the second immunization and stimulated with inactivated PPRV Nigeria 75/1 (10 μ μg/mL). Cells producing interleukin 2 (IL-2), IL-4, IL-10, or interferon γ (IFN-γ) were identified using enzyme-linked immunospot assay (ELISpot) kits (Mabtech AB, Stockholm, Sweden; R&D Systems, Minneapolis, MN, United States) according to the manufacturer's instructions. Spot-forming cells (SFCs) were counted using an automated ELISpot reader (AID ELISPOT reader-iSpot, AID GmbH, GER).

Enzyme-Linked Immunosorbent Assay for PPRV-Specific Antibody and Cytokine

Mouse sera obtained 2 weeks following the third immunization were analyzed for PPRV-specific IgG, IgG1, and IgG2a. Antibody titers were measured using an indirect enzyme-linked immunosorbent assay (ELISA), as previously described (Yan et al., 2019). Purified inactive PPRV (Nigeria 75/1) was used as the coating antigen at a concentration of 2 mg/mL, and the optical density value was recorded at 450 nm absorbance.

To determine antibody responses to the F and H protein of PPRV, an indirect ELISA was developed using purified F and H proteins produced in house from either the virulent Tibet/30 strain or Nigeria 75/1 vaccine strain. Briefly, 96-well flat-bottomed plates were coated with purified F and H proteins (0.5 μg/well) overnight at 4°C and all subsequent steps performed as previously described (Yan et al., 2019). Total IgG was detected using a similar method: 96-well plates were coated with 0.05 μg purified inactivated PPRV (Nigeria 75/1), and horseradish peroxidase (HRP)-conjugated rabbit anti-goat IgG diluted 1:10,000 in PBST (Thermo Fisher Scientific, United States) used as the secondary antibody.

Cytokine responses in goats and sheep were evaluated using commercially available ELISA kits for goat or sheep IL-2, IL-4, IL-10, and IFN-γ (Cusabio, Burlington, NC, United States). The reagents, samples, and standards were prepared according to the manufacturer's protocol.

Data Analysis

Figures were generated using GraphPad Prism 8.0 software (GraphPad Company, SanDiego, CA, United States). Differences between means were evaluated using the one-way analysis of variance (ANOVA) or two-way ANOVA and were deemed significant at $P \leq 0.05$.

RESULTS

Generation and Identification of PPRV VLPs

The M, F, and H genes derived from either the PPRV virulent Tibet/30 or Nigeria 75/1 vaccine strain were cloned into a modified pFastBacDual plasmid, which could carry three exogenous genes under the control of a p10 and two pH promoters, respectively, as shown in **Figure 1A**. Recombinant bacmid was obtained after homologous reorganization in competent DH10bac cells, and rBVs were rescued in Sf9 insect cells following bacmid transfection. Subsequent infection of High Five insect cells with the two rBVs yielded PPRV VLPs derived from the virulent Tibet/30 strain and Nigeria 75/1 vaccine strain, respectively. Expression of the PPRV M, F, and H proteins was confirmed by IFA and WB (**Figures 1B–I,Q**). Furthermore, transmission electron microscopy revealed that the morphology of the VLPs resembled that of authentic PPRV containing spikes on the particle surface (**Figures 1J,K,N**). In addition, removal of residual baculovirus following purification by ultracentrifugation using a sucrose density gradient was confirmed by transmission electron microscopy (**Figures 1L,O**). Lastly, immunoelectron microscopy suggested that the two major PPRV immunogenic glycoproteins F and H, respectively, were incorporated into the VLPs (**Figures 1M,P**) and confirmed by WB (**Figure 1Q**).

Characterization of the Humoral Immune Response to PPRV VLPs in Mice

To evaluate the immunogenicity of the PPRV VLPs, mice were vaccinated with 50 μg PPRV Tibet/30 or Nigeria 75/1 VLPs and boosted 2 and 4 weeks after primary vaccination, after which VNA titers were determined using a microneutralization assay to assess the humoral immune response. At 2 weeks

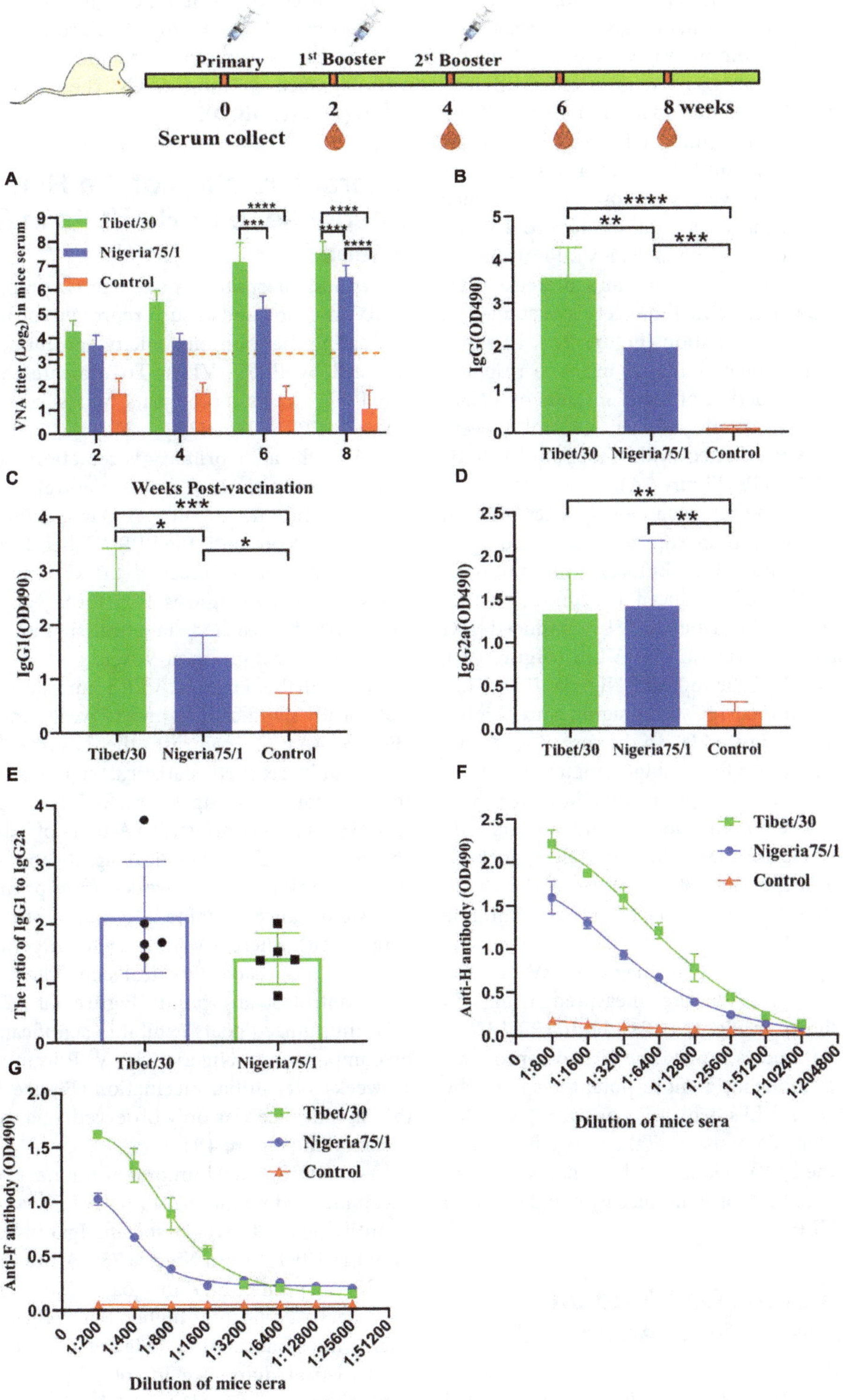

FIGURE 2 | Virus-like particle immunization induces humoral immune response in mice. Mice were immunized thrice via s.c. route at 2 weeks' interval with PPRV Tibet/30 VLPs, PPRV Nigeria 75/1 VLPs, or PBS, all with equal volume of adjuvant. Serum samples were collected 2, 4, 6, and 8 weeks after primary vaccination. **(A)** VNA titers were measured by virus neutralization assay. Dotted line represented antibody titers greater than 10, indicating positive serum conversion. **(B–D)** The specific anti-PPRV serum IgG and isotype responses were detected by ELISA. The serum dilution factor was 5,000. Serum IgG **(B)**, IgG1 **(C)**, and IgG2a **(D)**, responses were determined 6 weeks after the primary immunization. **(E)** The IgG1/IgG2a ratio was calculated. **(F,G)** Serum was collected from mouse 6 weeks after the primary immunization for analyzing F- and H-specific antibodies by ELISA. Data were depicted as the means ± SD for seven mice from each group and were analyzed by one- or two-way ANOVA (*P < 0.05, **P < 0.01, ***P < 0.001, ****P < 0.0001).

after primary vaccination, VNA titers from both the PPRV Tibet/30 and Nigeria 75/1 VLP-vaccinated groups exceeded 10 (**Figure 2A**), the standard minimum value as defined by the OIE, required for protection in goats immunized with live-attenuated PPRV Nigeria 75/1 (OIE, 2008; Yan et al., 2019). In the case of the Tibet/30 VLP-immunized group, VNA titers continued to increase to 2^5–2^6 and 2^7–2^8 at 4 and 6 weeks after primary vaccination, respectively, and those levels sustained at 2^7–2^8 at 8 weeks after primary vaccination (**Figure 2A**). By comparison, VNA titers from the Nigeria 75/1 VLP-immunized group increased to 2^3–2^4 and 2^5–2^6 four and 6 weeks after primary vaccination respectively and those levels sustained at 2^6–2^7 8 weeks after primary vaccination (**Figure 2A**). In short, both PPRV VLPs elicited a potent humoral immune response in mice, resulting in the production of high amounts of VNAs, however, VNA titers were significantly higher at 6 and 8 weeks after vaccination in mice vaccinated with Tibet/30 VLPs by comparison to Nigeria 75/1 VLPs (**Figure 2A**).

To further evaluate the humoral immune responses induced by the two PPRV VLPs, antigen-specific total IgG and IgG1 and IgG2a titers were determined by ELISA. While both the Tibet/30 and Nigeria 75/1 VLPs induced the production of PPRV-specific IgG in mice, the Tibet/30 VLPs induced IgG titers significantly higher than Nigeria 75/1 VLPs (**Figure 2B**). Furthermore, both the PPRV Tibet/30 and Nigeria 75/1 VLP-vaccinated groups exhibited total IgG titers significantly higher than the PBS control group (**Figure 2B**). In the case of IgG1, the trend was similar to that observed for total IgG (**Figure 2C**). Both VLPs significantly upregulated IgG2a production; however, there was no significant difference among Tibet/30 and Nigeria 75/1 VLP-vaccinated groups (**Figure 2D**). The relatively high ratio of IgG1 to IgG2a for both the Tibet/30 and Nigeria 75/1 VLP-vaccinated mice suggested the activation of T_H2-type immune response (**Figure 2E**).

Lastly, antibodies against the two major PPRV surface glycoproteins namely H and F were measured using an established ELISA. As shown in **Figures 2F,G**, both PPRV VLPs induced high levels of antibodies toward the H and F proteins, with the Tibet/30 VLPs inducing a more potent response by comparison to Nigeria 75/1 VLPs, which is consistent with the results obtained from the VNA assay. Taken together, these data demonstrate that the PPRV Tibet/30 VLPs elicited a more significant humoral immune response in mice by comparison to the PPRV Nigeria 75/1 VLPs.

Characterization of the Cell-Mediated Immune Response in Mice Vaccinated With PPRV VLPs

To investigate whether PPRV VLPs could elicit a cell-mediated immune response in mice, the activation of PPRV-specific IL-2, IL-4, IL-10, and IFN-γ in splenocytes were evaluated by ELISpot assays. The results demonstrated that the Tibet/30 VLPs elicited the activation of mouse splenocytes with significantly more SFCs for IL-2, IL-4, IL-10, and IFN-γ by comparison to the PBS control group (**Figure 3**). Although the Nigeria 75/1 VLPs exhibited significantly higher numbers of IL-2 and IFN-γ SFCs compared to the PBS control group, no significant difference was observed for IL-4 and IL-10 (**Figure 3**). Furthermore, the Tibet/30 VLPs appeared to be superior at eliciting IL-4 and IFN-γ production with significantly more SFCs when compared to Nigeria 75/1 VLPs (**Figures 3B,D**).

Characterization of the Humoral Immune Response to PPRV VLPs in Goats and Sheep

Goats and sheep are among the two most susceptible hosts to PPRV infection and as such represent the ideal animal models for evaluating the immunogenicity and humoral immune response induced by PPRV VLPs. To evaluate the immunogenicity of the PPRV VLPs, both goats and sheep were vaccinated with 300 μg PPRV Tibet/30 or Nigeria 75/1 VLPs and boosted 3 and 6 weeks after primary vaccination, after which VNA titers were determined using a microneutralization assay to assess the humoral immune response. At 3 weeks after primary vaccination, VNA titers from both the PPRV Tibet/30 and Nigeria 75/1 VLP-vaccinated groups exceeded the OIE standard of 10 for both goats and sheep (**Figures 4A,B**). In goats, VNA titers gradually increased and reached statistical significance by comparison to the PBS control group at 9 weeks after primary vaccination, in the case of the Tibet/30 VLP-immunized group and remained statistically significant 12 and 15 weeks after primary vaccination (**Figure 4A**). In contrast, the Nigeria 75/1 VLP-immunized group only reached statistical significance by comparison to the PBS control group 15 weeks following primary vaccination (**Figure 4A**). In contrast, VNA titers of Tibet/30 VLP-vaccinated sheep only reached statistical significance by comparison to the PBS control group 12 weeks after primary vaccination with this significance sustained 15 weeks after primary vaccination (**Figure 4B**), whereas VNA titers for Nigeria 75/1 VLP-vaccinated sheep did not reach statistical significance by comparison to the PBS control at any point (**Figure 4B**). Furthermore, Tibet/30 VLP-immunized goats exhibited significantly higher VNA titers by comparison to Nigeria 75/1 VLP-immunized goats 9, 12, and 15 weeks after initial vaccination (**Figure 4A**), whereas in sheep this significance was only observed 12 and 15 weeks after initial vaccination (**Figure 4B**).

As in mice, the humoral immune responses in goats and sheep induced by the two PPRV VLPs were further evaluated by quantifying total antigen-specific IgG titers by ELISA. Although both the Tibet/30 and Nigeria 75/1 VLPs induced the production of PPRV-specific IgG in goats, the Tibet/30 VLPs induced IgG titers significantly higher than Nigeria 75/1 VLPs 9 weeks after initial vaccination (**Figure 4C**). In contrast, there was no statistical difference in total IgG among sheep vaccinated with either the Tibet/30 or Nigeria 75/1 PPRV VLPs, which may be attributed to the lower susceptibility of sheep to PPRV (**Figure 4D**). Additionally, in both goats and sheep, total IgG levels for both the PPRV Tibet/30 and Nigeria 75/1 VLP-vaccinated groups were significantly higher than the PBS control group (**Figures 4C,D**).

Furthermore, all animals developed high levels of PPRV-specific antibodies against the two major PPRV surface

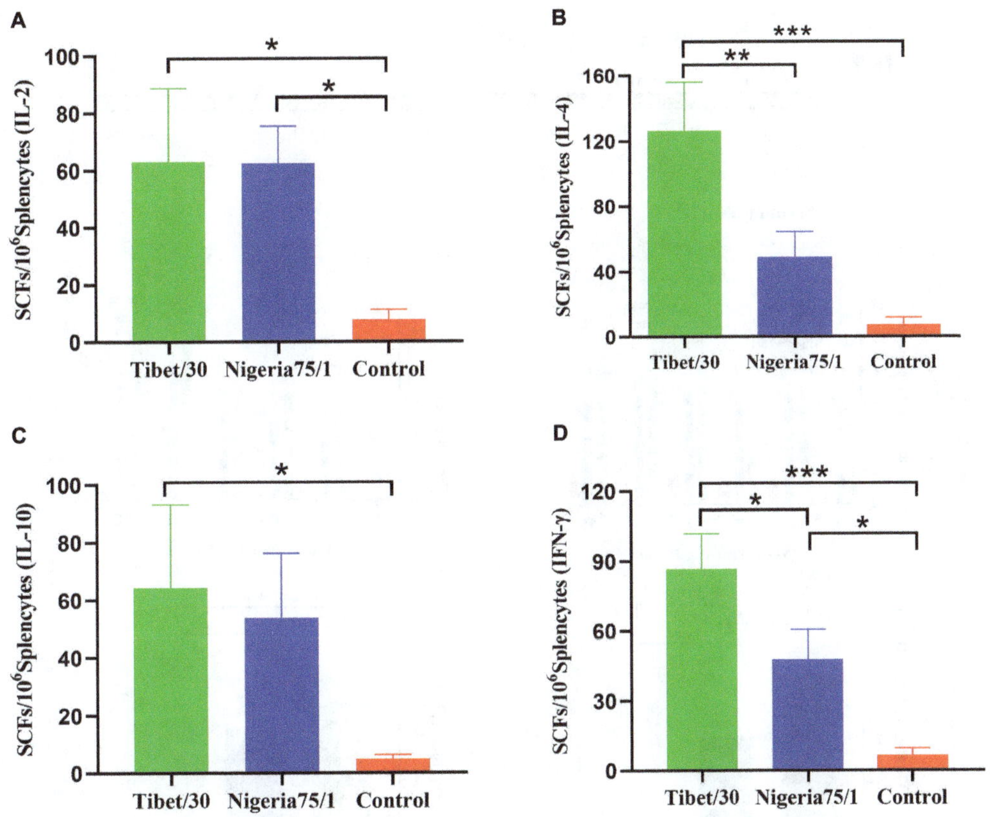

FIGURE 3 | Virus-like particle immunization induces cell-mediated immune response in mice. Splenocytes from mice were stimulated with inactivated PPRV 2 weeks after the third immunization. Splenocytes producing IL-2 **(A)**, IL-4 **(B)**, IL-10 **(C)**, or IFN-γ **(D)** were identified by ELISpot. Data are depicted as the means ± SD of SFCs per million splenocytes from three mice in each group and were analyzed by one-way ANOVA (*$P < 0.05$, **$P < 0.01$, ***$P < 0.001$).

glycoproteins, namely, H and F, with the Tibet/30 VLPs yielding higher titers by comparison to Nigeria 75/1 VLPs in both goats and sheep (**Figures 4E–H**). In general, the humoral immune indicators evaluated suggest that sheep mounted a less robust humoral immune response than goats, which could possibly be attributed to their reduced susceptibility to PPRV infection. Overall, these data are in agreement with those observed in mice and suggest that although both PPRV VLPs elicited a strong humoral immune response in goats and sheep, the Tibet/30 VLPs were more effective at inducing this response by comparison to Nigeria 75/1 VLPs.

Characterization of the Cell-Mediated Immune Response in Goats and Sheep Vaccinated With PPRV VLPs

Cell-mediated immune responses were evaluated by quantifying the levels of secreted IL-2, IL-4, IL-10, and IFN-γ in the serum of PPRV VLP-vaccinated goats and sheep as well as control animals by ELISA. In both goats and sheep, all four cytokines were significantly elevated in animals vaccinated with the Tibet/30 VLPs by comparison to the PBS control group (**Figure 5**). Despite, both goats and sheep vaccinated with Nigeria 75/1 VLPs exhibiting elevated levels of all four cytokines, none with the exception of IL-2 in sheep, were significantly elevated by comparison to the PBS control group (**Figure 5**). None of the animals in either control group exhibited a pronounced cytokine response as expected (**Figure 5**). Furthermore, the levels of IL-4 and IFN-γ were significantly elevated in both goats and sheep vaccinated with Tibet/30 VLPs by comparison to Nigeria 75/1 VLPs (**Figures 5B,D**). In addition, IL-10 levels were significantly elevated in goats but not sheep vaccinated with Tibet/30 VLPs by comparison to Nigeria 75/1 VLPs (**Figure 5C**). In both animals, there was no statistical difference in the levels of IL-2 among Tibet/30 or Nigeria 75/1 VLP-vaccinated groups (**Figure 5A**). Taken together, these data indicate that both PPRV VLPs elicited a cell-mediated immune response in goats and sheep, with the Tibet/30 VLPs inducing an overall more pronounced response than Nigeria 75/1 VLPs.

DISCUSSION

The production of VLPs using a baculovirus/insect cell expression system has proven to be an efficient strategy for vaccine development. Several VLP-based vaccines have been licensed and commercialized, such as Engerix-B®, 2012 (GSK, March 2012) and Cervarix®, 2011 (GSK, July 2011) against

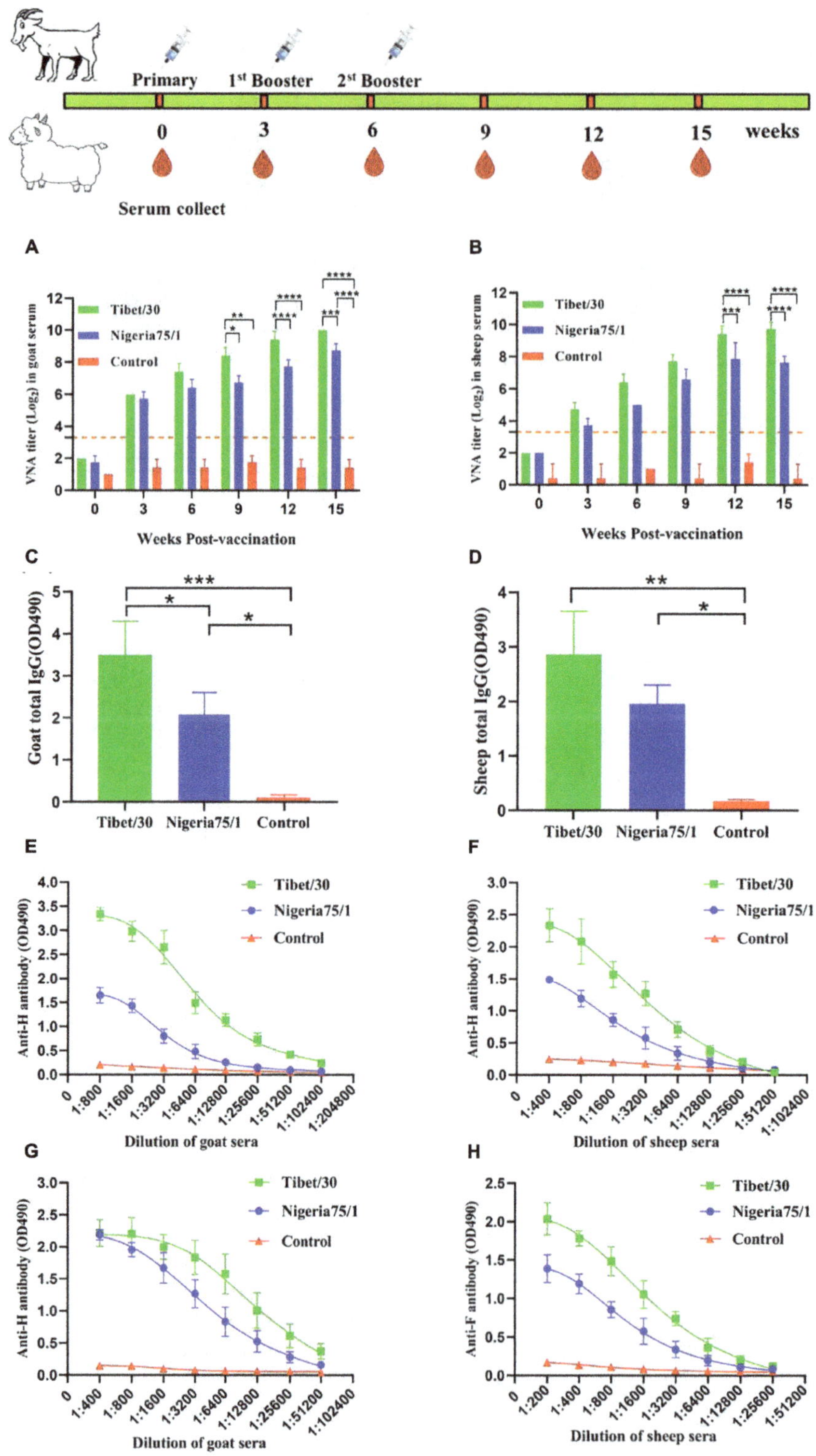

FIGURE 4 | Virus-like particle immunization induces humoral response in goats and sheep. Goats or sheep were immunized thrice via s.c. route at 3 weeks' interval with PPRV Tibet/30 VLPs, PPRV Nigeria 75/1 VLPs, or adjuvant. **(A,B)** VNA titers were measured at 3, 6, 9, 12, and 15 weeks after primary vaccination. Dotted lines represent antibody titers greater than 10, indicating positive serum conversion. **(C,D)** Total goat serum IgG **(C)** and total sheep serum IgG **(D)** responses were determined 9 weeks after the primary immunization. **(E–H)** Serum was collected from each goat or sheep 3 weeks after the second booster immunization for analyzing PPRV F- and H-specific antibodies by ELISA. Data are depicted as the means ± SD for three goats of sheep from each group and were analyzed by one-way or two-way ANOVA ($^{*}P < 0.05$, $^{**}P < 0.01$, $^{***}P < 0.001$, $^{****}P < 0.0001$).

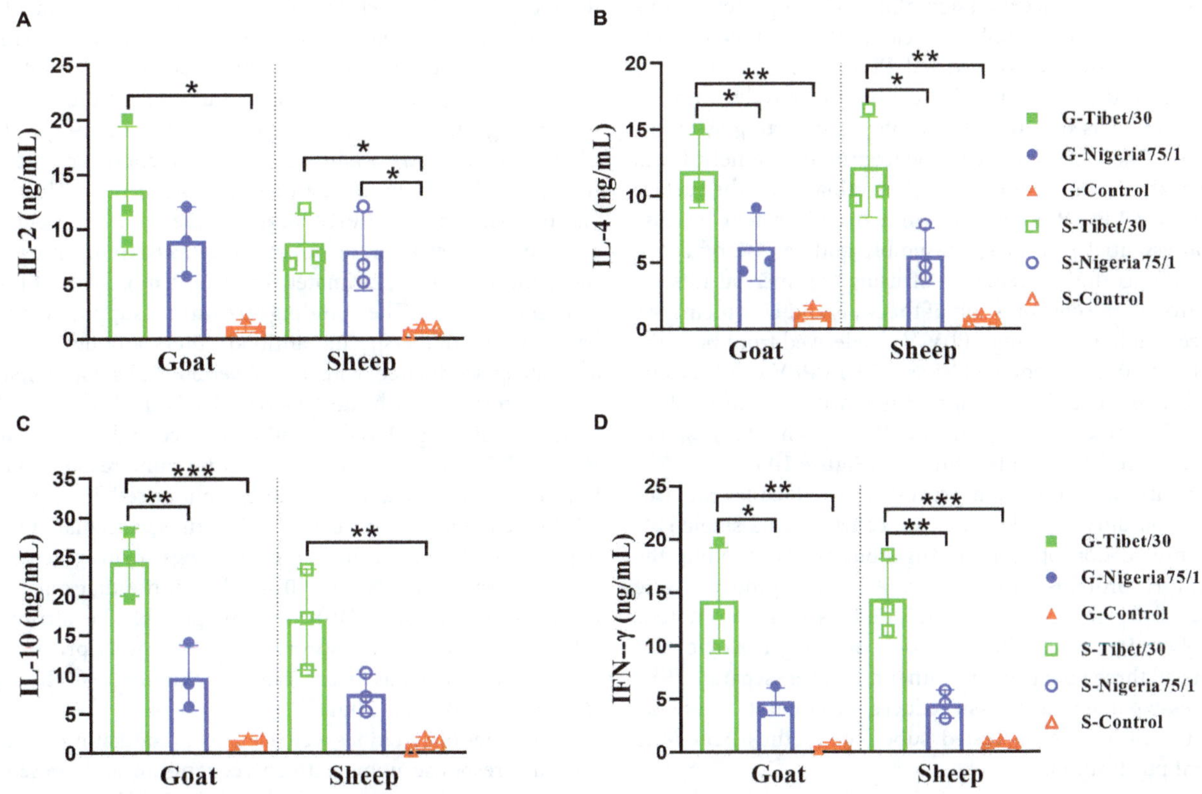

FIGURE 5 | Virus-like particle immunization induces significant cytokine response in goats and sheep. **(A–D)** Serum was collected 3 weeks after the second immunization from animals immunized with PPRV Tibet/30 VLPs, PPRV Nigeria 75/1 VLPs, or adjuvant and were analyzed for the production of IL-2 **(A)**, IL-4 **(B)**, IL-10 **(C)**, and IFN-γ **(D)**. Data are depicted as the means ± SD for three goats or sheep from each group and were analyzed by one-way ANOVA ($^{*}P < 0.05$, $^{**}P < 0.01$, $^{***}P < 0.001$).

hepatitis B virus and human papillomavirus, respectively, as well as the veterinary vaccine Porcilis® (Kushnir et al., 2012) against porcine circovirus type 2. Most often, VLPs are constructed using sequences derived from a virus vaccine strain due to its well-established immunogenicity. However, because of the lack of genetic material and certain structural proteins and/or the alteration of posttranslational glycosylation modifications, the immunogenicity of VLPs derived from a vaccine strain may not always be optimal. In this study, we constructed two PPRV VLP vaccine candidates derived from the sequences of either the virulent Tibet/30 or attenuated Nigeria 75/1 PPRV strains using a baculovirus system for the simultaneous coexpression of the codon-optimized M, F, and H proteins in insect cells. These VLPs were subsequently used to immunize mice, goats, and sheep and their immunogenicity compared by evaluating the magnitude of the humoral and cell-mediated immune responses they induced. Animal experiments demonstrated that both PPRV VLPs were capable of eliciting humoral and cell-mediated immune response in mice, goats, and sheep, with the Tibet/30 VLPs exhibiting a greater immunogenicity by comparison to the Nigeria 75/1 VLPs. Together, these data suggest that both PPRV VLPs represent suitable vaccine candidates for the control and eradication of PPR, with the Tibet/30 VLPs being the most promising candidate because of its greater immunogenicity. This conclusion also provides a way to improve VLP immunogenicity through the use of sequences derived from a PPRV strain rather than a vaccine strain.

A number of studies have previously explored the formation of PPRV VLPs and have demonstrated that coexpression of the PPRV M and N proteins are sufficient for the production of spikeless PPRV VLPs in insect cells. However, because of the lack of the PPRV H and F surface glycoproteins, which are the most immunological relevant determinants, these VLPs were unable to elicit an efficient protective immune response (Liu et al., 2014). On the other hand, coexpression of the N, M, F, and H proteins resulted in the successful assembly and release of PPRV VLPs in either Vero (Wang et al., 2017) or insect cells (Yan et al., 2019) and was capable of inducing strong humoral and cell-mediated immune responses in mice and goats (Yan et al., 2019). Furthermore, it has been demonstrated that expression of the M protein alone is sufficient for the assembly and release of PPRV VLPs; however, in the absence of M, no PPRV VLPs were released for any combination of N, H, and F proteins (Wang et al., 2017). While the expression of the F protein alone could support low levels of VLP assembly, no release was observed in the absence of M, further highlighting its crucial role as a structural protein in the assembly and release of VLPs (Wang et al., 2017). In contrast to the F protein, expression of the N or H proteins alone could neither support assembly nor release of VLPs (Wang et al., 2017). In our study, we constructed PPRV VLPs through the coexpression of the M, F, and H proteins respectively, with the M protein acting as the structural protein supporting assembly and release of the VLPs and the two glycoproteins, namely, F and H acting as the main immunogenic determinants on the surface of the PPRV VLPs. We chose to omit the N protein because of its non-essential role in the assembly and release of PPRV VLPs, as well as the convenience of using commercial kits for DIVA. Through the coexpression of the M, F, and H proteins, we were successful in generating PPRV VLPs derived from both the virulent Tibet/30 and attenuated Nigeria 75/1 PPRV strains, using a baculovirus/insect cell expression system, with the morphology of these VLPs resembling authentic PPRV containing spikes protruding from the particulate surfaces (**Figure 1A**).

To simplify the production process and reduce baculovirus contamination during purification, we constructed a single rBV carrying three codon-optimized exogenous genes encoding the M, F, and H proteins, respectively. All three proteins were expressed under the control of p10 and two pH promoters, respectively (**Figure 1**). This approach of using a single rBV expressing all three viral proteins rather than three separate rBVs each expressing one viral protein reduces the amount of residual baculovirus within the harvested supernatant, thus benefiting subsequent purification.

Peste des petits ruminants virus-like particles display antigenic epitopes in the correct conformation and in a highly repetitive manner, leading to crosslinking of B-cell immunoglobulin receptors (Bachmann and Zinkernagel, 1997; Grgacic and Anderson, 2006; Kushnir et al., 2012). This reaction stimulates B-cell proliferation and upregulation of both MHC class II and costimulatory molecules that allow for subsequent interactions with T-helper cells, which trigger immunoglobulin secretion, affinity maturation, and the long-lived memory B cells (Chackerian, 2007). Our results revealed that both PPRV VLPs were capable of eliciting a humoral immune response in mice, goats, and sheep, which resulted in the production of VNAs to titers sufficient for protection against PPRV infection. These data suggest that both the virulent Tibet/30 and vaccine Nigeria 75/1 PPRV strains share common neutralizing epitopes; however, those on the Tibet/30 strain appear to be more immunogenic, ultimately eliciting a more robust humoral immune response. These findings are further supported by higher levels of H- and F-specific antibody titers among mice, goats, and sheep vaccinated with the Tibet/30 VLPs as compared to those vaccinated with the Nigeria 75/1 VLPs. Additionally, the relatively high IgG1/IgG2a ratio in mice indicated that both PPRV VLPs elicited a T_H2-preferred immune response favoring humoral immunity and was more pronounced among Tibet/30 VLP-vaccinated animals compared to those vaccinated with the Nigeria 75/1 VLPs. Although these findings are in agreement with those observed by Li et al. (2014), they contradict our previous findings (Yan et al., 2019) and can possibly be attributed to differences in adjuvant and/or the lack of the N protein within the VLPs, which has been found to induce a CTL response (Mitra-Kaushik et al., 2001).

A number of cytokines were elevated, modulating an antiviral immune response upon antigen recognition and presentation. Analysis of ELISpot assays detecting IL-2–, IL-4–, IL-10–, and IFN-γ–secreting mouse splenocytes showed that the Tibet/30 VLP-vaccinated group exhibited significantly increased levels of all four cytokines as compared to the PBS control group. In contrast, mice vaccinated with the Nigeria 75/1 VLPs only demonstrated significantly increased levels of IL-2 and IFN-γ as compared to the PBS control group, with the levels of

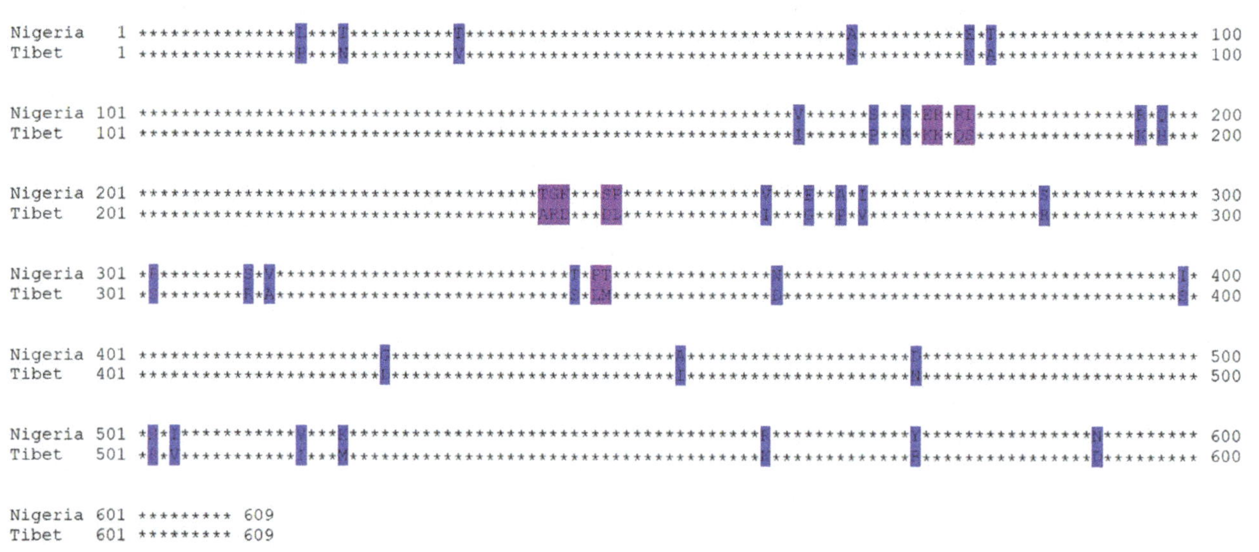

FIGURE 6 | Amino acid sequence alignment analyses of H protein. Homology of the PPRV H protein from PPRV Tibet/30 and Nigeria75/1 strains was analyzed using MEGA (Molecular Evolutionary Genetics Analysis) version 6.0. Capital letters represent the location of amino acid site mutations, and * represents the amino acid without difference between two strains.

IL-4 and IL-10, although slightly upregulated not reaching statistical significance. A similar trend was observed in both goats and sheep whereby all four cytokines were significantly elevated in animals vaccinated with the Tibet/30 VLPs by comparison to the PBS control group. Although both goats and sheep vaccinated with Nigeria 75/1 VLPs had elevated levels of all four cytokines, none with the exception of IL-2 in sheep were significantly elevated by comparison to the PBS control group. Interleukin 4 produced by T_H2 cells drives the maturation of B cells into plasma cells, resulting in antibody production, isotype switching, and affinity maturation (Fang et al., 2007). Interleukin 10, which is also secreted by T_H2 cells, inhibits the activation of T_H1 cells and ultimately their production of cytokines (Moore et al., 2001). Interestingly, IL-4 and IFN-γ levels were significantly elevated in mice, goats, and sheep vaccinated with Tibet/30 VLPs by comparison to Nigeria 75/1 VLPs. In addition, IL-10 levels were significantly elevated in goats but not sheep vaccinated with Tibet/30 VLPs by comparison to Nigeria 75/1 VLPs. Taken together, these data support the conclusion that the PPRV VLPs elicited a T_H2-preferred immune response favoring humoral immunity, which was more pronounced among Tibet/30 VLP-vaccinated animals compared with those vaccinated with Nigeria 75/1 VLPs. Overall the immune indicators in this study were more or less higher than those observed in our previous study and is likely due to the use of AddaVax as the adjuvant rather than Freund's complete adjuvant (Yan et al., 2019). AddaVax is a squalene-based oil-in-water nanoemulsion based on the formulation of MF95 that has been demonstrated to elicit both cellular and humoral immune responses and licensed in Europe for adjuvanted flu vaccines (Vesikari et al., 2011; Alving et al., 2012; Calabro et al., 2013).

A recent study by Hodgson et al. (2018) reported qualitative and quantitative differences in immunogenicity among PPRV lineages. To this effect, we set out to compare the immunogenicity of PPRV VLPs derived from PPRV strains of different lineages and virulence, namely, the lineage IV Tibet/30 virulent strain and the lineage II–attenuated Nigeria 75/1 vaccine strain. The PPRV lineage II Nigeria 75/1 strain was first isolated from a goat that succumbed to PPRV infection and later passaged on Vero cells to yield the first PPR-attenuated vaccine (Taylor and Abegunde, 1979; Diallo et al., 1989). The PPRV lineage IV Tibet/30 strain was isolated from a sick goat in July 2007 during the first outbreak of PPR in southwestern Tibet of China (Wang et al., 2009; Wu et al., 2016). The attenuated Nigeria 75/1 vaccine strain (lineage II) and virulent Tibet/30 strain (lineage IV) share 97, 96.5, and 92.9% similarity at the amino acid level for the M, F, and H proteins, respectively. The H protein of morbilliviruses is highly immunogenic and has been found to be a major inducer of both humoral and cell-mediated immune responses (Berhe et al., 2003). As such, the low homology in H proteins among the two PPRV strains under study could possibly account for the differences in immunogenicity observed for the two PPRV VLPs. The H protein of PPRV is a 609-residue type II integral membrane glycoprotein (Yu et al., 2017). The two PPRV strains under investigation differ by a total of 43 amino acids distributed among the N-terminal cytoplasmic tail (three mutants), stalk region (three mutants), and C-terminal globular head (37 mutants) containing the receptor binding site and immune epitopes, respectively (**Figure 6**; Colf et al., 2007; Yu et al., 2017). No mutants were observed in the transmembrane region of the PPRV H protein. B-cell epitope regions have been mapped to two discontinuous regions on the PPRV H protein from aa263-368 and aa538-609 (Renukaradhya et al., 2002). Interestingly, 11 mutants (25.6%) are located within aa263-368 and could possibly account for the differences in humoral immune responses observed among Tibet/30 and Nigeria 75/1 VLP-vaccinated animals. Frequent differences were also observed at aa163-179, the initial portion of head region N-terminal domain, and may represent a novel antigenic determinant. Lastly, differences in amino acids among the PPRV M and F proteins could also contribute to the differences in immunogenicity observed between the two PPRV VLPs by influencing the amount of antigenic proteins incorporated onto VLP surface, as well as the attachment and uptake rate of VLPs to host cells, which requires further investigation.

ETHICS STATEMENT

All live animal work was performed in accordance with guidelines from the Animal Welfare and Ethics Committee of the Changchun Veterinary Research Institute (Permit No. SCXK-2012-017). The environment and housing facilities satisfied the National Standards of Laboratory Animal Requirements (GB 14925-2001) of China.

AUTHOR CONTRIBUTIONS

FY, NF, CW, and YZ conceived the study and designed experiments. FY, EL, LL, and SZ performed the animal experiments. FY, EL, HW, GL, and NF performed *in vitro* experiments and analyzed data. FY, PH, HJ, and XZ interpreted the data. FY, EL, LL, and ZS wrote the manuscript. ZS, YG, and XX reviewed the manuscript.

FUNDING

This work was supported by grant from Wild Animal Epidemic Source Disease Surveillance Project of State Forestry Administration (21080611).

ACKNOWLEDGMENTS

We would like to thank Ms. Qi Wang for the excellent technical assistance with animal experiments.

REFERENCES

Alving, C. R., Peachman, K. K., Rao, M., and Reed, S. G. (2012). Adjuvants for human vaccines. *Curr. Opin. Immunol.* 24, 310–315. doi: 10.1016/j.coi.2012.03.008

Amarasinghe, G. K., Bao, Y., Basler, C. F., Bavari, S., Beer, M., Bejerman, N., et al. (2017). Taxonomy of the order Mononegavirales: update 2017. *Arch. Virol.* 162, 2493–2504. doi: 10.1007/s00705-017-3311-7

Bachmann, M. F., and Zinkernagel, R. M. (1997). Neutralizing antiviral B cell responses. *Annu. Rev. Immunol.* 15, 235–270. doi: 10.1146/annurev.immunol.15.1.235

Bailey, D., Banyard, A., Dash, P., Ozkul, A., and Barrett, T. (2005). Full genome sequence of peste des petits ruminants virus, a member of the *Morbillivirus* genus. *Virus Res.* 110, 119–124. doi: 10.1016/j.virusres.2005.01.013

Baron, M. D., Diallo, A., Lancelot, R., and Libeau, G. (2016). Peste des Petits Ruminants Virus. *Adv. Virus Res.* 95, 1–42. doi: 10.1016/bs.aivir.2016.02.001

Berhe, G., Minet, C., Le Goff, C., Barrett, T., Ngangnou, A., Grillet, C., et al. (2003). Development of a dual recombinant vaccine to protect small ruminants against peste-des-petits-ruminants virus and capripoxvirus infections. *J. Virol.* 77, 1571–1577. doi: 10.1128/jvi.77.2.1571-1577.2003

Calabro, S., Tritto, E., Pezzotti, A., Taccone, M., Muzzi, A., Bertholet, S., et al. (2013). The adjuvant effect of MF59 is due to the oil-in-water emulsion formulation, none of the individual components induce a comparable adjuvant effect. *Vaccine* 31, 3363–3369. doi: 10.1016/j.vaccine.2013.05.007

Cervarix® (2011). *Prescribing Information.* Brentford: GlaxoSmithKline.

Chackerian, B. (2007). Virus-like particles: flexible platforms for vaccine development. *Expert Rev. Vaccines* 6, 381–390. doi: 10.1586/14760584.6.3.381

Colf, L. A., Juo, Z. S., and Garcia, K. C. (2007). Structure of the measles virus hemagglutinin. *Nat. Struct. Mol. Biol.* 14, 1227–1228. doi: 10.1038/nsmb1342

Couacy-Hymann, E., Roger, F., Hurard, C., Guillou, J. P., Libeau, G., and Diallo, A. (2002). Rapid and sensitive detection of peste des petits ruminants virus by a polymerase chain reaction assay. *J. Virol. Methods* 100, 17–25. doi: 10.1016/s0166-0934(01)00386-x

Diallo, A., Barrett, T., Barbron, M., Subbarao, S. M., and Taylor, W. P. (1989). Differentiation of rinderpest and peste des petits ruminants viruses using specific cDNA clones. *J. Virol. Methods* 23, 127–136. doi: 10.1016/0166-0934(89)90126-2

Diallo, A., Minet, C., Le Goff, C., Berhe, G., Albina, E., Libeau, G., et al. (2007). The threat of peste des petits ruminants: progress in vaccine development for disease control. *Vaccine* 25, 5591–5597. doi: 10.1016/j.vaccine.2007.02.013

Engerix-B® (2012). *Prescribing Information.* Brentford: GlaxoSmithKline.

Fang, T. C., Yashiro-Ohtani, Y., Del Bianco, C., Knoblock, D. M., Blacklow, S. C., and Pear, W. S. (2007). Notch directly regulates Gata3 expression during T helper 2 cell differentiation. *Immunity* 27, 100–110. doi: 10.1016/j.immuni.2007.04.018

Forsyth, M. A., and Barrett, T. (1995). Evaluation of polymerase chain reaction for the detection and characterisation of rinderpest and peste des petits ruminants viruses for epidemiological studies. *Virus Res.* 39, 151–163. doi: 10.1016/0168-1702(95)00076-3

Gibbs, E. P., Taylor, W. P., Lawman, M. J., and Bryant, J. (1979). Classification of peste des petits ruminants virus as the fourth member of the genus *Morbillivirus*. *Intervirology* 11, 268–274. doi: 10.1159/000149044

Grgacic, E. V., and Anderson, D. A. (2006). Virus-like particles: passport to immune recognition. *Methods* 40, 60–65. doi: 10.1016/j.ymeth.2006.07.018

Haffar, A., Libeau, G., Moussa, A., Cecile, M., and Diallo, A. (1999). The matrix protein gene sequence analysis reveals close relationship between peste des petits ruminants virus (PPRV) and dolphin morbillivirus. *Virus Res.* 64, 69–75. doi: 10.1016/s0168-1702(99)00080-5

Hodgson, S., Moffat, K., Hill, H., Flannery, J. T., Graham, S. P., Baron, M. D., et al. (2018). Comparison of the immunogenicities and cross-lineage efficacies of live attenuated peste des petits ruminants virus vaccines PPRV/Nigeria/75/1 and PPRV/Sungri/96. *J. Virol.* 92:01471-18. doi: 10.1128/JVI.01471-18

Kumar, N., Maherchandani, S., Kashyap, S. K., Singh, S. V., Sharma, S., Chaubey, K. K., et al. (2014). Peste des petits ruminants virus infection of small ruminants: a comprehensive review. *Viruses* 6, 2287–2327. doi: 10.3390/v6062287

Kushnir, N., Streatfield, S. J., and Yusibov, V. (2012). Virus-like particles as a highly efficient vaccine platform: diversity of targets and production systems and advances in clinical development. *Vaccine* 31, 58–83. doi: 10.1016/j.vaccine.2012.10.083

Kwiatek, O., Ali, Y. H., Saeed, I. K., Khalafalla, A. I., Mohamed, O. I., Obeida, A. A., et al. (2011). Asian lineage of peste des petits ruminants virus Africa. *Emerg. Infect. Dis.* 17, 1223–1231. doi: 10.3201/eid1707.101216

Li, W., Jin, H., Sui, X., Zhao, Z., Yang, C., Wang, W., et al. (2014). Self-assembly and release of peste des petits ruminants virus-like particles in an insect cell-baculovirus system and their immunogenicity in mice and goats. *PLoS One* 9:e104791. doi: 10.1371/journal.pone.0104791

Liu, F., Li, J., Li, L., Liu, Y., Wu, X., and Wang, Z. (2018). Peste des petits ruminants in China since its first outbreak in 2007: a 10-year review. *Transbound Emerg. Dis.* 65, 638–648. doi: 10.1111/tbed.12808

Liu, F., Wu, X., Li, L., Liu, Z., and Wang, Z. (2014). Formation of peste des petits ruminants spikeless virus-like particles by co-expression of M and N proteins in insect cells. *Res. Vet. Sci.* 96, 213–216. doi: 10.1016/j.rvsc.2013.10.012

Liu, F., Wu, X., Zou, Y., Li, L., and Wang, Z. (2015). Peste des petits ruminants virus-like particles induce both complete virus-specific antibodies and virus neutralizing antibodies in mice. *J. Virol. Methods* 213, 45–49. doi: 10.1016/j.jviromet.2014.11.018

Mitra-Kaushik, S., Nayak, R., and Shaila, M. S. (2001). Identification of a cytotoxic T-cell epitope on the recombinant nucleocapsid proteins of Rinderpest and Peste des petits ruminants viruses presented as assembled nucleocapsids. *Virology* 279, 210–220. doi: 10.1006/viro.2000.0698

Moore, K. W., de Waal Malefyt, R., Coffman, R. L., and O'Garra, A. (2001). Interleukin-10 and the interleukin-10 receptor. *Annu. Rev. Immunol.* 19, 683–765. doi: 10.1146/annurev.immunol.19.1.683

Munir, M. (2015). *Peste des Petits Ruminants: An Introduction.* Berlin: Springer, 1–10.

OIE (2008). *Manual of Diagnostic Tests and Vaccines for Terrestrial Animals.* Paris: OIE.

OIE (2016). *Peste des Petits Ruminants Portal.* Availabe online at:https://www.oie.int/en/animal-health-in-the-world/ppr-portal/distribution/ (accessed April 9, 2019).

OIE, and FAO (2015). *Global Strategy for the Control and Eradication of PPR.* Paris: OIE.

Pohl, C., Duprex, W. P., Krohne, G., Rima, B. K., and Schneider-Schaulies, S. (2007). Measles virus M and F proteins associate with detergent-resistant membrane fractions and promote formation of virus-like particles. *J. Gen. Virol.* 88(Pt 4), 1243–1250. doi: 10.1099/vir.0.82578-0

Qi, Y., Kang, H., Zheng, X., Wang, H., Gao, Y., Yang, S., et al. (2015). Incorporation of membrane-anchored flagellin or *Escherichia coli* heat-labile enterotoxin B subunit enhances the immunogenicity of rabies virus-like particles in mice and dogs. *Front. Microbiol.* 6:169. doi: 10.3389/fmicb.2015.00169

Rahman, M. M., Shaila, M. S., and Gopinathan, K. P. (2003). Baculovirus display of fusion protein of Peste des petits ruminants virus and hemagglutination protein of Rinderpest virus and immunogenicity of the displayed proteins in mouse model. *Virology* 317, 36–49. doi: 10.1016/j.virol.2003.08.022

Renukaradhya, G. J., Sinnathamby, G., Seth, S., Rajasekhar, M., and Shaila, M. S. (2002). Mapping of B-cell epitopic sites and delineation of functional domains on the hemagglutinin-neuraminidase protein of peste des petits ruminants virus. *Virus Res.* 90, 171–185. doi: 10.1016/s0168-1702(02)00151-x

Sinnathamby, G., Renukaradhya, G. J., Rajasekhar, M., Nayak, R., and Shaila, M. S. (2001). Immune responses in goats to recombinant hemagglutinin-neuraminidase glycoprotein of Peste des petits ruminants virus: identification of a T cell determinant. *Vaccine* 19, 4816–4823. doi: 10.1016/s0264-410x(01)00210-9

Taylor, W. (2016). The global eradication of peste des petits ruminants (PPR) within 15 years–is this a pipe dream? *Trop. Anim. Health Prod.* 48, 559–567. doi: 10.1007/s11250-016-0993-x

Taylor, W. P., and Abegunde, A. (1979). The isolation of peste des petits ruminants virus from Nigerian sheep and goats. *Res. Vet. Sci.* 26, 94–96.

Vesikari, T., Knuf, M., Wutzler, P., Karvonen, A., Kieninger-Baum, D., Schmitt, H. J., et al. (2011). Oil-in-water emulsion adjuvant with influenza vaccine in young children. *N. Engl. J. Med.* 365, 1406–1416. doi: 10.1056/NEJMoa1010331

Wang, Q., Ou, C., Dou, Y., Chen, L., Meng, X., Liu, X., et al. (2017). M protein is sufficient for assembly and release of Peste des petits ruminants virus-like particles. *Microb. Pathog.* 107, 81–87. doi: 10.1016/j.micpath.2017.03.021

Wang, Z., Bao, J., Wu, X., Liu, Y., Li, L., Liu, C., et al. (2009). Peste des petits ruminants virus in Tibet, China. *Emerg. Infect. Dis.* 15, 299–301. doi: 10.3201/eid1502.080817

Wu, X., Liu, F., Li, L., Zou, Y., Liu, S., and Wang, Z. (2016). Major mutation events in structural genes of peste des petits ruminants virus through serial passages in vitro. *Virus Genes* 52, 422–427. doi: 10.1007/s11262-016-1317-y

Yan, F., Banadyga, L., Zhao, Y., Zhao, Z., Schiffman, Z., Huang, P., et al. (2019). Peste des petits ruminants virus-like particles induce a potent humoral and cellular immune response in goats. *Viruses* 11:918. doi: 10.3390/v11100918

Yu, R., Zhu, R., Gao, W., Zhang, M., Dong, S., Chen, B., et al. (2017). Fine mapping and conservation analysis of linear B-cell epitopes of peste des petits ruminants virus hemagglutinin protein. *Vet. Microbiol.* 208, 110–117. doi: 10.1016/j.vetmic.2017.07.008

14

Intradermal Immunization of EBOV VLPs in Guinea Pigs Induces Broader Antibody Responses Against GP than Intramuscular Injection

Ying Liu[1,2], Zhiyuan Wen[2,3], Ricardo Carrion Jr.[4], Jerritt Nunneley[4], Hilary Staples[4], Anysha Ticer[4], Jean L. Patterson[4], Richard W. Compans[2], Ling Ye[2] and Chinglai Yang[2]**

[1] State Key Laboratory of Food Nutrition and Safety, Institute of Health Biotechnology, College of Biotechnology, Tianjin University of Science and Technology, Tianjin, China, [2] Department of Microbiology and Immunology and Emory Vaccine Center, School of Medicine, Emory University, Atlanta, GA, United States, [3] Harbin Veterinary Research Institute, Harbin, China, [4] Texas Biomedical Research Institute, San Antonio, TX, United States

***Correspondence:**
Ling Ye
yling@emory.edu
Chinglai Yang
chyang@emory.edu

Ebolavirus (EBOV) infection in humans causes severe hemorrhagic fevers with high mortality rates that range from 30 to 80% as shown in different outbreaks. Thus the development of safe and efficacious EBOV vaccines remains an important goal for biomedical research. We have shown in early studies that immunization with insect cell-produced EBOV virus-like particles (VLPs) is able to induce protect vaccinated mice against lethal EBOV challenge. In the present study, we investigated immune responses induced by Ebola VLPs via two different routes, intramuscular and intradermal immunizations, in guinea pigs. Analyses of antibody responses revealed that similar levels of total IgG antibodies against the EBOV glycoprotein (GP) were induced by the two different immunization methods. However, further characterization showed that the EBOV GP-specific antibodies induced by intramuscular immunization were mainly of the IgG2 subtype whereas both IgG1 and IgG2 antibodies against EBOV GP were induced by intradermal immunization. In contrast, antibody responses against the EBOV matrix protein VP40 induced by intramuscular or intradermal immunizations exhibited similar IgG1 and IgG2 profiles. More interestingly, we found that the sites that the IgG1 antibodies induced by intradermal immunizations bind to in GP are different from those that bind to the IgG2 antibodies induced by intramuscular immunization. Further analyses revealed that sera from all vaccinated guinea pigs exhibited neutralizing activity against Ebola GP-mediated HIV pseudovirion infection at high levels. Moreover, all EBOV VLP-vaccinated guinea pigs survived the challenge by a high dose (1000 pfu) of guinea pig-adapted EBOV, while all control guinea pigs immunized with irrelevant VLPs succumbed to the challenge. The induction of both IgG1 and IgG2 antibody responses that recognized broader sites in GP by intradermal immunization of EBOV VLPs indicates that this approach may represent a more advantageous route of vaccination against virus infection.

Keywords: ebola, vaccine, intradermal immunization, antibody response, VLP

INTRODUCTION

Ebolavirus is a member of the filoviridae family, and infection by ebolavirus in humans and non-human primates (NHPs) results in onset of severe hemorrhagic fevers with high mortality rates (Feldmann and Geisbert, 2011; Li H. et al., 2015; Ye and Yang, 2015). Since their first identification in 1976, five different ebolavirus species have been isolated from outbreaks in humans or NHPs including Ebola virus (EBOV), Sudan virus (SUDV), Bundibugyo virus (BDBV), Tai Forest virus (TAFV), and Reston virus (RESTV), and these viruses differ significantly in their amino acid sequences by as much as 40% (Towner et al., 2008). Notably, the RESTV has been found only in non-human primates from the Philippines, whereas the other four filovirus species are only detected in tropical areas of the equator Africa, and studies in recent years have shown that the African green fruit bats may serve as the natural reservoir of these ebolaviruses (Leroy et al., 2005; Groseth et al., 2007). It is noted that in recent years ebolavirus infection of humans has become more frequent (Chowell and Nishiura, 2014). Of particular concern, the 2013–2016 EBOV outbreak that infected over 28000 human infections and resulted in over 11000 deaths. Moreover, the current ongoing 2018 Kivu outbreak has a mortality rate around 67% and has thus far resulted in over 2000 individuals killed. These large-scale outbreaks demonstrates that the serious threat of EOBV infection to public health is urgent and real. Furthermore, evidence also suggests that EBOV may also infect dogs during outbreaks in addition to infect humans and NHPs (Allela et al., 2005). On the other hand, RESTV has also been indicated to infect domestic pigs in Asia based on serological analyses (Barrette et al., 2009). Further, EBOV has been demonstrated to infect pigs in experimental settings with causing pathogenesis, and virus from infected pigs were shown to transmit to NHPs with no direct contact, demonstrating that this highly lethal virus may be capable of aerosol transmission from a infected host to another susceptible host (Reed et al., 2011; Weingartl et al., 2012). The potential of EBOV to cause non-pathogenic infection in domestic pigs poses a grave danger for these viruses to become endemic and infect humans through zoonotic transmission.

The high mortality rate of EBOV infection underscores the urgent need for an effective EBOV vaccine. A number of EBOV vaccine approaches have been explored in past studies, many of these vaccine strategies have been shown to be able to protect vaccinated animals against lethal EBOV challenge in small laboratory animal models with various efficacies (Yang et al., 2008; Marzi and Feldmann, 2014). Moreover, promising results have also been obtained with viral vector-based vaccine strategies in the NHP model for protection against lethal EBOV challenge, which include recombinant adenovirus replicons (Sullivan et al., 2006), VSV (Jones et al., 2005), parainfluenza virus (Bukreyev et al., 2007), Rabies virus (Blaney et al., 2013), VRP (Herbert et al., 2013), as well as a replication defective EBOV (Marzi et al., 2015) vaccines. In addition to viral vector-based vaccines, EBOV virus-like particles (VLPs) and other protein-based subunit vaccines have been shown to induce protective immune responses against lethal EBOV infection of NHPs (Warfield et al., 2007; Swenson et al., 2008). Of these, recombinant adenovirus replicons and recombinant VSV based vaccines have been evaluated in a number of Phase I clinical trials and shown to be safe and immunogenic (Ewer et al., 2016; Regules et al., 2017). More recently, a Phase III clinical trial was conducted in Guinea with a the recombinant VSV-based vaccine that expresses EBOV GP, and this vaccine was found to be highly effective in preventing EBOV infection of people with high risks to EBOV infections (Henao-Restrepo et al., 2015). The success of the recombinant VSV/EBOV vaccine in the Phase III trial showed that an effective vaccine can control the EBOV epidemics. Nonetheless, the efficacy of viral vector-based EBOV vaccines may be hampered by the pre-existing immunity in the affected area to these viral vectors. Further, immunization by such vaccines may also induce strong immune responses against the vector and therefore dampen their ability to induce immune responses in boosting immunizations for achieving durable protection or in subsequent vaccination of high risk personnel against another filovirus in future outbreaks. Thus, development of vaccine strategies to overcome the limitations of viral vector-based vaccines is still in need.

Among the different EBOV vaccine strategies, VLPs are a subunit vaccine platform that has been shown to protect EBOV infection in NHPs. In early studies, both EBOV and Marburg virus VLPs have been evaluated in different animal models and shown to be effective in eliciting protecting vaccinated animals against lethal challenge (Warfield and Aman, 2011), demonstrating that this vaccine strategy is able to control and prevent filovirus infection. We have shown in our previous studies that EBOV VLPs produced in insect cells by the recombinant baculovirus expression system are able to stimulate dendritic cells to secret various cytokines, and neutralizing antibodies against infection mediated by the EBOV GP are induced in vaccinated animals immunized with these VLPs (Ye et al., 2006). We further demonstrated that immunization with the EBOV VLP vaccines produced from insect cells completely protected mice against lethal challenge by a high dose of mouse-adapted EBOV (Sun et al., 2009). In this study, we investigated immune responses elicited by EBOV VLPs in guinea pigs via different routes, through intramuscular (IM) and intradermal (ID) injection respectively, and showed that immunization by EBOV VLPs produced in insect cells effectively induced neutralizing antibodies against EBOV GP and conferred complete protection against lethal challenge by guinea pig-adapted EBOV. Further, we found that by IM immunization, the EBOV VLPs induced both IgG1 and IgG2 antibodies against EBOV GP in guinea pigs, as compared to the dominant IgG2 antibody responses induced by IM immunizations. More interestingly, we show that the IgG1 antibodies induced by ID immunizations against GP bind to different targets from those recognized by the IgG2 antibodies induced by IM immunizations, demonstrating the potential advantage of ID immunization in eliciting broader antibody responses against infection by EBOV.

MATERIALS AND METHODS

Virus and Biosafety

The stock for guinea pig-adapted EBOV was produced and titered in Vero E6 cells. All experiments with live EBOV were conducted in the BSL-4 facility at the Texas Biomedical Research Institute (TxBiomed), San Antonio, TX, United States.

Cells and Antibodies

Spodoptera frugiperda Sf9 cells were maintained in SF-900 II serum-free medium with penicillin/streptomycin. The polyclonal rabbit serum against EBOV was a gift from Dr. P. Rollin (CDC). JC53BL cells (Wei et al., 2003), which express β-galactosidase and luciferase under a *tat*-activated promoter, was obtained from NIH AID Reagents and Reference Program, and maintained in DMEM plus 10% fetal calf serum (FCS). HeLa cells and 293T cells were obtained from ATCC and maintained in DMEM plus 10% FCS.

Production and Characterization of Ebola VLPs Produced in Insect Cells

Construction and production of recombinant baculoviruses (rBVs) that express EBOV GP and VP40 (designated as rBV-GP and rBV-VP40 respectively) has been described previously (Ye et al., 2006; Sun et al., 2009). For VLP production, Sf9 cells were grown in suspension and then infected with by rBV-GP and rBV-VP40 at the MOIs (multiplicity of infection) of 5 and 2 per cell for each virus. Cell culture medium was harvested at 48 h post-infection and clarified by centrifugating at 1500 RPM for 10 min in a 50 ml conical tube, and the supernatant was then concentrated through Quickstand filtration system (GE). Subsequently, VLPs were further purified through a discontinuous sucrose gradient (10–50%), concentrated again by ultra-centrifugation, and then resuspended in PBS with a concentration of 1 ug/ul (protein/volume) (Ye et al., 2006). Purified EBOV VLPs were analyzed by Western blot using rabbit serum against EBOV to detect viral VP40 and GP proteins, analyzed by electron microscopy to examine the morphology and integrity of VLPs, and analyzed by quantitative enzyme-linked immunosorbent assay (ELISA) to quantify the levels of GP proteins in VLP preparations (Sun et al., 2009). As a control antigen for vaccination, SIVgag VLPs were produced by expressing the SIV Gag protein in Sf9 cells using the recombinant baculovirus expression system and SIVgag VLPs were purified through a sucrose gradient similarly as described above and characterized as shown in previous studies (Ye et al., 2006).

Immunization of Guinea Pigs and Sample Collection

Female Hartley guinea pigs (~250 g in body weight) were obtained from the Charles River Laboratory and housed at the Division of Animal Research of Emory University. Twelve guinea pigs were divided into three groups with four animals per group. Two groups of guinea pigs were vaccinated by IM or ID injection first with 50 ug of EBOV VLPs two times and then boosted again with 200 ug EBOV VLPs at 4-week intervals. The control group guinea pigs were vaccinated with SIVgag VLPs (n = 4) of the same dose as an irrelevant VLP control. For ID injection, VLPs were delivered by using the Mantoux method to four sites (25 to 50 ul per site based on vaccine dose) of the shaved posterior-abdomen skin of guinea pigs under kentamine/xylazine anaesthetization. Blood samples were collected from cranial vena cava under anesthesia at 1 week prior to the first immunization and 2 weeks after the second and third immunizations, and stored at −80°C until being used in analyses.

Detection of GP and VP40 Antigen-Specific Antibodies

Antibodies against EBOV GP and VP40 antigens were detected in serum samples from each guinea pig by ELISA. The His-tagged EBOV GP was produced by infecting HeLa cells with a recombinant vaccinia virus that expresses the EBOV GP-histag protein, and the GP-histag protein secreted into the medium of infected HeLa cells was purified using a Ni-NTA agarose bead-based higtag protein purification kit following established protocols (Sun et al., 2009). The His-tagged EBOV VP40 (VP40-histag) was expressed in bacteria DH5a using plasmid DNA vector pBlusscript IIKS under the T7 promoter, and purified using Ni-NTA agarose bead-based histag protein purification kit following manufacturer's protocols. For ELISA analysis of serum samples, a microtiter plate (Maxisorb, Nunc) was coated overnight at 4°C with purified His-tagged EBOV GP or VP40 at a concentration of 2 ug/ml. Plates were then washed with PBST prior to blocking with 200 ul per well 2% BSA/PBST for 1 h at 37°C. Serum samples from vaccinated guinea pigs were serially diluted and then added to the wells of the microtiter plates that were coated and blocked and then incubated at room temperature for 2 h, and the bound antibodies specific for EBOV proteins were detected with horseradish peroxidase-labeled goat against guinea pig IgG, IgG1, or IgG2 antibodies (Bethyl Lab, Inc.). The wells were then washed and added with TMB (Sigma) at 50 ul per well to develop color, and the enzymatic reaction was stopped with addition of 50 ul per well of hydrochloric acid (0.2N), and afterward the absorbance value at 450 nm of each well was read in an ELISA reader (Bio-Tek Instruments, Inc., Winooski, VT, United States). Serial dilutions of purified guinea pig IgG (EQUITECH-BIO, Inc.) with known concentrations were used to generate a standard curve, which was used to calculate the concentrations of EBOV GP or VP40-specific antibodies in serum samples and the antibody concentrations of these antibodies were expressed as the amount of antibodies in 1 ml of serum (ng/ml).

Blocking ELISA

Blocking ELISA was employed to investigate whether IgG2 antibodies induced by IM injection of EBOV VLPs will affect binding of IgG1 antibodies induced by ID injection of EBOV VLPs to GP. Briefly, microtiter plates were coated o/n at 4°C with purified His-tagged GP as coating antigens at a reduced concentration of 0.5 ug/ml. Plates were then washed with PBST prior to blocking with 200 ul per well 2% BSA/PBST for 1 h at 37°C, and then added with 1:400 dilution of sera from each individual guinea pig vaccinated by IM injection of EBOV VLPs, sera from naïve guinea pigs, or PBST only for 2 h at room temperature. This serum dilution (1:400) has been pre-determined to saturate binding of the amount of coated His-tagged GP antigens. The plates were then washed again and then incubated with sera from individual guinea pigs that had been vaccinated by ID injection of EBOV VLPs or SIVgag VLPs (Control). After incubation for 2 h at room temperature, the plates were washed and the bound IgG1 antibodies were detected with horseradish peroxidase-labeled goat against guinea pig IgG1 secondary antibodies (Bethyl Lab, Inc.). The wells were added with 50 ul per well of TMB (Sigma) to develop color and the color reaction was stopped with addition of 50 ul per well of hydrochloric acid (0.2N), and afterward the absorbance value at 450 nm of each well was read in an ELISA reader (Bio-Tek Instruments, Inc., Winooski, VT, United States).

Analysis of Sera Neutralizing Activity With Pseudovirus

The levels of neutralizing antibodies against EBOV GP were detected by a single-round infectivity assay that we have developed in early studies (Mohan et al., 2012, 2015). Briefly, EBOV GP-HIV pseudovirions were produced by transfecting 293T-cells with and HIV backbone plasmid (Env-defective) and together with a DNA plasmid expressing EBOV GP in pCAGGS using the transfection reagent Fugene HD (Roche). At 48 h post-transfection, pseudovirions in the medium from transfected cells were harvested, clarified, and filtered using a 0.45 micron filter, and then titrated in JC53BL cells (Wei et al., 2003), which express β-galactosidase and luciferase under a *tat*-activated promoter. Neutralization assays were then carried out as described in our previous studies (Li W. et al., 2015). Briefly, pseudoviruses were fisrt incubated with serial dilutions of heat-inactivated serum samples for 1 h at 37°C, which were supplemented with heat-inactivated sera from naïve mouse (Innovative Research) to 5% of the total volume. The serum-pseudovirion mixtures were then added to JC53 cells that have been grown to 50% confluenvy in a 96-well plate and incubated at 37°C for 48 h. Afterward, the level of luciferase activity in each well were detected by a kit (Sigma), neutralization was calculated by measuring the percent decrease in luciferase activity in sample wells compared to virus-only control wells. The serum neutralizing activity is calculated with the formula: [(luciferase activity in control well − luciferase activity in sample well)/luciferase activity in control well × 100%], and is expressed as the percentage reduction of virus titers in sample wells compared to the titers in control wells. Statistical analysis of serum antibody responses between ID and IM vaccinated guinea pigs was performed by a Student's *t*-test.

Lethal Challenge by Guinea Pig-Adapted EBOV

EBOV challenge study was conducted in the ABSL-4 facility at Texas Biomedical Research Institute (San Antonio, TX, United States). Guinea pigs were challenged at 22 weeks after the third vaccination by intraperitoneal injection with 1000 plaque-forming units (pfu) of guinea pig-adapted EBOV. After challenge, guinea pigs were monitored at least twice daily for weight loss and disease symptoms, and animals that exhibited severe disease signs and lost significant levels of body weight (over 25%) were sacrificed in compliance with IACUC guidelines.

RESULTS

Comparison of Antibody Responses Induced by EBOV VLPs Through Intradermal and Intramuscular Immunization Routes

In our previous studies, we showed that mice were effectively protected by two intramuscular immunizations with 50 ug EBOV VLPs produced in insect cells (Sun et al., 2009). To investigate the immunogenicity of insect cell-produced EBOV VLPs in guinea pigs via different immunization routes, we first vaccinated guinea pigs (groups of 4) with 50 ug EBOV VLPs by IM or ID injection as outlined in **Figure 1A**. The control group animals received immunization by 50 ug SIVgag VLPs that were similarly produced in insect cells by IM or ID injection (2 animals each route). As outlined in **Figure 1A**, blood samples were first collected at 2 weeks after the second immunization and then analyzed for antibodies against EBOV GP. As shown in **Figure 1B** (gray columns), antibodies against EBOV GP were readily detected in sera from guinea pigs after two immunizations with 50 ug EBOV VLPs by both IM and ID injections. However, the levels of anti-GP antibodies were relatively low at about 3000 ng/ml for the IM group and 2500 ng/ml for the ID groups respectively. Further, analysis of sera neutralizing activity showed that these sera failed to reduce GP-pseudovirion infection by more than 50% at 1:100 dilution (data not shown).

Based on these results, we decided to give one additional boosting immunization using 200 ug EBOV VLPs or SIVgag VLPs for the control group by IM or ID injection respectively as outlined in **Figure 1A**, and collected blood samples at 2 weeks after the third immunization to analyze the levels of antibodies against GP. As shown in **Figure 1B** (black columns), the levels of antibody responses against GP increased significantly to about 25000 ng/ml by more than eightfold for both IM and ID immunization groups after the additional boosting immunization. The neutralizing activity of sera from vaccinated guinea pigs was then determined by a pseudovirion neutralization assay. As shown in **Figure 2**, sera from guinea pigs vaccinated by EBOV VLPs via either IM or ID injection exhibited significant levels of neutralizing activity against EBOV GP mediated pseudovirion infection, with the average 50% neutralization titers reaching above 1:800 and 1:1600 dilutions for the IM and ID immunization groups respectively. However, analysis by a Student's *t*-test showed that the differences in neutralizing activity between serum samples from guinea pigs in the IM and ID immunization groups at all four serum dilutions (1:200, 1:400, 1:800, and 1:1600) are not statistically significant ($p > 0.05$).

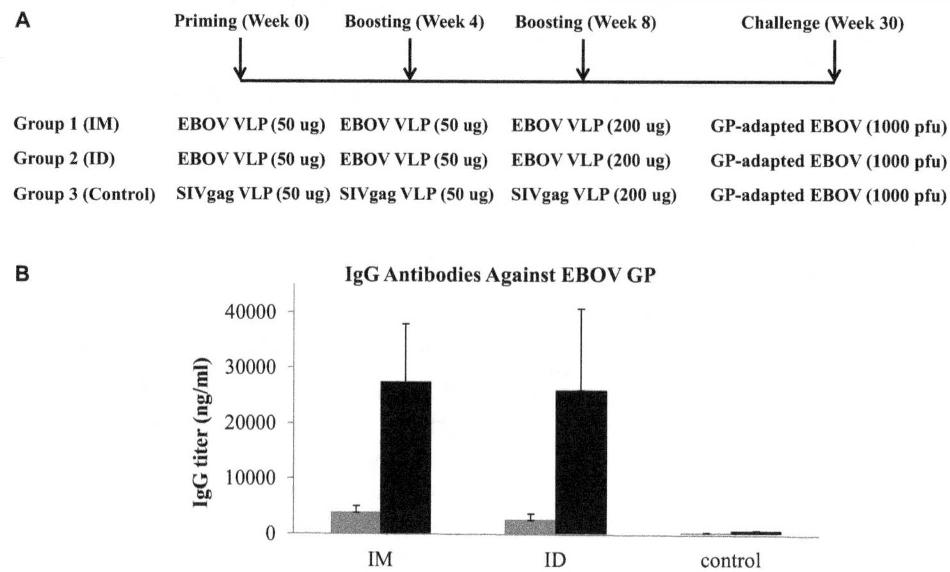

FIGURE 1 | (A) Schematic diagram of immunization and challenge study design. Female Hartley guinea pigs (groups of 4) were vaccinated with EBOV VLPs or control SIVgag VLPs at 4-week intervals via different immunization routes as presented. Blood samples were collected at 2 weeks after the second and third immunizations and guinea pigs were challenged at 22 weeks after the final immunization by 1000 pfu of guinea pig-adapted EBOV. **(B)** Antibody responses against GP induced by IM or ID injection of EBOV VLPs. The levels of antibody response against EBOV GP induced by VLP vaccines in guinea pigs were measured by ELISA using purified His-tagged GP as coating antigen. Antibody concentration was determined from a standard curve and expressed as ng/ml of IgG against GP in serum samples collected after the second and third immunizations. Results reported are the means and standard deviations for samples from individual animals of each group. Gray columns, antibody levels in sera from vaccinated collected at 2 weeks after the second immunization; black columns, antibody levels in sera from vaccinated collected at 2 weeks after the third immunization.

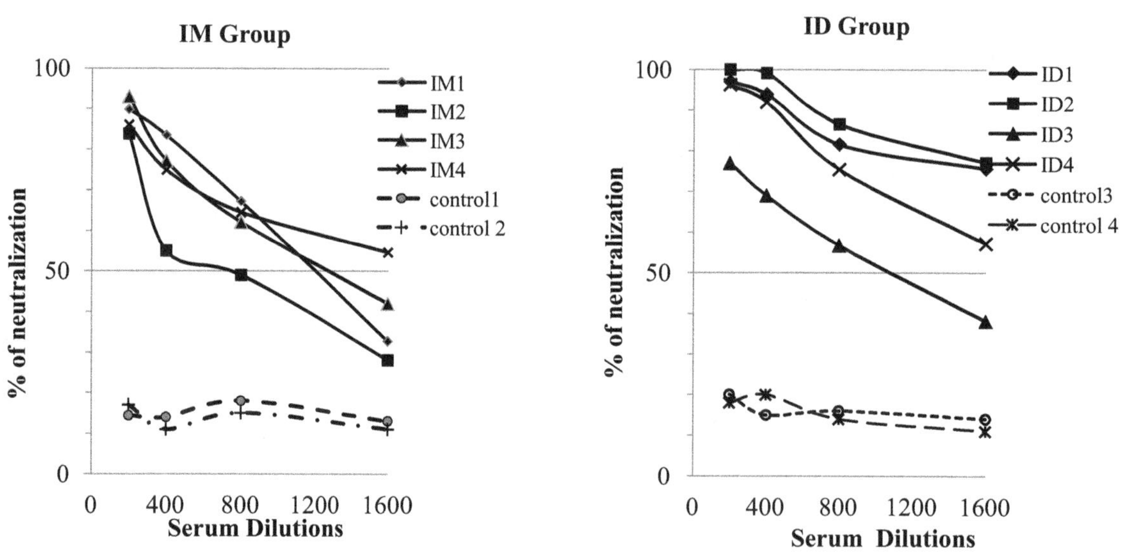

FIGURE 2 | Neutralization of GP-mediated pseudovirion infection by sera from vaccinated guinea pigs. Neutralizing activity of immune sera collected after the third immunization was determined by a pseudovirion neutralization assay. Serial twofold dilutions of sera were inbubated with 500 pfu of GP-pseudotyped virus at 37°C for 1 h, the mixtures were then added to JC53 cells seeded in a 96-well plate and incubated at 37°C for 2 days. Neutralization was measured as decrease in luciferase expression compared to virus-only controls after 48 h as described in Materials and Methods. Results reported are the percentage of pseudovirion neutralization by samples from individual animals of each group at the indicated dilutions. Statistical comparison of serum neutralizing activities at each dilution was performed by a Student's *t*-test, and was found to be not statistically significant ($p > 0.05$).

Immunization Routes Affect the Profiles of Antibody Responses Against GP Induced by EBOV VLPs

We further characterized the levels of IgG1 and IgG2 subclass antibodies against GP induced by IM or ID immunization with EBOV VLPs for comparison. As shown in **Figure 3**, immunization by IM or ID injection of EBOV VLPs induced similar levels of IgG2 antibodies against GP in guinea pigs ($p > 0.05$). On the other hand, ID immunization by EBOV VLPs induced significantly higher levels of IgG1 antibodies against GP than IM immunization ($p < 0.05$). To investigate whether such differences might also be observed for other vaccine antigens in EBOV VLPs, we further determined the levels of IgG1 and IgG2 antibodies against EBOV matrix protein VP40 in EBOV VLPs for comparison. As shown in **Figure 4**, similar levels of both IgG1 and IgG2 antibodies against EBOV VP40 were induced by immunization through IM or ID injection of EBOV VLPs in guinea pigs ($p > 0.05$). Further, it is also notable that the levels of IgG1 antibodies against GP are only about one-third of the levels of IgG2 antibodies by ID immunization and about one-tenth of the levels of IgG2 antibodies by IM injection. In contrast, the levels of IgG1 and IgG2 antibodies against VP40 are similar in both IM and ID immunization groups. Taken together, these results show that the antibody profiles induced by IM and ID immunization of EBOV VLPs in guinea pigs are different only for the GP antigen but not for VP40.

Based on the different levels of IgG1 antibodies against GP induced by ID and IM injection, we carried out blocking ELISA to determine whether the IgG1 and IgG2 antibodies against GP may target similar or different epitopes. Briefly, microtiter plates were coated with a limited amount of purified His-tagged GP protein at 0.05 ug per well. After blocking, the wells were treated with sera from guinea pigs vaccinated by IM injection of EBOV VLPs at 1:400 dilutions, a dilution that has been pre-determined to saturate binding of the amount of coated GP antigen. The controls were added with the same dilution of sera from control group guinea pigs or no sera as indicated. After incubating with the first antibody, the plate was washed and then added with sera from guinea pigs vaccinated by ID injection of EBOV VLPs or from control group guinea pigs at 1:400 dilutions as indicated, followed by addition of HRP-conjugated secondary antibody against guinea pig IgG1 to determine the levels of IgG1 antibodies bound to GP for comparison. The results in **Figure 5** show that pre-incubation with sera from IM-vaccinated guinea pigs did not affect the binding of IgG1 antibodies in sera from ID-vaccinated guinea pigs to GP as compared to pre-incubation with sera from control guinea pigs or no sera. Further, without the addition of sera from ID-vaccinated guinea pigs, only low levels of IgG1 antibodies against GP in sera from IM-vaccinated guinea pigs were detected. These results suggest that the interaction of IgG1 antibodies to EBOV GP elicited by ID injection of EBOV VLPs is not affected by pre-blocking of the GP antigen by GP-specific antibodies from IM-vaccinated guinea pigs that are predominantly of the IgG2 subclass, suggesting that the IgG1 antibodies induced by ID immunization may target different epitopes in GP from those targeted by IgG2 antibodies induced by IM immunization with EBOV VLPs.

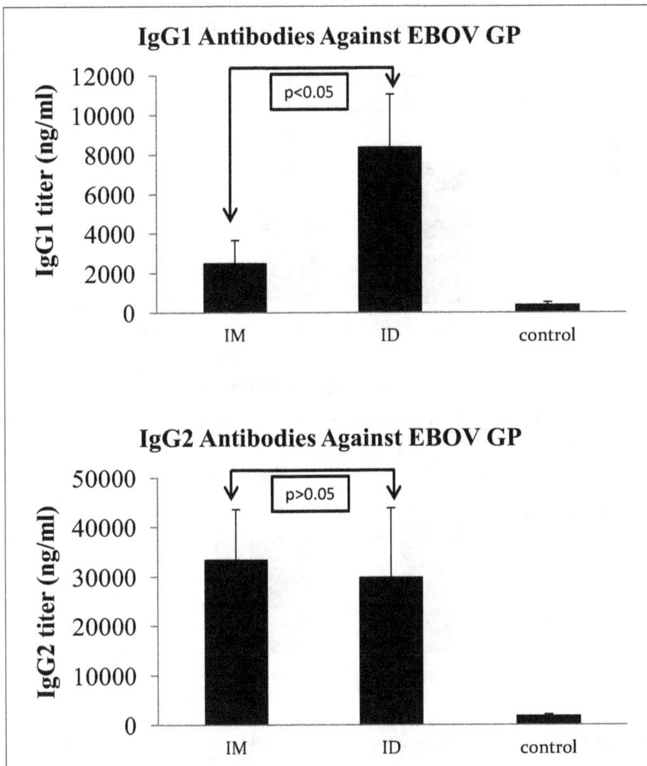

FIGURE 3 | Analysis of IgG1 and IgG2 subclass antibody responses against GP induced by IM and ID injection of EBOV VLPs in guinea pigs. Guinea pig sera collected after the third immunization were analyzed for IgG1 and IgG2 subclass antibody responses against GP by ELISA using purified His-tagged GP as coating antigen. The concentrations of IgG1 and IgG2 antibodies against GP were determined from a standard curve and expressed as ng/ml of GP-specific antibodies in sera. Results reported are the means and standard deviations for samples from individual animals of each group. Statistical comparison of antibody levels against EBOV GP was performed by a Student's *t*-test, and shown in each graph.

Protection of Guinea Pigs Against Lethal EBOV Challenge

After the third immunization, the guinea pigs were transferred to the Texas Biomedical Research Institute to evaluate the protective efficacy of EBOV VLP vaccination against lethal EBOV challenge in the ABSL-4 facility. As shown in **Figure 1**, vaccinated guinea pigs as well as the control group were infected by 1000 pfu of guinea pig-adapted EBOV at 22 weeks after the final immunization, and then observed daily for disease symptoms, weight changes, and body temperatures. As shown in **Figure 6**, all control group animals that received SIV Gag VLPs by either IM or ID injection succumbed to challenge with progressive weight losses and died by day 6 post-challenge. In contrast, all animals that had been vaccinated by EBOV VLPs by either IM or ID injection survived the challenge with no significant change in body weight over 24 days post-challenge. These results show that immunization by either IM or ID injection of EBOV VLPs

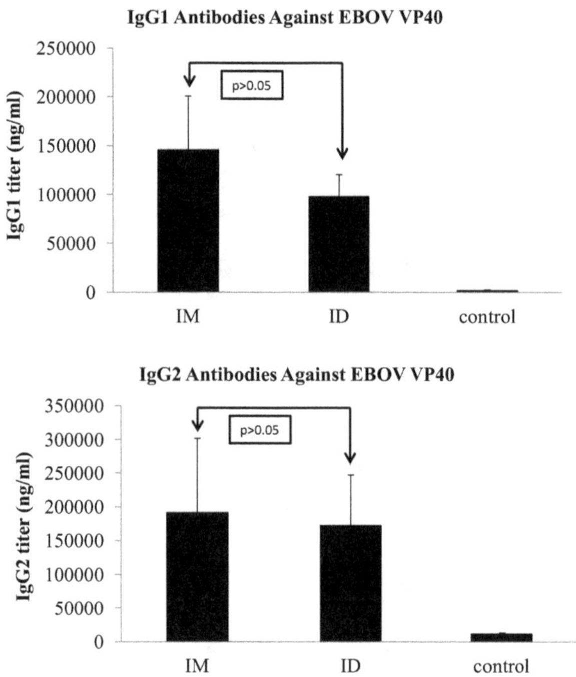

FIGURE 4 | Induction of similar levels of IgG1 and IgG2 subclass antibody responses against VP40 induced by IM and ID injection of EBOV VLPs in guinea pigs. Guinea pig sera collected after the third immunization were analyzed for IgG1 and IgG2 subclass antibody responses against VP40 by ELISA using purified His-tagged VP40 as coating antigen. The concentrations of IgG1 and IgG2 antibodies against VP40 were determined from a standard curve and expressed as ng/ml of VP40-specific antibodies in sera. Results reported are the means and standard deviations for samples from individual animals of each group. Statistical comparison of antibody levels against EBOV GP was performed by a Student's *t*-test, and shown in each graph.

effectively protected vaccinated animals against a high dose lethal challenge by guinea pig-adapted EBOV.

DISCUSSION

In the present study, we compared the effect of two different immunization routes, IM and ID injections respectively, on the immunogenicity and protective efficacy of insect cell-derived EBOV VLPs in the guinea pig model. Our results showed that EBOV VLPs administered via both IM and ID routes induced similar levels of antibody responses against EBOV GP and vaccinated were completely protected against a high dose lethal challenge by guinea pig-adapted EBOV. Of particular interest, we observed that while immunization with EBOV VLPs by IM or ID injection induced similar levels of IgG2 subclass antibodies against GP, the levels of IgG1 subclass antibodies against EBOV GP induced by ID immunization were significantly higher than the levels induced by IM immunizations. In contrast, immunization by both IM and ID routes induced similar levels of IgG1 and IgG2 antibody responses against VP40, the EBOV matrix protein in VLPs. Moreover, by further analyses, we observed that binding of IgG1 antibodies induced by ID injection

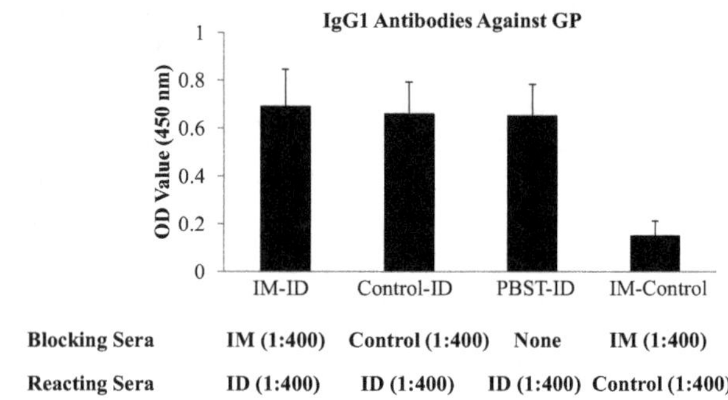

FIGURE 5 | Binding of IgG1 from ID immunized guinea pigs to GP was not affected by pre-incubation with sera from IM immunized guinea pigs. Microtiter plates coated with His-tagged GP were first incubated with 1:400 dilutions of sera from guinea pigs vaccinated by IM injection of EBOV VLPs (IM-ID and IM-Control), IM or ID injection of SIVgag VLPs (Control-ID), or PBST with no sera (Control-ID) as indicated for 2 h at room temperature. The plates were then washed and incubated with 1:400 dilution of sera from guinea pigs vaccinated by ID injection of EBOV VLPs (IM-ID, Control-ID, and PBST-ID) or SIVgag VLPs (IM-Control) for 2 h at room temperature. The plates were washed again and the levels of IgG1 antibodies bound to each well were determined by incubating with horseradish peroxidase-labeled goat against guinea pig IgG1 antibodies and expressed as OD values for comparison. Results reported are the means and standard deviations for samples from paired animals of each group.

of EBOV VLPs was not blocked by sera from IM-vaccinated animals, indicating that such IgG1 antibodies may react to different epitopes in GP from those recognized by antibodies induced by IM immunization, which are predominantly of the IgG2 subclass.

In addition to serving as a protective barrier, skin has also long been known to be an important part of the immune system (Bos and Kapsenberg, 1993). The first human vaccine, vaccinia, is administered by the ID route. Skin dermis is enriched with dermal DCs as well as Langerhans cells that are professional antigen presenting cells for immune surveillance (Flacher et al., 2006). In early studies, it has also been shown that influenza vaccines delivered by ID injection are safe and immunogenic in children (Rendtorff et al., 1959). However, due to the technical difficulty of ID injection by the conventional Mantoux method as well as the small volume of vaccines that can be delivered by this route, ID injection is not widely practiced for current vaccine delivery with the exception of the BCG vaccination against Tuberculosis. More recent studies showed that administration of influenza vaccines through ID immunization required reduced vaccine doses for eliciting similar levels of immune responses as IM delivery of influenza vaccines (Kenney et al., 2004; Chiu et al., 2007). In recent studies, new technologies are being development for vaccine delivery through the ID route. A new needle-syringe device that only exposed the tip of the needle has recently been designed for easier ID injection of influenza vaccines (Laurent et al., 2007; Holland et al., 2008), and this approach has now been approved for ID delivery of seasonal influenza vaccines. Moreover, microneedles are also under development for ID delivery of vaccines (Gill et al., 2014). Recent studies have shown that ID delivery of influenza vaccines using microneedles is

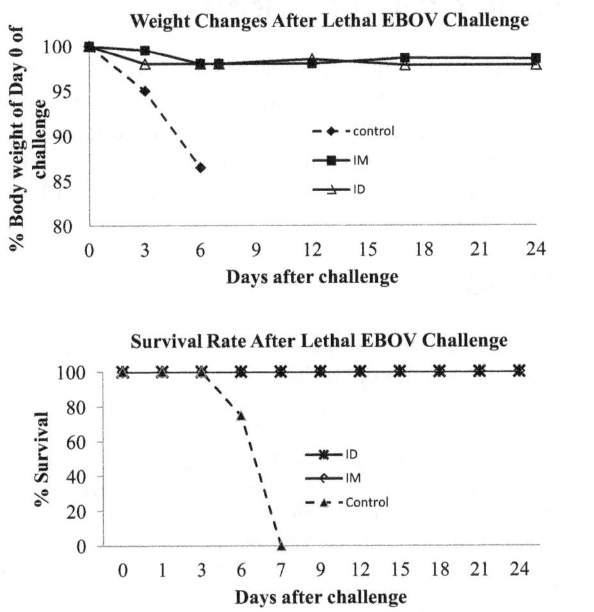

FIGURE 6 | Guinea pigs immunized by EBOV VLPs are protected against a high dose lethal challenge. As outlined in **Figure 1**, guinea pigs were challenged by i.p. injection of 1000 pfu guinea pig-adapted EBOV at 22 weeks after the third immunization. Guinea pigs were monitored daily and weighed on indicated days post-challenge for recording of weight changes after challenge, and animals that exhibit substantial weight loss and signs of severe disease were sacrificed in accordance with IACUC guidelines.

superior to the conventional IM immunization approach for inducing antibody responses to confer long lasting protection against influenza virus infection in mice (Koutsonanos et al., 2012). We have in recent studies shown that ID delivery of adjuvanted EBOV GP or sGP protein subunit vaccines by microneedles was able to induce strong antibody responses against EBOV GP similarly to IM immunizations, and provided complete protection against lethal challenge in mice (Liu et al., 2018a,b). Our results from this study demonstrated that ID injection of EBOV VLPs is as effective as IM injection for eliciting immune responses in guinea pigs that are protective against lethal EBOV challenge. Further, by analyzing antibody responses after immunizations, we found that while similar levels of IgG2 antibodies against GP were induced by both IM and ID injections, ID immunization of EBOV VLPs induced significantly higher levels of IgG1 antibodies against GP than IM immunization. Moreover, our results from blocking ELISA studies show that the IgG1 antibodies induced by ID injection recognize different epitopes from the IgG2 antibodies induced by IM injection. These findings indicate that antigens delivered to dermal sites may be processed differently by local antigen presenting cells that leads to more comprehensive presentation of different epitopes for induction of immune responses. Future studies to determine the targets in GP recognized by IgG1 antibodies induced by ID immunization will reveal whether such antibodies may contribute to the control of virus infection either directly or in synergy with IgG2 antibodies and provide more effective protection against EBOV infection.

In contrast to antibody responses against GP, we found that the immunization by IM or ID injection of EBOV VLPs induced similar levels of both IgG1 and IgG2 antibodies against VP40, the EBOV matrix protein that directs the formation of VLPs. Further, the levels of IgG1 and IgG2 antibody subclasses against VP40 are also similar in animals vaccinated by EBOV VLPs through either IM or ID injection, whereas antibodies against GP are predominantly of the IgG2 subclass regardless of the immunization routes. These results indicate that induction of enhanced IgG1 antibody responses by ID immunization of EBOV VLPs is specific for the GP antigen but not the VP40 antigen, even when these antigens are delivered in the same VLP vaccine complex. The functional properties of guinea pig IgG1 and IgG2 antibodies are still poorly understood. However, in an early study, it was found that the IgG2 antibodies activate complement through the classical pathway whereas the IgG1 antibodies activate complement through the alternative pathway (Togashi and Tozawa, 1982). In this respect, it seems that guinea IgG1 and IgG2 antibodies resemble more closely to mouse IgG1 or IgG2a antibodies respectively (Lucisano Valim and Lachmann, 1991; Seino et al., 1993). As such, by comparing the IgG1/IgG2 antibody ratios induced by EBOV VLPs in guinea pigs in this study, it seems that the antibody response against GP is biased toward to the Th1 type whereas the antibody response against VP40 would suggest a balanced Th1/Th2 type. These results indicate that the Th1/Th2 paradigm as demonstrated by IgG1 and IgG2 antibody ratios after vaccination may be antigen specific, underscoring the need of more comprehensive analyses for understanding the mechanism as well as correlates of vaccine-induced immune response against virus infection.

CONCLUSION

We show in this study that the EBOV VLPs produced by the recombinant baculoviruses from insect cells are able to provide effective protection against lethal challenge in the guinea pig model by both IM and ID immunizations. In comparison to IM immunization, ID immunization of EBOV VLPs was able to elicit enhanced IgG1 antibodies against epitopes in EBOV GP that were not recognized by the IgG2 antibodies induced by IM immunization. However, additional studies are needed to understand the underlying mechanism for this observation and to identify the targets recognized by the IgG1 antibodies induced by ID immunizations. Moreover, studies to determine the targets of the antibodies of different IgG subclasses induced by vaccination through different routes will further advance our understanding of the protection against EBOV infection by vaccine-induced immune responses. It will also be of interest to determine the effect of different adjuvant on the epitope breadth as well as subclass switching of antibody responses induced by ID immunizations in comparison with the conventional IM immunization approach. In particular, it will be of interest to determine if the use of an adjuvant will enhance or suppress induction of antibody responses to the subdominant epitopes in a vaccine antigen, and if subclass switching for dominant and subdominant epitopes will be similarly or differently affected by the use of an adjuvant. Moreover, optimization of EBOV VLPs or other subunit vaccines by ID immunization using novel microneedle vaccine delivery technologies will further reveal the potential of this vaccination approach for protection against infection by EBOV as well as other viral pathogens.

ETHICS STATEMENT

The animal study was reviewed and approved by the Institutional Animal Care and Usage Committee (IACUC) of Emory University and the Institutional Animal Care and Usage Committee (IACUC) of TxBiomed Research Institute.

AUTHOR CONTRIBUTIONS

YL, LY, and ZW conducted production and characterization of EBOV VLP vaccines, immunization studies, and analyses of immune responses. RC, JN, HS, AT, and JP conducted EBOV challenge studies. LY, RWC, and CY contributed to experimental design and data analysis. YL, LY, and CY contributed to manuscript preparation.

FUNDING

This study was supported by Public Service Grant AI093406 from the National Institutes of Health.

REFERENCES

Allela, L., Boury, O., Pouillot, R., Delicat, A., Yaba, P., Kumulungui, B., et al. (2005). Ebola virus antibody prevalence in dogs and human risk. *Emerg. Infect. Dis.* 11, 385–390. doi: 10.3201/eid1103.040981

Barrette, R. W., Metwally, S. A., Rowland, J. M., Xu, L., Zaki, S. R., Nichol, S. T., et al. (2009). Discovery of swine as a host for the *Reston ebolavirus*. *Science* 325, 204–206. doi: 10.1126/science.1172705

Blaney, J. E., Marzi, A., Willet, M., Papaneri, A. B., Wirblich, C., Feldmann, F., et al. (2013). Antibody quality and protection from lethal Ebola virus challenge in nonhuman primates immunized with rabies virus based bivalent vaccine. *PLoS Pathog.* 9:e1003389. doi: 10.1371/journal.ppat.1003389

Bos, J. D., and Kapsenberg, M. L. (1993). The skin immune system: progress in cutaneous biology. *Immunol. Today* 14, 75–78. doi: 10.1016/0167-5699(93)90062-p

Bukreyev, A., Rollin, P. E., Tate, M. K., Yang, L., Zaki, S. R., Shieh, W. J., et al. (2007). Successful topical respiratory tract immunization of primates against Ebola virus. *J. Virol.* 81, 6379–6388. doi: 10.1128/jvi.00105-07

Chiu, S. S., Peiris, J. S., Chan, K. H., Wong, W. H., and Lau, Y. L. (2007). Immunogenicity and safety of intradermal influenza immunization at a reduced dose in healthy children. *Pediatrics* 119, 1076–1082. doi: 10.1542/peds.2006-3176

Chowell, G., and Nishiura, H. (2014). Transmission dynamics and control of Ebola virus disease (EVD): a review. *BMC Med.* 12:196. doi: 10.1186/s12916-014-0196-0

Ewer, K., Rampling, T., Venkatraman, N., Bowyer, G., Wright, D., and Lambe, T. (2016). A monovalent chimpanzee adenovirus Ebola vaccine boosted with MVA. *N. Engl. J. Med.* 374, 1635–1646. doi: 10.1056/NEJMoa1411627

Feldmann, H., and Geisbert, T. W. (2011). Ebola haemorrhagic fever. *Lancet* 377, 849–862. doi: 10.1016/S0140-6736(10)60667-8

Flacher, V., Bouschbacher, M., Verronese, E., Massacrier, C., Sisirak, V., Berthier-Vergnes, O., et al. (2006). Human Langerhans cells express a specific TLR profile and differentially respond to viruses and Gram-positive bacteria. *J. Immunol.* 177, 7959–7967. doi: 10.4049/jimmunol.177.11.7959

Gill, H. S., Kang, S. M., Quan, F. S., and Compans, R. W. (2014). Cutaneous immunization: an evolving paradigm in influenza vaccines. *Expert Opin. Drug Deliv.* 11, 615–627. doi: 10.1517/17425247.2014.885947

Groseth, A., Feldmann, H., and Strong, J. E. (2007). The ecology of Ebola virus. *Trends Microbiol.* 15, 408–416.

Henao-Restrepo, A. M., Longini, I. M., Egger, M., Dean, N. E., Edmunds, W. J., Camacho, A., et al. (2015). Efficacy and effectiveness of an rVSV-vectored vaccine expressing Ebola surface glycoprotein: interim results from the Guinea ring vaccination cluster-randomised trial. *Lancet* 386, 857–866. doi: 10.1016/S0140-6736(15)61117-5

Herbert, A. S., Kuehne, A. I., Barth, J. F., Ortiz, R. A., Nichols, D. K., Zak, S. E., et al. (2013). Venezuelan equine encephalitis virus replicon particle vaccine protects nonhuman primates from intramuscular and aerosol challenge with *Ebolavirus*. *J. Virol.* 87, 4952–4964. doi: 10.1128/JVI.03361-12

Holland, D., Booy, R., De Looze, F., Eizenberg, P., McDonald, J., Karrasch, J., et al. (2008). Intradermal influenza vaccine administered using a new microinjection system produces superior immunogenicity in elderly adults: a randomized controlled trial. *J. Infect. Dis.* 198, 650–658. doi: 10.1086/590434

Jones, S. M., Feldmann, H., Stroher, U., Geisbert, J. B., Fernando, L., Grolla, A., et al. (2005). Live attenuated recombinant vaccine protects nonhuman primates against Ebola and Marburg viruses. *Nat. Med.* 11, 786–790. doi: 10.1038/nm1258

Kenney, R. T., Frech, S. A., Muenz, L. R., Villar, C. P., and Glenn, G. M. (2004). Dose sparing with intradermal injection of influenza vaccine. *N. Engl. J. Med.* 351, 2295–2301. doi: 10.1056/nejmoa043540

Koutsonanos, D. G., Vassilieva, E. V., Stavropoulou, A., Zarnitsyn, V. G., Esser, E. S., Taherbhai, M. T., et al. (2012). Delivery of subunit influenza vaccine to skin with microneedles improves immunogenicity and long-lived protection. *Sci. Rep.* 2:357. doi: 10.1038/srep00357

Laurent, P. E., Bonnet, S., Alchas, P., Regolini, P., Mikszta, J. A., Pettis, R., et al. (2007). Evaluation of the clinical performance of a new intradermal vaccine administration technique and associated delivery system. *Vaccine* 25, 8833–8842. doi: 10.1016/j.vaccine.2007.10.020

Leroy, E. M., Kumulungui, B., Pourrut, X., Rouquet, P., Hassanin, A., Yaba, P., et al. (2005). Fruit bats as reservoirs of Ebola virus. *Nature* 438, 575–576. doi: 10.1038/438575a

Li, H., Ying, T., Yu, F., Lu, L., and Jiang, S. (2015). Development of therapeutics for treatment of Ebola virus infection. *Microbes Infect.* 17, 109–117. doi: 10.1016/j.micinf.2014.11.012

Li, W., Ye, L., Carrion, R. Jr., Mohan, G. S., Nunneley, J., Staples, H., et al. (2015). Characterization of immune responses induced by Ebola virus glycoprotein (GP) and truncated GP isoform DNA vaccines and protection against lethal Ebola virus challenge in mice. *J. Infect. Dis.* 212(Suppl. 2), S398–S403. doi: 10.1093/infdis/jiv186

Liu, Y., Ye, L., Lin, F., Gomaa, Y., Flyer, D., and Carrion, R. (2018a). Intradermal immunization by Ebola virus GP subunit vaccines using microneedle patches protects mice against lethal EBOV challenge. *Sci. Rep* 8:11193. doi: 10.1038/s41598-018-29135-w

Liu, Y., Ye, L., Lin, F., Gomaa, Y., Flyer, D., and Carrion, R. (2018b). Intradermal vaccination with adjuvanted Ebola virus soluble glycoprotein subunit vaccine by microneedle patches protects mice against lethal Ebola virus challenge. *J. Infect. Dis* 218, S545–S552. doi: 10.1093/infdis/jiy267

Lucisano Valim, Y. M., and Lachmann, P. J. (1991). The effect of antibody isotype and antigenic epitope density on the complement-fixing activity of immune complexes: a systematic study using chimaeric anti-NIP antibodies with human Fc regions. *Clin. Exp. Immunol.* 84, 1–8. doi: 10.1111/j.1365-2249.1991.tb08115.x

Marzi, A., and Feldmann, H. (2014). Ebola virus vaccines: an overview of current approaches. *Expert Rev. Vaccines* 13, 521–531. doi: 10.1586/14760584.2014.885841

Marzi, A., Halfmann, P., Hill-Batorski, L., Feldmann, F., Shupert, W. L., Neumann, G., et al. (2015). Vaccines. An Ebola whole-virus vaccine is protective in nonhuman primates. *Science* 348, 439–442. doi: 10.1126/science.aaa4919

Mohan, G. S., Li, W., Ye, L., Compans, R. W., and Yang, C. (2012). Antigenic subversion: a novel mechanism of host immune evasion by Ebola virus. *PLoS Pathog.* 8:e1003065. doi: 10.1371/journal.ppat.1003065

Mohan, G. S., Ye, L., Li, W., Monteiro, A., Lin, X., Sapkota, B., et al. (2015). Less is more: Ebola virus surface glycoprotein expression levels regulate virus production and infectivity. *J. Virol.* 89, 1205–1217. doi: 10.1128/JVI.01810-14

Reed, D. S., Lackemeyer, M. G., Garza, N. L., Sullivan, L. J., and Nichols, D. K. (2011). Aerosol exposure to *Zaire ebolavirus* in three nonhuman primate species: differences in disease course and clinical pathology. *Microbes Infect.* 13, 930–936. doi: 10.1016/j.micinf.2011.05.002

Regules, J. A., Beigel, J. H., Paolino, K. M., Voell, J., Castellano, A. R., Hu, Z., et al. (2017). A recombinant vesicular stomatitis virus Ebola vaccine. *N. Engl. J. Med.* 376, 330–341. doi: 10.1056/NEJMoa1414216

Rendtorff, R. C., Walker, L. C., Rowland, M. E., and Packer, H. (1959). Intradermal immunization against Asian influenza in children. *J. Am. Med. Assoc.* 170, 524–528.

Seino, J., Eveleigh, P., Warnaar, S., van Haarlem, L. J., van Es, L. A., and Daha, M. R. (1993). Activation of human complement by mouse and mouse/human chimeric monoclonal antibodies. *Clin. Exp. Immunol.* 94, 291–296. doi: 10.1111/j.1365-2249.1993.tb03446.x

Sullivan, N. J., Geisbert, T. W., Geisbert, J. B., Shedlock, D. J., Xu, L., Lamoreaux, L., et al. (2006). Immune protection of nonhuman primates against Ebola virus with single low-dose adenovirus vectors encoding modified GPs. *PLoS Med.* 3:e177. doi: 10.1371/journal.pmed.0030177

Sun, Y., Carrion, R. Jr., Ye, L., Wen, Z., Ro, Y. T., and Brasky, K. (2009). Protection against lethal challenge by Ebola virus-like particles produced in insect cells. *Virology* 383, 12–21. doi: 10.1016/j.virol.2008.09.020

Swenson, D. L., Wang, D., Luo, M., Warfield, K. L., Woraratanadharm, J., Holman, D. H., et al. (2008). Vaccine to confer to nonhuman primates complete protection against multistrain Ebola and Marburg virus infections. *Clin. Vaccine Immunol.* 15, 460–467. doi: 10.1128/CVI.00431-07

Togashi, H., and Tozawa, H. (1982). Neutralization of sendai virus by the IgG subclass antibodies of the guinea pig. *Microbiol. Immunol.* 26, 821–829. doi: 10.1111/j.1348-0421.1982.tb00228.x

Towner, J. S., Sealy, T. K., Khristova, M. L., Albarino, C. G., Conlan, S., Reeder, S. A., et al. (2008). Newly discovered Ebola virus associated with hemorrhagic fever outbreak in Uganda. *PLoS Pathog.* 4:e1000212. doi: 10.1371/journal.ppat.1000212

Warfield, K. L., and Aman, M. J. (2011). Advances in virus-like particle vaccines for filoviruses. *J. Infect. Dis.* 204(Suppl. 3), S1053–S1059. doi: 10.1093/infdis/jir346

Warfield, K. L., Swenson, D. L., Olinger, G. G., Kalina, W. V., Aman, M. J., and Bavari, S. (2007). Ebola virus-like particle-based vaccine protects nonhuman primates against lethal Ebola virus challenge. *J. Infect. Dis.* 196(Suppl. 2), S430–S437.

Wei, X., Decker, J. M., Wang, S., Hui, H., Kappes, J. C., Wu, X., et al. (2003). Antibody neutralization and escape by HIV-1. *Nature* 422, 307–312.

Weingartl, H. M., Embury-Hyatt, C., Nfon, C., Leung, A., Smith, G., and Kobinger, G. (2012). Transmission of Ebola virus from pigs to non-human primates. *Sci. Rep.* 2:811. doi: 10.1038/srep00811

Yang, C., Ye, L., and Compans, R. W. (2008). Protection against filovirus infection: virus-like particle vaccines. *Expert Rev. Vaccines* 7, 333–344. doi: 10.1586/14760584.7.3.333

Ye, L., Lin, J., Sun, Y., Bennouna, S., Lo, M., Wu, Q., et al. (2006). Ebola virus-like particles produced in insect cells exhibit dendritic cell stimulating activity and induce neutralizing antibodies. *Virology* 351, 260–270. doi: 10.1016/j.virol.2006.03.021

Ye, L., and Yang, C. (2015). Development of vaccines for prevention of Ebola virus infection. *Microbes Infect.* 17, 98–108. doi: 10.1016/j.micinf.2014.12.004

15

Discovery of Retro-1 Analogs Exhibiting Enhanced Anti-Vaccinia Virus Activity

Lalita Priyamvada[1], Philip Alabi[2], Andres Leon[2], Amrita Kumar[3], Suryaprakash Sambhara[3], Victoria A. Olson[1], Jason K. Sello[2] and Panayampalli S. Satheshkumar[1]**

[1] Poxvirus and Rabies Branch, Centers for Disease Control and Prevention, Atlanta, GA, United States, [2] Department of Chemistry, Brown University, Providence, RI, United States, [3] Immunology and Pathogenesis Branch, Influenza Division, Centers for Disease Control and Prevention, Atlanta, GA, United States

***Correspondence:**
Jason K. Sello
Jason_sello@brown.edu
Panayampalli S. Satheshkumar
xdv3@cdc.gov

Orthopoxviruses (OPXVs) are an increasing threat to human health due to the growing population of OPXV-naive individuals after the discontinuation of routine smallpox vaccination. Antiviral drugs that are effective as postexposure treatments against variola virus (the causative agent of smallpox) or other OPXVs are critical in the event of an OPXV outbreak or exposure. The only US Food and Drug Administration-approved drug to treat smallpox, Tecovirimat (ST-246), exerts its antiviral effect by inhibiting extracellular virus (EV) formation, thereby preventing cell–cell and long-distance spread. We and others have previously demonstrated that host Golgi-associated retrograde proteins play an important role in monkeypox virus (MPXV) and vaccinia virus (VACV) EV formation. Inhibition of the retrograde pathway by small molecules such as Retro-2 has been shown to decrease VACV infection *in vitro* and to a lesser extent *in vivo*. To identify more potent inhibitors of the retrograde pathway, we screened a large panel of compounds containing a benzodiazepine scaffold like that of Retro-1, against VACV infection. We found that a subset of these compounds displayed better anti-VACV activity, causing a reduction in EV particle formation and viral spread compared to Retro-1. PA104 emerged as the most potent analog, inhibiting 90% viral spread at 1.3 μM with a high selectivity index. In addition, PA104 strongly inhibited two distinct ST-246-resistant viruses, demonstrating its potential benefit for use in combination therapy with ST-246. These data and further characterizations of the specific protein targets and *in vivo* efficacy of PA104 may have important implications for the design of effective antivirals against OPXV.

Keywords: viral inhibitor, poxvirus, antiviral agent, retrograde transport, vaccinia virus, Retro-1, retrograde inhibitor, ST-246

INTRODUCTION

The *Orthopoxvirus* (OPXV) genus contains several human pathogens of public health concern, including variola virus (the causative agent of smallpox), monkeypox virus (MPXV), cowpox virus, and vaccinia virus (VACV, the virus that formulates the smallpox vaccine) (Fenner and Nakano, 1988). While smallpox has been eradicated, other OPXVs continue to pose a threat to human health due to the lack of protective immunity post the cessation of routine smallpox vaccination (Durski et al., 2018). In particular, the incidence of MPXV has been on the rise due to several recent outbreaks in West and Central Africa after a long hiatus in reported epidemics (Durski et al., 2018). There is also a risk of MPXV infections spreading outside the endemic region through travel or the importation of infected animals, as seen in several recent cases (Reed et al., 2004; Vaughan et al., 2018; Angelo et al., 2019; Erez et al., 2019). In addition, the identification of several new OPXVs over the past decade demonstrates the ongoing circulation and maintenance of these viruses in animal reservoirs, and highlights the need for surveillance and development of better diagnostic assays and therapeutics (Hoffmann et al., 2015; Vora et al., 2015; Springer et al., 2017; Lanave et al., 2018).

OPXVs are large double-stranded DNA viruses that have a complex life cycle, replicate in the cytoplasm of infected cells, and generate two distinct virion forms: mature virus (MV) and extracellular virus (EV), differentiated based on the number of membranes surrounding the central DNA core (Condit et al., 2006). Mature viruses consist of a viral core and a single viral membrane and harbor all the necessary proteins required for virus binding and entry. Although infectious, MVs remain inside an infected cell until lysis (Smith et al., 2002). A proportion of MVs undergo double-membrane wrapping to generate wrapped virus (WV), which can stay attached to the infected cell (cell-associated virus) or exit the cell (EV) (Smith et al., 2002; Moss, 2006). Although EV particles constitute only 1–10% of MVs, they are essential for cell-to-cell and long-distance viral spread and therefore play an important role in OPXV pathogenesis (Payne, 1980; Blasco and Moss, 1992; Engelstad and Smith, 1993). VACV mutants that fail to generate EVs produce small plaques *in vitro* and are attenuated *in vivo*, even in severely immunodeficient animal models (Blasco and Moss, 1991; Engelstad and Smith, 1993; Wolffe et al., 1993; Grosenbach et al., 2010).

The importance of EV formation for VACV pathogenesis is further highlighted by the fact that pharmacological intervention is efficacious in suppressing infection. At present, tecovirimat (ST-246) is the only US Food and Drug Administration-approved antiviral available for postexposure treatment against smallpox. ST-246 targets the viral envelope protein F13 required for EV formation, thereby decreasing viral spread and infection-induced pathology (Yang et al., 2005; Grosenbach et al., 2011). However, prolonged treatment of ST-246 can lead to the generation of drug-resistant viruses due to mutations in the F13L gene, as documented in a progressive vaccinia (PV) patient in 2009 (Lederman et al., 2012). A single amino acid mutation in F13L may overcome the therapeutic effect of the drug, reinforcing the need for additional therapeutic candidates that are safe and effective against OPXVs.

In our efforts to develop new therapeutic strategies, we focused on the peculiar dependence of OPXVs on the retrograde transport pathway for EV formation. While several viruses (Simian virus 40, papillomavirus, and influenza) rely on retrograde transport for entry into a cell, OPXVs require retrograde transport for EV membrane wrapping, and consequently viral egress (Spooner et al., 2006; Harrison et al., 2016; Sivan et al., 2016). We and others have previously demonstrated that impeding the retrograde pathway by targeting the Golgi-associated retrograde protein complex can greatly reduce EV yield with minimal impact on MV formation in VACV and MPXV (Harrison et al., 2016; Realegeno et al., 2017). Treatment with small molecule inhibitors of the retrograde pathway such as Retro-1 and Retro-2 significantly decreased EV formation *in vitro* by preventing the trafficking of the viral protein F13, which is required for membrane wrapping (Harrison et al., 2016; Sivan et al., 2016). However, initial characterizations of the antiviral efficacy of Retro-2 *in vivo* yielded underwhelming results, with treated mice showing marginal improvement in signs of clinical disease and comparable lung viral titers compared to untreated mice (Harrison et al., 2016). Additionally, better clinical scores were only observed in animals pretreated with Retro-2, and not in mice treated only postinfection (Harrison et al., 2016). Given the highly selective, potent anti-VACV activities of Retro-1 and Retro-2 *in vitro*, we were interested in structurally optimizing these small molecule inhibitors to identify novel antivirals with greater inhibitory effect compared to the parent compounds *in vitro*, as well as better *in vivo* therapeutic efficacy.

To this end, we screened a diverse collection of greater than 80 compounds sharing a benzodiazepine scaffold like Retro-1 for efficacy in *in vitro* anti-VACV assays. These efforts led to the identification of a potent antiviral we have named PA104. Like Retro-1 and Retro-2, PA104 can potently inhibit EV formation and VACV spread, while minimally impacting MV yield and causing little to no cytotoxicity. We also show that the reduction in viral spread by PA104 is attributable to inhibition of EV formation as evidenced by lack of virus secreted in media and impaired actin tail formation in infected cells. It is particularly noteworthy that PA104 also inhibits viral spread of two distinct ST-246-resistant viruses, establishing its potential for use in postexposure treatment in combination with ST-246. These observations warrant further investigation of PA104 and its efficacy as an antiviral agent.

MATERIALS AND METHODS

Viruses, Cell Lines, and Inhibitors

Vaccinia virus WR-GFP, VACV WR A4-YFP, VACV WR-Luc, and VACV IHDJ stocks were grown in BSC40 cells with Dulbecco modified eagle medium (DMEM) containing 2% fetal bovine serum (FBS). Two ST-246-resistant viruses were used in this study, each containing distinct mutations in the F13L gene: the first (A290V) was isolated from a 2009 human PV case (Lederman et al., 2012) and thereafter passaged in our laboratory, and the second (N267D) was provided by SIGA Technologies (Smith et al., 2011). These two viruses will hereby be referred to as RV1 and RV2, respectively. All viral stocks were titered by plaque assay prior to use in experiments. BSC40 and HeLa cell lines were passaged in DMEM with 10% FBS and 10 units/mL of penicillin and 100 μg/mL of streptomycin (penicillin–streptomycin). For all experiments involving viral infection, DMEM containing 2% FBS, hereby referred to as "DMEM-2," was used as a diluent or culture media.

The novel compounds in this study were synthesized in-house using diversity-oriented synthetic approaches. Our synthetic approach involved two different six- and four-step synthetic schemes that were utilized (based on synthetic limitations: cost, the scope of reactions, readily available starting materials) at different stages of the SAR. The specific retrosynthetic disconnections that were effected to access these molecules are shown below. The exact details of these reaction modules/improvisations and navigations of synthetic constraints will be presented in a subsequent publication. Meanwhile, additional information about the compounds can be made available upon request.

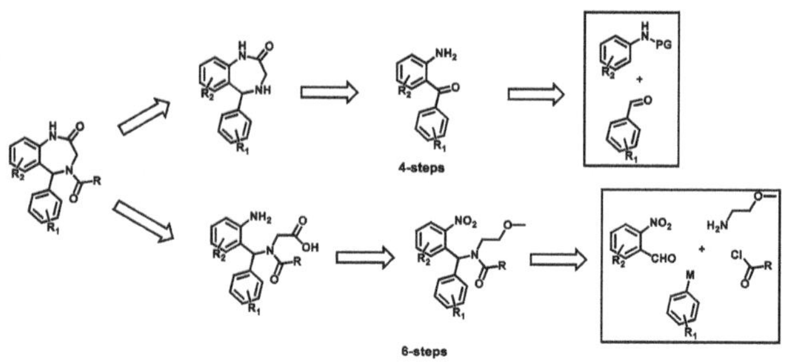

Viral Spread Assay

The viral spread assay was performed as previously described (Cryer et al., 2017). A serial dilution series of retrograde inhibitor compounds was mixed 1:1 (vol/vol) with VACV-WR-GFP virus diluted in DMEM-2 at multiplicity of infection (MOI) 0.3. The mixture was transferred to black 96-well, clear-bottom plates (06-443-2; Corning, NY, United States) containing HeLa cells. Each plate included four to eight wells of the following controls: uninfected cells, no treatment (virus only), and virus + AraC (cytosine arabinoside, 40 μg/mL), and each dilution series was tested in duplicate. The cells were infected with the virus + compound mixture at 37°C for 24 h. Following infection, the cells were washed once with phosphate-buffered saline (PBS) and fixed with 4% paraformaldehyde for 15 min at room temperature (RT). Cells were then washed with PBS and stained with 4',6-diamidino-2-phenylindole (DAPI) for nuclei visualization for 10 min at RT. The plates were imaged using the ArrayScan XTI High Content Screen (HCS) reader, and the percentage of GFP and DAPI positive cells was quantified using the HCS Studio Cell Analysis software as previously described (Johnson et al., 2008). Total viral spread and viral spread for each compound were measured as shown below:

$$Total\ viral\ spread = \%GFP^{+}_{virus\ only} - \%GFP^{+}_{AraC}$$

$$Viral\ spread\ for\ compound = \frac{\%GFP^{+}_{Compound} - \%GFP^{+}_{AraC}}{Total\ viral\ spread}$$

Viral spread data were analyzed using a non-linear regression (curve fit) with the sigmoidal dose-response variable slope equation to determine the concentrations required for 50% inhibition (IC_{50}) and 90% inhibition (IC_{90}) of viral spread relative to the no treatment control. Analyses were performed using GraphPad Prism software (GraphPad Software, v7, San Diego, CA, United States). Values were determined based on two or more replicates from two independent experiments.

Cytotoxicity Assay

The potential cytotoxic effects of the retrograde inhibitor compounds were tested at a range of concentrations spanning 400–0.3 μM. HeLa cells seeded in 96-well plates were infected with a mixture of VACV WR (MOI 0.01) and serially diluted compounds at 37°C for 24 h. Each concentration was tested in duplicate. Supernatants were collected, and the levels of extracellular lactate dehydrogenase (LDH) released in the supernatants were quantified using the LDH Cytotoxicity Assay Kit (88953; Thermo Scientific Pierce, Waltham, MA, United States) as per the manufacturer's instructions. Cytotoxicity data were analyzed using a non-linear regression (curve fit) with the sigmoidal dose–response variable slope equation to determine the concentrations required for 50% LDH signal (CC_{50}) relative to the positive control (lysed cells). This analysis was performed using GraphPad Prism software (GraphPad Software, v7). Values were determined based on two or more replicates from two independent experiments.

Entry Assay

BSC40 cells were infected with VACV WR-Luc virus at MOI 3 for 1 h at RT. After infection, cells were washed three times with PBS to remove unbound virus. Retrograde inhibitor compounds diluted to 2.5 μM in DMEM-2 were added to cells and incubated at 37°C for 2 h. All compounds were tested in duplicate. Reporter lysis buffer was added to the wells to lyse cells, and luciferase activity was measured using the Luciferase Assay System (Promega, Madison, WI, United States) according to manufacturer's instructions. Luciferase activity was measured using an ENSPIRE plate reader (PerkinElmer, Waltham, MA, United States).

MV and EV Quantification

BSC40 cells were infected with VACV IHDJ virus at MOI 3 for 1 h at RT. The infected cells were washed three times with DMEM-2 to remove excess virus, and retrograde inhibitor compounds were then added to the cells at a concentration of 2.5 μM. Each compound was tested in triplicate, and the cells were incubated with the compounds for 24 h at 37°C. Supernatants were collected and frozen down to determine EV yield. To measure MV yield, cells were washed three times with PBS to remove any EV particles, collected using a cell scraper, and freeze-thawed three times to release MV particles. Extracellular virus and MV yield was quantified by titering the supernatants and cells, respectively, by plaque assay. The percent EV formation and EV inhibition were determined as follows:

$$\%EV\ formation = \frac{EV\ yield}{(EV\ yield + MV\ yield)}$$

$$\%EV\ Inhibition\ for\ compound = 100 - \frac{\%EV\ formation_{Compound}}{\%EV\ formation_{Virus\ only}}$$

Statistical significance was measured using a one-way analysis of variance (ANOVA) test. MV end EV yields in the presence of the retrograde inhibitor compounds and ST-246 were compared to the virus only control using *post hoc* Sidak multiple-comparisons test.

Effect on ST-246-Resistant Viruses

BSC40 cells seeded in 12-well plates were infected with approximately 100 plaque forming units (pfu) of VACV WR, RV1, or RV2 for 1 h at 37°C. The virus was removed and compounds PA24, PA63, and PA104 were added to the cells at a concentration of 10 μM, and ST-246 at 2 μM diluted in DMEM containing 2% carboxymethylcellulose. After a 72-h incubation with the inhibitors at 37°C, the cells were stained with crystal violet (CV) containing 4% paraformaldehyde for 15 min at RT. Post-CV staining, the plates were washed with water and imaged.

Confocal Imaging

BSC40 cells were seeded in 24-well glass- bottom tissue culture plates (MatTek Corporation, Ashland, MA, United States) and infected with VACV WR A4-YFP (MOI 1) for 1 h at 37°C. The virus was removed, and compounds PA24, PA63, and PA104 were added to the cells at a concentration of 10 μM. After a 24-h incubation with the inhibitors at 37°C, cells were washed with PBS and fixed with 4% paraformaldehyde for 15 min at RT. Cells were stained with Alexa Flour 594 Phalloidin (ThermoFisher, Waltham, MA, United States) for actin visualization and with DAPI for nuclei visualization. After staining, cells were mounted with Prolong Gold Antifade Mounting media (Molecular Probes, Eugene, OR, United States) and imaged using the LSM 710 inverted confocal microscope (Zeiss, Oberkochen, Germany). Virus-loaded actin tails in infected cells were counted for each condition (number of cells counted per condition ranging between 5 and 9) and compared for statistical significance using a one-way ANOVA test.

Isolation of ST246-Resistant Virus From PV Case

BSC40 cells were infected with serially diluted culture material isolated from a 2009 PV patient (Lederman et al., 2012) in the presence or absence of ST-246. Plaques observed in the presence of ST-246 were picked and reconstituted in DMEM-2. Plaque purification was performed by serially passaging single plaques grown in the presence of ST-246 four times. The isolated virus was grown in a six-well plate of BSC40 cells to create an RV1 viral

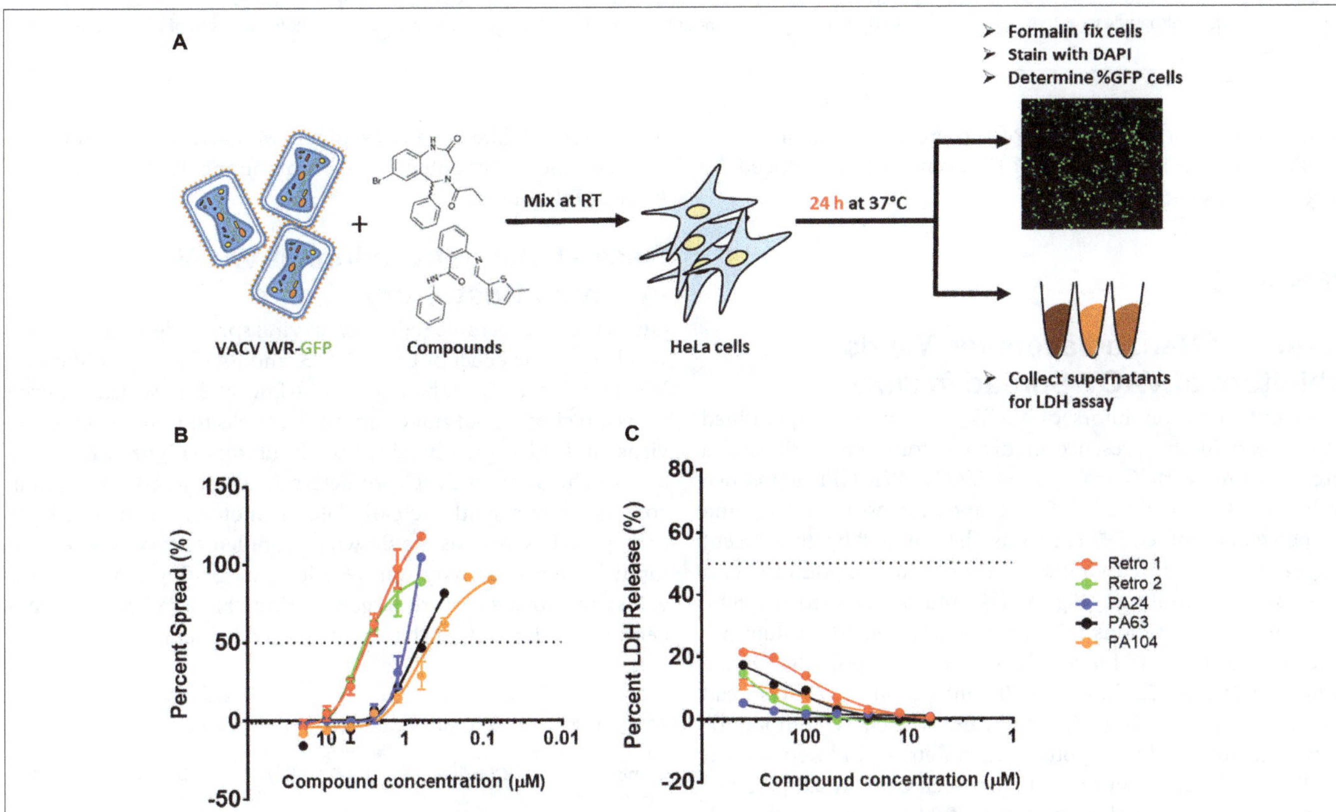

FIGURE 1 | Structural analogs of Retro-1 can inhibit VACV spread with minimal cytotoxicity. **(A)** Schematic representation of steps used to determine viral spread and cellular toxicity in the presence of Retro-1 analogs. The virus spread and cytotoxicity assays were performed twice for each compound, in duplicate. **(B)** Representative graph showing percent viral spread in the presence of a serial dilution series of five retrograde inhibitors. Values plotted represent the average of two independent experiments. **(C)** Representative graph showing percent LDH release in the presence of a serial dilution series of five retrograde inhibitors. Values plotted represent the average ± SEM from two independent experiments.

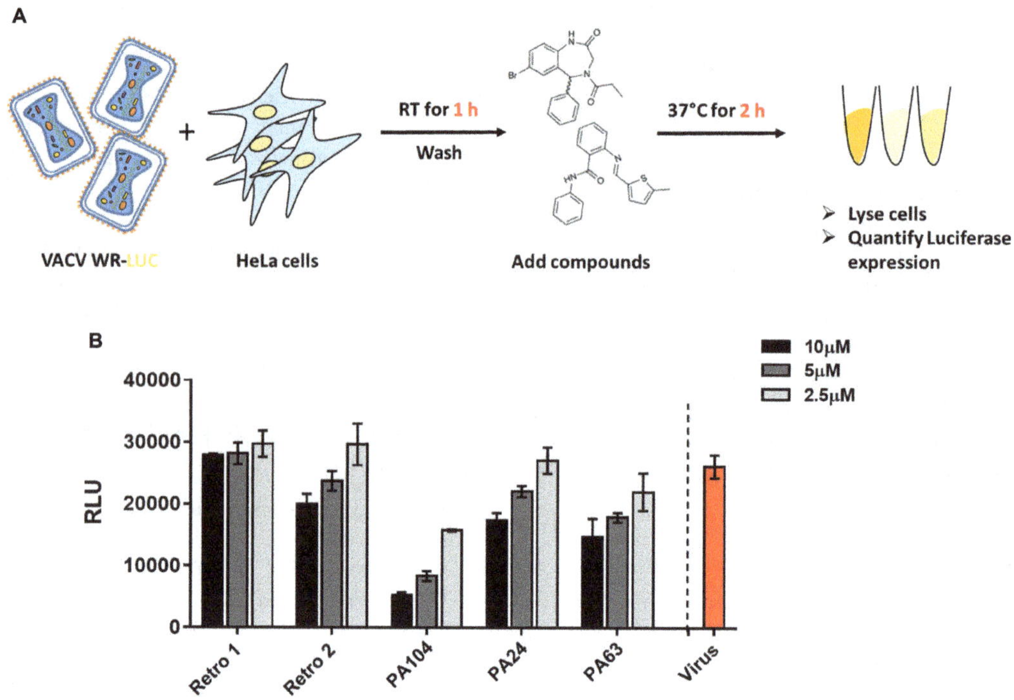

FIGURE 2 | Effect of Retro-1 analogs on early stages of VACV infection. **(A)** Schematic representation of VACV entry assay. **(B)** Relative light units (RLUs) in the presence of select retrograde inhibitors diluted to 2.5 μM (light gray), 5 μM (dark gray), and 10 μM (black). Values plotted represent the average of two independent experiments.

stock. To confirm the presence of the previously characterized A290V mutation in RV1, the F13L gene was sequenced by Sanger sequencing.

RESULTS

Screen of Benzodiazepines Yields Inhibitors of VACV Spread *in vitro*

To identify new inhibitors of VACV infection, we quantified viral spread in the presence of diverse compounds sharing a core structure with Retro-1 using VACV WR-GFP as shown in **Figure 1A**. A total of 83 compounds were tested, and the percentage of GFP^+ cells was determined by fluorescent imaging. We measured viral spread for each compound over a range of concentrations (**Figure 1B**) and determined the 50% inhibitory concentrations (IC_{50}) for all and the 90% inhibitory concentrations (IC_{90}) for a subset of the compounds. Of the compounds tested, 52 showed > 50% inhibition of VACV spread at concentrations ≤ 10 μM. Within this subset, 17 compounds showed greater inhibitory potency than Retro-1 and Retro-2 and had IC_{50} and IC_{90} values ranging between 0.5 and 2.0 μM and between 1.3 and 5.2 μM, respectively (**Table 1**, data not shown). In addition to examining their effect on viral spread, we also assessed the cellular cytotoxicity of a subset of compounds by measuring cell-released LDH levels (**Figure 1C**). We observed that a majority of potently inhibitory compounds exhibited low cytotoxicity even at 400 μM. Based on the viral spread screen of the Retro-1 like benzodiazepines, we narrowed our focus to three of the most potent VACV inhibitors: PA24, PA63, and PA104 (**Table 1**).

Retro-1 Derivatives Inhibit VACV Infection Post-entry

Given the considerable reduction in viral spread described earlier, we checked the effect of PA24, PA63, and PA104 on VACV entry. We infected cells with VACV WR-Luc at RT, which allowed virus attachment but not entry, washed cells to remove unbound virus, and subsequently added the inhibitors (**Figure 2A**). After a 2-h incubation at 37°C, we determined luciferase expression, controlled by a synthetic early/late promoter, as a surrogate for early protein synthesis. As shown in **Supplementary Figure S1A**, input luciferase activity was very low, suggesting that the RLU values in our assay were largely attributable to viral entry and gene expression, rather than prepackaged luciferase.

TABLE 1 | Inhibitory and cytotoxic activities of select compounds.

Compound	IC50 (μM)	IC90 (μM)	CC50 (μM)	SI
ST-246	0.04	0.1	>400	>10000
Retro 1	3.0	7.2	>400	>135
Retro 2	2.2	5.5	>400	>194
PA104	0.5	1.3	>400	>800
PA63	0.7	1.7	>400	>570
PA24	1.0	1.8	>400	>400

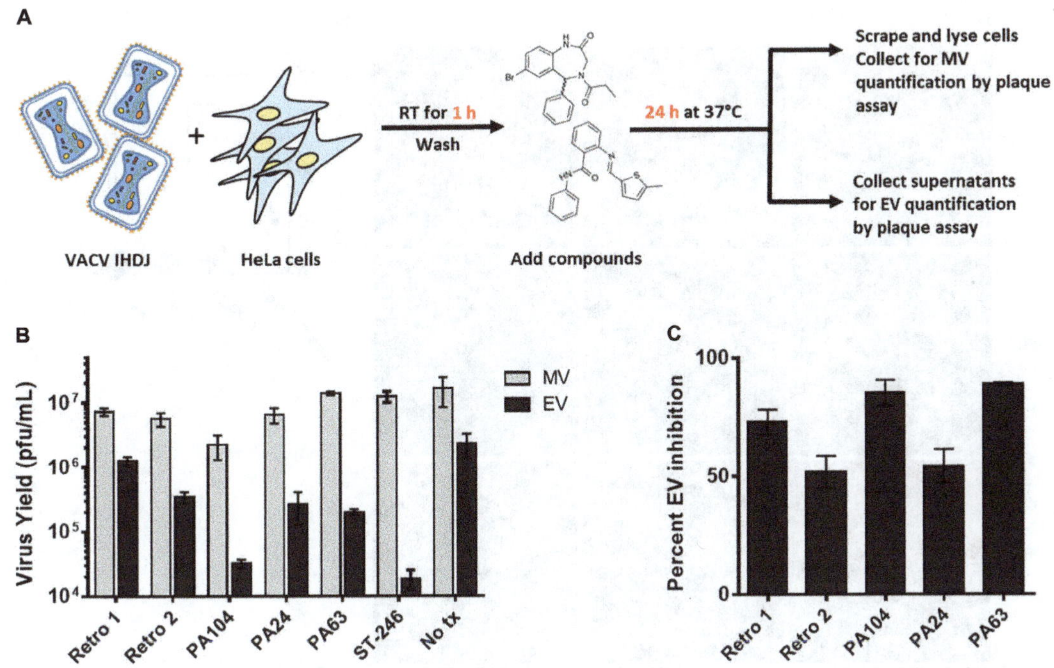

	Retro 1	Retro 2	PA104	PA24	PA63	ST-246
MV	ns	ns	ns	ns	ns	ns
EV	ns	*	**	**	**	**

FIGURE 3 | Reduced EV formation in the presence of Retro-1 analogs. **(A)** Schematic representation of assay used to determine MV and EV yield in the presence of Retro-2 and Retro-1 analogs. **(B)** Mature virus (light gray) and EV (black) yield (pfu/mL) in the presence of 2.5 μM retrograde inhibitors. Values represent the average of three replicates. The results of one-way analysis of variance and *post hoc* Sidak multiple-comparisons test comparing the three replicates ($n = 3$) of each compound to no treatment control are tabulated below graph: ns = not significant, $^{*}p \leq 0.05$ and $^{**}p \leq 0.005$. **(C)** Percent inhibition of EV formation in the presence of 2.5 μM retrograde inhibitors. Values calculated based upon yield data shown in **(B)**. Values in both **(B)** and **(C)** represent average ± SEM.

We observed that PA24 and PA63 did not markedly decrease viral entry at the lower concentrations tested, corroborating the findings of a previous study that tested Retro-1 and Retro-2 (Sivan et al., 2016) (**Figure 2B**). While a higher concentration (10 μM) of PA24 and PA63 reduced viral entry, for PA104 a decrease in viral entry was observed at all three concentrations tested (**Figure 2B**). To exclude the possibility that these compounds affect the enzymatic activity of luciferase, we added different concentrations of PA104 to lysed VACV WR-Luc-infected cells just before the addition of the substrate. We found no difference in luciferase activity between the treatment groups (**Supplementary Figure S1B**). Together, these data demonstrate that potent retrograde inhibitors may inhibit virus entry at high concentrations.

Reduced EV Yield in the Presence of Retro-1 Derivatives

Previous studies have shown that Retro-1 and Retro-2 can inhibit the retrograde pathway and cause a reduction in EV particle formation during VACV and MPXV infection (Harrison et al., 2016; Sivan et al., 2016). To confirm that the decrease in viral spread observed earlier was attributable to a reduction in EV but not MV particle production, we infected cells with VACV IHDJ, a VACV strain that produces a relatively higher proportion of EV particles (**Figure 3A**). We observed that at 2.5 μM all three compounds significantly decreased EV yield compared to control (**Figure 3B**). While none of the three compounds significantly affected MV formation, a small reduction in MV yield was observed in case of PA104 (**Figure 3B**). We hypothesize that this reduction in MV production could be due to effects on viral entry (**Figure 2B**). The reduction in EV yield among the compounds tested ranged between 54 and 89% (**Figure 3C**).

PA104 Strongly Suppresses Actin Tail Formation in VACV-Infected Cells

The double-membrane wrapping of MVs and subsequent formation of EVs in an infected cell triggers the polymerization of actin. This results in the formation of actin tails that can propel the EV particles to neighboring cells, causing cell-to-cell spread (Smith et al., 2002). Since we had observed a decrease

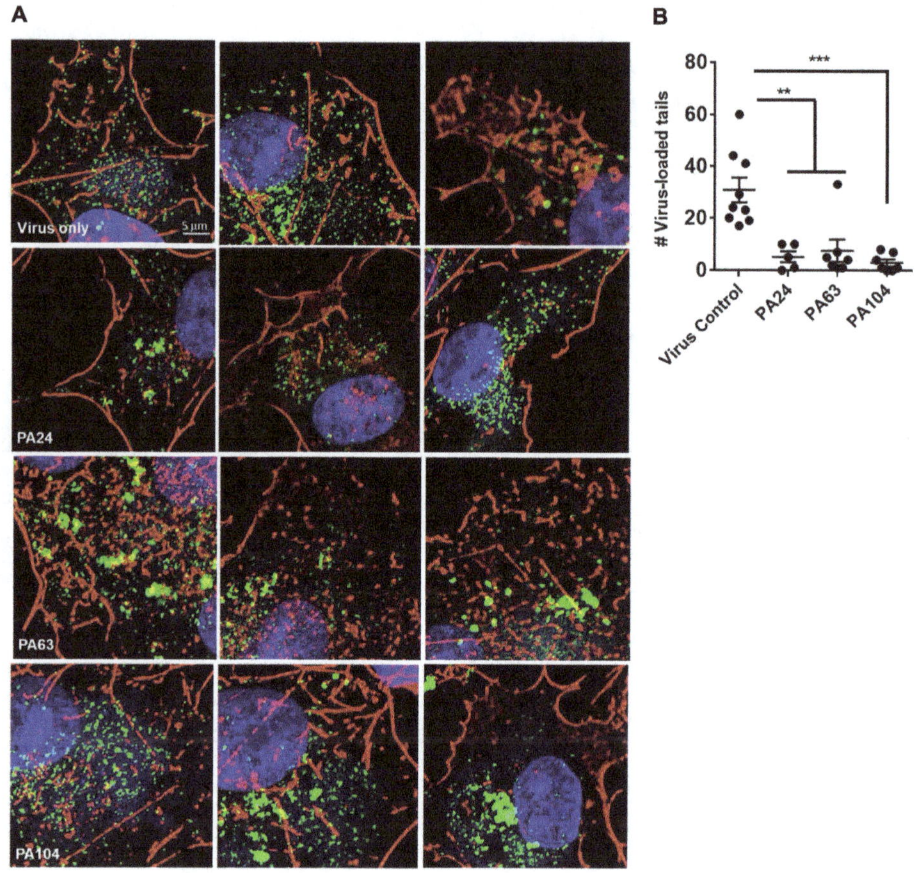

FIGURE 4 | Inhibition of EV formation visualized by actin staining. **(A)** Confocal microscopy images of cells infected with VACV WR A4-YFP virus in the presence or absence of Retro-1 analogs PA63, PA24, and PA104. Few to no virus-loaded actin tails observed in the presence of Retro-1 analogs in comparison to virus-only treatment. Nuclei, actin, and VACV are stained blue, red, and green, respectively. Scale bars represent 5 µm. **(B)** Average number of virus-loaded actin tails per cell for each treatment. For each condition, virus-loaded actin tails from five to nine cells were counted (virus control: 9, PA24: 5, PA63: 9, and PA104: 7). Each dot represents one cell, and the average ± SEM for all four conditions are shown. Results of one-way analysis of variance and *post hoc* Tukey multiple-comparisons test comparing the four treatments are described: $^{**}p \leq 0.005$ and $^{***}p \leq 0.0005$.

in both viral spread and EV yield in the presence of Retro-1 analogs, we were interested in testing the effect of these compounds on the appearance of virus-loaded actin tails within cells. To this end, we infected cells with VACV in the presence or absence of PA24, PA63, and PA104 and visualized actin-associated virus particles using confocal microscopy. In the absence of the Retro-1 inhibitors, infected cells had several actin tails loaded with VACV at the tips (the viral particles appear as green dots due to the fusion of GFP with the core protein A4), which is characteristic of VACV infection (**Figure 4** and **Supplementary Figure S2**). On the other hand, in all three inhibitor conditions, actin aggregates appeared shorter and did not resemble the clearly defined tails observed in the untreated control (**Figure 4A**). We enumerated the virus-loaded actin tails for each condition and found a significant decrease in virus-loaded tails in the presence of PA24, PA63, and PA104 (**Figure 4B**). In case of PA104, the reduction in actin tail staining was the most significant compared to the virus control. These data corroborate the results shown in **Figures 3B,C**, demonstrating that fewer virus-loaded actin tails appear in the presence of retrograde inhibitors, which results in a lower EV yield overall.

PA104 Potently Inhibits the Spread of ST-246-Resistant Viruses

ST-246, targets F13, a peripheral viral membrane protein, interfering with its intracellular localization (Yang et al., 2005). However, mutations in F13L gene can cause viral resistance to ST-246 as demonstrated previously (Yang et al., 2005; Lederman et al., 2012; Duraffour et al., 2015). To investigate whether the potent anti-VACV compounds identified in this study could inhibit ST-246–resistant virus, we infected cells with two different ST-246-resistant viruses in the presence of 10 µM PA104, PA24, and PA63. The two viruses used contained distinct resistance-conferring mutations; the first, hereby referred to as RV1, was isolated from the lesions of a PV patient by serial plaque purification in the presence of ST-246 (Lederman et al., 2012). We sequenced the F13L gene of our isolated RV1 and found the previously reported resistance mutation A290V (**Figure 5A**).

A

```
ACAM    MWPFASVPAGAKCRLVETLPENMDFRSDHLTTFECFNEIITLAKKYIYIASFCCNPLSTT 60
RV1     ------------------------------------------------------------ 60
RV2     ------------------------------------------------------------ 60
        ************************************************************

ACAM    RGALIFDKLKEASEKGIKIIVLLDERGKRNLGELQSHCPDINFITVNIDKKNNVGLLLGC 120
RV1     ------------------------------------------------------------ 120
RV2     ------------------------------------------------------------ 120
        ************************************************************

ACAM    FWVSDDERCYVGNASFTGGSIHTIKTLGVYSDYPPLATDLRRRFDTFKAFNSAKNSWLNL 180
RV1     ------------------------------------------------------------ 180
RV2     ------------------------------------------------------------ 180
        ************************************************************

ACAM    CSAACCLPVSTAYHIKNPIGGVFFTDSPEHLLGYSRDLDTDVVIDKLRSAKTSIDIEHLA 240
RV1     ------------------------------------------------------------ 240
RV2     ------------------------------------------------------------ 240
        ************************************************************

ACAM    IVPTTRVDGNSYYWPDIYNSIIEAAINRGVKIRLLVGNWDKNDVYSMATARSLDALCVQN 300
RV1     -------------------------------------------------V---------- 300
RV2     --------------------------D--------------------------------- 300
        **************************:**********************.**********

ACAM    DLSVKVFTIQNNTKLLIVDDEYVHITSANFDGTHYQNHGFVSFNSIDKQLVSEAKKIFER 360
RV1     ------------------------------------------------------------ 360
RV2     ------------------------------------------------------------ 360
        ************************************************************

ACAM    DWVSSHSKSLKI    372
RV1     ---------       369
RV2     ------------    369
        *********
```

B

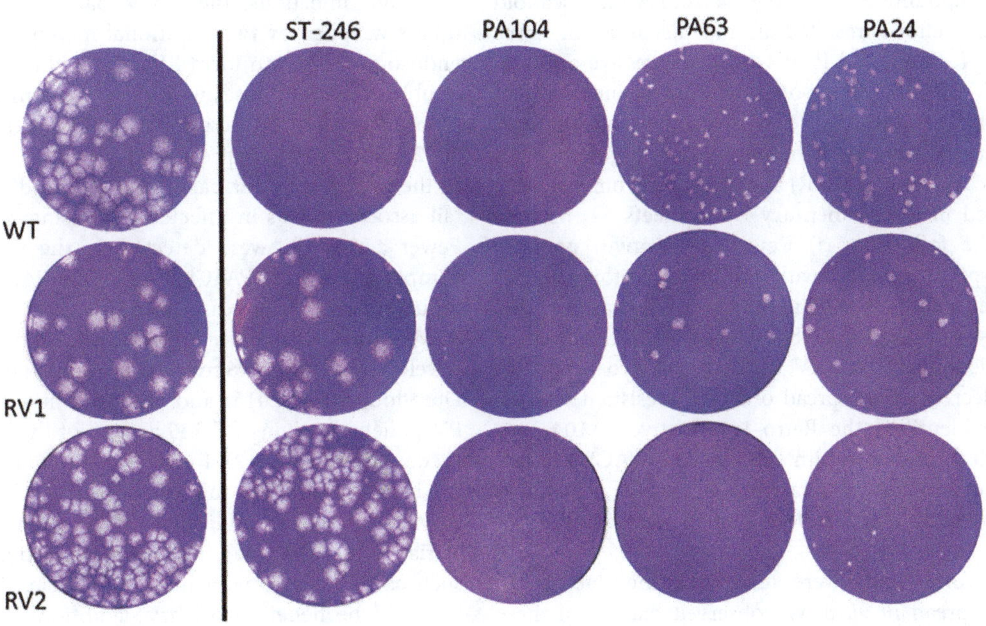

FIGURE 5 | Retro-1 analogs PA104, PA24, and PA63 inhibit viral spread of ST-246-resistant VACV. **(A)** RV1 and RV2 sequence alignments showing preserved A290V and N267D mutations, respectively. Amino acid alignment of F13 of lab-grown RV1 viral isolates and RV2 compared to published ACAM strain (Lederman et al., 2012). **(B)** Plaque assay images showing observable decrease in viral plaque size of RV1 and RV2 virus in the presence of 10 μM PA104, PA24, and PA63.

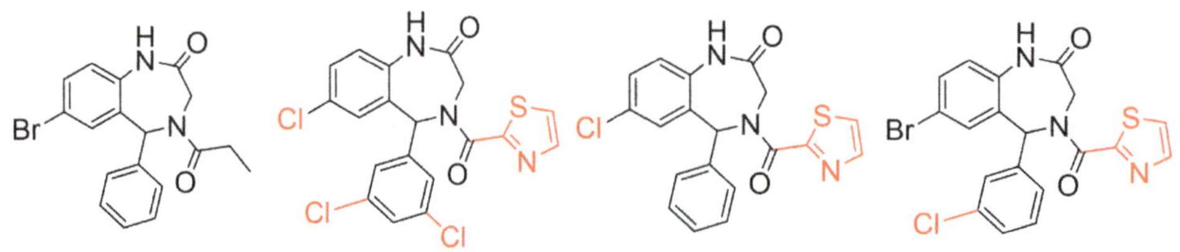

Retro1 PA24 PA63 PA104

FIGURE 6 | Structural modifications in PA104, PA24, and PA63. All modifications made to the original Retro-1 structure shown in red.

The second virus, hereby referred to as RV2, was acquired from SIGA Technologies and contains the N267D resistance mutation (Smith et al., 2011).

While both the ST-246-resistant viruses formed large plaques in the presence or absence of 2 μM ST-246, a concentration of ST-246 over 50-fold higher than its IC50 value, treatment with PA104, PA24, and PA63 caused a considerable reduction in viral plaque size. As shown in **Figure 5B**, all three compounds substantially reduced the size of RV2 plaques. For RV1, on the other hand, PA104 was markedly more effective in reducing viral spread than PA24 and PA63 (**Figure 5B**). Overall, these data show that retrograde inhibitors can block EV formation and spread of ST-246-resistant VACV.

DISCUSSION

In this study, we describe the screening and characterization of a panel of compounds sharing the benzodiazepine scaffold of Retro-1. These efforts resulted in the discovery of three compounds, PA24, PA63, and PA104, with impressive antiviral activity against VACV, the most potent and promising of which is PA104. The structural differences between these analogs and their parent Retro-1 have been highlighted in **Figure 6**, and nuclear magnetic resonance (NMR) and mass spectrometry (MS) data are provided in **Supplementary Data Sheets S1, S2**. We demonstrated the following: (i) Retro-1 derivatives potently inhibit VACV spread *in vitro* with minimal cytotoxicity. (ii) The inhibitory effect was predominantly at a late stage of viral replication. (iii) EV formation is the main target of the analogs, which have little impact on MV yield. (iv) Retro-1 analogs can effectively decrease viral spread of ST-246-resistant viruses. In addition, we identified the Retro-1 derivative PA104 as a promising antiviral candidate with superior anti-VACV efficacy compared to the previously characterized Retro-1 and Retro-2, low cellular toxicity, and potent activity against ST-246-resistant viruses.

In total, 83 compounds were tested for their ability to decrease VACV spread *in vitro*. We observed that 17 of these compounds had comparable or more potent anti-VACV activity than Retro-1 and Retro-2 (IC_{50} and IC_{90} values $\leq$ Retro-1 and Retro-2). We focused on three compounds with high potency and low cytotoxicity, PA24, PA63, and PA104, and subsequently tested their impact on VACV entry and EV/MV yield. The most potent inhibitor of VACV spread, PA104, caused an observable reduction in luciferase activity even at 2.5 μM. In contrast, PA24 and PA63 only appeared to affect entry at higher concentrations. All three compounds tested minimally impacted MV yield while considerably reducing EV yield, except for PA104, which caused a small reduction in MV yield in addition to decreasing EV formation. The spread assay, entry assay, and MV/EV yield data together suggest that while the main mechanism of viral inhibition by Retro-1 derivatives is the inhibition of EV particle formation, select compounds such as PA104 may impact viral entry when present at concentrations greater than their effective inhibitory concentrations. These findings aligned well with previous characterizations of Retro-1 and Retro-2 activity *in vitro* (Harrison et al., 2016; Sivan et al., 2016).

Vaccinia virus replicates in the cytoplasm of the infected cells, resulting in the formation of infectious, single-membrane MV particles at the site of replication (Condit et al., 2006). Although infectious, these MV particles remain intracellular unless wrapped by two additional membranes of post-Golgi or endosomal origin to form EVs. Once the outer layer of the EV double membrane fuses with the plasma membrane, an EV can be propelled out of the infected cell by actin tails (Smith et al., 2002). Because viral spread and EV yield were greatly reduced in the presence of our panel of compounds, we visualized actin tail-associated EVs in infected cells using confocal microscopy. Fewer actin tails were detected in the presence of all three compounds tested, PA104, PA63, and PA24, with the greatest reduction observed in case of PA104.

We and others have previously reported the spontaneous development of ST-246 resistance, both *in vitro* (Yang et al., 2005; Duraffour et al., 2015) and clinically in a smallpox-vaccinated PV patient receiving ST-246 as part of their treatment regimen (Lederman et al., 2012). In healthy individuals, it is possible that the immune response might overcome such resistant viruses, if they arise. However, additional interventions may be required for at-risk groups that cannot mount a protective immune response, such as individuals with immune deficiencies. For such cases, it would be beneficial to have additional antiviral candidates that can be administered in combination with ST-246 and can suppress ST-246-resistant viruses. We tested the inhibitory potential of PA104, PA63, and PA24 against two different ST-246-resistant viruses and found that all three compounds reduced viral spread of both viruses, as determined by a reduction in viral plaque size. Interestingly, while RV2 was substantially inhibited by all three Retro-1 compounds, RV1 appeared to be less efficiently inhibited by PA24 and PA63. These differences in the levels of viral inhibition by the same compounds could potentially be caused by additional uncharacterized mutations in other genes, or strain differences between the viruses; whereas RV1 was an Acambis strain of VACV, RV2 was a Western Reserve strain. Nevertheless, PA104 treatment resulted in maximal inhibition of plaque size for wild-type as well as RV1 and RV2 ST-246-resistant viruses. We hypothesize that its superior capacity to inhibit these viruses compared to PA24 and PA63 could be due to its ability to target multiple steps of VACV infection, including viral entry and MV formation, in addition to EV formation (**Figures 2, 3**).

In all, given its high SI (>800), submicromolar effective concentration, and potent inhibition of ST-246-resistant viruses, PA104 emerges as a promising candidate for future *in vivo* exploration. Further, PA104 targets a host-specific process rather than a viral protein, offering two additional advantages. First, the absence of a direct viral target reduces the probability of viral resistance to the compound (Lin and Gallay, 2013; Kaufmann et al., 2018). Second is the possibility of broad-range applicability to other viruses and non-viral pathogens that utilize the retrograde pathway for entry or egress. We and others have previously shown that Retro-2 and its analogs can reduce *Leishmania*, polyomavirus, and papillomavirus infections, as well as inhibit Shiga toxin trafficking in cells (Noel et al., 2013; Carney et al., 2014; Craig et al., 2017). Recent reports have also investigated the effect of Retro-2 derivatives on HSV2 infections (Dai et al., 2018). A majority of these studies have focused primarily on Retro-2 derivatives, and at present, less is understood about the antipathogenic potential of Retro-1 and its derivatives. To our knowledge, this is the first study to provide an in-depth, large-scale characterization of the inhibitory potential of compounds structurally related to Retro-1. As the retrograde pathway plays an important role for several pathogens and toxins, further characterization of compounds such as PA104 and exploration of their *in vivo* activity could have important implications for the design of broad-spectrum therapeutics that have immense public health benefits. An in-depth structure-activity relationship study of PA104 and other structural analogs of Retro-1 is in progress and will be reported in due course.

AUTHOR CONTRIBUTIONS

LP, JS, and PS contributed to the conception and design of the study. PA, AL, and JS designed and generated the benzodiazepine scaffold-containing compounds. LP and PS performed poxvirus experiments and wrote the first draft of the manuscript. AK and SS performed confocal imaging experiments. LP, PA, VO, JS, and PS edited the manuscript. All authors contributed to the manuscript revision and read and approved the submitted version.

FUNDING

The study was supported by the CDC Intramural Research and Biomedical Advanced Research and Developmental Authority (BARDA) and an ORISE Postdoctoral Fellowship (LP) and funding from Brown University (JS).

ACKNOWLEDGMENTS

We thank Dr. Bernard Moss, Dr. Jan Carette, and SIGA Technologies for reagents, and Dr. Jinxin Gao for his help with F13 sequencing. The findings and conclusions in this report are those of the authors and do not necessarily represent the official position of the Centers for Disease Control and Prevention.

SUPPLEMENTARY MATERIAL

FIGURE S1 | Validation of luciferase-based viral entry assay. **(A)** Minimal input luciferase activity after 5 min infection at RT. Luciferase activity in cells infected for 5 min at RT was significantly lower than infection for 2 h at 37°C. **** indicates an unpaired *t*-test *p*-value < 0.0001. **(B)** PA104 does not impact luciferase enzyme activity. No difference observed in RLU values in the presence of three concentrations of PA104. Both graphs show mean values ± SEM.

FIGURE S2 | Fewer virus-loaded actin tails in the presence of Retro-1 inhibitors. Confocal microscopy images of cells infected with VACV WR A4-YFP virus in the presence or absence of Retro-1 analogs PA63, PA24, and PA104. Lower magnification images of cells pictured in **Figure 4**. Scale bars represent 10 μm and white boxes indicate the area within each cell that was magnified to create **Figure 4**.

DATA SHEET S1 | NMR and MS data for PA104, PA24, and PA63.

REFERENCES

Angelo, K. M., Petersen, B. W., Hamer, D. H., Schwartz, E., and Brunette, G. (2019). Monkeypox transmission among international travellers-serious monkey business?. *J. Travel Med.* 26:taz002.

Blasco, R., and Moss, B. (1991). Extracellular vaccinia virus formation and cell-to-cell virus transmission are prevented by deletion of the gene encoding the 37,000-Dalton outer envelope protein. *J. Virol.* 65, 5910–5920.

Blasco, R., and Moss, B. (1992). Role of cell-associated enveloped vaccinia virus in cell-to-cell spread. *J. Virol.* 66, 4170–4179.

Carney, D. W., Nelson, C. D., Ferris, B. D., Stevens, J. P., Lipovsky, A., Kazakov, T., et al. (2014). Structural optimization of a retrograde trafficking inhibitor that protects cells from infections by human polyoma- and papillomaviruses. *Bioorg. Med. Chem.* 22, 4836–4847. doi: 10.1016/j.bmc.2014.06.053

Condit, R. C., Moussatche, N., and Traktman, P. (2006). In a nutshell: structure and assembly of the vaccinia virion. *Adv. Virus Res.* 66, 31–124.

Craig, E., Huyghues-Despointes, C. E., Yu, C., Handy, E. L., Sello, J. K., and Kima, P. E. (2017). Structurally optimized analogs of the retrograde trafficking inhibitor Retro-2cycl limit Leishmania infections. *PLoS Negl. Trop. Dis.* 11:e0005556. doi: 10.1371/journal.pntd.0005556

Cryer, M., Lane, K., Greer, M., Cates, R., Burt, S., Andrus, M., et al. (2017). Isolation and identification of compounds from Kalanchoe pinnata having human alphaherpesvirus and vaccinia virus antiviral activity. *Pharm. Biol.* 55, 1586–1591. doi: 10.1080/13880209.2017.1310907

Dai, W., Wu, Y., Bi, J., Wang, J., Wang, S., Kong, W., et al. (2018). Antiviral effect of Retro-2.1 against Herpes simplex virus type 2 in vitro. *J. Microbiol. Biotechnol.* 28, 849–859. doi: 10.4014/jmb.1712.12052

Duraffour, S., Lorenzo, M. M., Zoller, G., Topalis, D., Grosenbach, D., Hruby, D. E., et al. (2015). ST-246 is a key antiviral to inhibit the viral F13L phospholipase, one of the essential proteins for orthopoxvirus wrapping. *J. Antimicrob. Chemother.* 70, 1367–1380. doi: 10.1093/jac/dku545

Durski, K. N., Mccollum, A. M., Nakazawa, Y., Petersen, B. W., Reynolds, M. G., Briand, S., et al. (2018). Emergence of Monkeypox - West and Central Africa, 1970-2017. *MMWR Morb. Mortal. Wkly. Rep.* 67, 306–310. doi: 10.15585/mmwr.mm6710a5

Engelstad, M., and Smith, G. L. (1993). The vaccinia virus 42-kDa envelope protein is required for the envelopment and egress of extracellular virus and for virus virulence. *Virology* 194, 627–637.

Erez, N., Achdout, H., Milrot, E., Schwartz, Y., Wiener-Well, Y., Paran, N., et al. (2019). Diagnosis of imported monkeypox Israel, 2018. *Emerg. Infect. Dis.* 25, 980–983. doi: 10.3201/eid2505.190076

Fenner, F., and Nakano, J. H. (1988). "Poxviridae: the poxviruses," in *Laboratory Diagnosis of Infectious Diseases Principles and Practice: VOLUME II Viral, Rickettsial, and Chlamydial Diseases*, eds E. H. Lennette, P. Halonen, and F. A. Murphy (New York, NY: Springer New York), 177–210.

Grosenbach, D. W., Berhanu, A., King, D. S., Mosier, S., Jones, K. F., Jordan, R. A., et al. (2010). Efficacy of ST-246 versus lethal poxvirus challenge in immunodeficient mice. *Proc. Natl. Acad. Sci. U.S.A.* 107, 838–843. doi: 10.1073/pnas.0912134107

Grosenbach, D. W., Jordan, R., and Hruby, D. E. (2011). Development of the small-molecule antiviral ST-246 as a smallpox therapeutic. *Future Virol.* 6, 653–671.

Harrison, K., Haga, I. R., Pechenick Jowers, T., Jasim, S., Cintrat, J. C., Gillet, D., et al. (2016). Vaccinia virus uses retromer-independent cellular retrograde transport pathways to facilitate the wrapping of intracellular mature virions during virus morphogenesis. *J. Virol.* 90, 10120–10132. doi: 10.1128/JVI.01464-16

Hoffmann, D., Franke, A., Jenckel, M., Tamosiunaite, A., Schluckebier, J., Granzow, H., et al. (2015). Out of the reservoir: phenotypic and genotypic characterization of a novel cowpox virus isolated from a common vole. *J. Virol.* 89, 10959–10969. doi: 10.1128/JVI.01195-15

Johnson, M. C., Damon, I. K., and Karem, K. L. (2008). A rapid, high-throughput vaccinia virus neutralization assay for testing smallpox vaccine efficacy based on detection of green fluorescent protein. *J. Virol. Methods* 150, 14–20. doi: 10.1016/j.jviromet.2008.02.009

Kaufmann, S. H. E., Dorhoi, A., Hotchkiss, R. S., and Bartenschlager, R. (2018). Host-directed therapies for bacterial and viral infections. *Nat. Rev. Drug Discov.* 17, 35–56. doi: 10.1038/nrd.2017.162

Lanave, G., Dowgier, G., Decaro, N., Albanese, F., Brogi, E., Parisi, A., et al. (2018). Novel Orthopoxvirus and lethal disease in cat. *Italy. Emerg. Infect. Dis* 24, 1665–1673. doi: 10.3201/eid2409.171283

Lederman, E. R., Davidson, W., Groff, H. L., Smith, S. K., Warkentien, T., Li, Y., et al. (2012). Progressive vaccinia: case description and laboratory-guided therapy with vaccinia immune globulin ST-246, and CMX001. *J. Infect. Dis.* 206, 1372–1385. doi: 10.1093/infdis/jis510

Lin, K., and Gallay, P. (2013). Curing a viral infection by targeting the host: the example of cyclophilin inhibitors. *Antiviral Res.* 99, 68–77. doi: 10.1016/j.antiviral.2013.03.020

Moss, B. (2006). Poxvirus entry and membrane fusion. *Virology* 344, 48–54.

Noel, R., Gupta, N., Pons, V., Goudet, A., Garcia-Castillo, M. D., Michau, A., et al. (2013). N-methyldihydroquinazolinone derivatives of Retro-2 with enhanced efficacy against Shiga toxin. *J. Med. Chem.* 56, 3404–3413. doi: 10.1021/jm4002346

Payne, L. G. (1980). Significance of extracellular enveloped virus in the in vitro and in vivo dissemination of vaccinia. *J. Gen. Virol.* 50, 89–100.

Realegeno, S., Puschnik, A. S., Kumar, A., Goldsmith, C., Burgado, J., Sambhara, S., et al. (2017). Monkeypox virus host factor screen using haploid cells identifies essential role of GARP complex in extracellular virus formation. *J. Virol.* 91:e00011-17.

Reed, K. D., Melski, J. W., Graham, M. B., Regnery, R. L., Sotir, M. J., Wegner, M. V., et al. (2004). The detection of monkeypox in humans in the Western Hemisphere. *N. Engl. J. Med.* 350, 342–350.

Sivan, G., Weisberg, A. S., Americo, J. L., and Moss, B. (2016). Retrograde transport from early endosomes to the trans-Golgi network enables membrane wrapping and egress of vaccinia virus virions. *J. Virol.* 90, 8891–8905. doi: 10.1128/JVI.01114-16

Smith, G. L., Vanderplasschen, A., and Law, M. (2002). The formation and function of extracellular enveloped vaccinia virus. *J. Gen. Virol.* 83, 2915–2931. doi: 10.1099/0022-1317-83-12-2915

Smith, S. K., Self, J., Weiss, S., Carroll, D., Braden, Z., Regnery, R. L., et al. (2011). Effective antiviral treatment of systemic orthopoxvirus disease: ST-246 treatment of prairie dogs infected with monkeypox virus. *J. Virol.* 85, 9176–9187. doi: 10.1128/JVI.02173-10

Spooner, R. A., Smith, D. C., Easton, A. J., Roberts, L. M., and Lord, J. M. (2006). Retrograde transport pathways utilised by viruses and protein toxins. *Virol. J.* 3:26.

Springer, Y. P., Hsu, C. H., Werle, Z. R., Olson, L. E., Cooper, M. P., Castrodale, L. J., et al. (2017). Novel Orthopoxvirus Infection in an Alaska Resident. *Clin. Infect. Dis.* 64, 1737–1741. doi: 10.1093/cid/cix219

Vaughan, A., Aarons, E., Astbury, J., Balasegaram, S., Beadsworth, M., Beck, C. R., et al. (2018). Two cases of monkeypox imported to the United Kingdom, September 2018. *Euro. Surveill.* 23, doi: 10.2807/1560-7917.ES.2018.23.38.1800509

Vora, N. M., Li, Y., Geleishvili, M., Emerson, G. L., Khmaladze, E., Maghlakelidze, G., et al. (2015). Human infection with a zoonotic orthopoxvirus in the country of Georgia. *N. Engl. J. Med.* 372, 1223–1230. doi: 10.1056/NEJMoa1407647

Wolffe, E. J., Isaacs, S. N., and Moss, B. (1993). Deletion of the vaccinia virus B5R gene encoding a 42-kilodalton membrane glycoprotein inhibits extracellular virus envelope formation and dissemination. *J. Virol.* 67, 4732–4741.

Yang, G., Pevear, D. C., Davies, M. H., Collett, M. S., Bailey, T., Rippen, S., et al. (2005). An orally bioavailable antipoxvirus compound (ST-246) inhibits extracellular virus formation and protects mice from lethal orthopoxvirus Challenge. *J. Virol.* 79, 13139–13149.

16

Broadly Protective Strategies Against Inflluenza Viruses: Universal Vaccines and Therapeutics

*Olivia A. Vogel[1] and Balaji Manicassamy[2]**

[1] Department of Microbiology, The University of Chicago, Chicago, IL, United States, [2] Department of Microbiology and Immunology, The University of Iowa, Iowa City, IA, United States

***Correspondence:**
Balaji Manicassamy
balaji-manicassamy@uiowa.edu

Influenza virus is a respiratory pathogen that can cause disease in humans, with symptoms ranging from mild to life-threatening. The vast majority of influenza virus infections in humans are observed during seasonal epidemics and occasional pandemics. Given the substantial public health burden associated with influenza virus infection, yearly vaccination is recommended for protection against seasonal influenza viruses. Despite vigilant surveillance for new variants and careful selection of seasonal vaccine strains, the efficacy of seasonal vaccines can vary widely from year to year. This often results in lowered protection within the population, regardless of vaccination status. In order to broaden the protection afforded by seasonal influenza vaccines, the National Institute of Allergy and Infectious Diseases (NIAID) has deemed the development of a universal influenza virus vaccine to be a priority in influenza virus vaccine research. This universal vaccine would provide protection against all influenza virus strains, eliminating the need for the yearly reformulations of seasonal influenza vaccines. In addition to universal influenza vaccine efforts, substantial progress has been made in developing novel influenza virus therapeutics that utilize broadly neutralizing antibodies to provide protection against influenza virus infection and to mitigate disease outcomes during infection. In this review, we discuss various approaches toward the goal of improving influenza virus vaccine efficacy through a universal influenza virus vaccine. We also address the novel methods of discovery and utilization of broadly neutralizing antibodies to improve influenza disease outcomes.

Keywords: influenza, universal influenza vaccine, vaccine, influenza therapeutics, immunization

INTRODUCTION

Influenza viruses are a significant public health burden worldwide, causing yearly epidemics and occasional pandemics. Infection with influenza virus causes acute upper respiratory disease in humans that can potentially lead to hospitalization or death. In addition to the morbidity and mortality associated with influenza virus infection, the yearly economic burden of influenza virus infections in the United States is estimated to be around $11.2 billion (Putri et al., 2018). Given the considerable impact of influenza virus infection in communities worldwide, significant attention has been focused on preventing influenza virus infection and spread of the virus through vaccination within the population as well as with other public health measures.

Influenza viruses are members of the *Orthomyxoviridae* family of viruses, which are characterized by segmented, negative sense, single-stranded RNA genome. Of the influenza virus types, influenza A and B are the only types that are known to cause disease in humans. In addition to humans, influenza A viruses can infect a broad variety of species including pigs, horses, and birds (Webster et al., 1995). In nature, influenza A viruses are maintained in water fowls, which are the main reservoir for influenza A (Webster et al., 1995). Influenza A viruses can be further classified into different subtypes based on the two major viral surface glycoproteins, hemagglutinin (HA) and neuraminidase (NA) (Fields et al., 2013). For influenza A viruses, there are 18 known HA subtypes that fall into two phylogenetic groups (Group 1 or Group 2); like HA, the 11 NA subtypes also fall within two phylogenetic groups. These phylogenetic groups are composed of viruses that are derived from a common ancestor. Unlike influenza A viruses, the diversity of influenza B viruses is limited and is categorized into two lineages, B/Yamagata and B/Victoria (Rota et al., 1990). Despite the limited diversity, influenza B viruses evolve to escape immunity and remain in circulation in humans; thus, necessitating yearly updates of the influenza B virus strains included in the seasonal vaccine.

IMMUNOLOGICAL RESPONSES TO INFLUENZA VIRUS INFECTION

Influenza viruses predominantly infect and replicate in the epithelial cells lining the upper respiratory tract. Viral infection is initiated by the binding of viral surface glycoprotein HA to host sialic acid residues followed by internalization of the virus through endocytosis (Fields et al., 2013). Subsequently, the fusion of the viral membrane with the endosomal membrane releases the viral genomic RNA into the cytoplasm, and the RNA is then imported into the nucleus for replication (Fields et al., 2013). The initial innate immune responses against influenza virus infection are activated by the sensing of viral RNA by pattern recognition receptors such as the retinoic acid-inducible gene-I (RIG-I) and Toll-Like Receptor 7 (TLR7) (Iwasaki and Pillai, 2014). Additional innate sensing pathways also contribute to robust innate responses against influenza virus infection (Iwasaki and Pillai, 2014). Ultimately, the activation of these innate sensing pathways leads to the production of interferon and cytokines/chemokines critical for efficient activation of adaptive immune responses (B- and T-cell responses) that help control and clear infection.

Studies in humans and mice demonstrate the importance of T-cell responses in clearing primary influenza virus infection and mounting robust recall responses in subsequent infection. The importance of T-cell responses was highlighted by a study following 342 healthy adults in the UK during the 2009 H1N1 pandemic, which determined that illness was less severe in individuals with higher frequencies of pre-existing T cells to conserved CD8 epitopes (Sridhar et al., 2013). The importance of $CD8^+$ T cells during influenza virus infection was further highlighted in adoptive transfer experiments in which mice were given $CD8^+$ effector cells. After infection, viral replication was reduced in the lungs of recipient mice compared to mice that did not receive $CD8^+$ T cells (Yap et al., 1978; Lukacher et al., 1984; Hamada et al., 2009, 2013). Additionally, mice receiving $CD8^+$ T cells also displayed increased recruitment of NK cells, macrophages, and B cells after infection (Hamada et al., 2013). These results further highlight the importance of mounting $CD8^+$ immune responses during infection. More recently, $CD4^+$ T cells have also been shown to have an important role in clearing influenza infection, with the lack of $CD4^+$ T cells correlating with reduced viral clearance (Belz et al., 2002). As with $CD8^+$ T cells, adoptive transfer of $CD4^+$ memory T cells in mice was associated with greater protection during influenza infection (McKinstry et al., 2012).

The mucosal antibody response is an important feature in determining the ability of the host to efficiently clear viral infections. Mucosal antibody responses are more effective in preventing subsequent infection rather than primary viral infection. The three main immunoglobulin (Ig) isotypes induced during influenza infection are IgG, IgA, and IgM. Secretory IgA antibodies are generated early during infection and can act as an indicator of acute influenza infection (Rothbarth et al., 1999). Additionally, secretory IgA antibodies have been associated with greater protection in the upper respiratory tract while also providing cross-reactive protection against different influenza virus strains (Tamura et al., 1990; Asahi et al., 2002; Renegar et al., 2004; Ainai et al., 2013). IgM antibodies are also generated during primary infection and have been shown to have a role in complement mediated virus neutralization (Rothbarth et al., 1999; Fernandez Gonzalez et al., 2008). In contrast to serum IgA antibodies, serum IgG antibodies are associated with protection in the lower respiratory tract as well as providing strain-specific protection (Tamura et al., 1990).

CURRENT SEASONAL INFLUENZA VACCINES

The composition of seasonal influenza virus vaccines is based on the strains currently propagating in the human population. Presently, there are two influenza A virus strains (H1N1 and H3N2) and two influenza B virus lineages circulating in humans, with only one influenza B strain from each type circulating as the predominant strain during influenza season. However, as it is impossible to predict the predominant strain for a given season, the majority of the current seasonal influenza vaccines are composed of all four strains. The selection of influenza strains for incorporation into seasonal vaccines is based on surveillance of circulating strains by WHO influenza centers as well as on an assessment of which strains will likely become the predominant strain in human populations (Gerdil, 2003). Once the vaccine strains have been selected by the WHO committee, seasonal vaccine production can begin and requires roughly 6 months for the commonly used inactivated vaccine to be produced and distributed (Gerdil, 2003).

There are four types of seasonal influenza virus vaccines currently licensed for use in humans: inactivated, live attenuated, recombinant protein, and cell-based vaccines. A vast majority of the influenza virus vaccines administered in humans are split inactivated vaccines, which are produced in embryonated chicken eggs. For split inactivated vaccines, vaccine strains are individually grown in the allantoic cavity of embryonated chicken eggs and inactivated by treatment with formalin or β-propriolactone (Gerdil, 2003). Once purified, virus particles are then split using ether and detergent to reduce the level of viral ribonucleoproteins, which cause reactogenicity at the site of injection (Gerdil, 2003). The individual vaccine components are mixed in a standardized manner to ensure an inclusion of 15 μg of HA per strain (Sridhar et al., 2015). Inactivated vaccine is administered intramuscularly to stimulate the systemic immune response, producing mainly IgG antibodies and low amounts of IgA antibodies (Clements et al., 1986). Similar to inactivated vaccines, live attenuated influenza vaccines (LAIVs) are grown in embryonated eggs. LAIV strains are generated using a reverse genetics approach to incorporate HA and NA genes from circulating influenza strains into a cold-adapted, attenuated influenza virus backbone (Sridhar et al., 2015). Cold adaption of the LAIV backbone ensures that the replication of the vaccine strain does not occur at temperatures above 33°C, allowing for replication in the upper respiratory tract but not in the lower respiratory tract (Sridhar et al., 2015). LAIV, which is administered intranasally to mimic natural infection, stimulates robust IgA and IgG responses in the upper respiratory tract (Clements et al., 1986). LAIV has also been shown to elicit T-cell mediated responses in vaccinated children (He et al., 2006; Hoft et al., 2011). While both inactivated vaccine virus strains and LAIV viruses are grown in embryonated eggs, this poses a challenge in the event of egg shortages and for immunization of individuals with egg allergies. Recombinant protein vaccines and cell culture-based influenza vaccines have been developed to overcome limitations of egg-based vaccines. Currently, there is only one recombinant vaccine, named Flublok®, approved for use by the US Food and Drug Administration (FDA). Flublok® still contains HA protein antigens representing the selected influenza strains for the current season, but it is produced in insect cells (Cox and Hollister, 2009). In contrast to embryonated egg-based vaccines, manufacturing of Flublok® takes approximately 2 months and can be administered in individuals with egg allergies, providing an advantage over traditional seasonal egg-based vaccines (Cox and Hollister, 2009). In regard to cell-based vaccines, Flucelvax® is a licensed quadrivalent inactivated vaccine that is grown in a mammalian cell line and can avoid any potential egg-based mutations (Lamb, 2019). As with Flublok®, Flucelvax® can be administered to individuals with egg allergies and requires a shorter production time than egg-grown vaccines.

CHALLENGES FOR CURRENT SEASONAL VACCINES

Yearly vaccination with split, inactivated influenza vaccines is still one of the most popular and efficient means of protection against seasonal influenza viruses. Prior to 2012, influenza vaccines were trivalent and contained only one influenza B virus in the vaccine. This often resulted in inadequate protection against influenza B virus, due to mismatches between the circulating influenza B virus lineage and the influenza B virus lineage chosen for vaccine incorporation (Tisa et al., 2016). To avoid issues with influenza B virus lineage mismatches, a quadrivalent inactivated vaccine that contains both influenza B virus lineages was developed (Tisa et al., 2016). Despite these improvements to the seasonal influenza virus vaccines, the effectiveness of seasonal influenza vaccines can vary greatly, depending on how closely the vaccine strains match the circulating strains. In fact, there are several instances in the recent past where seasonal vaccines failed to provide protection against antigenically drifted strains (David et al., 2005; Halloran et al., 2007; Skowronski et al., 2007). Furthermore, yearly vaccines do not provide protection against novel influenza virus strains introduced from zoonotic reservoirs, causing significant morbidity and mortality due to lack of immunity in the general population.

The types of immune responses elicited by different seasonal influenza vaccines also impact the degree and the longevity of protection. As mentioned previously, inactivated vaccines administered intramuscularly elicit production of serum IgG antibodies but fail to induce antibody and T-cell responses in the respiratory mucosa. As such, this type of vaccine provides strain-specific protection but can leave individuals vulnerable to infection by new variant strains. Preclinical studies indicate that intranasal administration of inactivated vaccines induces robust responses in the respiratory mucosa. LAIV administered intranasally closely mimics natural infection and stimulates robust IgA and IgG antibody responses; however, this vaccine failed to provide adequate protection against influenza A(H1N1) pdm09 during the 2013–2014 and 2015–2016 seasons (Grohskopf et al., 2016, 2018). This inadequate protection prompted the Advisory Committee on Immunization Practices (ACIP) to recommend against administration of this vaccine for the 2016–2017 and 2017–2018 seasons (Grohskopf et al., 2016, 2017). Later, the manufacturer determined that the reduced protection associated with the LAIV was most likely due to reduced replicative fitness of the A/California and A/Bolivia (H1N1)pdm09 LAIV strains (Ambrose et al., 2016). Currently, the quadrivalent LAIV has incorporated a new influenza A(H1N1)pdm09-like virus that provides better protection and is recommended again for use (Grohskopf et al., 2018). While the LAIV has been demonstrated to provide robust protection in younger children, responses to LAIV vaccination in preimmune adults are likely limited due to immune-mediated restriction of LAIV replication prior to induction of effective immunity.

A vast majority of seasonal influenza vaccines are manufactured in eggs. Occasionally, during vaccine production, egg adaptive mutations can arise that alter the antigenicity of the virus and, as a result, can reduce vaccine effectiveness against circulating strains. H3N2 strains in particular have been associated with increased egg-based mutations that result in reduced antigenicity of the vaccine strain, negatively impacting the protection afforded by the vaccine (Skowronski et al., 2014; Wu et al., 2017, 2019; Zost et al., 2017). Consequently, egg grown vaccines must be monitored to ensure that the vaccine strain incorporated into the vaccine matches the seed strain chosen at the start of manufacturing. The risk of adaptive mutations and reduced antigenicity is mitigated in recombinant protein vaccines, which are grown in insect cells, or by producing the vaccine strains in mammalian cell lines. However, the cost associated with large-scale production of cell-culture grown vaccine strains remains high as compared to ones produced in eggs (Barr et al., 2018).

Another alternative to egg grown vaccine approaches involves the use of DNA and mRNA vaccines. While none are currently approved for use, DNA and mRNA vaccines can be manufactured synthetically, allowing for quicker production times than egg and cell-culture grown vaccines (Stachyra et al., 2014; Kanekiyo et al., 2019) Furthermore, DNA and mRNA vaccine approaches do not induce the anti-vector immune responses that can be elicited with viral vector-based vaccine approaches (Kanekiyo et al., 2019). DNA vaccines have also shown promise as a method of vaccine priming (Ledgerwood et al., 2011). In fact, several of the universal vaccination methods described in this review utilize DNA prime-boost vaccination to improve immune responses. Likewise, mRNA-based vaccines show potential as an alternative vaccination approach. An example of an mRNA-based approach includes RNActive® vaccines. RNActive® vaccines are mRNA vaccines complexed with protamine, which allow for the mRNA to acts as a "self-adjuvant" through interaction with TLR7 (Kallen et al., 2013). An RNActive® vaccine encoding the full-length PR8 HA has been shown to induce IgG antibodies against PR8 HA and provide protection against homologous PR8 viral challenge (Petsch et al., 2012). Furthermore, transfer of serum from PR8 HA mRNA-vaccinated mice to unvaccinated recipient mice provided protection against PR8 infection (Petsch et al., 2012). Together, these different vaccination approaches have the potential for improving upon yearly influenza virus vaccines as well as in the development of universal influenza virus vaccines.

An additional consideration for seasonal influenza vaccines is the ability to provide protection among older adults, who are often at higher risk for influenza infection. The usual dosage of 15 µg HA antigen per vaccine strain in seasonal inactivated vaccines is insufficient to induce protection in older adults. To address this concern, a new vaccine named Fluzone® was developed to improve serum antibody responses in older adults. Fluzone® is a trivalent, inactivated split-virus vaccine that contains 60 µg of HA for each influenza strain included in the vaccine (Robertson et al., 2016). This dosage is four times that of standard inactivated vaccines and has been shown to increase protection in older adults, providing a promising alternative for this high-risk group (Robertson et al., 2016).

The most significant challenge for the seasonal influenza vaccine production strategy involves ensuring that the vaccine strains match the dominant circulating strains in the population. There have been significant efforts to improve upon methods of monitoring and identifying newly evolved influenza strains worldwide, including the incorporation of modeling techniques such as antigenic cartography (Ampofo et al., 2015). Despite these efforts, the screening process is imperfect, and as result, it is not unusual to see the emergence of a variant strain after selection of another strain for vaccine production. Neutralizing antibodies induced upon vaccination predominantly target the highly immunogenic head domain of HA and provide potent protection against matching strains by blocking virus attachment to cells (Knossow et al., 2002). Consequently, these highly immunogenic regions in the head domain are prone to high mutation rates due to immune selection pressure from neutralizing antibodies. In a circulating strain, accumulation of mutations in the head domain over time leads to changes in antigenic properties (antigenic drift) and can render vaccine-induced immunity ineffective against them. In addition, these variant strains can cause epidemics in populations lacking immunity to the newly evolved strain (Fields et al., 2013). Antigenic drift is the major driving force behind the need to reformulate influenza vaccines each year and poses a significant challenge for vaccine development. Furthermore, seasonal influenza virus vaccines fail to provide protection against the novel strains transmitted from zoonotic reservoirs.

Given the considerable public health consequences associated with a lack of sufficient protection against seasonal and pandemic influenza stains, the National Institute of Allergy and Infectious Diseases (NIAID) has prioritized the development of a universal influenza vaccine that can afford protection against a broad variety of influenza viruses (Erbelding et al., 2018). Currently, the majority of universal influenza vaccine research efforts are aimed at inducing immunity against the highly conserved regions on the influenza surface proteins or internal proteins of influenza viruses as means to induce universal protection against all influenza virus strains (**Figure 1**).

UNIVERSAL INFLUENZA VACCINE APPROACHES

Hemagglutinin-Directed

The influenza virus surface protein HA is one of the major targets of the immune system. HA is synthesized as a precursor HA0 that is proteolytically processed into HA1 and HA2 subunits, which remain attached through a disulfide bond. Three HA molecules form a trimeric rod-shaped molecule that is composed of a long fibrous stem formed by the HA2 trimer and a globular head formed by the HA1 trimer (Fields et al., 2013). The globular head domain of HA contains the receptor binding pocket, which facilitates virus attachment to the host cell surface sialic acids (Wilson et al., 1981; Rogers et al., 1983). Once the bound virus is internalized through endocytosis, HA undergoes conformational changes under low pH conditions that allow HA2 to initiate the fusion of the viral and endosomal membranes (Skehel et al., 1982; Bullough et al., 1994). This process enables the release of the viral genomic contents into the cytoplasm. The HA1 region is highly immunogenic, more flexible to accommodate mutations than HA2 and displays a high degree of variability among influenza virus strains. Conversely, the HA2 region is highly conserved among different influenza virus subtypes and is more structurally constrained in its ability to accommodate mutations.

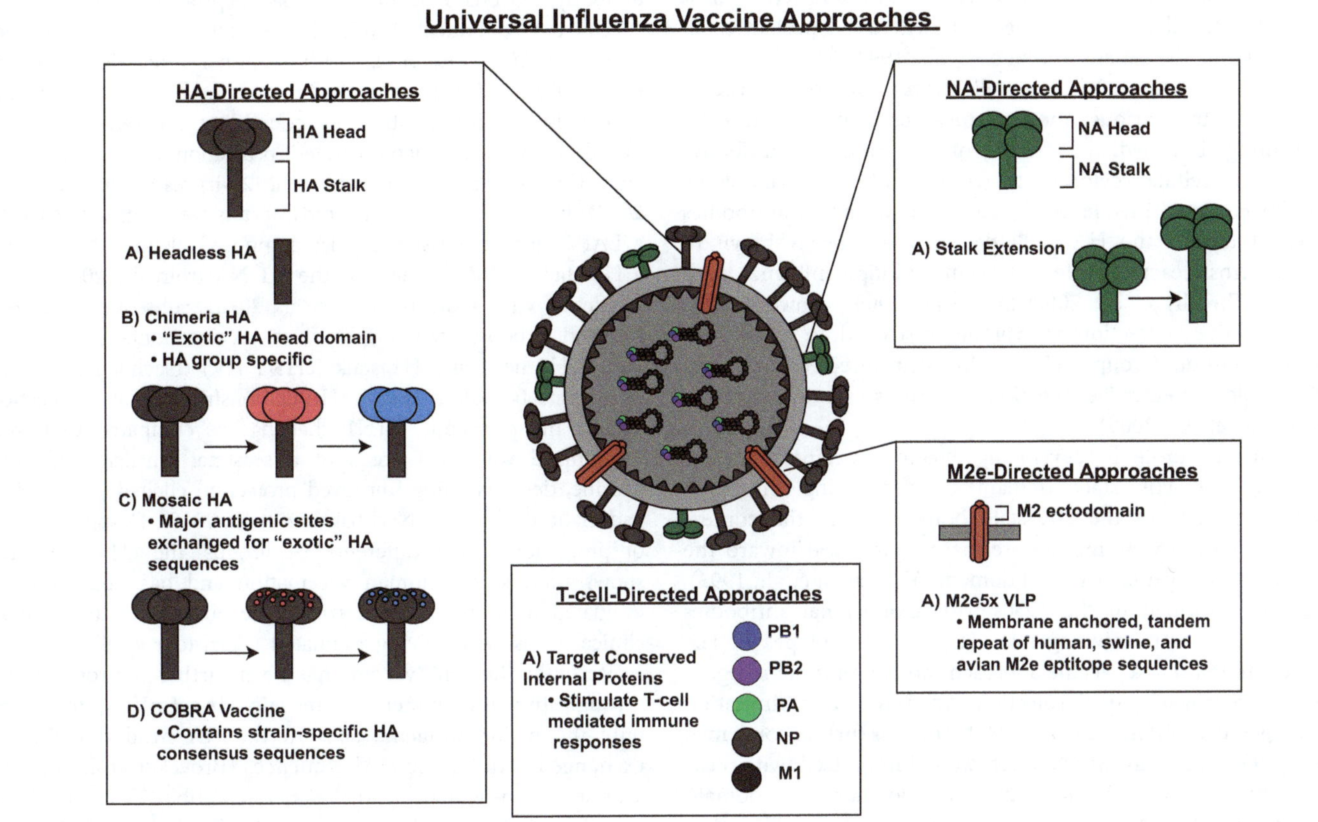

FIGURE 1 | A schematic representation of various preclinical approaches for a universal influenza vaccine.

As described above, the antigenic variation of the HA1 domain and its resulting antigenic drift is the major reason for reformulating seasonal influenza vaccines with new strains every year. To address this challenge, several vaccine strategies based on conserved sequences in HA have been developed. Once such approach involves a novel computational-based antigen design methodology. This approach, termed computationally optimized broadly reactive antigen (COBRA), was used to generate a consensus H5 HA sequence by aligning 129 unique HA sequences from clade 2 H5N1 viruses isolated from 2004 to 2006 (Giles and Ross, 2011). Following alignment, the most common amino acid at each position was selected to generate a consensus sequence for the COBRA H5 HA (Giles and Ross, 2011). This newly generated COBRA H5 HA was confirmed to exhibit normal HA activity, including receptor binding and particle fusion (Giles and Ross, 2011). The efficacy of this COBRA H5 HA was evaluated in virus-like particle (VLP) based vaccination and challenge studies (Giles and Ross, 2011). Following vaccination of mice and ferrets, the COBRA H5N1 VLP vaccines induced increased hemagglutinin inhibition titers and provided enhanced protection against lethal challenge with different clade 2 H5N1 viruses when compared to a VLP vaccine containing an HA derived from a primary isolate (Giles and Ross, 2011). The improved efficacy of COBRA vaccine approaches have been supported by studies in a non-human primate model (cynomolgus macaques) with the COBRA HA H5N1 VLPs (Giles et al., 2012). The sera from vaccinated macaques demonstrated hemagglutinin inhibition titers against a wider range of H5N1 strains than animals vaccinated with contemporary H5N1 HA VLPs (Giles et al., 2012). In addition, vaccinated macaques were protected against viral challenge as well as exhibiting reduced lung inflammation (Giles et al., 2012). Following the same methodology used for the generation of COBRA HA H5N1 VLPs, COBRA HA H3N2 and COBRA HA H1N1 VLPS have been generated using consensus sequences from both modern and historical H3N2 and H1N1 strains. These COBRA VLP vaccines provided broad protection against a wide range of H3N2 and H1N1 strains (Carter et al., 2016; Wong et al., 2017). Recently, the COBRA H1 and H3 antigens, along with the AF03 adjuvant (squalene-in-water emulsion), induced protective responses in ferrets, with ferrets exhibiting decreased viral shedding (Allen et al., 2018). By generating more broadly reactive HAs, the COBRA approach provides an intriguing solution to overcome the challenges posed by antigenic drift of circulating strains, as COBRA-based seasonal vaccine has the potential to provide protection even during mismatch. However, as protection afforded by COBRA vaccines is only against specific HA subtypes, COBRA vaccines still fall short of serving as a true universal influenza vaccine.

To generate broadly protective immune responses against multiple influenza virus strains, several research groups developing universal influenza vaccines have targeted the highly conserved stalk domain of HA. Antibodies directed against the HA stalk domain have been shown to be protective in both mice and humans (Okuno et al., 1993; Throsby et al., 2008; Ekiert et al., 2009). The stalk-specific antibodies provide protection by various mechanisms, including by directly preventing HA-mediated fusion or by inducing antibody-dependent cellular cytotoxicity (ADCC; Ekiert et al., 2009; DiLillo et al., 2014; He et al., 2016). Importantly, antibodies directed toward the HA stalk domain have been shown to provide cross-reactive protection against multiple influenza virus strains (Throsby et al., 2008; Sui et al., 2009). However, this cross-reactive protection is typically restricted to HAs from the same group, Group 1 HA-specific stem-directed antibodies are unable to neutralize infection by viruses carrying Group 2 HAs (Sui et al., 2009).

A major hurdle in developing effective vaccine strategies targeting the HA stalk domain is overcoming the poor immunogenicity of the HA stalk domain, as in the context of full-length HA, antibodies are mainly produced toward the highly immunogenic HA head domain (Vareckova et al., 1993). Studies performed in the 1980s with monoclonal antibodies that were cross reactive against H1 and H2 subtypes of HA demonstrated that a vaccine approach targeting the stem region of HA can provide broad protection and overcome the limitation of antigenic drift (Graves et al., 1983). This was further confirmed in a 1996 study in which mice were immunized with cells overexpressing an HA that lacked the globular head domain (Sagawa et al., 1996). Following challenge with H1N1, mice that were immunized with the headless HA exhibited increased survival compared to mice immunized with full length HA expressing cells (Sagawa et al., 1996). These studies underscore the potential immunogenicity of the HA stalk in the absence of the HA head domain.

In recent years, vaccine approaches have attempted to enhance exposure of the HA stalk domain to the immune system using HAs that lack the dominant head domain (Steel et al., 2010; Impagliazzo et al., 2015). These "headless" HAs were incorporated onto VLPs for vaccination (Steel et al., 2010; Impagliazzo et al., 2015). Nanoparticles have also been used as a method to improve HA stalk exposure during vaccination, using either HAs lacking the head domain or full-length HAs (Kanekiyo et al., 2013; Yassine et al., 2015). Vaccination in mice and ferrets demonstrated that these nanoparticle-based approaches provided cross-reactive protection following viral challenge with different influenza A virus strains (Kanekiyo et al., 2013; Yassine et al., 2015). Interestingly, when ferrets were immunized with the nanoparticle vaccine containing a full-length HA fused to ferritin, both HA stem and receptor binding site-specific antibodies were detected, demonstrating the utility of this approach in generating more broadly immunogenic HA-based vaccines (Kanekiyo et al., 2013).

Another method of improving exposure of the HA stalk domain involves the generation of chimeric HAs (cHA) that express the head domain from one virus strain and the stalk domain of another. This method involves sequential immunization with constructs that express the same stalk domain but different "exotic" head domains, thereby specifically stimulating stalk-directed antibody responses to induce broader protection than strain-specific HA head directed antibodies generated by seasonal vaccines (Hai et al., 2012; Pica et al., 2012; Krammer et al., 2013; Margine et al., 2013; Nachbagauer et al., 2017; Liu et al., 2019). Sequential vaccination of mice with cHA containing the same H1 stem but different heads demonstrated protection against challenge from Group 1 viruses but not Group 2 viruses (Krammer et al., 2013). In a recent preclinical study, ferrets were immunized with a LAIV virus expressing a cHA composed of an H8 head and a H1 stalk (cH8/1) as well as the N1 NA from the 2009 H1N1 pandemic virus (Nachbagauer et al., 2018). Subsequently, ferrets received a boost with a split virus vaccine containing a cHA with a H5 head and H1 stalk (cH5/1 IIV) (Nachbagauer et al., 2018). Ferrets vaccinated with cHA demonstrated greater protection against the pandemic H1N1 challenge as compared to ferrets immunized with two doses of a seasonal trivalent influenza vaccine, demonstrating improved protection elicited by the cHA vaccination approach (Nachbagauer et al., 2018). Despite the lack of protection across different HA groups, the cHA approach shows promise for human vaccination and has been recently evaluated in human clinical trials. The outcome of the human clinical trials is still being evaluated (Bernstein et al., 2019).

Recently, the cHA vaccine has been further improved upon through the development of mosaic HAs (mHA), in which only the major antigenic sites in the HA head domain are exchanged with "exotic HA" sequences (Broecker et al., 2019a). This strategy was developed to generate antibodies against both the stalk domain and epitopes in the head domain that fall outside the major antigenic sites (Broecker et al., 2019a). Sequential vaccination with inactivated mHA viruses induced cross-reactive antibodies to both the stalk domain and the head domain (Broecker et al., 2019a). Additionally, transfer of sera from vaccinated mice into naïve mice provided protection against viral challenge with reassortment viruses containing PR8 internal proteins with HA and NA from different H3N2 strains as compared to the seasonal inactivated quadrivalent vaccine (Broecker et al., 2019a). These results indicate that the mHA approach also has potential to provide broader protection than current seasonal vaccines.

An important challenge for HA stalk-directed vaccines is whether these vaccine strategies are capable of providing protection against strains from both HA groups. As described above, HA stalk-directed antibodies often provide HA group-specific protection. While the ability to provide protection against a broad range of influenza virus strains within a given HA subtype is a vast improvement over approved seasonal vaccines, this still falls short of providing universal influenza virus protection. Another important consideration involves providing protection for both influenza A and B virus strains. While the HA stalk-directed approaches described above demonstrate protection against influenza A viruses, protection against influenza B strains is not always addressed. A truly universal vaccine should be able to provide protection against both influenza A and B strains. Therefore, current universal vaccine research should be cognizant of the need to elicit protection for both types of influenza viruses. Antibodies targeting the HA stalk domain have been shown to be protective against influenza B strains, with the human monoclonal antibody CR9114 demonstrating protection against lethal challenge from both influenza A and B strains (Dreyfus et al., 2012). Recently, the mHA approach was used in an attempt to generate a universal influenza B vaccine that could provide protection against a wide range of influenza B virus lineages (Sun et al., 2019). To generate the influenza B mHA, the major antigenic sites were replaced with "exotic" influenza A sequences (Sun et al., 2019). Immunization of mice involved a DNA primer followed by two mHA protein boosts (Sun et al., 2019). Importantly, mice vaccinated with the influenza B mHA demonstrated improved survival following lethal challenge with different influenza B strains (Sun et al., 2019). While this study does not provide evidence for protection against influenza A strains, it further serves to highlight the potential for vaccination approaches that improve upon the breadth of protection provided by the current seasonal vaccination strategies. It would be interesting to examine whether combining influenza A mHAs and influenza B mHAs into a single vaccine might provide even greater protection for both influenza A and B strains than the current inactivated quadrivalent vaccine.

Neuraminidase-Directed

The second major surface protein for influenza A virus is the NA protein, which has an important role in facilitating virus release from the host cell. The sialidase or neuraminidase activity of NA helps cleave the terminal sialic acids from glycans and thereby facilitate virion release from infected cells (Fields et al., 2013). NA has been an important target for the development of antiviral drugs, such as oseltamivir (Tamiflu®) and zanamivir, both of which target the enzymatic activity of NA and are effective against both influenza A and B virus strains. Mutations that render NA resistant to the aforementioned drugs have been reported. While NA is also capable of undergoing antigenic changes, these changes occur at a much slower rate than those observed with HA (Kilbourne et al., 1990). Given the relatively conserved nature of NA, there have been several potential vaccine candidates developed that target NA in order to generate improved influenza vaccines.

Unlike HA antibodies, NA antibodies do not neutralize infection, but they have been shown to inhibit NA enzymatic activity as well as reduce viral titers in mouse models (Rott et al., 1974). In addition, NA antibodies have been shown to be protective in both chickens and humans (Murphy et al., 1972; Clements et al., 1986; Webster et al., 1988). In humans, antibodies against NA have been associated with decreased viral shedding and shortened duration of symptoms (Maier et al., 2019). Recent studies have highlighted the importance of examining neuraminidase inhibition titers as well as hemagglutinin inhibition titers as a measure of influenza disease severity, suggesting that NA-based protection should be an important consideration when developing new influenza vaccines (Monto et al., 2015; Memoli et al., 2016).

There have been several approaches taken to develop NA-based vaccines, including use of recombinant NA proteins, DNA plasmid-based NA expression, and NA incorporation onto VLPs to boost NA-directed antibody responses (Sandbulte et al., 2007; Easterbrook et al., 2012; Liu et al., 2015; Job et al., 2018). Recently, a recombinant modified vaccinia virus Ankara (MVA) vector was used to express either HA or NA from three different H7 viruses. Following vaccination with a MVA vector expressing N3 NA, mice were protected against challenge with H7N3 (Meseda et al., 2018). Likewise, a passive transfer of sera from MVA-N3 vaccinated mice into naive mice demonstrated protection against H7N3 infection (Meseda et al., 2018) In contrast, mice that received sera from the MVA-N7 vaccine were not protected against challenge with H7N3 despite the vaccine containing an NA from the same subtype as N3, suggesting that further optimization of this vaccine approach is required to elicit broader NA-based protection (Meseda et al., 2018). Another NA vaccine approach involved the use of recombinant baculovirus VLPs expressing the N1 NA from A/California/04/2009 (N1 VLP) (Kim et al., 2019). The N1 VLP vaccine elicited NA inhibition activity for H1N1, H5N1, and H3N2 (Kim et al., 2019). Additionally, the N1 VLP vaccine provided protection in mice against challenge with H1N1, H5N1, and H3N2 (Kim et al., 2019). This suggests that the N1 VLP vaccine has the potential to confer protection against different influenza strains with different N1 subtype NAs (Kim et al., 2019). Additional studies in animal models that more closely recapitulate human influenza infection, like ferrets, are necessary to further examine the efficacy of this vaccine, but this study does provide more evidence for the importance of considering NA-based immune responses for influenza vaccines.

An important challenge in inducing NA directed immune responses involves overcoming the immunodominance of HA over NA. In an attempt to subvert the HA immunodominance, a recent study generated two recombinant influenza viruses based on the H1N1 stain A/Puerto Rico/8/1934 (PR8) in which the NA stalk domain was extended by 15–30 amino acids (Broecker et al., 2019b). Using formalin-inactivated viruses expressing wildtype NA or the extended NA, the authors demonstrated that the extended NA stalk induced higher anti-NA IgG responses than the unmodified NA in mice (Broecker et al., 2019b). Similarly, extension of the NA stalk from H3N2 virus increased NA-specific antibody responses (Broecker et al., 2019b). While additional challenge studies need to be performed, the NA stalk extension approach offers an interesting solution to improving the immunogenicity of NA.

As with HA-directed vaccination approaches, these NA-directed approaches do not always demonstrate that protection elicited by the vaccine extends to both NA groups. Another consideration for NA-directed vaccines involves whether these approaches can provide robust protection in humans. As stated previously, NA-directed antibodies do not neutralize infection, and antibodies against NA have been shown to reduce the duration of symptoms in humans. As a result, more studies demonstrating protection in humans or models that more accurately reflect human influenza virus infection are necessary to demonstrate the protection these NA-based methods can provide.

M2 Ectodomain-Directed

The third surface protein on the influenza virion is the M2 protein. M2 is encoded by the M segment, which encodes

M1 from unspliced mRNA and M2 protein by mRNA splicing (Fields et al., 2013). M2 forms homotetramers and possesses ion channel activity that allows for acidification of the inside of the virion during endocytosis and facilitates the dissociation of the matrix protein M1 from viral ribonucleoprotein complexes (Fields et al., 2013). The M2 ectodomain (M2e), which is the exposed portion of the M2 protein found on the virion membrane, is highly conserved among influenza strains (Ito et al., 1991). Additionally, M2e-directed antibodies have been detected during influenza infection and have been shown to be protective in both mice and ferrets (Black et al., 1993; Neirynck et al., 1999; Zharikova et al., 2005; El Bakkouri et al., 2011). Importantly, like NA-directed antibodies, M2 antibodies do not prevent infection but instead reduce disease severity and control the spread of infection (Mozdzanowska et al., 1999; Grandea et al., 2010). Given the conserved nature of M2e and the protection demonstrated with M2e-directed antibodies, M2e has become a target for universal influenza vaccine approaches.

As with NA and the HA stalk, M2e-directed immune responses must overcome the highly immunogenic HA head domain. In addition, while M2 is abundantly expressed on the cell surface of infected cells, M2 is less abundant on the virion itself, a challenge for eliciting robust immune responses in LAIV approaches due to the reduced availability of M2 on the LAIV virion (Lamb et al., 1985; Zebedee and Lamb, 1988). Previous attempts to improve M2e-directed immune responses involved the use of several viral vectors including papaya mosaic virus (PapMV) carrying M2e, HPV VLPs conjugated to the M2 protein, or VLPs derived from the RNA phage Qβ that display the M2e protein (Ionescu et al., 2006; Bessa et al., 2008; Denis et al., 2008). These M2e-based vaccines elicited M2 specific antibody responses and protected mice against influenza A virus challenge, highlighting the importance of M2e mediated protection and the importance of considering the M2e protein when formulating universal influenza vaccines (Ionescu et al., 2006; Bessa et al., 2008; Denis et al., 2008). Another approach to improve M2e antibody responses involved expressing a membrane anchored tandem repeat of M2e epitope sequences of human, swine, and avian origin on recombinant baculovirus VLPs (M2e5x VLP) (Kim et al., 2013; Kang et al., 2019). The M2e5x VLPs induced M2e-specific antibody responses against H1N1, H3N2, and H5N1 and conferred protection in mice against both H1N1 and H3N2 challenges (Kim et al., 2013). Recently, combinatorial vaccination with both M2e5x VLPs and HA-VLPs generated higher antibody titers, reduced lung inflammation, and provided improved protection against lethal challenge with H5N1 as compared to M2e5x VLP alone (Kang et al., 2019). While this study did not address whether these responses were greater than with HA-VLP vaccination alone, this study demonstrated the utility of combinatorial vaccination approaches to induce broader protection. The M2e5x approach was taken a step further by supplementing an attenuated pandemic A/Netherlands/602/09 LAIV with M2e5x VLPs (Lee et al., 2019). This strategy showed improved protection from morbidity and mortality in mice following viral challenge as compared to vaccination with LAIV alone (Lee et al., 2019). Importantly, incorporating LAIV into this approach allowed for induction of T-cell responses, providing an additional layer of protection against influenza viruses in the respiratory tract (Lee et al., 2019). As with NA-directed approaches, the question remains whether M2e vaccines are able to provide meaningful protection in humans when M2e directed antibodies are only shown to reduce disease severity. Likewise, the modest protection provided by M2e vaccines is a limitation for this vaccination approach as is the breadth of influenza strain protection. While M2e vaccination approaches may not provide as strong of protection as other methods, an exciting possibility for M2e approaches involves the inclusion of M2e into other vaccine strategies. This approach should be considered in the development of other vaccines to enhance the immunogenicity and protection against a broader range of influenza viruses.

T-Cell-Directed

In comparison to the surface glycoproteins of influenza virus, the internal proteins show higher degrees of conservation among influenza viruses and are often targeted by the antigen-specific $CD8^+$ cytotoxic T cells and $CD4^+$ helper T lymphocytes. Given the importance of T cells in protection against influenza virus infection, vaccines stimulating influenza specific T-cell immunity have been explored as a promising avenue for improving influenza vaccine efficacy and developing a universal influenza vaccine.

Most T-cell-directed vaccine approaches involve targeting conserved internal influenza proteins or other highly conserved epitopes that stimulate T-cell-mediated immune responses. One such vaccine approach involved recombinantly expressing one B-cell epitope and two T-cell epitopes from H3 influenza strains in the flagellin of the *Salmonella* vaccine strain (Ben-Yedidia et al., 1999). After demonstrating the majority of the transplanted human cells in their human/mouse radiation chimeras were $CD8^+$ and $CD4^+$ cells, the recombinant vaccine was shown to elicit virus-specific antibodies and improved viral clearance after lethal challenge (Ben-Yedidia et al., 1999). In order to develop a more broadly protective vaccine, another study sought to identify conserved T-cell reactive regions by analyzing sequences from human and zoonotic influenza A and B viral proteins (Stoloff and Caparros-Wanderley, 2007). The internal proteins M1, NP, and PB1 and the surface protein M2 were found to contain conserved T-cell reactive regions, with M2 and PB1 sharing conserved sequences in both influenza A and B isolates (Stoloff and Caparros-Wanderley, 2007). Mice immunized with an antigen preparation comprised of the six conserved T-cell reactive regions, named FLU-v displayed increased $CD8^+$ T-cell responses and improved survival following challenge with PR8 (Stoloff and Caparros-Wanderley, 2007). While this study did not determine whether the vaccine provides protection against challenge with influenza B infection, it does further demonstrate the importance of stimulating $CD8^+$ T cells to generate protection against influenza infection. This vaccine is currently undergoing phase 2 clinical trials (Bernstein et al., 2019). Another conserved epitope vaccine undergoing clinical trials involving conserved T-cell and B-cell epitopes is the Multimeric-001 vaccine, which consists of nine conserved epitopes of HA, NP, and M1 from influenza A and B viruses (Atsmon et al., 2012). Healthy human volunteers vaccinated with the Multimeric-001 vaccine exhibited increased IgG titers against the Multimeric-001 vaccine component as well as increased IL-2 and IFNγ secretion (Atsmon et al., 2012). Additionally, sera from vaccinated subjects showed increased complement mediated lysis of infected MDCK cells (Atsmon et al., 2012). This measure was incorporated as an alternative to the hemagglutinin inhibition assay, which they were unable to use because the vaccine lacked the antigenic sites for neutralizing antibodies (Atsmon et al., 2012). While this study shows promise for inducing broad protection in humans, further challenge studies are needed to determine the efficacy of this vaccine.

As with the other vaccine approaches, there have been attempts to generate T-cell-based influenza vaccines through the use of viral vectors. One approach currently in clinical trials involves the use of a modified vaccinia virus Ankara (MVA) that encodes influenza proteins NP and M1 (MVA – NP + M1) (Berthoud et al., 2011; Lillie et al., 2012). A phase 1 clinical trial demonstrated that individuals vaccinated with the MVA – NP + M1 vaccine exhibited increased T-cell responses as measured by IFNγ ELISPOT, with the majority of them being antigen-specific T cells (Berthoud et al., 2011). Next, a phase 2a clinical trial was conducted in which volunteers vaccinated with the MVA – NP + M1 exhibited less severe symptoms and reduced viral shedding after challenge with A/Wisconsin/67/2005 (H3N2) (Lillie et al., 2012). This study was performed with a limited number of human volunteers, but it does highlight another promising avenue for stimulating T-cell-based protection against influenza.

Recently, another viral vector-based vaccine approach has been described using the live-attenuated vaccinia Wyeth backbone expressing HA, NA, M1, M2, and NP from H5N1 along with IL-15 as an adjuvant (Poon et al., 2009). In a mouse model, this vaccine was shown to be protective against both Group 1 and Group 2 HA viruses, including H7N9, H3N2, H1N1, and H7N7 (Valkenburg et al., 2014). Following depletion of $CD4^+$ T cells at the time of vaccination or challenge, vaccinated mice showed reduced survival, suggesting that $CD4^+$ T cells are required for this vaccine-mediated protection (Valkenburg et al., 2018). This vaccine also stimulated increased production of H5-specific $CD4^+$ and $CD8^+$ T cells from human PBMCs, highlighting its potential for protection in humans as well (Valkenburg et al., 2018). Together, these studies illustrate the importance of stimulating T-cell-based immunity for influenza virus protection.

Challenges to Universal Vaccine Development

An important question when discussing universal vaccine development involves defining the criteria for a successful universal influenza vaccine. Would a universal vaccine provide protection against all influenza A and B strains? Only influenza A or B? Or would the vaccine only provide universal protection within particular HA or NA subtypes? The route of administration should also be considered, especially when determining the durability of protection provided by the vaccine. Furthermore, many of the universal vaccine strategies described above require sequential vaccinations or boosters in order to achieve protection. Considering that individuals may be less likely to return to complete their vaccination regimens, this approach may have a negative impact on vaccine effectiveness from a public health standpoint. Likewise, sequential vaccination regimens with components that change at each booster vaccination may increase the likelihood of error during administration.

While the universal vaccine approaches described above demonstrate novel methods of improving protection against influenza virus infection, a concern that is often overlooked involves the degree to which pre-existing immunity impacts the antibody response to influenza infection and vaccination. This is true for all of the vaccination approaches, including HA, NA, M2e, and T-cell-directed approaches. This concept, referred to as "original antigenic sin," suggests that the first influenza virus variant an individual encounters impacts the immune response to subsequent influenza virus variants (Henry et al., 2018). While controversial, the concept that previous influenza virus exposure impacts antibody responses to influenza vaccination remains an important consideration for vaccine development (Henry et al., 2018). This can also be an important determinant in LAIV approaches, where pre-existing immunity can impact LAIV replication. It is important to note that most of the animal studies done to validate these vaccination approaches are done in naïve animals that lack any previous influenza virus exposure. While unavoidable, this serves to highlight the importance of experiments that more accurately recapitulate the complexity of pre-existing antibody responses in humans as well as thorough clinical trials in order to fully assess the potential for new vaccines to provide broad and long-lasting protection within the population.

THERAPEUTIC APPROACH: BROADLY NEUTRALIZING ANTIBODIES

While vaccination remains the most efficient method to provide protection against influenza virus infection, there is also significant interest in developing more broadly protective therapeutic methods for prevention and treatment of influenza virus infection. A growing area of interest involves utilizing broadly neutralizing antibodies to protect against influenza virus infection. As with influenza vaccines, a significant focus on broadly neutralizing antibody research revolves around the development of HA stem targeting antibodies, in particular antibodies that neutralize both Group 1 and Group 2 influenza virus HAs. Despite the fact that the majority of neutralizing antibodies targeting the HA stem only protect against Group 1 or Group 2 HAs, HA targeting antibodies capable of neutralizing both phylogenetic groups have been identified (Corti et al., 2011; Joyce et al., 2016). Further improvements in broadly neutralizing antibody discovery have enabled the development of novel therapies, several of which are currently in different stages of clinical trials. For example, one study was able to identify four broadly neutralizing influenza A antibodies through the activation and enrichment of human peripheral blood mononuclear cells from vaccinated donors (Nakamura et al., 2013). Of these four antibodies, two were able to neutralize both Group 1 and Group 2 influenza A viruses while also improving the survival of mice and ferrets that received the antibody 72 h post infection (Nakamura et al., 2013). Interestingly, co-administration of oseltamivir and the antibody after lethal challenge significantly improved the survival of mice as compared to either therapy alone, demonstrating a potential avenue for improving current therapies through co-administration of both antivirals and neutralizing antibodies (Nakamura et al., 2013). Using a novel antibody design approach, another broadly neutralizing HA antibody, VIS410, was engineered and shown to bind both Group 1 and Group 2 HAs (Tharakaraman et al., 2015). Experiments in mice demonstrated that VIS410 improved survival when administered either prophylactically or 48 h post infection (Tharakaraman et al., 2015). These studies also demonstrated improved protection when co-administered with oseltamivir (Tharakaraman et al., 2015). When administered post infection, VIS401-treated mice showed reduced clinical symptoms of influenza virus infection, including decreased viral spread and reduced damage in the lungs (Baranovich et al., 2016). VIS401 is currently under clinical trials. MEDI8852 is another broadly neutralizing antibody targeting the HA stem that has been shown to interact with both Group 1 and Group 2 HAs (Kallewaard et al., 2016). Even when administered 4 days post lethal virus challenge, MEDI8852 treatment improved survival of mice and protected against several different influenza A virus strains (Kallewaard et al., 2016). Similar results were observed in ferrets, with MEDI8852 providing protection against lethal challenge when administered up to 3 days post infection, further underscoring the therapeutic potential of this antibody (Kallewaard et al., 2016). In addition to several HA targeting monoclonal antibodies, a M2e targeting antibody, TCN-032, is currently in clinical trials (Ramos et al., 2015). Healthy human volunteers infected with H3N2 and treated with TCN-032 exhibited reduced viral shedding and reduced clinical symptoms (Ramos et al., 2015). While the broadly neutralizing antibodies in these studies show promise in providing protection in humans, the studies fail to address the potential for the development of escape mutants that are able to evade antibody neutralization following treatment with these antibodies. Studies examining whether prolonged treatment with these antibodies leads to resistance are important in determining whether these therapeutics can truly provide meaningful protection for a wide range of individuals. Together, these studies underscore the potential for utilizing broadly neutralizing antibodies to improve clinical outcomes of influenza virus infection.

CONCLUSIONS

Significant resources have been invested into the development of universal influenza virus vaccines and improved therapeutics for the treatment of influenza virus infection. Many universal influenza virus vaccine candidates focus on targeting conserved epitopes of influenza, including either the three influenza surface proteins or highly conserved internal proteins. In doing so, these approaches attempt to elicit broader protection against several strains of influenza as opposed to the strain-specific protection provided by current seasonal influenza vaccines. In attempting to generate a truly universal vaccine, which would offer protection against all influenza strains, these approaches have also highlighted innovative methods for improving current vaccination approaches. By providing protection for a broader range of influenza strains, these approaches have the potential to reduce the need for yearly vaccine reformulations. While influenza strains should still be closely monitored, broader protection against more influenza strains could aid in improving yearly vaccine efficacy. The development and discovery of broadly neutralizing antibodies also illustrate the important contributions these therapeutics can offer in preventing and improving disease outcomes associated with influenza virus infection. Additionally, these studies have provided an insight into novel combinatorial approaches, as seen with studies combining M2e5x VLPs and HA-VLPs to improve vaccine immunogenicity or by combining broadly neutralizing antibodies with current antivirals to improve recovery from influenza virus infection (Nakamura et al., 2013; Tharakaraman et al., 2015; Kang et al., 2019). While the ultimate goal of developing a truly universal influenza virus vaccine has yet to be achieved, the progress made in pursuit of this goal shows the exciting promise of these new approaches for improving influenza disease outcomes and as well as the public health burden associated with inefficient protection against influenza virus infection.

AUTHOR CONTRIBUTIONS

All authors listed have made a substantial, direct and intellectual contribution to the work, and approved it for publication.

FUNDING

OV is supported by the NIH Molecular and Cellular Biology training program at the University of Chicago (T32GM007183). BM is supported by NIAID grants (R01AI123359 and R01AI127775).

ACKNOWLEDGMENTS

We would like to thank Dr. Michael Rebagliati for critical reading of the manuscript.

REFERENCES

Ainai, A., Tamura, S., Suzuki, T., van Riet, E., Ito, R., Odagiri, T., et al. (2013). Intranasal vaccination with an inactivated whole influenza virus vaccine induces strong antibody responses in serum and nasal mucus of healthy adults. *Hum. Vaccin. Immunother.* 9, 1962–1970. doi: 10.4161/hv.25458

Allen, J. D., Ray, S., and Ross, T. M. (2018). Split inactivated COBRA vaccine elicits protective antibodies against H1N1 and H3N2 influenza viruses. *PLoS One* 13:e0204284. doi: 10.1371/journal.pone.0210043

Ambrose, C. S., Bright, H., and Mallory, R. (2016). Letter to the editor: potential causes of the decreased effectiveness of the influenza A(H1N1)pdm09 strain in live attenuated influenza vaccines. *Euro Surveill.* 21, pii: 30394. doi: 10.2807/1560-7917.ES.2016.21.45.30394

Ampofo, W. K., Azziz-Baumgartner, E., Bashir, U., Cox, N. J., Fasce, R., Giovanni, M., et al. (2015). Strengthening the influenza vaccine virus selection and development process: report of the 3rd WHO informal consultation for improving influenza vaccine virus selection held at WHO headquarters, Geneva, Switzerland, 1-3 April 2014. *Vaccine* 33, 4368–4382. doi: 10.1016/j.vaccine.2015.06.090

Asahi, Y., Yoshikawa, T., Watanabe, I., Iwasaki, T., Hasegawa, H., Sato, Y., et al. (2002). Protection against influenza virus infection in polymeric Ig receptor knockout mice immunized intranasally with adjuvant-combined vaccines. *J. Immunol.* 168, 2930–2938. doi: 10.4049/jimmunol.168.6.2930

Atsmon, J., Kate-Ilovitz, E., Shaikevich, D., Singer, Y., Volokhov, I., Haim, K. Y., et al. (2012). Safety and immunogenicity of multimeric-001--a novel universal influenza vaccine. *J. Clin. Immunol.* 32, 595–603. doi: 10.1007/s10875-011-9632-5

Baranovich, T., Jones, J. C., Russier, M., Vogel, P., Szretter, K. J., Sloan, S. E., et al. (2016). The Hemagglutinin stem-binding monoclonal antibody VIS410 controls influenza virus-induced acute respiratory distress syndrome. *Antimicrob. Agents Chemother.* 60, 2118–2131. doi: 10.1128/AAC.02457-15

Barr, I. G., Donis, R. O., Katz, J. M., McCauley, J. W., Odagiri, T., Trusheim, H., et al. (2018). Cell culture-derived influenza vaccines in the severe 2017–2018 epidemic season: a step towards improved influenza vaccine effectiveness. *NPJ Vaccines* 3, 1–5. doi: 10.1038/s41541-018-0079-z

Belz, G. T., Wodarz, D., Diaz, G., Nowak, M. A., and Doherty, P. C. (2002). Compromised influenza virus-specific CD8(+)-T-cell memory in CD4(+)-T-cell-deficient mice. *J. Virol.* 76, 12388–12393. doi: 10.1128/JVI.76.23.12388-12393.2002

Ben-Yedidia, T., Marcus, H., Reisner, Y., and Arnon, R. (1999). Intranasal administration of peptide vaccine protects human/mouse radiation chimera from influenza infection. *Int. Immunol.* 11, 1043–1051. doi: 10.1093/intimm/11.7.1043

Bernstein, D. I., Guptill, J., Naficy, A., Nachbagauer, R., Berlanda-Scorza, F., Feser, J., et al. (2019). Immunogenicity of chimeric haemagglutinin-based, universal influenza virus vaccine candidates: interim results of a randomised, placebo-controlled, phase 1 clinical trial. *Lancet Infect. Dis.* 20, 80–92. doi: 10.1016/S1473-3099(19)30393-7

Berthoud, T. K., Hamill, M., Lillie, P. J., Hwenda, L., Collins, K. A., Ewer, K. J., et al. (2011). Potent CD8+ T-cell immunogenicity in humans of a novel heterosubtypic influenza A vaccine, MVA-NP+M1. *Clin. Infect. Dis.* 52, 1–7. doi: 10.1093/cid/ciq015

Bessa, J., Schmitz, N., Hinton, H. J., Schwarz, K., Jegerlehner, A., and Bachmann, M. F. (2008). Efficient induction of mucosal and systemic immune responses by virus-like particles administered intranasally: implications for vaccine design. *Eur. J. Immunol.* 38, 114–126. doi: 10.1002/eji.200636959

Black, R. A., Rota, P. A., Gorodkova, N., Klenk, H. D., and Kendal, A. P. (1993). Antibody response to the M2 protein of influenza A virus expressed in insect cells. *J. Gen. Virol.* 74, 143–146. doi: 10.1099/0022-1317-74-1-143

Broecker, F., Liu, S. T. H., Suntronwong, N., Sun, W., Bailey, M. J., Nachbagauer, R., et al. (2019a). A mosaic hemagglutinin-based influenza virus vaccine candidate protects mice from challenge with divergent H3N2 strains. *NPJ Vaccines* 31, 1–9. doi: 10.1038/s41541-019-0126-4

Broecker, F., Zheng, A., Suntrongwong, N., Sun, W., Bailey, M. J., Krammer, F., et al. (2019b). Extending the stalk enhances immunogenicity of the influenza virus neuraminidase. *J. Virol.* 93, 1–12. doi: 10.1128/JVI.00840-19

Bullough, P. A., Hughson, F. M., Skehel, J. J., and Wiley, D. C. (1994). Structure of influenza haemagglutinin at the pH of membrane fusion. *Nature* 371, 37–43. doi: 10.1038/371037a0

Carter, D. M., Darby, C. A., Lefoley, B. C., Crevar, C. J., Alefantis, T., Oomen, R., et al. (2016). Design and characterization of a computationally optimized broadly reactive hemagglutinin vaccine for H1N1 influenza viruses. *J. Virol.* 90, 4720–4734. doi: 10.1128/JVI.03152-15

Clements, M. L., Betts, R. F., Tierney, E. L., and Murphy, B. R. (1986). Serum and nasal wash antibodies associated with resistance to experimental challenge with influenza A wild-type virus. *J. Clin. Microbiol.* 24, 157–160. doi: 10.1128/JCM.24.1.157-160.1986

Corti, D., Voss, J., Gamblin, S. J., Codoni, G., Macagno, A., Jarrossay, D., et al. (2011). A neutralizing antibody selected from plasma cells that binds to group 1 and group 2 influenza A hemagglutinins. *Science* 333, 850–856. doi: 10.1126/science.1205669

Cox, M. M., and Hollister, J. R. (2009). FluBlok, a next generation influenza vaccine manufactured in insect cells. *Biologicals* 37, 182–189. doi: 10.1016/j.biologicals.2009.02.014

David, S., Skowronski, D., Tweed, S., Tuk, T., Danderfer, G., Li, Y., et al. (2005). Epidemiologic profile of a new H3N2 variant of influenza A mismatched to vaccine, 2003-2004 influenza season. *Can. Commun. Dis. Rep.* 31, 21–31. Available at: https://www.canada.ca/en/public-health/services/reports-publications/canada-communicable-disease-report-ccdr/monthly-issue/2005-31/epidemiologic-profile-a-new-h3n2-variant-influenza-a-mismatched-vaccine-2003-2004-influenza-season.html

Denis, J., Acosta-Ramirez, E., Zhao, Y., Hamelin, M. E., Koukavica, I., Baz, M., et al. (2008). Development of a universal influenza A vaccine based on the M2e peptide fused to the papaya mosaic virus (PapMV) vaccine platform. *Vaccine* 26, 3395–3403. doi: 10.1016/j.vaccine.2008.04.052

DiLillo, D. J., Tan, G. S., Palese, P., and Ravetch, J. V. (2014). Broadly neutralizing hemagglutinin stalk-specific antibodies require FcγR interactions for protection against influenza virus in vivo. *Nat. Med.* 20, 143–151. doi: 10.1038/nm.3443

Dreyfus, C., Laursen, N. S., Kwaks, T., Zuijdgeest, D., Khayat, R., Ekiert, D. C., et al. (2012). Highly conserved protective epitopes on influenza B viruses. *Science* 337, 1343–1348. doi: 10.1126/science.1222908

Easterbrook, J. D., Schwartzman, L. M., Gao, J., Kash, J. C., Morens, D. M., Couzens, L., et al. (2012). Protection against a lethal H5N1 influenza challenge by intranasal immunization with virus-like particles containing 2009 pandemic H1N1 neuraminidase in mice. *Virology* 432, 39–44. doi: 10.1016/j.virol.2012.06.003

Ekiert, D. C., Bhabha, G., Elsliger, M. A., Friesen, R. H., Jongeneelen, M., Throsby, M., et al. (2009). Antibody recognition of a highly conserved influenza virus epitope. *Science* 324, 246–251. doi: 10.1126/science.1171491

El Bakkouri, K., Descamps, F., De Filette, M., Smet, A., Festjens, E., Birkett, A., et al. (2011). Universal vaccine based on ectodomain of matrix protein 2 of influenza A: Fc receptors and alveolar macrophages mediate protection. *J. Immunol.* 186, 1022–1031. doi: 10.4049/jimmunol.0902147

Erbelding, E. J., Post, D. J., Stemmy, E. J., Roberts, P. C., Augustine, A. D., Ferguson, S., et al. (2018). A universal influenza vaccine: the strategic plan for the National Institute of Allergy and Infectious Diseases. *J. Infect. Dis.* 218, 347–354. doi: 10.1093/infdis/jiy103

Fernandez Gonzalez, S., Jayasekera, J. P., and Carroll, M. C. (2008). Complement and natural antibody are required in the long-term memory response to influenza virus. *Vaccine* 26(Suppl. 8), I86–I93. doi: 10.1016/j.vaccine.2008.11.057

Fields, B. N., Knipe, D. M., and Howley, P. M. (2013). *Fields virology*. Philadelphia: Lippincott-Raven Publishers.

Gerdil, C. (2003). The annual production cycle for influenza vaccine. *Vaccine* 21, 1776–1779. doi: 10.1016/S0264-410X(03)00071-9

Giles, B. M., Crevar, C. J., Carter, D. M., Bissel, S. J., Schultz-Cherry, S., Wiley, C. A., et al. (2012). A computationally optimized hemagglutinin virus-like particle vaccine elicits broadly reactive antibodies that protect nonhuman primates from H5N1 infection. *J. Infect. Dis.* 205, 1562–1570. doi: 10.1093/infdis/jis232

Giles, B. M., and Ross, T. M. (2011). A computationally optimized broadly reactive antigen (COBRA) based H5N1 VLP vaccine elicits broadly reactive antibodies in mice and ferrets. *Vaccine* 29, 3043–3054. doi: 10.1016/j.vaccine.2011.01.100

Grandea, A. G. III, Olsen, O. A., Cox, T. C., Renshaw, M., Hammond, P. W., Chan-Hui, P. Y., et al. (2010). Human antibodies reveal a protective epitope that is highly conserved among human and nonhuman influenza A viruses. *Proc. Natl. Acad. Sci. USA* 107, 12658–12663. doi: 10.1073/pnas.0911806107

Graves, P. N., Schulman, J. L., Young, J. F., and Palese, P. (1983). Preparation of influenza virus subviral particles lacking the HA1 subunit of hemagglutinin: unmasking of cross-reactive HA2 determinants. *Virology* 126, 106–116. doi: 10.1016/0042-6822(83)90465-8

Grohskopf, L. A., Sokolow, L. Z., Broder, K. R., Olsen, S. J., Karron, R. A., Jernigan, D. B., et al. (2016). Prevention and control of seasonal influenza with vaccines. *MMWR Recomm. Rep.* 65, 1–54. doi: 10.15585/mmwr.rr6505a1

Grohskopf, L. A., Sokolow, L. Z., Broder, K. R., Walter, E. B., Bresee, J. S., Fry, A. M., et al. (2017). Prevention and control of seasonal influenza with vaccines: recommendations of the advisory committee on immunization practices — United States, 2017–18 influenza season. *MMWR Recomm. Rep.* 66, 1–20. doi: 10.15585/mmwr.rr6602a1

Grohskopf, L. A., Sokolow, L. Z., Fry, A. M., Walter, E. B., and Jernigan, D. B. (2018). Update: ACIP recommendations for the use of quadrivalent live attenuated influenza vaccine (LAIV4) - United States, 2018-19 influenza season. *MMWR Morb. Mortal. Wkly Rep.* 67, 643–645. doi: 10.15585/mmwr.mm6722a5

Hai, R., Krammer, F., Tan, G. S., Pica, N., Eggink, D., Maamary, J., et al. (2012). Influenza viruses expressing chimeric hemagglutinins: globular head and stalk domains derived from different subtypes. *J. Virol.* 86, 5774–5781. doi: 10.1128/JVI.00137-12

Halloran, M. E., Piedra, P. A., Longini, I. M. Jr., Gaglani, M. J., Schmotzer, B., Fewlass, C., et al. (2007). Efficacy of trivalent, cold-adapted, influenza virus vaccine against influenza A (Fujian), a drift variant, during 2003-2004. *Vaccine* 25, 4038–4045. doi: 10.1016/j.vaccine.2007.02.060

Hamada, H., Bassity, E., Flies, A., Strutt, T. M., Garcia-Hernandez Mde, L., McKinstry, K. K., et al. (2013). Multiple redundant effector mechanisms of CD8+ T cells protect against influenza infection. *J. Immunol.* 190, 296–306. doi: 10.4049/jimmunol.1200571

Hamada, H., Garcia-Hernandez Mde, L., Reome, J. B., Misra, S. K., Strutt, T. M., McKinstry, K. K., et al. (2009). Tc17, a unique subset of CD8 T cells that can protect against lethal influenza challenge. *J. Immunol.* 182, 3469–3481. doi: 10.4049/jimmunol.0801814

He, X. S., Holmes, T. H., Zhang, C., Mahmood, K., Kemble, G. W., Lewis, D. B., et al. (2006). Cellular immune responses in children and adults receiving inactivated or live attenuated influenza vaccines. *J. Virol.* 80, 11756–11766. doi: 10.1128/JVI.01460-06

He, W., Tan, G. S., Mullarkey, C. E., Lee, A. J., Lam, M. M. W., Krammer, F., et al. (2016). Epitope specificity plays a critical role in regulating antibody-dependent cell-mediated cytotoxicity against influenza A virus. *Proc. Natl. Acad. Sci. USA* 113, 11931–11936. doi: 10.1073/pnas.1609316113

Henry, C., Palm, A. E., Krammer, F., and Wilson, P. C. (2018). From original antigenic sin to the universal influenza virus vaccine. *Trends Immunol.* 39, 70–79. doi: 10.1016/j.it.2017.08.003

Hoft, D. F., Babusis, E., Worku, S., Spencer, C. T., Lottenbach, K., Truscott, S. M., et al. (2011). Live and inactivated influenza vaccines induce similar humoral responses, but only live vaccines induce diverse T-cell responses in young children. *J. Infect. Dis.* 204, 845–853. doi: 10.1093/infdis/jir436

Impagliazzo, A., Milder, F., Kuipers, H., Wagner, M. V., Zhu, X., Hoffman, R. M., et al. (2015). A stable trimeric influenza hemagglutinin stem as a broadly protective immunogen. *Science* 349, 1301–1306. doi: 10.1126/science.aac7263

Ionescu, R. M., Przysiecki, C. T., Liang, X., Garsky, V. M., Fan, J., Wang, B., et al. (2006). Pharmaceutical and immunological evaluation of human papillomavirus viruslike particle as an antigen carrier. *J. Pharm. Sci.* 95, 70–79. doi: 10.1002/jps.20493

Ito, T., Gorman, O. T., Kawaoka, Y., Bean, W. J., and Webster, R. G. (1991). Evolutionary analysis of the influenza A virus M gene with comparison of the M1 and M2 proteins. *J. Virol.* 65, 5491–5498. doi: 10.1128/JVI.65.10.5491-5498.1991

Iwasaki, A., and Pillai, P. S. (2014). Innate immunity to influenza virus infection. *Nat. Rev. Immunol.* 14, 315–328. doi: 10.1038/nri3665

Job, E. R., Ysenbaert, T., Smet, A., Christopoulou, I., Strugnell, T., Oloo, E. O., et al. (2018). Broadened immunity against influenza by vaccination with computationally designed influenza virus N1 neuraminidase constructs. *NPJ Vaccines* 3:55. doi: 10.1038/s41541-018-0093-1

Joyce, M. G., Wheatley, A. K., Thomas, P. V., Chuang, G. Y., Soto, C., Bailer, R. T., et al. (2016). Vaccine-induced antibodies that neutralize group 1 and group 2 influenza A viruses. *Cell* 166, 609–623. doi: 10.1016/j.cell.2016.06.043

Kallen, K. J., Heidenreich, R., Schnee, M., Petsch, B., Schlake, T., Thess, A., et al. (2013). A novel, disruptive vaccination technology: self-adjuvanted RNActive((R)) vaccines. *Hum. Vaccin. Immunother.* 9, 2263–2276. doi: 10.4161/hv.25181

Kallewaard, N. L., Corti, D., Collins, P. J., Neu, U., McAuliffe, J. M., Benjamin, E., et al. (2016). Structure and function analysis of an antibody recognizing all influenza A subtypes. *Cell* 166, 596–608. doi: 10.1016/j.cell.2016.05.073

Kanekiyo, M., Ellis, D., and King, N. P. (2019). New vaccine design and delivery technologies. *J. Infect. Dis.* 219, S88–S96. doi: 10.1093/infdis/jiy745

Kanekiyo, M., Wei, C. J., Yassine, H. M., McTamney, P. M., Boyington, J. C., Whittle, J. R., et al. (2013). Self-assembling influenza nanoparticle vaccines elicit broadly neutralizing H1N1 antibodies. *Nature* 499, 102–106. doi: 10.1038/nature12202

Kang, H. J., Chu, K. B., Lee, D. H., Lee, S. H., Park, B. R., Kim, M. C., et al. (2019). Influenza M2 virus-like particle vaccination enhances protection in combination with avian influenza HA VLPs. *PLoS One* 14:e0216871. doi: 10.1371/journal.pone.0216871

Kilbourne, E. D., Johansson, B. E., and Grajower, B. (1990). Independent and disparate evolution in nature of influenza A virus hemagglutinin and neuraminidase glycoproteins. *Proc. Natl. Acad. Sci. USA* 87, 786–790.

Kim, K. H., Lee, Y. T., Park, S., Jung, Y. J., Lee, Y., Ko, E. J., et al. (2019). Neuraminidase expressing virus-like particle vaccine provides effective cross protection against influenza virus. *Virology* 535, 179–188. doi: 10.1016/j.virol.2019.07.008

Kim, M. C., Song, J. M., Eunjo, O., Kwon, Y. M., Lee, Y. J., Compans, R. W., et al. (2013). Virus-like particles containing multiple M2 extracellular domains confer improved cross-protection against various subtypes of influenza virus. *Mol. Ther.* 21, 485–492. doi: 10.1038/mt.2012.246

Knossow, M., Gaudier, M., Douglas, A., Barrere, B., Bizebard, T., Barbey, C., et al. (2002). Mechanism of neutralization of influenza virus infectivity by antibodies. *Virology* 302, 294–298. doi: 10.1006/viro.2002.1625

Krammer, F., Pica, N., Hai, R., Margine, I., and Palese, P. (2013). Chimeric hemagglutinin influenza virus vaccine constructs elicit broadly protective stalk-specific antibodies. *J. Virol.* 87, 6542–6550. doi: 10.1128/JVI.00641-13

Lamb, Y. N. (2019). Cell-based quadrivalent inactivated influenza virus vaccine (flucelvax((R)) tetra/flucelvax quadrivalent((R))): a review in the prevention of influenza. *Drugs* 79, 1337–1348. doi: 10.1007/s40265-019-01176-z

Lamb, R. A., Zebedee, S. L., and Richardson, C. D. (1985). Influenza virus M2 protein is an integral membrane protein expressed on the infected-cell surface. *Cell* 40, 627–633. doi: 10.1016/0092-8674(85)90211-9

Ledgerwood, J. E., Wei, C. J., Hu, Z., Gordon, I. J., Enama, M. E., Hendel, C. S., et al. (2011). DNA priming and influenza vaccine immunogenicity: two phase 1 open label randomised clinical trials. *Lancet Infect. Dis.* 11, 916–924. doi: 10.1016/S1473-3099(11)70240-7

Lee, Y. T., Kim, K. H., Ko, E. J., Kim, M. C., Lee, Y. N., Hwang, H. S., et al. (2019). Enhancing the cross protective efficacy of live attenuated influenza virus vaccine by supplemented vaccination with M2 ectodomain virus-like particles. *Virology* 529, 111–121. doi: 10.1016/j.virol.2019.01.017

Lillie, P. J., Berthoud, T. K., Powell, T. J., Lambe, T., Mullarkey, C., Spencer, A. J., et al. (2012). Preliminary assessment of the efficacy of a T-cell-based influenza vaccine, MVA-NP+M1, in humans. *Clin. Infect. Dis.* 55, 19–25. doi: 10.1093/cid/cis327

Liu, W. C., Lin, C. Y., Tsou, Y. T., Jan, J. T., and Wu, S. C. (2015). Cross-reactive neuraminidase-inhibiting antibodies elicited by immunization with recombinant neuraminidase proteins of H5N1 and pandemic H1N1 influenza A viruses. *J. Virol.* 89, 7224–7234. doi: 10.1128/JVI.00585-15

Liu, W. C., Nachbagauer, R., Stadlbauer, D., Solorzano, A., Berlanda-Scorza, F., Garcia-Sastre, A., et al. (2019). Sequential immunization with live-attenuated chimeric Hemagglutinin-based vaccines confers Heterosubtypic immunity against influenza A viruses in a preclinical ferret model. *Front. Immunol.* 10:756. doi: 10.3389/fimmu.2019.00756

Lukacher, A. E., Braciale, V. L., and Braciale, T. J. (1984). In vivo effector function of influenza virus-specific cytotoxic T lymphocyte clones is highly specific. *J. Exp. Med.* 160, 814–826. doi: 10.1084/jem.160.3.814

Maier, H. E., Nachbagauer, R., Kuan, G., Ng, S., Lopez, R., Sanchez, N., et al. (2019). Pre-existing anti-neuraminidase antibodies are associated with shortened duration of influenza A (H1N1)pdm virus shedding and illness in naturally infected adults. *Clin. Infect. Dis.* 1–8. doi: 10.1093/cid/ciz639 [Epub ahead of print].

Margine, I., Krammer, F., Hai, R., Heaton, N. S., Tan, G. S., Andrews, S. A., et al. (2013). Hemagglutinin stalk-based universal vaccine constructs protect against group 2 influenza A viruses. *J. Virol.* 87, 10435–10446. doi: 10.1128/JVI.01715-13

McKinstry, K. K., Strutt, T. M., Kuang, Y., Brown, D. M., Sell, S., Dutton, R. W., et al. (2012). Memory CD4+ T cells protect against influenza through multiple synergizing mechanisms. *J. Clin. Invest.* 122, 2847–2856. doi: 10.1172/JCI63689

Memoli, M. J., Shaw, P. A., Han, A., Czajkowski, L., Reed, S., Athota, R., et al. (2016). Evaluation of antihemagglutinin and antineuraminidase antibodies as correlates of protection in an influenza A/H1N1 virus healthy human challenge model. *MBio* 7:e00417-16. doi: 10.1128/mBio.00417-16

Meseda, C. A., Atukorale, V., Soto, J., Eichelberger, M. C., Gao, J., Wang, W., et al. (2018). Immunogenicity and protection against influenza H7N3 in mice by modified vaccinia virus ankara vectors expressing influenza virus hemagglutinin or neuraminidase. *Sci. Rep.* 8:5364. doi: 10.1038/s41598-018-23712-9

Monto, A. S., Petrie, J. G., Cross, R. T., Johnson, E., Liu, M., Zhong, W., et al. (2015). Antibody to influenza virus neuraminidase: an independent correlate of protection. *J. Infect. Dis.* 212, 1191–1199. doi: 10.1093/infdis/jiv195

Mozdzanowska, K., Maiese, K., Furchner, M., and Gerhard, W. (1999). Treatment of influenza virus-infected SCID mice with nonneutralizing antibodies specific for the transmembrane proteins matrix 2 and neuraminidase reduces the pulmonary virus titer but fails to clear the infection. *Virology* 254, 138–146. doi: 10.1006/viro.1998.9534

Murphy, B. R., Kasel, J. A., and Chanock, R. M. (1972). Association of serum anti-neuraminidase antibody with resistance to influenza in man. *N. Engl. J. Med.* 286, 1329–1332. doi: 10.1056/NEJM197206222862502

Nachbagauer, R., Krammer, F., and Albrecht, R. A. (2018). A live-attenuated prime, inactivated boost vaccination strategy with chimeric hemagglutinin-based universal influenza virus vaccines provides protection in ferrets: a confirmatory study. *Vaccines* 6, 1–11. doi: 10.3390/vaccines6030047

Nachbagauer, R., Liu, W. C., Choi, A., Wohlbold, T. J., Atlas, T., Rajendran, M., et al. (2017). A universal influenza virus vaccine candidate confers protection against pandemic H1N1 infection in preclinical ferret studies. *NPJ Vaccines* 2:26. doi: 10.1038/s41541-017-0026-4

Nakamura, G., Chai, N., Park, S., Chiang, N., Lin, Z., Chiu, H., et al. (2013). An in vivo human-plasmablast enrichment technique allows rapid identification of therapeutic influenza A antibodies. *Cell Host Microbe* 14, 93–103. doi: 10.1016/j.chom.2013.06.004

Neirynck, S., Deroo, T., Saelens, X., Vanlandschoot, P., Jou, W. M., and Fiers, W. (1999). A universal influenza A vaccine based on the extracellular domain of the M2 protein. *Nat. Med.* 5, 1157–1163. doi: 10.1038/13484

Okuno, Y., Isegawa, Y., Sasao, F., and Ueda, S. (1993). A common neutralizing epitope conserved between the hemagglutinins of influenza A virus H1 and H2 strains. *J. Virol.* 67, 2552–2558. doi: 10.1128/JVI.67.5.2552-2558.1993

Petsch, B., Schnee, M., Vogel, A. B., Lange, E., Hoffmann, B., Voss, D., et al. (2012). Protective efficacy of in vitro synthesized, specific mRNA vaccines against influenza A virus infection. *Nat. Biotechnol.* 30, 1210–1216. doi: 10.1038/nbt.2436

Pica, N., Hai, R., Krammer, F., Wang, T. T., Maamary, J., Eggink, D., et al. (2012). Hemagglutinin stalk antibodies elicited by the 2009 pandemic influenza virus as a mechanism for the extinction of seasonal H1N1 viruses. *Proc. Natl. Acad. Sci. USA* 109, 2573–2578. doi: 10.1073/pnas.1200039109

Poon, L. L., Leung, Y. H., Nicholls, J. M., Perera, P. Y., Lichy, J. H., Yamamoto, M., et al. (2009). Vaccinia virus-based multivalent H5N1 avian influenza vaccines adjuvanted with IL-15 confer sterile cross-clade protection in mice. *J. Immunol.* 182, 3063–3071. doi: 10.4049/jimmunol.0803467

Putri, W., Muscatello, D. J., Stockwell, M. S., and Newall, A. T. (2018). Economic burden of seasonal influenza in the United States. *Vaccine* 36, 3960–3966. doi: 10.1016/j.vaccine.2018.05.057

Ramos, E. L., Mitcham, J. L., Koller, T. D., Bonavia, A., Usner, D. W., Balaratnam, G., et al. (2015). Efficacy and safety of treatment with an anti-m2e monoclonal antibody in experimental human influenza. *J. Infect. Dis.* 211, 1038–1044. doi: 10.1093/infdis/jiu539

Renegar, K. B., Small, P. A. Jr., Boykins, L. G., and Wright, P. F. (2004). Role of IgA versus IgG in the control of influenza viral infection in the murine respiratory tract. *J. Immunol.* 173, 1978–1986. doi: 10.4049/jimmunol.173.3.1978

Robertson, C. A., DiazGranados, C. A., Decker, M. D., Chit, A., Mercer, M., and Greenberg, D. P. (2016). Fluzone(R) high-dose influenza vaccine. *Expert Rev. Vaccines* 15, 1495–1505. doi: 10.1080/14760584.2016.1254044

Rogers, G. N., Paulson, J. C., Daniels, R. S., Skehel, J. J., Wilson, I. A., and Wiley, D. C. (1983). Single amino acid substitutions in influenza haemagglutinin change receptor binding specificity. *Nature* 304, 76–78. doi: 10.1038/304076a0

Rota, P. A., Wallis, T. R., Harmon, M. W., Rota, J. S., Kendal, A. P., and Nerome, K. (1990). Cocirculation of two distinct evolutionary lineages of influenza type B virus since 1983. *Virology* 175, 59–68. doi: 10.1016/0042-6822(90)90186-U

Rothbarth, P. H., Groen, J., Bohnen, A. M., de Groot, R., and Osterhaus, A. D. (1999). Influenza virus serology--a comparative study. *J. Virol. Methods* 78, 163–169. doi: 10.1016/S0166-0934(98)00174-8

Rott, R., Becht, H., and Orlich, M. (1974). The significance of influenza virus neuraminidase in immunity. *J. Gen. Virol.* 22, 35–41. doi: 10.1099/0022-1317-22-1-35

Sagawa, H., Ohshima, A., Kato, I., Okuno, Y., and Isegawa, Y. (1996). The immunological activity of a deletion mutant of influenza virus haemagglutinin lacking the globular region. *J. Gen. Virol.* 77, 1483–1487. doi: 10.1099/0022-1317-77-7-1483

Sandbulte, M. R., Jimenez, G. S., Boon, A. C., Smith, L. R., Treanor, J. J., and Webby, R. J. (2007). Cross-reactive neuraminidase antibodies afford partial protection against H5N1 in mice and are present in unexposed humans. *PLoS Med.* 4:e59. doi: 10.1371/journal.pmed.0040059

Skehel, J. J., Bayley, P. M., Brown, E. B., Martin, S. R., Waterfield, M. D., White, J. M., et al. (1982). Changes in the conformation of influenza virus hemagglutinin at the pH optimum of virus-mediated membrane fusion. *Proc. Natl. Acad. Sci. USA* 79, 968–972.

Skowronski, D. M., Janjua, N. Z., De Serres, G., Sabaiduc, S., Eshaghi, A., Dickinson, J. A., et al. (2014). Low 2012-13 influenza vaccine effectiveness associated with mutation in the egg-adapted H3N2 vaccine strain not antigenic drift in circulating viruses. *PLoS One* 9:e92153. doi: 10.1371/journal.pone.0092153

Skowronski, D. M., Masaro, C., Kwindt, T. L., Mak, A., Petric, M., Li, Y., et al. (2007). Estimating vaccine effectiveness against laboratory-confirmed influenza using a sentinel physician network: results from the 2005-2006 season of dual A and B vaccine mismatch in Canada. *Vaccine* 25, 2842–2851. doi: 10.1016/j.vaccine.2006.10.002

Sridhar, S., Begom, S., Bermingham, A., Hoschler, K., Adamson, W., Carman, W., et al. (2013). Cellular immune correlates of protection against symptomatic pandemic influenza. *Nat. Med.* 19, 1305–1312. doi: 10.1038/nm.3350

Sridhar, S., Brokstad, K. A., and Cox, R. J. (2015). Influenza vaccination strategies: comparing inactivated and live attenuated influenza vaccines. *Vaccines* 3, 373–389. doi: 10.3390/vaccines3020373

Stachyra, A., Gora-Sochacka, A., and Sirko, A. (2014). DNA vaccines against influenza. *Acta Biochim. Pol.* 61, 515–522. doi: 10.18388/abp.2014_1873

Steel, J., Lowen, A. C., Wang, T. T., Yondola, M., Gao, Q., Haye, K., et al. (2010). Influenza virus vaccine based on the conserved hemagglutinin stalk domain. *MBio* 1, 1–9. doi: 10.1128/mBio.00018-10

Stoloff, G. A., and Caparros-Wanderley, W. (2007). Synthetic multi-epitope peptides identified in silico induce protective immunity against multiple influenza serotypes. *Eur. J. Immunol.* 37, 2441–2449. doi: 10.1002/eji.200737254

Sui, J., Hwang, W. C., Perez, S., Wei, G., Aird, D., Chen, L. M., et al. (2009). Structural and functional bases for broad-spectrum neutralization of avian and human influenza A viruses. *Nat. Struct. Mol. Biol.* 16, 265–273. doi: 10.1038/nsmb.1566

Sun, W., Kirkpatrick, E., Ermler, M., Nachbagauer, R., Broecker, F., Krammer, F., et al. (2019). Development of influenza B universal vaccine candidates using the "mosaic" Hemagglutinin approach. *J. Virol.* 93, 1–17. doi: 10.1128/JVI.00333-19

Tamura, S., Funato, H., Hirabayashi, Y., Kikuta, K., Suzuki, Y., Nagamine, T., et al. (1990). Functional role of respiratory tract haemagglutinin-specific IgA antibodies in protection against influenza. *Vaccine* 8, 479–485. doi: 10.1016/0264-410X(90)90250-P

Tharakaraman, K., Subramanian, V., Viswanathan, K., Sloan, S., Yen, H. L., Barnard, D. L., et al. (2015). A broadly neutralizing human monoclonal antibody is effective against H7N9. *Proc. Natl. Acad. Sci. USA* 112, 10890–10895. doi: 10.1073/pnas.1502374112

Throsby, M., van den Brink, E., Jongeneelen, M., Poon, L. L., Alard, P., Cornelissen, L., et al. (2008). Heterosubtypic neutralizing monoclonal antibodies cross-protective against H5N1 and H1N1 recovered from human IgM+ memory B cells. *PLoS One* 3:e3942. doi: 10.1371/journal.pone.0003942

Tisa, V., Barberis, I., Faccio, V., Paganino, C., Trucchi, C., Martini, M., et al. (2016). Quadrivalent influenza vaccine: a new opportunity to reduce the influenza burden. *J. Prev. Med. Hyg.* 57, E28–E33. doi: 10.15167/2421-4248/jpmh2016.57.1.600

Valkenburg, S. A., Li, O. T. W., Li, A., Bull, M., Waldmann, T. A., Perera, L. P., et al. (2018). Protection by universal influenza vaccine is mediated by memory CD4 T cells. *Vaccine* 36, 4198–4206. doi: 10.1016/j.vaccine.2018.06.007

Valkenburg, S. A., Li, O. T., Mak, P. W., Mok, C. K., Nicholls, J. M., Guan, Y., et al. (2014). IL-15 adjuvanted multivalent vaccinia-based universal influenza vaccine requires CD4+ T cells for heterosubtypic protection. *Proc. Natl. Acad. Sci. USA* 111, 5676–5681. doi: 10.1073/pnas.1403684111

Vareckova, E., Mucha, V., Ciampor, F., Betakova, T., and Russ, G. (1993). Monoclonal antibodies demonstrate accessible HA2 epitopes in minor subpopulation of native influenza virus haemagglutinin molecules. *Arch. Virol.* 130, 45–56. doi: 10.1007/BF01318995

Webster, R. G., Reay, P. A., and Laver, W. G. (1988). Protection against lethal influenza with neuraminidase. *Virology* 164, 230–237. doi: 10.1016/0042-6822(88)90640-X

Webster, R. G., Sharp, G. B., and Claas, E. C. (1995). Interspecies transmission of influenza viruses. *Am. J. Respir. Crit. Care Med.* 152, S25–S30. doi: 10.1164/ajrccm/152.4_Pt_2.S25

Wilson, I. A., Skehel, J. J., and Wiley, D. C. (1981). Structure of the haemagglutinin membrane glycoprotein of influenza virus at 3 A resolution. *Nature* 289, 366–373. doi: 10.1038/289366a0

Wong, T. M., Allen, J. D., Bebin-Blackwell, A. G., Carter, D. M., Alefantis, T., DiNapoli, J., et al. (2017). Computationally optimized broadly reactive hemagglutinin elicits hemagglutination inhibition antibodies against a panel of H3N2 influenza virus cocirculating variants. *J. Virol.* 91, 1–19. doi: 10.1128/JVI.01581-17

Wu, N. C., Lv, H., Thompson, A. J., Wu, D. C., Ng, W. W. S., Kadam, R. U., et al. (2019). Preventing an antigenically disruptive mutation in egg-based H3N2 seasonal influenza vaccines by mutational incompatibility. *Cell Host Microbe* 25, 836–844.e5. doi: 10.1016/j.chom.2019.04.013

Wu, N. C., Zost, S. J., Thompson, A. J., Oyen, D., Nycholat, C. M., McBride, R., et al. (2017). A structural explanation for the low effectiveness of the seasonal influenza H3N2 vaccine. *PLoS Pathog.* 13:e1006682. doi: 10.1371/journal.ppat.1006682

Yap, K. L., Ada, G. L., and McKenzie, I. F. (1978). Transfer of specific cytotoxic T lymphocytes protects mice inoculated with influenza virus. *Nature* 273, 238–239. doi: 10.1038/273238a0

Yassine, H. M., Boyington, J. C., McTamney, P. M., Wei, C. J., Kanekiyo, M., Kong, W. P., et al. (2015). Hemagglutinin-stem nanoparticles generate heterosubtypic influenza protection. *Nat. Med.* 21, 1065–1070. doi: 10.1038/nm.3927

Zebedee, S. L., and Lamb, R. A. (1988). Influenza A virus M2 protein: monoclonal antibody restriction of virus growth and detection of M2 in virions. *J. Virol.* 62, 2762–2772. doi: 10.1128/JVI.62.8.2762-2772.1988

Zharikova, D., Mozdzanowska, K., Feng, J., Zhang, M., and Gerhard, W. (2005). Influenza type A virus escape mutants emerge in vivo in the presence of antibodies to the ectodomain of matrix protein 2. *J. Virol.* 79, 6644–6654. doi: 10.1128/JVI.79.11.6644-6654.2005

Zost, S. J., Parkhouse, K., Gumina, M. E., Kim, K., Diaz Perez, S., Wilson, P. C., et al. (2017). Contemporary H3N2 influenza viruses have a glycosylation site that alters binding of antibodies elicited by egg-adapted vaccine strains. *Proc. Natl. Acad. Sci. USA* 114, 12578–12583. doi: 10.1073/pnas.1712377114

17

The Underlying Mechanism of 3-Hydroxyphthalic Anhydride-Modified Bovine Beta-Lactoglobulin to Block Human Papillomavirus Entry into the Host Cell

Chen Hua[1†], Yun Zhu[2], Congquan Wu[3†], Lulu Si[1], Qian Wang[1], Long Sui[3*] and Shibo Jiang[1*]*

[1]Key Laboratory of Medical Molecular Virology (MOE/NHC/CAMS), School of Basic Medical Sciences, Fudan-Jinbo Functional Protein Joint Research Center, Fudan University, Shanghai, China, [2]National Laboratory of Biomacromolecules, Institute of Biophysics, Chinese Academy of Sciences, Beijing, China, [3]Medical Center for Diagnosis and Treatment of Cervical Disease, Obstetrics and Gynecology Hospital, Fudan University, Shanghai, China

***Correspondence:**
Yun Zhu
zhuyun@ibp.ac.cn
Long Sui
suilong@fudan.edu.cn
Shibo Jiang
shibojiang@fudan.edu.cn

We have previously demonstrated that 3-hydroxyphthalic anhydride (3HP)-modified bovine beta-lactoglobulin (3HP-β-LG) is highly effective in inhibiting entry of pseudovirus (PsV) of high- and low-risk human papillomavirus (HPV) into the target cell. Intravaginally applied 3HP-β-LG-containing vaginal gel could significantly inhibit HPV infection and reduce viral load in the cervical region. However, we still do not understand the underlying molecular mechanism by which 3HP-β-LG is able to inhibit HPV infection. Here, though, we showed that 3HP-β-LG did not inactivate HPV PsV, but rather blocked entry of HPV PsV into the target cell *via* its interaction with virus, not cell. It bound to the positively charged region in the HPV L1 protein, suggesting that 3HP-β-LG binds to HPV L1 protein through the interaction between the negatively charged region in 3HP-β-LG and the positively charged region in HPV L1 protein, thus competitively blocking the binding of HPV to the receptor on the basement membrane in vaginal mucosa. Although 3HP-modified chicken ovalbumin (3HP-OVA) also carries high net negative charges, it exhibited no anti-HPV activity, suggesting that the interaction between 3HP-modified protein and HPV L1 protein relies on both electrostatic and matchable conformation of the binding sites in both proteins. When topically applied, 3HP-β-LG did not enter the host cell or blood circulation. These findings suggest that 3HP-β-LG targets HPV L1 protein and blocks HPV entry into the host cell, thus being safe and effective for topical application in the treatment of HPV infection.

Keywords: 3HP-β-LG, human papillomavirus, virus entry inhibition, L1 protein, mechanism of action

INTRODUCTION

Cervical cancer is the second most common cancer among women in China (Chen et al., 2016). Almost all these cases result from the persistent infection of human papillomavirus (HPV) (Bosch et al., 2002). HPVs are a large viral family consisting of about 200 different types (Bernard et al., 2010). Among them, 18 types have high oncogenic properties, and these are regarded as the high-risk types, such as HPV16, HPV18, and HPV58. The high-risk types of HPV have relatively low self-clearance rate compared to the low-risk types of HPV (Safaeian et al., 2008). To prevent the infection of these high-risk HPVs and the occurrence of cervical cancer, several prophylactic vaccines, like Cervarix, Gardasil, and Gardasil 9 (Deschuyteneer et al., 2010; McCormack, 2014), have been developed and approved for marketing in many countries. However, no therapeutic vaccines or drugs have been approved for clinical use to treat HPV-infected patients.

HPV is a non-enveloped, double-stranded DNA virus. Its capsid is made up of two proteins, major protein L1 and minor protein L2. They are both involved in receptor binding and viral entry. Analysis of the atomic structure of native $T = 7$ HPV virus-like particle (VLP) reveals that 72 L1 pentamers form the icosahedral shell of HPV (Baker et al., 1991; Li et al., 2016). The L1 pentamer strongly binds to HPV receptors, such as heparan sulfate proteoglycans (HSPGs), on the basement membrane to mediate viral entry and infection (Kines et al., 2009). The highly potent neutralizing antibodies elicited by HPV vaccines were found to bind to the L1 protein and prevent HPV infection (Li et al., 2018). Thus, the L1 pentamer is regarded as the most important target for development of antiviral agents against HPV infection.

Viral entry inhibitors represent a class of antiviral agents that inhibit virus infection by blocking virus entry into the host cells. Jiang et al. reported the first peptide-based HIV entry inhibitor, SJ-2176, in 1993 (Jiang et al., 1993) and the first HIV entry inhibitor-based anti-HIV drug, enfuvirtide, was approved by U.S. FDA for clinical use in 2003 (Dando and Perry, 2003). Later, Jiang and colleagues have reported that anhydride-modified proteins such as 3-hydroxyphthalic anhydride (3HP)-modified proteins are potent virus entry inhibitors against a number of enveloped viruses, such as HIV (Neurath et al., 1996), herpes simplex virus (HSV) (Neurath et al., 1996), and Ebola virus (EBOV) (Li et al., 2017). In 2012, Jiang's group reported that 3HP-modified bovine beta-lactoglobulin (3HP-β-LG) could also inhibit entry into the target cell of the pseudovirus (PsV) of non-enveloped virus, HPV (high-risk HPV16 and HPV18, and low-risk HPV6) (Lu et al., 2013). In the clinical trial, the topical application of vaginal gel containing 3HP-β-LG was proven to be very safe and highly effective in suppressing HPV infection and reducing viral load in vaginal mucosa (Guo et al., 2016a,b). However, we still do not understand the molecular mechanism by which 3HP-β-LG inhibits HPV infection. In this study, we found that while 3HP-β-LG could not inactivate HPV PsV, it was effective in inhibiting HPV PsV entry into the host cell *via* its interaction with virus, not the cell. Unlike β-LG, 3HP-β-LG could bind with L1 protein and the peptides derived from the positively charged region in the HPV L1 protein, suggesting that 3HP-β-LG inhibits HPV infection by binding, *via* its negatively charged region, to L1 protein, and thus competitively blocking HPV binding to the receptor on the basement membrane in vaginal mucosa, which then inhibits HPV from entering and replicating in the host cell. We have also shown that topically applied 3HP-β-LG does not enter the host cell and blood circulation. Therefore, the 3HP-β-LG-containing formulations can be safely used in vagina for treatment of HPV infection and prevention of cervical cancer development.

MATERIALS AND METHODS

Reagents

3-Hydroxyphthalic anhydride (HP), 2,4,6-trinitrobenzenesulfonic acid (TNBS), human serum albumin (HSA), β-lactoglobulin (β-LG), chicken ovalbumin (OVA), and bovine serum albumin (BSA) were purchased from Sigma. Horseradish peroxidase (HRP)-conjugated goat anti-human IgA and IgE antibodies were purchased from Abcam (UK). HRP-conjugated rabbit anti-mouse IgG antibody was purchased from Dako (Denmark). The HPV16- and HPV-58-L1/L2-expressing plasmids and Luciferase pCLucf plasmid were kindly provided by Dr. John Schiller at the Laboratory of Cellular Oncology, National Cancer Institute, NIH, MD, USA.

Chemical Modification and Characterization of Anhydride-Modified Proteins

Anhydride-modified proteins were produced as previously described (Lu et al., 2013). Briefly, each kind of protein was dissolved with 0.1 M phosphate buffer (pH 8.5) at a final concentration of 20 mg/ml. Afterward, protein solutions were mixed with anhydrides (HP at 1 M in DMSO) to a final concentration of 60 mM by the addition of five equal aliquots at 20-min intervals, while the pH was adjusted to 9.0 with 4 M NaOH after each mixing. All mixtures were kept at 25°C for two more hours and then dialyzed against PBS.

3-Hydroxyphthalic Anhydride Modified Bovine Beta-Lactoglobulin-Mediated Inhibition Against Human Papillomavirus Pseudovirus Entry Into HeLa or HaCaT Cells

The HPV pseudovirus was produced as previously described[1]. Briefly, 293 T cells, which had been seeded in a 10-cm culture dish (4×10^6 cells) at 16 h before transfection, were transfected with a mixture of HPV16-L1/L2-expressing plasmid (p16sheLL) and pCLucf plasmid for HPV16 PsV, or a mixture of HPV58-L1/L2-expressing plasmid (p58sheLL) and pCLucf plasmid for HPV58 PsV, using VigoFect (Vigorous Biotechnology Corp.). The cells were suspended in 0.5 ml of lysis buffer and incubated for 24 h at 37°C with slow rotation. The lysate was cooled on ice for 5 min, mixed with 5 M NaCl solutions to adjust the concentration of NaCl to 0.85 M, and further kept on ice for 10 min. Then, the lysate was centrifuged at 5,000 × *g* for 10 min at 4°C, and quantified for the concentration of L1/L2 capsid protein levels. To remove aggregates, the pseudovirion stock was filtered before use for the neutralization assay. The

[1]http://home.ccr.cancer.gov/lco/default.asp

inhibitory activity of 3HP-β-LG against HPV PsV entry into HeLa or HaCaT cells was detected as previously described (Surviladze et al., 2012; Kwak et al., 2014). Briefly, HeLa or HecCatT cells were seeded at 1.5 × 10^4 cells in 100 μl of 10% FBS DMEM (DMEM-10) per well in a 96-well plate, followed by a culture at 37°C overnight. 3HP-β-LG or β-LG was serially diluted in DMEM and incubated with 100 μl of HPV PsV (equal to 35 ng L1). Mixtures were added to HeLa or HaCaT cells and incubated at 37°C for 16 h. After replacement of the culture supernatants with free medium and culture for additional 72 h, cells were lysed for measurement of luciferase activity, according to the manufacturer's manual (Promega, Madison, WI, USA).

Enzyme-Linked Immunosorbent Assay

3HP-β-LG diluted in PBS was coated onto all wells of a 96-well polystyrene plate (Corning, USA) at 4°C overnight. After blocking with protein-free blocking buffer (Thermo Fisher Scientific, USA), HPV L1 (type16 or 18) protein at 1 μg/ml was added into the wells for 50 μl/well, and the plate was incubated at 37°C for 1 h. After washing with PBST three times, mouse anti-HPV L1 (type16 or 18) antibody (Abcam, UK) was added at a 1: 1,000 dilution. After incubation at 37°C for 1 h and washing again, HRP-conjugated rabbit anti-mouse IgG antibody (Dako, Denmark) was added for 1 h. After washing and adding tetramethylbenzidine (Sigma, USA), the absorbance was measured at 450 nm. Similar protocols were used for detection of 3HP-β-LG in the serum of rhesus monkeys and 3HP-β-LG-specific IgA and IgE in the vaginal swab eluates, which were leftover samples from the clinical trials for evaluating the *in vivo* safety and efficacy of the intravaginally applied 3HP-β-LG-containing vaginal gels (Registry No.: ChiCTR-TRC-12002016) (Guo et al., 2016a,b).

Isothermal Titration Calorimetry for Measurement of the Binding Ability of 3-Hydroxyphthalic Anhydride Modified Bovine Beta-Lactoglobulin and Beta-Lactoglobulin to Peptides

Two positively charged peptides of HPV L1 protein, L1-I (residues 474–488: LKAKPKFTLGKRKAT) and L1-II (residues 493–505: STSTTAKRKKRKL), were synthesized by a standard solid-phase Fmoc method as previously reported (He et al., 2007). The peptide solution (1 mM) was prepared in 50 mM phosphate buffer (pH 7.4) and added into the titration sample cells. 3HP-β-LG and β-LG were also dissolved in phosphate buffer to 50 μM and then added to the titration needle. Isothermal titration calorimetry (ITC) analysis was carried out at constant temperature of 18°C with stirring speed of 1,000 rev/min. Each titration volume was 2 μl, and the titration interval was 60 s for the first drop and 120 s for the others.

Time-of-Addition Assay

HeLa cells were plated in a 96-well plate (for 1.0 × 10^5/well) overnight. Then, cells were incubated with 3HP-β-LG at a final concentration of 15 μg/ml at 0.5 h before or 0, 0.5, 1, 2, 4, 8, 12, 24, and 48 h after addition of HPV PsV (equal to 36 ng L1), followed by an incubation at 37°C for 16 h. After replacement of culture supernatant with fresh medium and an incubation for additional 72 h, cells were lysed to determine the entry inhibition ratio, according to the manufacturer's manual (Promega).

Cell Wash Assay

HeLa cells in 96-well plates were preincubated with 100 μl of 3HP-β-LG (5 μM) or β-LG (5 μM) at 37°C for 1 h and then washed with DMEM three times before addition of HPV PsV. For the control, 3HP-β-LG- or β-LG-pretreated HeLa cells were not washed before HPV PsV was added. HPV PsV entry into HeLa cells was detected as described above.

Temperature Shift Assay

The plated HeLa cells and 3HP-β-LG mixture were both prechilled at 4°C for 30 min. Then, the cells were incubated with the 3HP-β-LG mixture at 4°C for 12 h. After washing with cold PBS buffer twice, the cells were further incubated at 37°C for 72 h. Then the cells were lysed to determine luciferase activity, according to the luciferase assay system manual (Promega, USA).

Experiment on Rhesus Macaques

The experiment on rhesus macaques was conducted under ethical guidelines and approved by the Ethics Committee of the Institute of Laboratory Animal Science, Chinese Academy of Medical Sciences and Peking Union Medical College (approval number: ILAS-VL-2015-001). In brief, the rhesus macaques were randomly divided into treatment group and control group. In the treatment group, vaginal gel containing 3HP-β-LG (1.8 mg per dose) was dispersed into carbomer gel and administered intravaginally or rectally. In the control group, only carbomer gel was applied. Then, 2 ml of blood was collected before or after injection at −1 h, 0 h, 30 min, 1 h, 2 h, 3 h, 6 h, 12 h, and 24 h. The serum was separated after condensation.

Immunofluorescence Staining

To determine whether 3HP-β-LG could enter into HeLa or 293 T cells, cells (1 × 10^5) were seeded onto coverslips in a 6-well plate. Then, 3HP-β-LG (0.5 μg/ml) was added for 12 h. Then, the supernatant was replaced with DMEM containing 2% FBS. After 24 days, the cells were fixed by 4% paraformaldehyde (PFA; Sigma-Aldrich, St. Louis, MO), perforated by 0.2% Triton X-100, and blocked with 3% BSA (Amresco, LLC, Solon, OH). Next, cells were incubated overnight with anti-3HP-β-LG mAb or anti-β-actin mAb (1:1,000) at 4°C. After five washes, the cells were incubated with Alexa Fluor 488-labeled donkey anti-mouse IgG (1, 1,000, Thermo Fisher Scientific, Wilmington, DE, USA) at room temperature for 1h. After five washes, the coverslips were sealed with Prolong Gold Antifade reagent with 4,6-diamidino-2-phenylindole (Thermo Fisher Scientific) and scanned with the Leica SP8 confocal microscope.

RESULTS

3-Hydroxyphthalic Anhydride Modified Bovine Beta-Lactoglobulin Is the Most Potent Anhydride-Modified Protein Against Human Papillomavirus Entry Into the Target Cell

Our previous studies have shown that 3-hydroxyphthalic anhydride-modified bovine beta-lactoglobulin (3HP-β-LG) is a promising HPV entry inhibitor against entry of PsV of both high-risk and low-risk HPV types (Lu et al., 2013). This inhibitory activity was attributed to the interaction of the increased net negative charges on β-LG after 3-hydroxyphthalic anhydride modification (Lu et al., 2013). One may ask whether all proteins with increased net negative charges can inhibit HPV entry into the target cell. To answer this question, we compared the inhibitory activity of 3HP-β-LG with that of 3-hydroxyphthalic anhydride-modified human serum albumin (3HP-HSA) and 3-hydroxyphthalic anhydride-modified chicken ovalbumin (3HP-OVA) against entry of HPV16 PsV into HeLa cells, using the unmodified β-LG, HSA, and OVA as controls. As shown in **Figure 1A**, 3HP-β-LG exhibited potent anti-HPV activity in a dose-dependent manner with an IC_{50} (the half maximal inhibitory concentration) of 0.59 μg/ml, which is more potent than that of 3HP-HSA (IC_{50}: 2.28 μg/ml). 3HP-OVA and all three unmodified proteins at the concentration as high as 10 μg/ml showed no significant inhibitory activity against HPV16 PsV entry into the target cell. These results confirm that not all, just some, proteins, such as β-LG and HSA, modified by 3-hydroxyphthalic anhydride gain the ability to inhibit HPV infection.

In our previous studies, we proved the antiviral activity of 3HP-β-LG against entry of the high-risk HPV types 16 and 18 and low-risk HPV type 6 into the target cell (Lu et al., 2013). Aside from these three representative HPV types worldwide, another important high-risk type, HPV58, is found with high incidence in China. To determine whether 3HP-β-LG is also effective against HPV58, we constructed the HPV58 pseudovirus and tested its sensitivity to 3HP-β-LG (control: β-LG). As shown in **Figure 1B**, 3HP-β-LG could also inhibit HPV58 PsV entry into the target cell in a dose-dependent manner (IC_{50} of 0.28 μg/ml), confirming that 3HP-β-LG has broad-spectrum anti-HPV activity.

Considering that the HaCaT cells express abundant integrin and heparan sulfate proteoglycan (HSPG), the receptors for HPV (Aksoy et al., 2014; Kumar et al., 2014) and act as target cells for HPV infection, we also evaluated the inhibitory activity of 3HP-β-LG against HPV16 and HPV58 PsV entry into HaCaT cells. As shown in **Figures 1C,D**, 3HP-β-LG was also effective

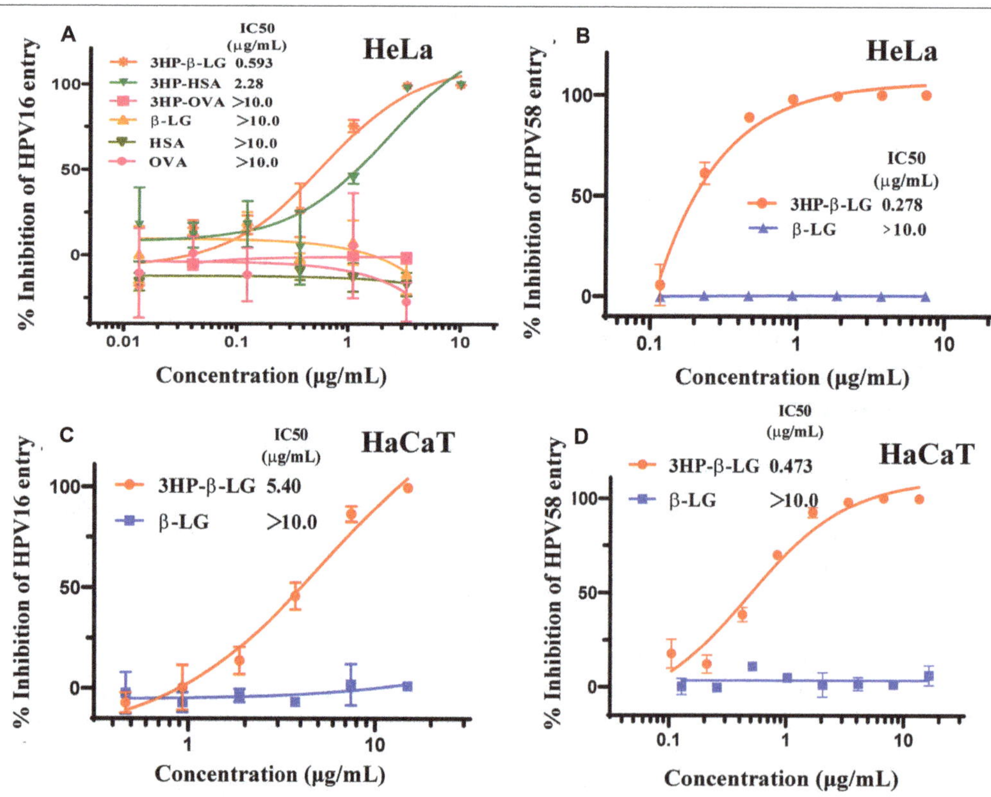

FIGURE 1 | Anti-HPV activities of anhydride-modified proteins. **(A)** Inhibition of anhydride-modified proteins on entry of HPV16 PsV into HeLa cells. Protein candidates include human serum albumin (HSA), β-lactoglobulin (β-LG), and chicken ovalbumin (OVA). **(B)** Inhibition of 3HP-β-LG on entry of HPV58 PsV into HeLa cells. **(C)** Inhibition of 3HP-β-LG on entry of HPV16 PsV into HaCaT cells. **(D)** Inhibition of 3HP-β-LG on entry of HPV58 PsV into HaCaT cells. Each sample was tested in triplicate, and the experiment was repeated twice. Data from a representative experiment are presented as mean ± standard deviation (SD).

against entry of HPV16 and HPV58 PsV into HaCaT cells, suggesting that 3HP-β-LG acts on the virus, rather than the target cell.

3-Hydroxyphthalic Anhydride Modified Bovine Beta-Lactoglobulin Binds to the L1 Protein and the Peptides Derived From the Positively Charged Residue-Enriched Region in Human Papillomavirus L1 Protein

As we proposed before, 3HP-β-LG inhibited HPV PsV entry into the target cell possibly through the binding of the negatively charged residues in 3HP-β-LG with the positively charged residues in a protein on the surface of the viral particle, thereby blocking the interaction between viral protein and receptor on the target cell (Lu et al., 2013). However, it is still unclear which protein on the virus surface may be involved in this interaction. The most abundant protein on the HPV particle is L1 protein. Here we detected the interaction between 3HP-β-LG and HPV L1 protein by ELISA. As shown in **Figures 2Aa,Ab**, 3HP-β-LG could strongly bind to the L1 protein of both HPV16 and HPV18, while the unmodified β-LG protein could not.

The C-terminal positively charged region of HPV L1 was proved to regulate the binding of HPV to the receptor (Sibbet et al., 2000; Bousarghin et al., 2003). This region was exposed on the viral surface, and involved in the binding to cell surface receptors or neutralizing antibodies. Therefore, we synthesized two positively charged peptides in this region of L1 protein, L1-I (residues 474–488) and L1-II (residues 493–505). The binding ability of 3HP-β-LG and β-LG to these peptides was measured by isothermal titration calorimetry (ITC). As shown in **Figure 2B**, β-LG had no obvious binding to L1-I or L1-II peptide, while 3HP-β-LG showed high binding ability against both L1-I (binding constant K_a value equals 2.31 × 10^5/M) and L1-II (binding constant K_a value equals 1.04 × 10^5/M). These results suggested that 3HP-β-LG may bind to the positively charged sites in the C-terminal region of L1 protein on the HPV surface to block the interaction between the viral particle and cell receptor.

3-Hydroxyphthalic Anhydride Modified Bovine Beta-Lactoglobulin Did Not Inactivate Human Papillomavirus Pseudovirus, but, Instead, Blocked Entry of Human Papillomavirus Pseudovirus Into the Target Cell *via* Its Inaction With Virus, Not Cells

To determine whether 3HP-β-LG could inactivate HPV PsV, we incubated HPV PsV with 3HP-β-LG at room temperature

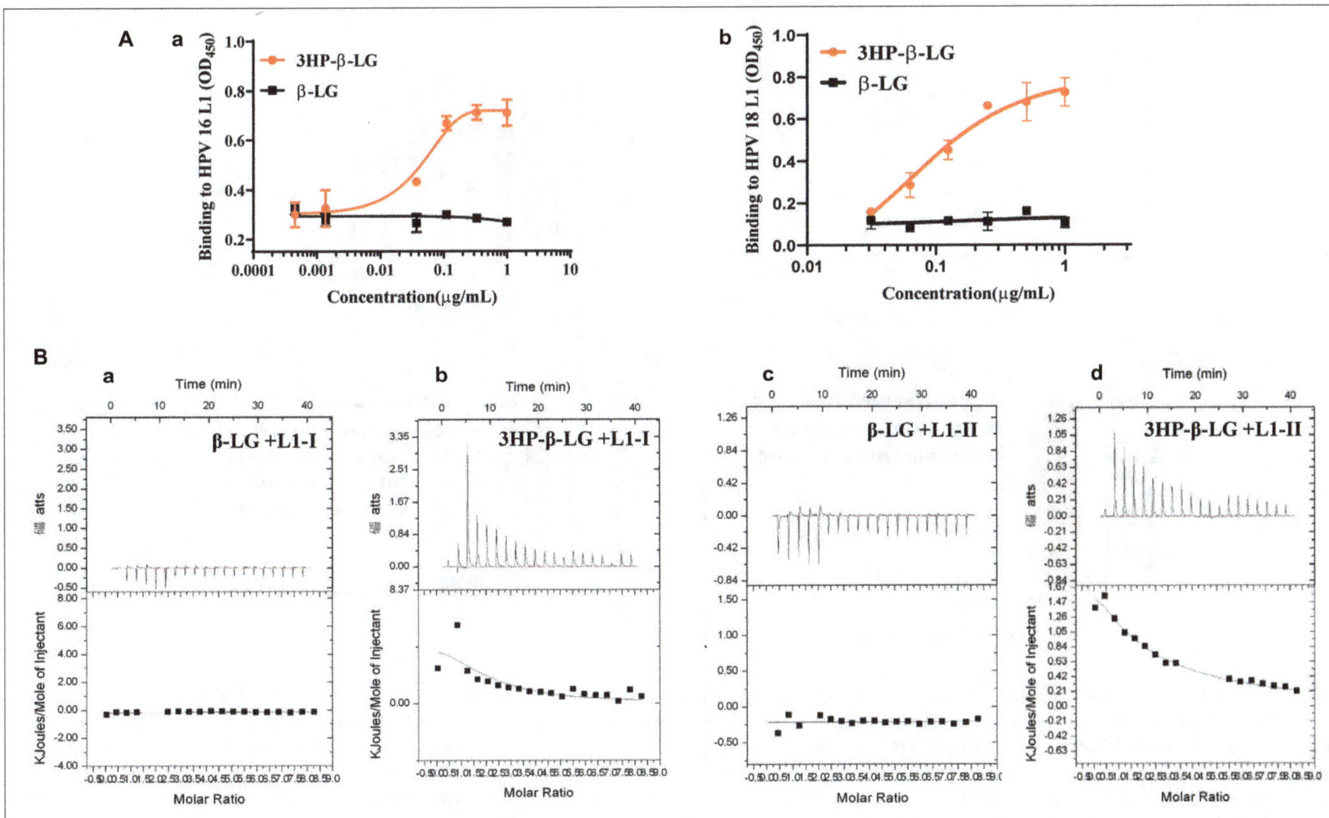

FIGURE 2 | Interaction of 3HP-β-LG with HPV L1 protein and with peptides derived from the positively charged region in the HPV L1 protein. **(A)** Binding of 3HP-β-LG (control: β-LG) with L1 protein of HPV16 **(a)** and HPV18 **(b)** in ELISA. Each sample was tested in triplicate, and the experiment was repeated twice. Data from a representative experiment are presented as mean ± SD. **(B)** Binding of 3HP-β-LG (control: β-LG) with L1–1 peptide **(a** and **b)** or L1-II peptide **(c** and **d)** derived from the region of residues 474–488 (LKAKPKFTLGKRKAT) or region of residues 493–505 (STSTTAKRKKRKL) of HPV16, respectively, in ITC.

for 2 h and then removed 3HP-β-LG by PEG-8000 precipitation. As shown in **Figure 3A**, the treated virus could still infect the target host cell with no reduced activity, compared the control virus (DMEM- or β-LG-treated), suggesting that the binding between 3HP-β-LG and HPV PsV may be noncovalent and reversible so that 3HP-β-LG cannot permanently inactive the virus.

HPV entry into the host cell takes more than 10 h, a relatively slow process compared to other viruses (Aksoy et al., 2017), which provides a long window period for an entry inhibitor to bind with the viral protein responsible for interaction with the receptor on the target cell and block viral entry. Here, we performed a time-addition assay to pinpoint the window of functional 3HP-β-LG blocking of HPV entry into the target cell. As shown in **Figure 3B**, 3HP-β-LG (15 μg/ml) could fully inhibit HPV16 PsV entry when it was added to the cells 0.5 h before and 0.5, 1, 2, 4, and 8 h after addition of HPV16 PsV, respectively, while about 70, 10, and 5% of HPV16 PsV entry were blocked when 3HP-β-LG was added to the cells 12, 24, and 48 h after addition of HPV16 PsV, respectively (**Figure 3B**). This result suggests that during this relatively long period of entry process (Aksoy et al., 2017), the entry inhibitor 3HP-β-LG remains sufficiently active to inhibit HPV PsV entry into the target cell.

To confirm the functional stage of 3HP-β-LG in blocking viral entry, we used a temperature shift assay to slow down the viral infection process. At 4°C, HPV PsV could bind to cell receptors, but could not fully enter the cytoplasm because the speeds of membrane fusion and cytoskeletal transformation are largely reduced at such low temperature. We incubated HPV PsV and HeLa cells at 4°C for 12 h so that HPV could bind to the cell surface. Then we washed away the unbound HPV before shifting the cells to 37°C for further 72 h of incubation. When 3HP-β-LG was added into the cells at the beginning and then removed by washing, no viral entry occurred (**Figure 3C**). This proved that 3HP-β-LG blocked the attachment between PsV and cell receptor at the earliest stage of infection. To determine whether 3HP-β-LG could also bind to the receptor on the target cell surface to block HPV entry, we incubated HeLa cells with 3HP-β-LG (control: β-LG) at 37°C for 1 h. The cells were washed with DMEM to remove the unbound proteins, or not washed (as control), before addition of HPV PsV. Under the washing conditions, HPV PsV entry into the HeLa cells was not blocked, while under the non-washing conditions, HPV PsV entry into the HeLa cells was effectively blocked. No inhibition was observed in the β-LG control groups, no matter whether the β-LG-treated HeLa cells were

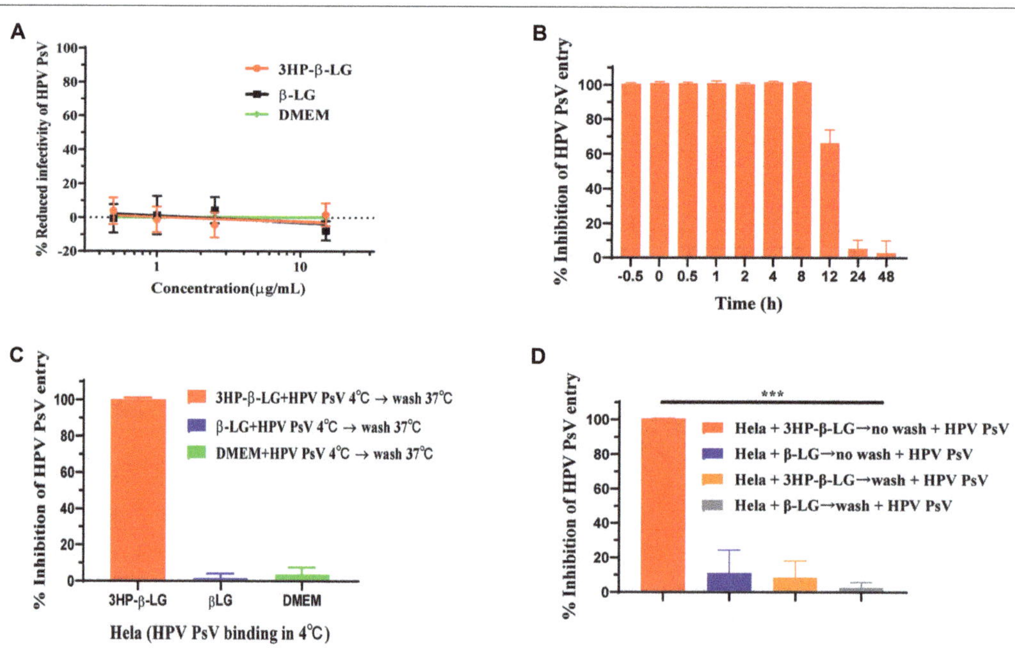

FIGURE 3 | 3HP-β-LG inhibited HPV PsV entry by targeting virus, not cells. **(A)** 3HP-β-LG was unable to inactivate HPV PsV. HPV PsV was incubated with 3HP-β-LG (control: β-LG) at room temperature for 2 h and then separated by PEG-8000 to analyze its entry activity. The DMEM-treated virus was taken as negative control. **(B)** 3HP-β-LG blocked HPV PsV entry into the target cell. HeLa cells were incubated with HPV PsV, while 3HP-β-LG (15 μg/ml) was added at different time points (−0.5, 0, 0.5, 1, 2, 4, 8, 12, 24, and 48 h) to analyze the inhibitory activity. **(C)** 3HP-β-LG blocked HPV PsV entry by targeting virus. Temperature shift assay for anti-HPV activity of 3HP-β-LG (control: β-LG). Diluted 3HP-β-LG or β-LG at 15 μg/ml was mixed with HPV PsV and prechilled at 4°C for 30 min; then they were added to HeLa cells for 12 h. After washing twice, the cells were further incubated at 37°C for 72 h and then analyzed for fluorescent integrated density. **(D)** 3HP-β-LG inhibited HPV PsV entry by targeting the virus, not the host cell. HeLa cells were incubated with 3HP-β-LG (control: β-LG) at 37°C for 1 h with/without washing by DMEM before addition of HPV PsV. Each sample was tested in triplicate, and the experiment was repeated twice. Data from a representative experiment are presented as mean ± SD. Asterisks represent significant differences. ***$p < 0.001$.

washed or not washed (**Figure 3D**). These results suggest that 3HP-β-LG inhibition of HPV PsV entry into HeLa cells does not result from its binding to HPV's receptor on the host cell.

3-Hydroxyphthalic Anhydride Modified Bovine Beta-Lactoglobulin Could Not Penetrate Into the Cell and the Vaginally Applied 3-Hydroxyphthalic Anhydride Modified Bovine Beta-Lactoglobulin Did Not Enter Into the Blood Circulation

To determine whether intravaginally applied 3HP-β-LG could enter into epithelial cells, we incubated HeLa cells and 293 T cells with 3HP-β-LG for 24 h and then washed the cells three times using PBS. The cells were stained with mouse anti-3HP-β-LG antibody or anti-β-actin antibody, as a control, and Alexa Fluor 488-labeled donkey anti-mouse IgG. Different from the anti-β-actin antibody-treated cells that showed strong fluorescence signals, anti-3HP-β-LG antibody-treated cells displayed no significant fluorescence signals inside or outside the cells (**Figure 4**). These results indicate that 3HP-β-LG could neither enter into the cell nor bind the cell surface proteins, including the receptor(s) for HPV.

To investigate whether the topically applied 3HP-β-LG enters the blood circulation, a carbomer gel with or without 3HP-β-LG was topically administered in the vagina or anus of rhesus macaques. Their blood samples were collected at different time points before and after gel application. The concentration of 3HP-β-LG in the blood samples and that in the gel (as positive control) were quantified with ELISA using anti-3HP-β-LG mAb. As shown in **Figure 5**, no 3HP-β-LG was detected in the blood samples of rhesus macaques vaginally or rectally administered with carbomer gel with or without 3HP-β-LG, confirming that the topically applied 3HP-β-LG does not enter the blood circulation.

DISCUSSION

About 10–20% of acute HPV infections become persistent, leading to various forms of cancer (Shanmugasundaram and You, 2017), such as the cervical cancer. Although several multivalent prophylactic HPV vaccines have been used in clinics to prevent HPV infection and cervical cancer development, they have no effect against pre-existing HPV infection in middle-aged and elderly women, the population at high risk for cervical cancer. Therefore, it is essential to develop effective and safe therapeutic agents for treatment of HPV infection in order to reduce the morbidity of cervical cancer.

Viral entry inhibitors have been proven effective and safe for the treatment of viral infections (Jiang et al., 1993; Dando and Perry, 2003; Lu et al., 2016; Li et al., 2017; Su et al., 2019). We have previously reported that an HPV entry inhibitor, 3HP-β-LG, is highly effective in blocking the entry of HPV, both high- and low-risk types, into the host cell (Lu et al., 2013). In a randomized clinical trial, topical application of the vaginal gel containing 3HP-β-LG has shown excellent efficacy and safety to treat high-risk HPV infections (Guo et al., 2016a,b). However, how 3HP-β-LG inhibits HPV entry into the target cell is still unclear.

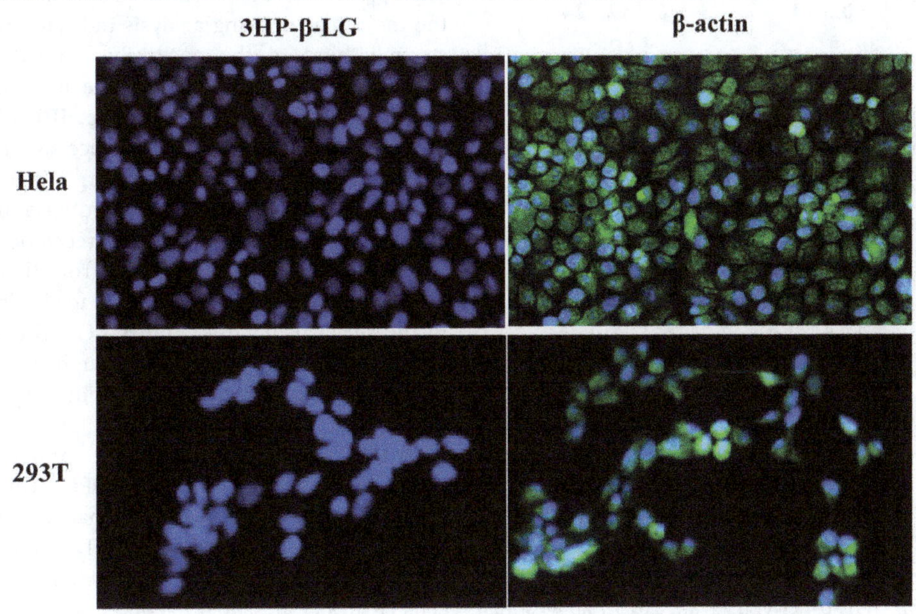

FIGURE 4 | 3HP-β-LG could not enter into the target cell. After incubation with HeLa and 293 T cells, 3HP-β-LG in the cells was detected by immunofluorescence assay using anti-3HP-β-LG mAb (green). β-actin was used as positive control. Cell nuclei were stained by 4,6-diamidino-2-phenylindole (blue).

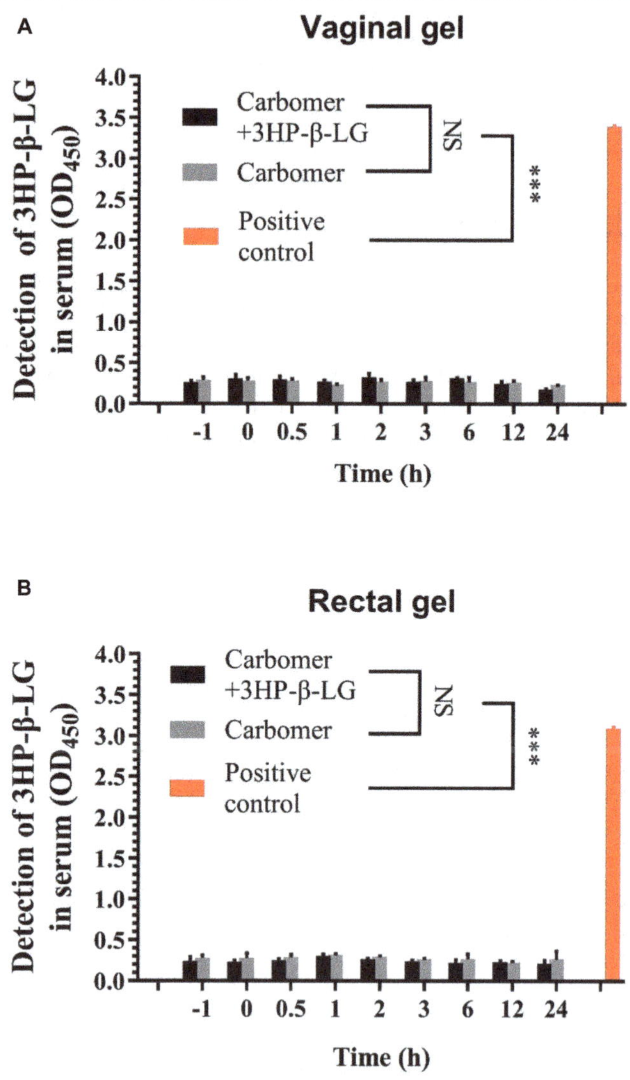

FIGURE 5 | 3HP-β-LG could not enter into blood circulation when applied through the vagina or anus. **(A)** Concentration of 3HP-β-LG in sera of monkeys through vaginal administration. **(B)** Concentration of 3HP-β-LG in sera of monkeys through rectal administration. 3HP-β-LG was formulated in a carbomer gel (1.8 mg/each) and administered through the vagina or anus of rhesus macaques. Their blood samples were collected at different time points before and after the application (–1 to 24 h). 3HP-β-LG in the blood samples was analyzed by ELISA. Each sample was tested in triplicate, and the experiment was repeated twice. Data from a representative experiment are presented as mean ± SD. The asterisks represent significant differences: $^{*}p < 0.05$; $^{**}p < 0.01$; $^{***}p < 0.001$.

In our previous study, we demonstrated that the inhibitory activity of 3HP-β-LG on HPV PsV entry into the target cell is closely correlated with the number of the positively charged lysine and arginine residues in 3HP-β-LG, as modified, *i.e.*, the net negative charges on 3HP-β-LG (Lu et al., 2013), suggesting that the negatively charged residues on 3HP-β-LG play an important role in 3HP-β-LG-mediated inhibition of HPV infection. As shown in **Figure 6A**, the unmodified bovine β-LG contains 18 positively charged residues (15 Lys and 3 Arg) and 26 negatively charged residues (16 Asp and 10 Glu) (Qin et al., 1999), thus having a net charge of –8. In 3HP-β-LG, 14 out of the 15 Lys and all 3 Arg were modified by 3HP at 6 mM (Lu et al., 2013), resulting in the neutralization of 17 of the 18 positive charges. Therefore, the net charge of 3HP-β-LG becomes –25, making 3HP-β-LG be active in binding to a viral protein with high positive net charges and inhibiting virus infection.

In this study, we demonstrated that 3HP-β-LG could strongly bind to the L1 protein on the HPV16 PsV, while the unmodified β-LG protein could not (**Figure 2A**). Using ITC analysis, we showed that unlike β-LG, 3HP-β-LG could strongly interact with the positively charged residue-enriched C-terminal regions (residues 474–488 and 493–505) of L1 protein, which is responsible for the attachment of the HPV particle to the host cell, possibly through its interaction with the cellular receptor(s).

One may argue that 3HP-β-LG may bind to any virus with high net positive charges on its surface protein and inhibit its infection. Indeed, 3HP-β-LG can also inhibit infection of simian immunodeficiency virus (SIV) (Wyand et al., 1999) and HSV (Neurath et al., 1996), but it is not effective against infection of MERS-CoV and VSV (unpublished data). In this study, we showed that 3HP-modified HSA (3HP-HSA) was also effective, while 3HP-modified OVA (3HP-OVA) was not effective in inhibiting HPV PsV entry (**Figure 1**), even though 3HP-OVA also contains high net negative charges on its surface. Thus, aside from having high net negative charges, these results suggest that the active site in 3HP-β-LG for binding to the viral protein must possess a conformation that fits with that in the corresponding site in the viral protein (**Figure 6B**), enabling 3HP-β-LG to strongly and closely interact with the viral protein to block HPV entry into the host cell. Indeed, the molecular docking analysis indicated that 3HP-β-LG could strongly bind to the positively charged region of HPV L1 protein, which is the binding site for the negatively charged HSPG receptor for HPV (**Figure 6B**). 3HP-β-LG has many more negative charges on the surface, and the interface between 3HP-β-LG and HPV-L1 is much larger than the HSPG molecule. Therefore, 3HP-β-LG can competitively bind to HPV L1 to block the binding of the HSPG receptor.

Based on the results obtained from this study, we proposed a mechanistic model of 3HP-β-LG for inhibiting HPV infection in the cervical mucosa (**Figure 6C**). The newly invaded HPV accesses the basal cell layer through micro lesions or breaks in the cervical epithelium and binds to the HSPG receptor on the basement membrane through interaction between the positively charged region in L1 protein of HPV and the negatively charged region in HSPG. This interaction results in a series of conformational changes in the capsid, which leads to protease digestion of L2 and exposure of its N terminus, thus initiating entry of HPV into to the epithelial cells (Kines et al., 2009; Pyeon et al., 2009). After HPV infects the epithelial cell, it gradually matures along with the host cell cycles and moves toward the top layer of epithelia, followed by eventual release from the epidermal cells. The newly released

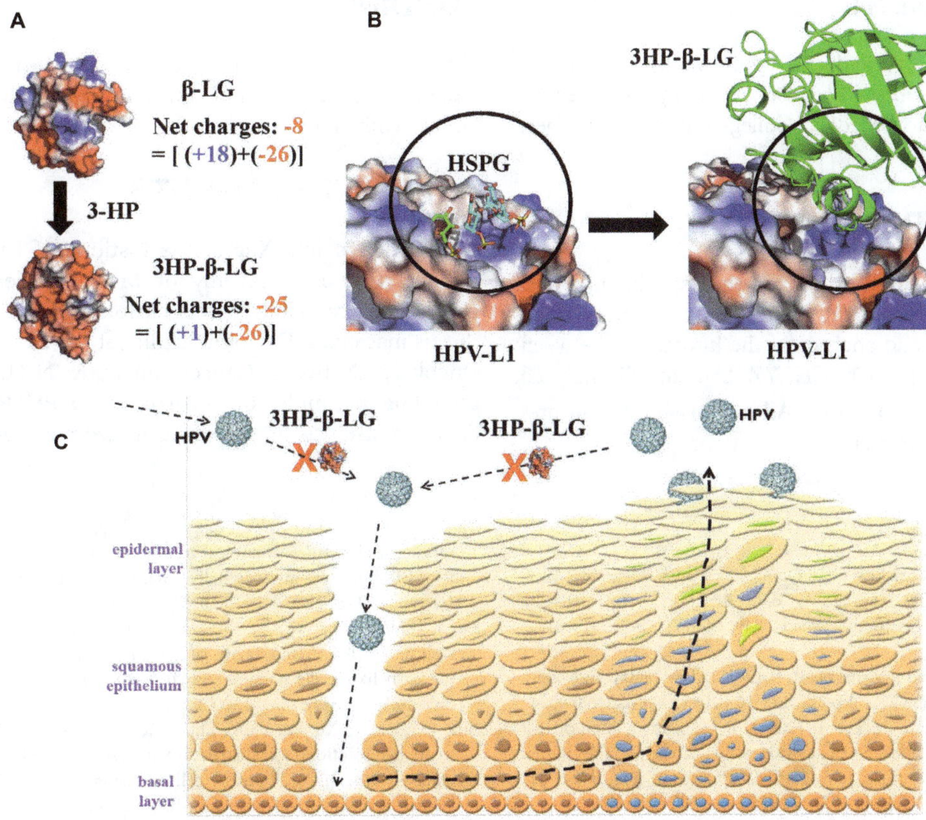

FIGURE 6 | Proposed mechanism by which 3HP-β-LG inhibits HPV infection in cervical mucosa. **(A)** The increased net negative charges on β-lactoglobulin after modification of the protein with 3-hydroxyphthalic anhydride. The structure of 3HP-β-LG was modeled by COOT (Emsley et al., 2010) using the crystal structure of β-LG (PDB entry: 1BEB). The structures were shown as an electrostatic surface by Pymol (Alexander et al., 2011). **(B)** Predicted interactions between HPV L1 pentamer and 3HP-β-LG. Crystal structure of HSPG-bound HPV L1 pentamer (PDB entry: 5W1O) was shown as electrostatic surface (Dasgupta et al., 2011), and the docking structure between HPV L1 and 3HP-β-LG was generated by AutoDock (Trott and Olson, 2010). **(C)** Schematic illustration showing how 3HP-β-LG inhibits HPV entry and infection. The newly invaded or newly released HPV particles access the basal layer through the mucosal lesion, or breaks, and bind to the HSPG receptor on the basement membrane, resulting in the entry of HPV into and replication in mucosal epithelial cells. 3HP-β-LG can bind with HPV L1 protein, through the electrostatic interaction between the negatively charged region in 3HP-β-LG and the positively charged region in L1 protein, to block the attachment of HPV to the HSPG receptor, resulting in inhibition of HPV infection in vaginal mucosa.

HPV particles access the basement membrane through micro lesions of the cervical epithelium and start another infection and replication cycle, gradually establishing persistent infection and promoting the development of cervical cancer.

3HP-β-LG that is topically applied in the vagina can bind to the L1 protein of the newly invaded or the newly released HPV and block the attachment of HPV to the basement membrane, thereby inhibiting the entry of HPV into the host cells for replication. After treatment with 3HP-β-LG for a certain period of time (e.g., 2 months), the newly produced HPV-free epithelial cells in the lower part of the mucosal epithelium are expected to move upward and push the HPV-infected cells away from the vaginal mucosa (this movement is accelerated during the menstrual period), making all layers of mucosal epithelium free of HPV infection.

Considering that the presence of micro lesions or breaks in the cervical epithelium, possibly caused by sexual activity, is the requirement for HPV to access the HSPG receptor on basement membrane (Bousarghin et al., 2003), combinational use of some biocompatible materials for mucosa wound healing, such as human collagen proteins (Hua et al., 2019), may have synergistic or complementary effects against HPV infection.

The results from the time-of-addition assay, cell washout assay, and virus inactivation indicate that 3HP-β-LG could interact with the virions, rather than the cells, to effectively block the entry of HPV PsV into the target cell, but could not inactivate the virions (**Figure 3**). These biological properties of 3HP-β-LG make it an ideal anti-HPV agent for topical application to treat HPV infection because it can interact with HPV particles on the vaginal mucosa and block the virions binding to the receptor, e.g., HSPG, on basement membrane. Since 3HP-β-LG cannot enter into the cell or the blood circulation, it is not expected to cause systemic toxicity to human or induce harmful 3HP-β-LG-specific antibodies. Therefore, the topical formulations containing 3HP-β-LG can be safely used to treat local HPV infection.

ETHICS STATEMENT

The animal study was reviewed and approved by Institute of Laboratory Animal Science, Chinese Academy of Medical Sciences and Peking Union Medical College (approval number: ILAS-VL-2015-001).

AUTHOR CONTRIBUTIONS

SJ, LSu, and YZ conceived and designed the experiments. CH, CW, LSi, and QW conducted the experiments. YZ performed the computer modeling and analysis of the interaction between 3HP-β-LG and HPV L1 protein. CH, YZ, LSu, and SJ analyzed the data and wrote the manuscript. All authors have read and approved the final manuscript.

FUNDING

This work was supported by an intramural fund of Fudan-Jinbo Functional Protein Joint Research Center, Fudan University.

ACKNOWLEDGMENTS

We thank Dr. Jing Xue at the Institute of Laboratory Animal Science, Chinese Academy of Medical Sciences and Peking Union Medical College for performing the experiments on rhesus macaques; Dr. John Schiller at the Laboratory of Cellular Oncology, National Cancer Institute, NIH, MD, USA for providing plasmids for constructing HPV PsV; and Yuhong Fu for assistance in preparing anhydrate-modified proteins.

REFERENCES

Aksoy, P., Abban, C. Y., Kiyashka, E., Qiang, W., and Meneses, P. I. (2014). Hpv16 infection of HaCaTs is dependent on beta4 integrin, and alpha6 integrin processing. *Virology* 449, 45–52. doi: 10.1016/j.virol.2013.10.034

Aksoy, P., Gottschalk, E. Y., and Meneses, P. I. (2017). Hpv entry into cells. *Mutat. Res. Rev. Mutat. Res.* 772, 13–22. doi: 10.1016/j.mrrev.2016.09.004

Alexander, N., Woetzel, N., and Meiler, J. (2011). Bcl::cluster: a method for clustering biological molecules coupled with visualization in the Pymol molecular graphics system. *IEEE Int. Conf. Comput. Adv. Bio. Med. Sci.* 2011, 13–18. doi: 10.1109/ICCABS.2011.5729867

Baker, T. S., Newcomb, W. W., Olson, N. H., Cowsert, L. M., Olson, C., and Brown, J. C. (1991). Structures of bovine and human papillomaviruses. Analysis by cryoelectron microscopy and three-dimensional image reconstruction. *Biophys. J.* 60, 1445–1456. doi: 10.1016/S0006-3495(91)82181-6

Bernard, H. U., Burk, R. D., Chen, Z., van Doorslaer, K., zur Hausen, H., and de Villiers, E. M. (2010). Classification of papillomaviruses (Pvs) based on 189 Pv types and proposal of taxonomic amendments. *Virology* 401, 70–79. doi: 10.1016/j.virol.2010.02.002

Bosch, F. X., Lorincz, A., Munoz, N., Meijer, C. J., and Shah, K. V. (2002). The causal relation between human papillomavirus and cervical cancer. *J. Clin. Pathol.* 55, 244–265. doi: 10.1136/jcp.55.4.244

Bousarghin, L., Touze, A., Combita-Rojas, A. L., and Coursaget, P. (2003). Positively charged sequences of human papillomavirus type 16 capsid proteins are sufficient to mediate gene transfer into target cells via the heparan sulfate receptor. *J. Gen. Virol.* 84, 157–164. doi: 10.1099/vir.0.18789-0

Chen, W., Zheng, R., Baade, P. D., Zhang, S., Zeng, H., Bray, F., et al. (2016). Cancer statistics in China, 2015. *CA Cancer J. Clin.* 66, 115–132. doi: 10.3322/caac.21338

Dando, T. M., and Perry, C. M. (2003). Enfuvirtide. *Drugs* 63, 2755–2766; discussion 67-8. doi: 10.2165/00003495-200363240-00005

Dasgupta, J., Bienkowska-Haba, M., Ortega, M. E., Patel, H. D., Bodevin, S., Spillmann, D., et al. (2011). Structural basis of oligosaccharide receptor recognition by human papillomavirus. *J. Biol. Chem.* 286, 2617–2624. doi: 10.1074/jbc.M110.160184

Deschuyteneer, M., Elouahabi, A., Plainchamp, D., Plisnier, M., Soete, D., Corazza, Y., et al. (2010). Molecular and structural characterization of the L1 virus-like particles that are used as vaccine antigens in Cervarix, the As04-adjuvanted Hpv-16 and -18 cervical cancer vaccine. *Hum. Vaccin.* 6, 407–419. doi: 10.4161/hv.6.5.11023

Emsley, P., Lohkamp, B., Scott, W. G., and Cowtan, K. (2010). Features and development of Coot. *Acta Crystallogr. D Biol. Crystallogr.* 66, 486–501. doi: 10.1107/S0907444910007493

Guo, X., Qiu, L., Wang, Y., Wang, Y., Meng, Y., Zhu, Y., et al. (2016a). Safety evaluation of chemically modified beta-lactoglobulin administered intravaginally. *J. Med. Virol.* 88, 1098–1101. doi: 10.1002/jmv.24439

Guo, X., Qiu, L., Wang, Y., Wang, Y., Wang, Q., Song, L., et al. (2016b). A randomized open-label clinical trial of an anti-Hpv biological dressing (Jb01-Bd) administered intravaginally to treat high-risk Hpv infection. *Microbes Infect.* 18, 148–152. doi: 10.1016/j.micinf.2015.10.004

He, Y., Liu, S., Jing, W., Lu, H., Cai, D., Chin, D. J., et al. (2007). Conserved residue Lys574 in the cavity of HIV-1 Gp41 coiled-coil domain is critical for six-helix bundle stability and virus entry. *J. Biol. Chem.* 282, 25631–25639. doi: 10.1074/jbc.M703781200

Hua, C., Zhu, Y., Xu, W., Ye, S., Zhang, R., Lu, L., et al. (2019). Characterization by high-resolution crystal structure analysis of a triple-helix region of human collagen type iii with potent cell adhesion activity. *Biochem. Biophys. Res. Commun.* 508, 1018–1023. doi: 10.1016/j.bbrc.2018.12.018

Jiang, S., Lin, K., Strick, N., and Neurath, A. R. (1993). HIV-1 inhibition by a peptide. *Nature* 365:113. doi: 10.1038/365113a0

Kines, R. C., Thompson, C. D., Lowy, D. R., Schiller, J. T., and Day, P. M. (2009). The initial steps leading to papillomavirus infection occur on the basement membrane prior to cell surface binding. *Proc. Natl. Acad. Sci. USA* 106, 20458–20463. doi: 10.1073/pnas.0908502106

Kumar, A., Jacob, T., Abban, C. Y., and Meneses, P. I. (2014). Intermediate heparan sulfate binding during Hpv-16 infection in Hacats. *Am. J. Ther.* 21, 331–342. doi: 10.1097/MJT.0000000000000054

Kwak, K., Jiang, R., Wang, J. W., Jagu, S., Kirnbauer, R., and Roden, R. B. (2014). Impact of inhibitors and L2 antibodies upon the infectivity of diverse alpha and beta human papillomavirus types. *PLoS One* 9:e97232. doi: 10.1371/journal.pone.0097232

Li, Z., Song, S., He, M., Wang, D., Shi, J., Liu, X., et al. (2018). Rational design of a triple-type human papillomavirus vaccine by compromising viral-type specificity. *Nat. Commun.* 9:5360. doi: 10.1038/s41467-018-07199-6

Li, Z., Yan, X., Yu, H., Wang, D., Song, S., Li, Y., et al. (2016). The C-terminal arm of the human papillomavirus major capsid protein is immunogenic and involved in virus-host interaction. *Structure* 24, 874–885. doi: 10.1016/j.str.2016.04.008

Li, H., Yu, F., Xia, S., Yu, Y., Wang, Q., Lv, M., et al. (2017). Chemically modified human serum albumin potently blocks entry of Ebola pseudoviruses and viruslike particles. *Antimicrob. Agents Chemother.* 61. doi: 10.1128/AAC.02168-16

Lu, L., Yang, X., Li, Y., and Jiang, S. (2013). Chemically modified bovine beta-lactoglobulin inhibits human papillomavirus infection. *Microbes Infect.* 15, 506–510. doi: 10.1016/j.micinf.2013.03.003

Lu, L., Yu, F., Cai, L., Debnath, A. K., and Jiang, S. (2016). Development of small-molecule HIV entry inhibitors specifically targeting Gp120 or Gp41. *Curr. Top. Med. Chem.* 16, 1074–1090. doi: 10.2174/1568026615666150901114527

McCormack, P. L. (2014). Quadrivalent human papillomavirus (types 6, 11, 16, 18) recombinant vaccine (Gardasil®): a review of its use in the prevention of premalignant anogenital lesions, cervical and anal cancers, and genital warts. *Drugs* 74, 1253–1283. doi: 10.1007/s40265-014-0255-z

Neurath, A. R., Jiang, S., Strick, N., Lin, K., Li, Y. Y., and Debnath, A. K. (1996). Bovine beta-lactoglobulin modified by 3-hydroxyphthalic anhydride blocks the Cd4 cell receptor for HIV. *Nat. Med.* 2, 230–234. doi: 10.1038/nm0296-230

Neurath, A. R., Li, Y. Y., Strick, N., and Jiang, S. (1996). A herpesvirus inhibitor from bovine whey. *Lancet* 347, 1703–1704. doi: 10.1016/S0140-6736(96)91539-1

Pyeon, D., Pearce, S. M., Lank, S. M., Ahlquist, P., and Lambert, P. F. (2009). Establishment of human papillomavirus infection requires cell cycle progression. *PLoS Pathog.* 5:e1000318. doi: 10.1371/journal.ppat.1000318

Qin, B. Y., Bewley, M. C., Creamer, L. K., Baker, E. N., and Jameson, G. B. (1999). Functional implications of structural differences between variants A and B of bovine beta-lactoglobulin. *Protein Sci.* 8, 75–83. doi: 10.1110/ps.8.1.75

Safaeian, M., Kiddugavu, M., Gravitt, P. E., Gange, S. J., Ssekasanvu, J., Murokora, D., et al. (2008). Determinants of incidence and clearance of high-risk human papillomavirus infections in rural Rakai, Uganda. *Cancer Epidemiol. Biomark. Prev.* 17, 1300–1307. doi: 10.1158/1055-9965.EPI-07-2678

Shanmugasundaram, S., and You, J. (2017). Targeting persistent human papillomavirus infection. *Viruses* 9, 229. doi: 10.3390/v9080229

Sibbet, G., Romero-Graillet, C., Meneguzzi, G., and Saveria Campo, M. (2000). Alpha6 integrin is not the obligatory cell receptor for bovine papillomavirus type 4. *J. Gen. Virol.* 81:1629. doi: 10.1099/0022-1317-81-2-327

Su, S., Rasquinha, G., Du, L., Wang, Q., Xu, W., Li, W., et al. (2019). A peptide-based HIV-1 fusion inhibitor with two tail-anchors and palmitic acid exhibits substantially improved in vitro and ex vivo anti-HIV-1 activity and prolonged in vivo half-life. *Molecules* 24, 1134. doi: 10.3390/molecules24061134

Surviladze, Z., Dziduszko, A., and Ozbun, M. A. (2012). Essential roles for soluble virion-associated heparan sulfonated proteoglycans and growth factors in human papillomavirus infections. *PLoS Pathog.* 8:e1002519. doi: 10.1371/journal.ppat.1002519

Trott, O., and Olson, A. J. (2010). AutoDock Vina: improving the speed and accuracy of docking with a new scoring function, efficient optimization, and multithreading. *J. Comput. Chem.* 31, 455–461. doi: 10.1002/jcc.21334

Wyand, M. S., Manson, K. H., Miller, C. J., and Neurath, A. R. (1999). Effect of 3-hydroxyphthaloyl-beta-lactoglobulin on vaginal transmission of simian immunodeficiency virus in rhesus monkeys. *Antimicrob. Agents Chemother.* 43, 978–980. doi: 10.1128/AAC.43.4.978

Permissions

All chapters in this book were first published by Frontiers; hereby published with permission under the Creative Commons Attribution License or equivalent. Every chapter published in this book has been scrutinized by our experts. Their significance has been extensively debated. The topics covered herein carry significant findings which will fuel the growth of the discipline. They may even be implemented as practical applications or may be referred to as a beginning point for another development.

The contributors of this book come from diverse backgrounds, making this book a truly international effort. This book will bring forth new frontiers with its revolutionizing research information and detailed analysis of the nascent developments around the world.

We would like to thank all the contributing authors for lending their expertise to make the book truly unique. They have played a crucial role in the development of this book. Without their invaluable contributions this book wouldn't have been possible. They have made vital efforts to compile up to date information on the varied aspects of this subject to make this book a valuable addition to the collection of many professionals and students.

This book was conceptualized with the vision of imparting up-to-date information and advanced data in this field. To ensure the same, a matchless editorial board was set up. Every individual on the board went through rigorous rounds of assessment to prove their worth. After which they invested a large part of their time researching and compiling the most relevant data for our readers.

The editorial board has been involved in producing this book since its inception. They have spent rigorous hours researching and exploring the diverse topics which have resulted in the successful publishing of this book. They have passed on their knowledge of decades through this book. To expedite this challenging task, the publisher supported the team at every step. A small team of assistant editors was also appointed to further simplify the editing procedure and attain best results for the readers.

Apart from the editorial board, the designing team has also invested a significant amount of their time in understanding the subject and creating the most relevant covers. They scrutinized every image to scout for the most suitable representation of the subject and create an appropriate cover for the book.

The publishing team has been an ardent support to the editorial, designing and production team. Their endless efforts to recruit the best for this project, has resulted in the accomplishment of this book. They are a veteran in the field of academics and their pool of knowledge is as vast as their experience in printing. Their expertise and guidance has proved useful at every step. Their uncompromising quality standards have made this book an exceptional effort. Their encouragement from time to time has been an inspiration for everyone.

The publisher and the editorial board hope that this book will prove to be a valuable piece of knowledge for researchers, students, practitioners and scholars across the globe.

List of Contributors

Daniela S. Rajão and Daniel R. Pérez
Department of Population Health, University of Georgia, Athens, GA, United States

Zhe Cong, Ling Tong, Aihua Su, Ting Chen, Qiang Wei, Jing Xue and Chuan Qin
Beijing Key Laboratory for Animal Models of Emerging and Remerging Infectious Diseases, NHC Key Laboratory of Human Disease Comparative Medicine, Institute of Laboratory Animal Science, Chinese Academy of Medical Sciences and Comparative Medicine Center, Peking Union Medical College, Beijing, China

Yuhong Wang
Department of Gerontology and Geriatrics, The First Affiliated Hospital of Harbin Medical University, Harbin, China

Rongrong Liu, Hongwei Ma, Ziyu Liu, Fanglin Zhang and Xingan Wu
Department of Microbiology, School of Basic Medicine, Fourth Military Medical University, Xi'an, China

Xia Jin
Scientific Research Center, Shanghai Public Health Clinical Center & Institutes of Biomedical Sciences, Key Laboratory of Medical Molecular Virology of Ministry of Education & Health, Shanghai Medical College, Fudan University, Shanghai, China
Viral Disease and Vaccine Translational Research Unit, CAS Key Laboratory of Molecular Virology and Immunology, Institut Pasteur of Shanghai, Chinese Academy of Sciences, Shanghai, China
Shanghai Public Health Clinical Center, Fudan University, Shanghai, China

Jiayi Shu
Scientific Research Center, Shanghai Public Health Clinical Center & Institutes of Biomedical Sciences, Key Laboratory of Medical Molecular Virology of Ministry of Education & Health, Shanghai Medical College, Fudan University, Shanghai, China
Viral Disease and Vaccine Translational Research Unit, Institut Pasteur of Shanghai, Chinese Academy of Sciences, Shanghai, China

Qiang Zhang
School of Biology and Basic Medical Sciences, Soochow University, Suzhou, China

Mingwei Han
Cadet Brigade, School of Basic Medicine, Fourth Military Medical University, Xi'an, China

Joseph Torresi
Department of Microbiology and Immunology, The Peter Doherty Institute for Infection and Immunity, University of Melbourne, Parkville, VIC, Australia

Kai Wang, Ling Ran, Zheng Niu, Zifei Kan, Yiling Zhang, Yang Yang, Luyi Xie, Shilei Huang, Qiuhan Yu, Di Wu and Zhenhui Song
Department of Microbiology and Immunology, College of Animal Science, Southwest University, Chongqing, China

Tao Yan
Department of Preventive Veterinary Medicine, Medical College of Animals, Xinjiang Agricultural University, Ürümqi, China

Jin Sun
Viral Disease and Vaccine Translational Research Unit, CAS Key Laboratory of Molecular Virology and Immunology, Institut Pasteur of Shanghai, Chinese Academy of Sciences, Shanghai, China

Gong Cheng and Senyan Du
Tsinghua-Peking Center for Life Sciences, School of Medicine, Tsinghua University, Beijing, China

Zhihang Zheng
Viral Disease and Vaccine Translational Research Unit, CAS Key Laboratory of Molecular Virology and Immunology, Institut Pasteur of Shanghai, Chinese Academy of Sciences, Shanghai, China
Institut Pasteur of Shanghai, Chinese Academy of Sciences, University of Chinese Academy of Sciences, Shanghai, China

Victoria M. W. Gould, Alethea V. Cope and John S. Tregoning
Mucosal Infection and Immunity, Section of Virology, Imperial College London, London, United Kingdom

James N. Francis, Katie J. Anderson and Bertrand Georges
Altimmune, London BioScience Innovation Centre, London, United Kingdom

Leiliang Zhang and Shan Gao
Institute of Basic Medicine, Shandong First Medical University & Shandong Academy of Medical Sciences, Jinan, China

Siqi Song
Institute of Basic Medicine, Shandong First Medical University & Shandong Academy of Medical Sciences, Jinan, China
School of Basic Medicine, Qingdao University, Qingdao, China

Rita M. Meganck
Curriculum in Genetics and Molecular Biology, The University of North Carolina at Chapel Hill, Chapel Hill, NC, United States

Longping V. Tse and Rachel L. Graham
Department of Epidemiology, The University of North Carolina at Chapel Hill, Chapel Hill, NC, United States

Ralph S. Baric
Department of Epidemiology, The University of North Carolina at Chapel Hill, Chapel Hill, NC, United States
Department of Microbiology and Immunology, The University of North Carolina at Chapel Hill, Chapel Hill, NC, United States

Thomas R. Fuerst and Brian G. Pierce
Institute for Bioscience and Biotechnology Research, University of Maryland, Rockville, MD, United States
Department of Cell Biology and Molecular Genetics, University of Maryland, College Park, MD, United States

Zhen-Yong Keck and Steven K. H. Foung
Department of Pathology, Stanford University School of Medicine, Stanford, CA, United States

Caroline de Souza Barros and Izabel Christina Nunes de Palmer Paixão
Laboratório de Virologia Molecular e Biotecnologia Marinha, Programa de Pós-graduação em Ciências e Biotecnologia, Departamento de Biologia Celular e Molecular, Instituto de Biologia, Universidade Federal Fluminense, Niterói, Brazil

Claudio Cesar Cirne-Santos
Laboratório de Virologia Molecular e Biotecnologia Marinha, Programa de Pós-graduação em Ciências e Biotecnologia, Departamento de Biologia Celular e Molecular, Instituto de Biologia, Universidade Federal Fluminense, Niterói, Brazil
Departamento de Ensino, Curso de Farmácia na Universidade Salgado de Oliveira, Niterói, Brazil

Caio Cesar Richter Nogueira
Laboratório de Virologia Molecular e Biotecnologia Marinha, Programa de Pós-graduação em Ciências e Biotecnologia, Departamento de Biologia Celular e Molecular, Instituto de Biologia, Universidade Federal Fluminense, Niterói, Brazil
Laboratório de Produtos Naturais de Algas Marinhas (ALGAMAR), Departamento de Biologia Marinha, Instituto de Biologia, Universidade Federal Fluminense, Niterói, Brazil

Renata Campos Azevedo, Kristie Aimi Yamamoto and Guilherme Louzada Silva Meira
Instituto de Microbiologia Paulo de Góes (IMPPG), Departamento de Virologia, Universidade Federal do Rio de Janeiro, Rio de Janeiro, Brazil

Zilton Farias Meira de Vasconcelos
Instituto Fernandes Figueira (IFF), Fundação Oswaldo Cruz (Fiocruz), Rio de Janeiro, Brazil

Norman Arthur Ratcliffe
Department of Biosciences, College of Science, Swansea University, Swansea, United Kingdom

Valéria Laneuville Teixeira
Laboratório de Produtos Naturais de Algas Marinhas (ALGAMAR), Departamento de Biologia Marinha, Instituto de Biologia, Universidade Federal Fluminense, Niterói, Brazil
Laboratório de Biologia e Taxonomia de Algas (LABIOTAL), Programa de Pós-graduação em Biodiversidade Neotropical, Instituto de Biociencias, Universidade Federal do Estado do Rio de Janeiro, Rio de Janeiro, Brazil

Davis Fernandes Ferreira
Instituto de Microbiologia Paulo de Góes (IMPPG), Departamento de Virologia, Universidade Federal do Rio de Janeiro, Rio de Janeiro, Brazil
Department of Molecular and Structural Biochemistry, North Carolina State University, Raleigh, NC, United States

Jonas Schmidt-Chanasit
Bernhard Nocht Institute for Tropical Medicine, WHO Collaborating Centre for Arbovirus and Haemorrhagic Fever Reference and Research, Hamburg, Germany

Mutsuyo Takayama-Ito and Masayuki Saijo
Department of Virology I, National Institute of Infectious Diseases, Tokyo, Japan

Feihu Yan, Yuwei Gao, Na Feng, Yongkun Zhao and Chengyu Wang
Key Laboratory of Jilin Province for Zoonosis Prevention and Control, Changchun Veterinary Research Institute, Chinese Academy of Agricultural Sciences, Changchun, China

Entao Li
Key Laboratory of Jilin Province for Zoonosis Prevention and Control, Changchun Veterinary Research Institute, Chinese Academy of Agricultural Sciences, Changchun, China
College of Veterinary Medicine, South China Agricultural University, Guangzhou, China

Ling Li
National Research Center for Exotic Animal Diseases, China Animal Health and Epidemiology Center, Qingdao, China

Zachary Schiffman
Department of Medical Microbiology and Infectious Diseases, University of Manitoba, Winnipeg, MB, Canada
National Microbiology Laboratory, Special Pathogens Program, Public Health Agency of Canada, Winnipeg, MB, Canada

Pei Huang
Key Laboratory of Jilin Province for Zoonosis Prevention and Control, Changchun Veterinary Research Institute, Chinese Academy of Agricultural Sciences, Changchun, China
College of Veterinary Medicine, Jilin Agricultural University, Changchun, China

Xianzhu Xia
Key Laboratory of Jilin Province for Zoonosis Prevention and Control, Changchun Veterinary Research Institute, Chinese Academy of Agricultural Sciences, Changchun, China
College of Veterinary Medicine, South China Agricultural University, Guangzhou, China
College of Veterinary Medicine, Jilin Agricultural University, Changchun, China

Shengnan Zhang
Key Laboratory of Jilin Province for Zoonosis Prevention and Control, Changchun Veterinary Research Institute, Chinese Academy of Agricultural Sciences, Changchun, China
College of Wildlife Resources, Northeast Forestry University, Harbin, China
College of Animal Science and Technology, Shihezi University, Shihezi, China

Hongli Jin and Xinghai Zhang
College of Veterinary Medicine, Jilin University, Changchun, China
Key Laboratory of Jilin Province for Zoonosis Prevention and Control, Changchun Veterinary Research Institute, Chinese Academy of Agricultural Sciences, Changchun, China

Hualei Wang
College of Veterinary Medicine, Jilin University, Changchun, China

Zhiyuan Wen
Department of Microbiology and Immunology and Emory Vaccine Center, School of Medicine, Emory University, Atlanta, GA, United States
Harbin Veterinary Research Institute, Harbin, China

Ying Liu
State Key Laboratory of Food Nutrition and Safety, Institute of Health Biotechnology, College of Biotechnology, Tianjin University of Science and Technology, Tianjin, China
Department of Microbiology and Immunology and Emory Vaccine Center, School of Medicine, Emory University, Atlanta, GA, United States

Richard W. Compans, Ling Ye and Chinglai Yang
Department of Microbiology and Immunology and Emory Vaccine Center, School of Medicine, Emory University, Atlanta, GA, United States

Ricardo Carrion Jr., Jerritt Nunneley, Hilary Staples, Anysha Ticer and Jean L. Patterson
Texas Biomedical Research Institute, San Antonio, TX, United States

Lalita Priyamvada, Victoria A. Olson and Panayampalli S. Satheshkumar
Poxvirus and Rabies Branch, Centers for Disease Control and Prevention, Atlanta, GA, United States

Philip Alabi, Andres Leon and Jason K. Sello
Department of Chemistry, Brown University, Providence, RI, United States

Amrita Kumar and Suryaprakash Sambhara
Immunology and Pathogenesis Branch, Influenza Division, Centers for Disease Control and Prevention, Atlanta, GA, United States

Balaji Manicassamy
Department of Microbiology and Immunology, The University of Iowa, Iowa City, IA, United States

Chen Hua, Lulu Si, Qian Wang and Shibo Jiang
Key Laboratory of Medical Molecular Virology (MOE/NHC/CAMS), School of Basic Medical Sciences, Fudan-Jinbo Functional Protein Joint Research Center, Fudan University, Shanghai, China

Yun Zhu
National Laboratory of Biomacromolecules, Institute of Biophysics, Chinese Academy of Sciences, Beijing, China

Congquan Wu and Long Sui
Medical Center for Diagnosis and Treatment of Cervical Disease, Obstetrics and Gynecology Hospital, Fudan University, Shanghai, China

Index

www.ingramcontent.com/pod-product-compliance
Lightning Source LLC
LaVergne TN
LVHW082145200926
848484LV00008B/2106
9798887405605